Current C A N C E R *Therapeutics*

John M. Kirkwood

Professor and Chief, Division of Medical Oncology, University of Pittsburgh School of Medicine
Chief, Melanoma Center, Pittsburgh Cancer Institute, Pittsburgh, Pennsylvania

Michael T. Lotze

Professor of Surgery, Molecular Genetics, and Biochemistry
Chief, Section of Surgical Oncology, University of Pittsburgh School of Medicine
Chief, Biotherapy Center, Pittsburgh Cancer Institute, Pittsburgh, Pennsylvania

Joyce M. Yasko

Professor, School of Nursing, University of Pittsburgh
Associate Director of Clinical Administration, Pittsburgh Cancer Institute, Pittsburgh, Pennsylvania

First Edition

Current Medicine

CURRENT MEDICINE
20 North Third Street
Philadelphia, PA 19106

MANAGING EDITOR: *Chris Baumle*
DEVELOPMENTAL EDITOR: *Kim Loretucci*
ART DIRECTOR: *Paul Fennessy*
DESIGN AND LAYOUT: *Robert LeBrun and Patrick Whelan*
ILLUSTRATION DIRECTOR: *Larry Ward*
ILLUSTRATORS: *Wiesia Langenfeld and Larry Ward*
PRODUCTION MANAGER: *David Myers*

ISBN: 1-878132-12-1
ISSN: 1074-2816

Manufactured in the United States of America
Printed by Princeton Academic Press, Inc.
5 4 3 2 1

SANJIV S. AGARWALA, MD
Instructor, Department of Medicine
University of Pittsburgh School of
  Medicine
Pittsburgh, Pennsylvania

MICHAEL B. ATKINS, MD
Associate Professor of Medicine
Division of Hematology/Oncology
New England Medical Center
Boston, Massachusetts

ROBERT R. BAHNSON, MD
Associate Professor of Surgery
Division of Urologic Surgery/
  Urologic Oncology
University of Pittsburgh School of
  Medicine
Pittsburgh, Pennsylvania

EDWARD D. BALL, MD
Professor of Medicine
University of Pittsburgh School
  of Medicine
Chief, Division of Hematology/
  Bone Marrow Transplantation
University of Pittsburgh Medical Center
Pittsburgh, Pennsylvania

JULIE K. BALTZ, PharmD
Clinical Research Pharmacist
Investigational Drug Branch
National Cancer Institute
Bethesda, Maryland

RUSSELL L. BASSER, MD
Melbourne Tumour Biology Branch
Ludwig Institute for Cancer Research
The Royal Melbourne Hospital
Victoria, Australia

MICHAEL E. BOZIK, MD
Fellow in Neuro-oncology
Brain Tumor Center
Pittsburgh Cancer Institute
Pittsburgh, Pennsylvania

SALLY E. CARTY, MD
Assistant Professor of Surgery
University of Pittsburgh School
  of Medicine
Pittsburgh, Pennsylvania

ROBERT J. DELAP, MD, PhD
Medical Officer, Oncology Group
Food and Drug Administration
Rockville, Maryland

MARC S. ERNSTOFF, MD
Associate Professor of Medicine
Section of Hematology/Oncology
Dartmouth Medical School
Director, Clinical Therapeutics
  Research Program
Norris Cotton Cancer Center
Lebanon, New Hampshire

RICHARD I. FISHER, MD
Professor of Medicine
Director, Section of Hematology/
  Oncology
Loyola University Medical Center
Maywood, Illinois

YUMAN FONG, MD
Assistant Professor of Surgery
  and Cell Biology and Anatomy
Cornell University Medical College
New York, New York

MARC B. GARNICK, MD
Vice President, Clinical Development
Genetics Institute
Associate Professor of Medicine
Harvard Medical College
Cambridge, Massachusetts

ELLEN R. GAYNOR, MD
Associate Professor of Medicine
Section of Hematology/Oncology
Loyola University Medical Center
Maywood, Illinois

MARK R. GILBERT, MD
Assistant Professor of Neurology,
  Medicine and Neurosurgery
University of Pittsburgh School
  of Medicine
Co-director, Brain Tumor Center
Pittsburgh Cancer Institute
Pittsburgh, Pennsylvania

MICHAEL D. GREEN, MD
Department of Clinical Hematology
  and Medical Oncology
The Royal Melbourne Hospital
Western Hospital
Victoria, Australia

R. ELIZABETH GREGORY, PharmD
Clinical Coordinator
The Johns Hopkins Oncology
  Center Pharmacy
Baltimore, Maryland

JEAN L. GREM, MD
Navy Medical Oncology Branch
National Cancer Institute
Bethesda, Maryland

STUART A. GROSSMAN, MD
Associate Professor of Oncology,
  Medicine and Neurosurgery
The Johns Hopkins School of Medicine
Director, Neuro-oncology
The Johns Hopkins Oncology Center
Baltimore, Maryland

J. MICHAEL HAMILTON, MD
Navy Medical Oncology Branch
National Cancer Institute
Bethesda, Maryland

JOHN A. HEANEY, MD
Professor of Surgery (Urology)
Chief, Section of Urology
Dartmouth Medical School
Norris Cotton Cancer Center
Lebanon, New Hampshire

I. CRAIG HENDERSON, MD
Professor of Medicine
Chief, Medical Oncology
University of California at San Francisco
San Francisco, California

ANN JAKUBOWSKI, MD, PhD
Assistant Attending Physician
Memorial Sloan-Kettering Cancer Center
New York, New York

V. CRAIG JORDAN, PhD, DSc
Professor of Cancer Pharmacology
Director, Breast Cancer Research
  Program
Northwestern University Medical School
Chicago, Illinois

KEN KOBAYASHI, MD
Fellow in Medicine
Section of Hematology/Oncology
The University of Chicago
The Pritzker School of Medicine
Chicago, Illinois

JOHN M. KIRKWOOD, MD
Professor and Chief
Division of Medical Oncology
University of Pittsburgh School of
  Medicine
Chief, Melanoma Center
Pittsburgh Cancer Institute
Pittsburgh, Pennsylvania

BARRY C. LEMBERSKY, MD
Assistant Professor of Medicine
Division of Medical Oncology
University of Pittsburgh School of
Medicine
Pittsburgh, Pennsylvania

JEFFREY P. LETZER, DO
Senior Fellow in Medicine
Section of Hematology/Oncology
Loyola University Medical Center
Maywood, Illinois

MICHAEL T. LOTZE, MD
Professor of Surgery, Molecular
Genetics, and Biochemistry
Chief, Section of Surgical Oncology
University of Pittsburgh School of
Medicine
Chief, Biotherapy Center
Pittsburgh Cancer Institute
Pittsburgh, Pennsylvania

STEPHEN F. LOWRY, MD
Professor of Surgery
Cornell University Medical College
New York, New York

DIANA MARAVICH MAY, PharmD
Chief of Clinical Services
Morris Pharmacy
Duke University Medical Center
Durham, North Carolina

ROSEMARY MAZANET, MD, PhD
Associate Director of Clinical Research
Amgen, Inc.
Thousand Oaks, California

JOSEPH MIRRO, JR., MD
Professor of Pediatrics
University of Pittsburgh School of
Medicine
Chief, Division of Pediatric
Hematology/Oncology
Children's Hospital of Pittsburgh
Pittsburgh, Pennsylvania

BOB MORGAN, RPh
Chief of Operations
Morris Pharmacy
Duke University Medical Center
Durham, North Carolina

CRAIG MOSKOWITZ, MD
Lymphoma Service
Memorial Sloan-Kettering
Cancer Center
New York, New York

JAMES L. MULSHINE, MD
Chief, Biomarkers and Prevention
Research Branch
National Cancer Institute
Bethesda, Maryland

MARTIN M. OKEN, MD
Medical Director
The Virginia Piper Cancer Institute
Abbott Northwestern Hospital
Minneapolis, Minnesota

CAROL S. PORTLOCK, MD
Acting Chief, Lymphoma Service
Memorial Sloan-Kettering Cancer
Center
New York, New York

MITCHELL C. POSNER, MD
Assistant Professor of Surgery
Section of Surgical Oncology
University of Pittsburgh School of
Medicine
Pittsburgh, Pennsylvania

JOHN H. RAAF, MD
Chief, Department of Surgery
Meridia Huron Hospital
Cleveland, Ohio

BLANCHE RASMUSSEN, PharmD
Cancer Center Pharmacist
University of Nebraska Medical Center
Omaha, Nebraska

ARTHUR R. RHODES, MD, MPH
Professor of Dermatology
University of Pittsburgh School of
Medicine
Pittsburgh, Pennsylvania

JOSHUA T. RUBIN, MD
Assistant Professor of Surgery
Section of Surgical Oncology
University of Pittsburgh School of
Medicine
Pittsburgh, Pennsylvania

SUSAN A. SAJER, MD
Associate Professor of Medicine
Division of Hematology/Oncology
New England Medical Center
Boston, Massachusetts

MARK P. SERALY, MD
Resident in Dermatology
University of Pittsburgh School of
Medicine
Pittsburgh, Pennsylvania

CHERYL A. STEELE, RN, MN, OCN, CS
Clinical Director of Outpatient Services
Pittsburgh Cancer Institute
Pittsburgh, Pennsylvania

ROGER STUPP, MD
Fellow in Medicine
Section of Hematology/Oncology
The University of Chicago
The Pritzker School of Medicine
Chicago, Illinois

MARGARET A. TEMPERO, MD
Associate Professor of Medicine
Section of Oncology and Hematology
University of Nebraska
Medical Center
Omaha, Nebraska

DEBASISH TRIPATHY, MD
Assistant Clinical Professor of Medicine
Division of Hematology and Oncology
University of California
at San Francisco
San Francisco, California

NICHOLAS J. VOGELZANG, MD
Professor of Medicine
Section of Hematology/Oncology
The University of Chicago
The Pritzker School of Medicine
Chicago, Illinois

EVERETT E. VOKES, MD
Associate Professor of Medicine
Section of Hematology/Oncology
The University of Chicago
The Pritzker School of Medicine
Chicago, Illinois

SCOTT WADLER, MD
Associate Professor of Medicine
Albert Einstein College of Medicine
Director, Gastrointestinal Oncology
Montefiore Medical Center
Bronx, New York

JOYCE M. YASKO, RN, PhD
Professor, School of Nursing
University of Pittsburgh
Associate Director of Clinical
Administration
Pittsburgh Cancer Institute
Pittsburgh, Pennsylvania

TABLE OF CONTENTS

ACKNOWLEDGMENTS

The editors thank each of the contributors to this volume, and especially our colleagues who took the time and effort to envision the new format that we had developed, often crystallizing as the volume came into being. We thank Nancy M. Patuc, who was the focal point of contact for all, and M. Linda Wastyn and Kim Loretucci, who assisted the authors and editors to develop this new work. We acknowledge the invaluable detailed review of our book by our two pharmacists, Carol Mathews, R.Ph. and Rowena A. Schwartz, Pharm. D.

Finally, our gratitude is to our children, spouses, friends, and colleagues who helped us to launch this effort—and without whom this work would lose its value.

PREFACE

The field of cancer medicine has given rise to a variety of surgical, medical, nursing, and other subspecialty handbooks. This volume, *Current Cancer Therapeutics*, presents an integrated interdisciplinary source for oncologists from the medical, surgical, and radiotherapy disciplines, as well as for oncology nurses, physician assistants, pharmacists, social workers, psychologists, and others concerned with cancer treatment. The major goal of this work is to present the most current information regarding the agents in current use, the protocols relevant to each of the malignant diseases, and the supportive care required to deliver advanced cancer therapy in a user-friendly, concise, and consistent format. The volume has been organized in accordance with the clinical decision-making process and for interdisciplinary use by oncologists and trainees at the bedside on the inpatient ward and in the outpatient clinic. The book has four sections:

1. The cytotoxic, biologic, and hormonal agents used to treat cancer.
2. The major malignancies and leading standard and developing protocols of treatment for each.
3. Administration of therapy: selection and use of vascular access devices.
4. Supportive care for the manifestations of cancer and toxicity of cancer therapy.

We have selected chapter authors who have vast clinical experience and who have developed innovative treatment plans through clinical research. The information provided is timely, clinically organized, and at the leading edge of the trial. We are very appreciative of the expertise and efforts on behalf of all contributors to *Current Cancer Therapeutics*. Inevitably, the design and development of a new book is an occasion for conflict and disagreement, but also for growth and learning. We not only survived the ordeal but thrived as each of us better understands the others' disciplines and we have become even more committed to interdisciplinary care. We hope this volume inspires others for interdisciplinary efforts in the clinic! We hope the volume will be of use to all who are engaged in the challenging and changing field of clinical oncology in the 1990s.

The biologic and chemical activities of the nitrogen mustards were studied extensively in the period between World Wars I and II. Although originally conceived as a possible war weapon because of their vesicant activity on the skin, eyes, and respiratory tract, the mustards were studied for their effects on lymphosarcomas in mice during World War II. This led to the start of clinical studies in 1942 and initiated the era of modern cancer chemotherapy [1].

MECHANISMS OF ACTION

Alkylating agents are polyfunctional compounds that have the ability to substitute alkyl groups for hydrogen ions. These compounds react with phosphate, amino, hydroxyl, sulfhydryl, carboxyl, and imidazole groups, which are part of the molecular makeup of the body. In neutral or alkaline solution, alkylators ionize and produce positively charged ions that attach to susceptible nuclear proteins—the most likely site of alkylation being the N-7 position of guanine. This alkylation reaction leads to abnormal base pairing, cleaving of the imidazole ring of guanine, cross-linking of DNA, depurination of DNA, interference with DNA replication, transcription of RNA, and the disruption of nucleic acid function. All these actions lead to an interruption in the normal cell functions of both cancerous and normal tissues [1,2].

The alkylating agents are cell cycle phase–nonspecific agents in that they exert their activity independent of the specific phase of the cell cycle. The nitrogen mustards and alkyl alkone sulfonates are most effective against cells in the G_1 or M phase. Nitrosoureas, nitrogen mustards, and aziridines impair progression from the G_1 and S phases to the M phase [1,2].

Table 1 gives the general mechanisms of action of each class of alkylating agent.

CLASSES OF ALKYLATING AGENTS

The alkylating agents are traditionally divided into five classes; however, the platinum-containing compounds have been added as a sixth class due to their ability to bind to DNA and produce cross-links in the DNA helix. The traditional classes of alkylators include the bischloroethylamines (nitrogen mustards), the aziridines (ethylenimines), the alkyl alkone sulfonates, the nitrosoureas, and the nonclassical alkylating agents [1]. Table 2 groups the alkylating agents by classes and includes the trade names, manufacturers, and dosage forms of the various agents.

Table 1. Mechanisms of Action of the Classes of Alkylating Agents

Class	Mechanism of Action
Bischloroethylamines	Interfere with DNA replication and RNA transcription
Aziridines	Interfere with DNA replication and RNA transcription
Alkyl alkone sulfonates	Interfere with DNA replication and RNA transcription
Nitrosoureas	Alkylation of DNA and RNA
Nonclassic alkylating agents	Alkylation; inhibition of DNA, RNA, and protein synthesis
Platinum compounds	Formation of interstrand and intrastrand DNA cross-links

FDA-APPROVED INDICATIONS

The alkylating agents are active against a wide variety of neoplastic diseases, with significant activity in the treatment of leukemias and lymphomas. This group of drugs is routinely used in the treatment of acute and chronic leukemias, Hodgkin's disease, non-Hodgkin's lymphoma, multiple myeloma, primary brain tumors, malignant melanoma, and carcinomas of the breast, ovaries, testes, lungs, bladder, cervix, head, and neck (Table 3).

TOXICITIES

The major toxicity common to all of the alkylating agents is myelosuppression (Table 4). Gastrointestinal adverse effects of variable severity occur commonly, and various organ toxicities are associated with specific compounds [3,4].

Leukopenia, thrombocytopenia, and anemia occur due to the effect of these drugs on the hematopoietic system. Hematologic toxicity is dose-related, cumulative, and can lead to treatment cycle delay and/or dosage reductions. Although the toxicity is usually reversible upon discontinuation of the alkylator, long-term administration can lead to severe and prolonged suppression of the bone marrow. The oral agents chlorambucil, melphalan, busulfan, lomustine, altretamine, and procarbazine have slower onsets of

Table 2. Classes of Alkylating Agents

Agent	Trade Name	Manufacturer	Dosage Forms
Bischloroethylamines (nitrogen mustards)			
Chlorambucil	Leukeran	Burroughs Wellcome	PO
Cyclophosphamide	Cytoxan	Bristol-Myers Oncology	PO, IV
	Neosar	Adria	IV
Ifosfamide	Ifex	Bristol-Myers Oncology	IV
Mechlorethamine	Mustargen	Merck & Co.	IV
Melphalan	Alkeran	Burroughs Wellcome	PO, IV
Uracil mustard	Uracil mustard	Upjohn	PO
Aziridines			
Thiotepa	Thiotepa	Immunex	IV
Alkyl alkone sulfonates			
Busulfan	Myleran	Burroughs Wellcome	PO
Nitrosoureas			
Carmustine	BiCNU	Bristol-Myers Oncology	IV
Lomustine	CeeNU	Bristol-Myers Oncology	PO
Streptozocin	Zanosar	Upjohn	IV
Nonclassic alkylating agents			
Altretamine	Hexalen	US Bioscience	PO
Dacarbazine	DTIC	Dome	IV
Procarbazine	Matulane	Roche	PO
Platinum compounds			
Carboplatin	Paraplatin	Bristol-Myers Oncology	IV
Cisplatin	Platinol	Bristol-Myers Oncology	IV

hematologic toxicity, taking anywhere from 3 to 6 weeks for decreases in blood counts to appear. Nadirs for the intravenously administered alkylators appear within 1 to 2 weeks and persist for 1 to 2 weeks after discontinuing drug therapy.

A complete blood count, including hematocrit, hemoglobin, platelets, and total and differential leukocyte counts should be obtained weekly throughout the treatment course to allow the physician to monitor for significant hematologic changes. Other serum chemistries such as BUN, creatinine, SGPT, SGOT, LDH, and bilirubin should be obtained at periodic intervals to monitor for adverse effects on liver and kidney function.

Patients being treated for lymphomas and leukemias who have high tumor burdens are especially subject to hyperuricemia. Hyperuricemia is caused by extensive purine catabolism, which accompanies rapid cellular destruction and is not a specific toxicity of the drug. Because hyperuricemia is associated with rapid tumor lysis, patients being treated with chlorambucil, cyclophosphamide, mechlorethamine, uracil mustard, busulfan, carboplatin, and cisplatin should have serum uric acid levels monitored throughout the course of therapy.

Treatment of severe hematologic toxicity includes supportive therapy with platelet and red blood cell transfusion, and appropriate antibiotics for febrile neutropenia. The use of a prophylactic colony-stimulating factor may be indicated. Patients who have elevated serum uric acid levels should be treated with allopurinol and advised to increase their oral fluid intake.

Antineoplastic agents, including the alkylators, are toxic to rapidly proliferating cells. Because the gastrointestinal mucosa turns over rapidly, it is susceptible to these agents. Nausea and vomiting are the most common adverse gastrointestinal effects seen with this group of drugs. Stomatitis and anorexia also occur. These adverse effects can lead to decreased nutritional intake.

The gastrointestinal effects can be minimized by including antiemetic agents as a part of the chemotherapy regimen and providing patients with orally or rectally administered antiemetics to use at home to combat delayed-onset emesis. Supportive care in the form of increased intake of fluids should also be part of the patient's care to prevent complications associated with dehydration due to loss of excessive fluid volume.

Hemorrhagic cystitis is a major toxicity of ifosphamide, as well as high-dose cyclophosphamide therapy, and is caused by an accumulation of the metabolite acrolein [5,6]. A urinalysis should be obtained and examined for microscopic hematuria prior to each course of treatment, especially with ifosfamide. To help prevent this complication, patients should be adequately hydrated prior to the start of the ifosfamide infusion. Mesna, a uroprotective agent, should be administered in an intravenous dosage equal to 20% of the ifosfhamide dosage at the time of ifosfamide administration and repeated 4 and 8 hours after each dose of ifosfamide. Other mesna dosing schedules may also be used in patients receiving either ifosfamide or high-dose cyclophosfamide. Patients receiving either of these therapies on an outpatient basis should be advised to increase their oral fluid intake and to void every 2 hours during the day and once at night on the days they receive their chemotherapy treatments to decrease the risk of hemorrhagic cystitis [7,8].

Table 4 lists the hematologic, gastrointestinal, and other major toxicities associated with the alkylating agents [9–12].

MECHANISMS OF RESISTANCE

Resistance to antineoplastic agents is the major cause of treatment failure for many cancer patients. Increasing dosages of drugs may be required although this may raise doses to levels where toxicities are prohibitive. Alternatively, changing the regimen to a non–cross-resistant drug or to a combination of drugs that will be effective against the particular neoplasm is possible. Resistance is either primary (natural) or acquired—*primary resistance* resulting when innate resistance is selected out from natural cell lines and *acquired resistance* resulting from drug-induced adaptation or muta-

Table 3. Approved Indications for Alkylating Agents

Agent	FDA-Approved Indications
Bischloroethylamines	
Chlorambucil	Chronic lymphocytic leukemia, malignant lymphomas, lymphosarcoma, giant follicular lymphoma, Hodgkin's disease
Cyclophosphamide	Acute lymphocytic leukmeia, acute myelocytic leukemia, chronic myelocytic leukemia, chronic lymphocytic leukemia, acute monocytic leukemia, Hodgkin's and non-Hodgkin's lymphoma, carcinoma of the breast and ovary, multiple myeloma, mycosis fungoides, Burkitt's lymphoma, neuroblastoma, retinoblastoma
Ifosfamide	Third-line therapy for germ-cell testicular tumors
Mechlorethamine	Palliative treatment of Stage III and IV Hodgkin's disease, lymphosarcoma, chronic myelocytic leukemia, chronic lymphocytic leukemia, polycythemia vera, mycosis fungoides, bronchogenic carcinoma, malignant effusions
Melphalan	Palliative treatment of multiple myeloma and non-resectable epithelial ovarian carcinoma
Uracil mustard	Palliative treatment of chronic lymphocytic leukemia, chronic myelocytic leukemia, non-Hodgkin's lymphomas, mycosis fungoides, early polycythemia vera
Aziridines	
Thiotepa	Intravesical treatment of tumors of the bladder
Alkyl alkone sulfonates	
Busulfan	Chronic myelogenous leukemia, severe thrombocytosis, polycythemia vera
Nitrosoureas	
Carmustine	Palliative treatment of primary and metastatic brain tumors, multiple myeloma, disseminated Hodgkin's disease, non-Hodgkin's lymphomas
Lomustine	Palliative treatment of primary and metastatic brain tumors, disseminated Hodgkin's disease
Streptozocin	Pancreatic islet cell carcinoma
Nonclassic alkylating agents	
Altretamine	Palliative treatment of advanced ovarian cancer
Dacarbazine	Malignant melanoma, Hodgkin's disease
Procarbazine	Advanced Hodgkin's disease
Platinum compounds	
Carboplatin	Advanced ovarian carcinoma
Cisplatin	Metastatic testicular tumors, metastatic ovarian tumors, advanced bladder carcinoma

tion of neoplastic cells. Acquired resistance may be due to decreased intracellular concentrations of the drug, increased degradation of the active compound, decreased conversion of the drug to the active form, changes in cellular metabolism and utilization of separate metabolic pathways, and increased activity or concentration of target enzymes within the cell. Among the alkylating agents, cross-resistance has been reported with carmustine and lomustine.

AREAS OF RESEARCH ACTIVITY

As oncologists strive to improve the treatment of cancer, research studies continue with many drugs being tried for possible new indications [13,14]. The alkylating agents, although among the oldest antineoplastic agents, have been and continue to be looked at for

possible new indications, both alone and in combination with other antineoplastic agents.

Among the alkylators, ifosfamide and dacarbazine are being examined in the treatment of soft tissue sarcomas. Mechlorethamine and carmustine have been studied for topical application in the treatment of mycosis fungoides. Cyclophosphamide is being studied in small cell lung carcinoma, renal cell carcinoma, and in carcinomas of the gastrointestinal tract, endometrium, testes, prostate, and bladder. Streptozocin has shown activity in metastatic carcinoid tumors and in metastatic colorectal cancer. Cisplatin has shown activity in metastatic squamous cell carcinomas of the head and neck and cervix and in non–small cell lung carcinoma.

High-dose chemotherapy is being used in the area of bone marrow transplant. Cyclophosphamide, carmustine, and thiotepa are among the alkylators being applied this way [15–20].

Table 4. Major Toxicities of the Alkylating Agents

Agent	Hematologic Toxicities	Gastrointestinal Toxicities	Other Toxicities
Bischloroethylamines			
Chlorambucil	Leukopenia, thrombocytopenia	Nausea, vomiting, diarrhea, gastric discomfort (doses > 20 mg)	Hyperuricemia*
Cyclophosphamide	Leukopenia, anemia, thrombocytopenia	Nausea, vomiting, anorexia	Hemorrhagic cystitis, alopecia, hyperuricemia*
Ifosfamide	Leukopenia, thrombocytopenia	Nausea, vomiting	Hemorrhagic cystitis, alopecia
Mechlorethamine	Leukopenia, anemia, thrombocytopenia, hemorrhagic diathesis	Nausea and vomiting (severe)	Thrombophlebitis, headache, weakness, hyperuricemia*
Melphalan	Leukopenia, thrombocytopenia	Nausea, vomiting (infrequently PO, more IV), mucositis	
Uracil mustard	Leukopenia, thrombocytopenia	Nausea and vomiting (severe), anorexia, diarrhea, epigastric distress	Hyperuricemia*
Aziridines			
Thiotepa	Leukopenia, anemia, thrombocytopenia	Nausea, vomiting, anorexia (infrequently), diarrhea	Pain at injection site, headache, dizziness
Alkyl alkone sulfonates			
Busulfan	Leukopenia, anemia, thrombocytopenia	Nausea, vomiting, diarrhea (infrequently)	Hyperuricemia*
Nitrosoureas			
Carmustine	Leukopenia, anemia, thrombocytopenia	Nausea and vomiting (severe)	Hepatotoxicity, pulmonary infiltrates
Lomustine	Leukopenia, anemia, thrombocytopenia with prolonged therapy	Nausea, vomiting	
Streptozocin	Mild-to-moderate leukopenia, anemia, thrombocytopenia	Nausea and vomiting (severe)	Nephrotoxicity, pain at injection site
Nonclassic alkylating agents			
Altretamine	Leukopenia, anemia, thrombocytopenia	Nausea, vomiting	Peripheral neuropathy
Dacarbazine	Leukopenia, thrombocytopenia	Nausea and vomiting (severe), anorexia	Pain at injection site, fever, myalgia, malaise
Procarbazine	Leukopenia, anemia, thrombocytopenia	Nausea, vomiting, anorexia, stomatitis	
Platinum compounds			
Carboplatin	Leukopenia, anemia, thrombocytopenia	Nausea, vomiting	Peripheral neuropathies, ototoxicity
Cisplatin	Leukopenia, anemia, thrombocytopenia	Nausea and vomiting (severe)	Nephrotoxicity, hypomagnesemia, hypocalcemia, hypokalemia, ototoxicity, peripheral neuropathy, hyperuricemia*

*Hyperuricemia is most often associated with leukemia and lymphoma patients who have a high tumor burden and is not necessarily an adverse effect of the drug.

REFERENCES

1. Gilman A, Rall T, Nies A, Palmer T (eds): *Goodman and Gilman's The Pharmacological Basis of Therapeutics*, 8th ed. 1990. New York: Pergamon Press. pp. 1202–1276.

2. Chabner BA, Collins JM (eds): *Cancer Chemotherapy: Principles and Practice.* 1990, Philadelphia: JB Lippincott.

3. Black DJ, Livingston RB: Antineoplastic drugs in 1990: A review (Part I). *Drugs* 1990, 39:489–501.

4. Black DJ, Livingston RB: Antineoplastic drugs in 1990: A review (Part II). *Drugs* 1990, 39:652–673.

5. Dorr RT: Ifosfamide and cyclophosphamide: Review and appraisal. 1992, 5–21.

6. Frasier LH, Kanekal S, Kehrer JP: Cyclophosphamide toxicity: Characterising and avoiding the problem. *Drugs* 1991, 42:781–795.

7. Dechant KL, Brogden RN, Pilkington T, *et al.*: Ifosfamide/mesna: A review of antineoplastic activity, pharmacokinetic properties, and therapeutic efficacy in cancer. *Drugs* 1991, 42:428–467.

8. Sanchiz F, Milla A: High-dose ifosfamide and mesna in advanced breast cancer. *Cancer Chem Pharm* 1990, 26(suppl):91–92.

9. Smith AC: The Pulmonary toxicity of nitrosoureas. *Pharm Ther* 1989, 41:443–460.

10. Wagstaff AJ, Ward A, Benfield P, *et al.*: Carboplatin. A preliminary review of its pharmacodynamic and pharmacokinetic properties and therapeutic efficacy in the treatment of cancer. *Drugs* 1990, 37:162–190.

11. Blachley JD, Hill JB: Renal and electrolyte disturbances associated with cisplatin. *Ann Intern Med* 1981, 95:628–632.

12. Finley RS, Fortner CL, Grove WR, *et al.*: Cisplatin nephrotoxicity: A summary of preventative interventions. *Drug Intell Clin Pharm* 1985, 19:362–367.

13. Bishop JF: Current experience with high-dose carboplatin therapy. *Sem Oncol* 1992, 19(suppl 2):150–154.

14. Calvert AH, Newell DR, Gore HE, *et al.*: Future directions with carboplatin: Can therapeutic monitoring, high dose administration, and hematologic support with growth factors expand the spectrum compared with cisplatin? *Sem Oncol* 1992, 19(suppl 2):155–163.

15. Ackland SP, Choike, Ratain MJ, *et al.*: Human plasma pharmacokinetics following administration of high-dose thiotepa and cyclophosphamide. *J Clin Oncol* 1988, 6:1192–1196.

16. Corden BJ, Fine RL, Ozols RF, *et al.*: Clinical pharmacology of high-dose cisplatin. *Cancer Chem Pharm* 1985, 14:38–41.

17. Henner WD, Peters WP, Eder JP, *et al.*: Pharmacokinetics and immediate effects of high-dose carmustine in man. *Cancer Treat Rep* 1986, 70:877–880.

18. Peters WP: Dose intensification using combination alkylating agents and autologous bone marrow support in the treatment of primary and metastatic breast cancer: A review of the Duke bone marrow transplant program experience. Effects of therapy on biology and kinetics of the residual tumor. Part B: Clinical aspects. 1990, 185–194.

19. Peters WP: High dose chemotherapy and autologous bone marrow support for breast cancer. *Important Advances in Oncology*. 1992, Philadelphia: JB Lippincott. pp. 135–150.

20. Rohaly J: The use of busulfan therapy in bone marrow transplantation. *Cancer Nurs* 1989, 12:144–152.

ALTRETAMINE

Altretamine (hexamethylmelamine) is an antineoplastic agent that is structurally similar to triethylenemelamine, a known alkylating agent. The mechanism of action is unknown. It has been postulated that altretamine may act as an alkylator or as an antimetabolite. Altretamine is activated via hepatic microsomal enzymes to cytotoxic intermediates, which may bind to microsomal proteins and DNA. The National Cancer Institute developed altretamine approximately 18 years ago, and the FDA approved the drug for marketing in 1991.

DOSAGE AND ADMINISTRATION

Ovarian cancer: 4–12 mg/kg po in divided daily doses for 21 to 90 d, **or** 240–320 mg/m² po in divided daily doses for 21 d; doses are repeated every 6 wk

SPECIAL PRECAUTIONS

Pregnant/nursing patients

TOXICITIES

GI: nausea and vomiting (50% to 70%) (dose-limiting); anorexia, abdominal cramps, diarrhea
Neurologic: paresthesias, numbness, sleep disturbances, confusion, hallucinations, seizures, Parkinsonian-like syndrome with ataxia (20% for all neurologic side effects)
Hematologic: mild leukopenia, thrombocytopenia
Dermatologic: alopecia, rash, pruritus

INDICATIONS

FDA-approved: advanced ovarian cancer; **clinical studies show activity in:** metastatic breast cancer, refractory lymphoma, pancreatic adenocarcinoma, and colorectal, cervical, and endometrial cancers, small cell and non–small cell lung cancer

PHARMACOKINETICS

Absorption—enhanced GI absorption with capsule, although oral absorption is extremely variable; **Peak plasma concentration**—0.5 to 3 hr after administration; **Distribution**—minimally protein bound and highly lipid-soluble, metabolites cross the blood–brain barrier; **Metabolism**—liver; **Elimination**—urine as metabolites, **Half-life**—3–10 hr

DRUG INTERACTIONS

Cimetidine, phenobarbital, monoamine oxidase inhibitors

RESPONSE RATES

Ovarian cancer—complete and partial response rates of 20–30%; in combination with cyclophosphamide, doxorubicin, or melphalan—rates ranging from 20–80%
Small cell and non–small cell lung cancer—response rates of 4–42% in combination, widely variable rates

PATIENT MONITORING

Monitor complete blood cell count during course; perform complete neurologic exam routinely

NURSING INTERVENTIONS

Monitor treatment tolerance, weight, nutritional status; give appropriate antiemetics (daily doses should be divided into a 4-times-a-day schedule); administer concomitant pyridoxine (100 mg) to reduce neurotoxicity

PATIENT INFORMATION

Patient should call physician immediately if intractable nausea and vomiting, unusual bruising or bleeding, or fever above 102°F occurs; report vomiting episodes that occur soon after taking oral dose; report symptoms of neurotoxicity

FORMULATION

Available as Hexalen®, Applied Analytical Industries, Wilmington, NC (distributed by US Bioscience, West Conshohocken, PA)
50-mg hard gelatin capsules. Stored at room temperature.

BUSULFAN

Busulfan is an oral alkylating agent that is cell cycle–nonspecific. It interferes with DNA replication and transcription of RNA and ultimately results in the disruption of nucleic acid function. Busulfan is primarily used to control chronic myelogenous leukemia because of its selective depression of granulocytopoiesis at low doses. At higher doses the effect on all three hematopoietic cell lines is increased.

DOSAGE AND ADMINISTRATION

Chronic myelogenous leukemia: 0.06 mg/kg or 1.8 mg/m^2 PO intermittently or continuously for adults and children

DOSAGE MODIFICATIONS: discontinue therapy if leukocyte count is ≤ 10,000/mm^3 and resume when leukocyte count reaches 50,000/mm^3

SPECIAL PRECAUTIONS

Life-threatening pancytopenia possible
Life-threatening hepatic veno-occlusive disease (rare, associated with very high doses)
Pregnant/nursing patients
Hypersensitivity to the drug
Chronic myelogenous leukemia

TOXICITIES

Hematologic: bone marrow suppression (dose related, usually reversible, but sometimes abruptly irreversible); severe leukopenia, anemia, thrombocytopenia (10 days after therapy); bone marrow fibrosis, chronic aplasia, secondary neoplasia (possible)
Pulmonary: bronchopulmonary dysplasia with a diffuse interstitial pulmonary fibrosis characterized by persistent cough, fever, rales, dyspnea ("busulfan lung") (rare, associated with long-term therapy)
Metabolic: hyperuricemia; Addison-like adrenal insufficiency syndrome (rare, occurring with long-term therapy)
Neurologic: dizziness, blurred vision, loss of consciousness, intermittent muscle twitching; myoclonic and generalized tonic-clonic seizures (especially with high doses, prophylactic anticonvulsant administration possible)
Infertility: ovarian suppression and amenorrhea with menopausal symptoms in premenopausal woman; ovarian fibrosis, atrophy; affected spermatogenesis, causing impotence, sterility, azoospermia, testicular atrophy
Miscellaneous: mild gynecomastia, cheilosis, glossitis, hepatic dysfunction, and cholestatic jaundice, porphyria cutanea tarda, melanoderma, urticaria, rashes, dryness of skin and mucous membranes, anhidrosis, alopecia, cataracts, hemorrhagic cystitis, fatigue (all rare); nausea, vomiting, diarrhea, anorexia, weight loss (infrequent)

INDICATIONS

FDA-approved: palliative treatment of chronic myelogenous leukemias; **clinical studies show activity in:** severe thrombocytosis and polycythemia vera; myelofibrosis; in marrow-ablative conditioning regimens prior to bone marrow transplant for malignant and nonmalignant conditions

PHARMACOKINETICS

Absorption—rapidly and completely absorbed from the GI tract within 0.5–2 hr after oral administration; **Distribution**—cleared rapidly from the plasma, distribution into the CSF or into breast milk unknown; **Metabolism**—liver; **Elimination:** urine metabolites (10–15% within 24 hr)

DRUG INTERACTIONS

Thioguanine, cytotoxic drugs

RESPONSE RATES

Previously untreated chronic myelogenous leukemia—response rates of 90% (less effective in patients without Philadelphia chromosome)

PATIENT MONITORING

Monitor complete blood count weekly (leukocyte count will generally not decrease for 10–15 d); monitor signs of persistent cough and progressive dyspnea; watch for symptoms of adrenal insufficiency (abrupt weakness, unusual fatigue, anorexia, weight loss, nausea and vomiting, melanoderma)

NURSING INTERVENTIONS

Monitor treatment tolerance, weight, and nutritional status; assure that appropriate lab tests are conducted

PATIENT INFORMATION

Patient should call physician immediately if unusual bruising or bleeding, fever > 102°F, sore throat, or other signs of infection occurs; inform physician of persistent cough or difficult breathing; avoid aspirin-containing products

FORMULATION

Available as Myleran®, Burroughs Wellcome Co., Research Triangle Park, NC
2-mg scored tablets containing additionally the inactive ingredients magnesium stearate and sodium chloride. Stored at room temperature.

CARBOPLATIN

Carboplatin is a second-generation platinum compound that may be classified as a nonclassical alkylating agent and is cell cycle–nonspecific. Carboplatin and cisplatin have similar spectrums of activity. This second-generation platinum is used primarily for the treatment of ovarian cancer, but it also has shown promise in the treatment of seminomas, squamous cell carcinomas of the head and neck, and small cell lung cancer. Carboplatin, "the kinder platinum," was developed in an attempt to decrease the severe side effects of cisplatin. Nephrotoxicity, ototoxicity, neurotoxicity, and dose-limiting nausea and vomiting are less severe with carboplatin than with cisplatin therapy. The major dose-limiting toxicity of carboplatin is myelosuppression.

Like cisplatin, carboplatin is a cytotoxic platinum complex that reacts with nucleophilic sites on DNA. This causes inter- and intrastrand cross-links and DNA-protein cross-links, which inhibit DNA, RNA, and protein synthesis.

DOSAGE AND ADMINISTRATION

With previous treatment: 240–270 mg/m^2 bolus every 4 wk or 240 mg/m^2 24-hr continuous infusion every 4–5 wk **or** 100 mg/m^2 weekly bolus for 4 consecutive wk with 2 wk of rest **or** 77 mg/m^2 bolus for 5 consecutive d every 4–6 wk
With no previous therapy: 350–450 mg/m^2 bolus every 4 wk or 320 mg/m^2 24-hr continuous infusion every 4–5 wk **or** 125 mg/m^2 weekly bolus for 4 consecutive wk with 2 wk of rest **or** 100 mg/m^2 bolus for 5 consecutive d every 4–6 wk. Intraperitoneal doses of 200–650 mg/m^2 have been used. High-dose carboplatin (800–2000 mg/m^2) has been used investigationally with and without bone marrow support. Administer with hydration to reduce nephrotoxicity.

DOSAGE MODIFICATIONS: if platelets are > 100,000 adjust dose to 125%; if platelets are < 50,000 adjust dose to 75% Renal dosage adjustment should only be used for initial therapy

SPECIAL PRECAUTIONS

Pregnant/nursing patients
Patients with severe allergic reactions to platinum-containing compounds or mannitol

TOXICITIES

Hematologic: thrombocytopenia (dose-limiting in 37–80% increased with age, renal impairment, concurrent and previous chemotherapy); leukopenia and anemia (27–38%); reversible myelosuppression but severity may be cumulative with repeated doses
GI: nausea and vomiting (mild and rarely dose-limiting, at administration and 6–12 hr after therapy)
Renal: nephrotoxicity caused by chronic tubular damage
Miscellaneous: mild alopecia, abnormal liver function tests, hepatotoxicity (doses > 200 mg/m^2), neurotoxicity, hypersensitivity, stomatitis, mucositis, flu-like syndrome

INDICATIONS

FDA-approved: initial and secondary treatment of advanced ovarian cancer; **clinical studies show activity in:** lung cancers, squamous cell cancers of the head and neck, GI cancer, testicular cancer

PHARMACOKINETICS

Absorption—when administered intraperitoneally, plasma concentrations are one fifth of peritoneal dose; **Distribution**—tissue concentrations detected in kidneys, liver, skin, ileum, very low concentrations in spleen, lung, muscle, heart, testes, brain, fat, bone marrow; **Protein binding**—10–18%, shortly after bolus administration, volume of distribution of 16 to 20 l; **Metabolism**—possibly metabolized into highly reactive diamine metabolites similar to cisplatin metabolites; **Elimination**—renal; **Half-life:** carboplatin 3 hr, free platinum 6 hr

DRUG INTERACTIONS

Nephrotoxic drugs

RESPONSE RATES

Ovarian cancer response rates of 25 to 28% with carboplatin alone in patients previously treated with cisplatin (intraperitoneal, 53%), responses of 85% in patients not previously treated with cisplatin, complete and partial response rates of 30 to 83% with combination therapy; Small cell lung cancer and non–small cell lung cancer—responses vary: 0 to 60% with small cell lung cancer, 50–77% in combination therapy; 40–56% in non–small cell lung cancer; Low response rates averaging 25% are reported when carboplatin is used alone in the treatment of squamous cell carcinoma of the head and neck—25%, 62–92% in combination therapy; Seminomatous testicular cancer—84–86% response rate

PATIENT MONITORING

Monitor complete blood count, particularly for leukopenia, thrombocytopenia, anemia; take serum chemistries routinely, especially serum creatinine; perform complete neurologic exam

NURSING INTERVENTIONS

Monitor treatment tolerance, weight, nutritional status, ensure appropriate lab tests are conducted to monitor leukopenia, thrombocytopenia, anemia, renal function; nausea and vomiting are usually mild to moderate; provide appropriate antiemetics; provide concurrent fluid hydration during carboplatin administration

PATIENT INFORMATION

Patient should call immediately if intractable nausea and vomiting, unusual bruising and bleeding, fever > 102°F occurs; avoid exposure to people with infections; continue hydration with water 1 or 2 d after therapy

FORMULATION

Available as Paraplatin®, Bristol-Myers Oncology Division, Princeton NJ; 50-mg, 150-mg, and 450-mg vials of sterile, lyophilized white powder containing equal parts carboplatin and mannitol. Stored at room temperature and protected from light.

CARMUSTINE

Carmustine is a nitrosourea derivative that has demonstrated cytotoxic activity against a wide variety of malignancies. As with other alkylating agents, carmustine is considered to be cell cycle–nonspecific. Active metabolites are responsible for the alkylation and carbamoylation activity that interferes with DNA, RNA, and protein synthesis. Cross-resistance between carmustine and lomustine has occurred.

Carmustine and its metabolites are distributed rapidly into the CSF. Nitrosureas as a class tend to be highly lipophilic, thus enhancing their ability to cross the blood–brain barrier and be used in the treatment of meningeal leukemias and brain tumors. The long-term use of nitrosureas has been associated with profound cumulative myelosuppression and renal failure (especially with methyl-CCNU, used investigationally only) with lesions similar to radiation-induced nephritis.

Topical preparations of carmustine have been used to treat mycosis fungoides (cutaneous T-cell lymphoma). Historically topical nitrogen mustard (mechlorethamine) has been used for mycosis fungoides. Its mechanism of action is unknown because the alkylating action of mechlorethamine is dissipated shortly after it is dissolved in water although the anti-T-cell lymphoma activity remains. The mechanism of action of topical carmustine is similarly unknown.

DOSAGE AND ADMINISTRATION

Advanced neoplasms: 30–200 mg/m^2 single slow infusion or divided into multiple infusions over 2–5 d every 6 wk. Repeated doses should not be given until WBC count is greater than 4000/mm^3 and platelet count is greater than 100,000/mm^3. Doses up to 600 mg/m^2 are used as a single agent or in combination therapy in autologous bone marrow transplant protocols for breast cancer and advanced neoplasms.

DOSAGE MODIFICATIONS: give 70% of dose if leukocytes drop to 2000–2900 or platelets to 25,000–74,999, give 50% of dose if leukocytes drop < 2000 or platelets < 25,000.

SPECIAL PRECAUTIONS

Prolonged myelosuppression
Pulmonary toxicity
Patients with hepatic and/or renal dysfunction
Children
Pregnant/nursing patients
Caution with administration—skin contact can cause hyperpigmentation

TOXICITIES

Hematologic: leukopenia (dose-limiting), thrombocytopenia (most severe effect), anemia, acute leukemias and bone marrow dysplasias
GI: common moderate-to-severe nausea and vomiting (acute and delayed), diarrhea, esophagitis, anorexia, dysphagia
Pulmonary: pulmonary infiltrates and/or fibrosis (possibly progressive and fatal with cumulative doses > 100 mg/m^2)
Hepatic: hepatotoxicity (mild and reversible) increasing with high doses
Miscellaneous: renal toxicity (rare); significant hypotension and tachycardia (with high doses, associated with intense flushing of face and upper chest); dementia (with high doses); burning at injection site
Topical application: severe dermatitis, petechiae, hyperpigmentation, telangiectasia, hypersensitivity reactions (rare); mild bone marrow depression (< 10%)

INDICATIONS

FDA-approved: palliative treatment of primary and metastatic brain tumors, multiple myeloma (in combination therapy), disseminated Hodgkin's disease and non-Hodgkin's lymphoma (in combination therapy); **clinical studies show activity in:** carcinoma of the lung, GI tract, and breast, Ewing's sarcoma, malignant melanoma, Burkitt's lymphoma, mycosis fungoides (topical application)

PHARMACOKINETICS

Absorption—not absorbed across the GI tract, apparent absorption of topical application; **Distribution**—cleared rapidly from the plasma, rapidly crosses blood–brain barrier, CSF concentrations of metabolites 15–70% of the concurrent plasma concentrations; **Protein binding**—77%; **Volume of distribution**—≥ 5.1 l/kg; **Metabolism**—liver; **Elimination**—urine (60–70%), lungs (6–7%); **Half-life**—22 min

DRUG INTERACTION

Cimetidine

RESPONSE RATES

Brain tumors—objective response rates in 50%; carmustine and prednisone in multiple myeloma—response rates of 39%, carmustine alone—response rate of 11%; advanced Hodgkin's disease refractory to other treatments—response rates of 50%; non-Hodgkin's lymphoma—28% response rate; solid tumors of the lung, breast, and GI tract—21% response rate; mycosis fungoides—5-yr survival rates of 30%

PATIENT MONITORING

Monitor complete blood cell count weekly for 6 to 8 wk after administration (leukopenia, thrombocytopenia, anemia); monitor renal, hepatic, and pulmonary status

NURSING INTERVENTIONS

Monitor treatment tolerance, weight, and nutritional status; educate patients about neutropenic precautions and self-care at home; wear gloves while administering and avoid contact with skin; do not mix with other drugs during IV administration; if pain occurs at infusion site, dilute solution further and/or slow infusion rate; if extravasation occurs, stop infusion immediately; give antiemetics as needed; minimize possible intense facial and upper chest flushing by slowing infusion and check blood pressure for significant hypotension

PATIENT INFORMATION

Patient should call immediately if sore throat, fever, or any unusual bruising or bleeding develops; avoid aspirin or nonsteroidal anti-inflammatory agents; avoid exposure to people with infections

FORMULATION

Available as BiCNU®, Bristol-Myers Oncology Division, Princeton, NJ; 100-mg vials. Stored at 2–8°C.

CHLORAMBUCIL

Chlorambucil is a bifunctional alkylating agent within the nitrogen mustard class. It is a cell cycle–nonspecific antineoplastic agent that is cytotoxic to nonproliferating cells. Its antineoplastic activity occurs from the formation of an unstable ethylene immonium ion, which then alkylates or binds with intracellular structures. The cytotoxicity of chlorambucil is due to cross-linking of strands of DNA and RNA and to inhibition of protein synthesis. Additionally, chlorambucil is metabolized to phenylacetic acid mustard, which is also a bifunctional alkylating agent. Phenylacetic acid mustard has shown antineoplastic activity in some human cell lines approximately equal to that of chlorambucil. Chlorambucil also has immunosuppressant activity. It has the slowest onset of activity and the least toxicity of the classic nitrogen mustard agents.

DOSAGE AND ADMINISTRATION

CLL, Hodgkin's disease, non-Hodgkin's lymphoma: initiation or short course— 0.1–0.2 mg/kg/d for 3–6 wk (4–10 mg daily) (single or divided doses) **or** intermittent, biweekly course—0.4 mg/kg (or 12 mg/m^2), increased by 0.1 mg/kg (or 3 mg/m^2) every 2 wk until effective or toxic dose is reached

DOSAGE MODIFICATIONS: with lymphocytic infiltration or hypoplasia of bone marrow, < 0.1 mg/kg/d dose is given

SPECIAL PRECAUTIONS

Possible life-threatening damage to the bone marrow (reduced dosage for patients with prior radiation or chemotherapy or depressed leukocyte or platelet counts)
History of seizures or hypersensitivity to the drug
Pregnant/nursing patients
Children

TOXICITIES

Hematologic: lymphopenia, leukopenia, neutropenia, thrombocytopenia; bone marrow suppression (can be reversible); acute leukemias and bone marrow dysplasias (with long-term therapy)
GI: nausea and vomiting (mild), diarrhea, oral ulceration, anorexia, abdominal pain
Hepatic: hepatotoxicity (jaundice, hepatic necrosis, cirrhosis—rare)
Pulmonary: bronchopulmonary dysplasia, pulmonary fibrosis (rare, with prolonged therapy), interstitial pneumonia
Reproductive: sterility in prepubertal and pubertal males (high incidence), azoospermia, amenorrhea
Neurologic: tremors, muscular twitching, confusion, agitation, ataxia, flaccid paresis, hallucinations (rare), seizures
Miscellaneous: drug fever, skin hypersensitivity, peripheral neuropathy, sterile cystitis, keratitis, hyperuricemia, uric acid nephropathy

INDICATIONS

FDA-approved: palliation for chronic lymphocytic leukemia (CLL), malignant lymphomas, lymphosarcoma, giant follicular lymphoma, Hodgkin's disease; **clinical studies show activity in:** hairy cell leukemia, acute histiocytosis X, autoimmune hepatic anemias, advanced breast cancer, nonseminomatous testicular carcinoma, multiple myeloma, mycosis fungoides, Wegener's granulomatosis, sarcoidosis, macroglobulinemia, polycythemia vera, ovarian cancer, nephrotic syndrome, thrombocythemia

PHARMACOKINETICS

Absorption—rapidly absorbed from the GI tract, peak plasma levels reached in 1 hr; **Oral bioavailability**—50%; **Distribution**—extensively protein-bound (99%); crosses the placenta; **Metabolism**— liver, producing active metabolites; **Elimination**— kidneys; **Half-life**—90 min (parent drug) and 145 min (acid)

DRUG INTERACTIONS

Barbiturates, probenecid, sulfinpyrazone, bone marrow depressants, immunosuppressants

RESPONSE RATES

CLL—gradual response over several months; malignant lymphomas—complete remissions in 10–15%, partial responses in 40–70%

PATIENT MONITORING

Monitor complete blood count at periodic intervals during therapy; take SGPT, SGOT, LDH, and serum uric acids levels prior to and during therapy; watch for leukopenia and thrombocytopenia (dosage determinants)

NURSING INTERVENTIONS

Monitor treatment tolerance, weight, nutritional status; administer antiemetics as necessary; educate patients about side effects, neutropenic precautions, and self-care at home; ensure adequate hydration and administer allopurinol if necessary to prevent hyperuricemia

PATIENT INFORMATION

Patient should call physician immediately if vomiting occurs shortly after dose is taken or if sore throat, fever, or any unusual bruising or bleeding develops; avoid aspirin or nonsteroidal anti-inflammatory agents; avoid exposure to people with infections

FORMULATION

Available as Leukeran®, Burroughs-Wellcome Co., Triangle Research Park, NC
2-mg, sugar-coated tablets in bottles. Stored in a well-closed, light-resistant container at 15–30°C.

CISPLATIN

Cisplatin was the first heavy metal compound shown to have antineoplastic activity. During phase I trials, cisplatin was nearly discarded due to its extreme gastrointestinal and renal toxicities. However responses reported with testicular cancer showed promise and researchers developed mechanisms to decrease toxicity.

The mechanism of action of cisplatin is similar to alkylating agents and it is therefore considered a nonclassic alkylator. The *cis*, not the *trans*, isomer of cisplatin is the active moiety. In the relatively high chloride concentrations of plasma, the cisplatin complex is un-ionized and able to pass through cell membranes. In the presence of low chloride concentrations intracellularly, the chloride ligands of the complex are displaced by water and produce the positively charged platinum compound, which is toxic and probably the active form of the drug. The *cis* isomer forms intra- and interstrand cross-links between guanine–guanine pairs of DNA and inhibits synthesis. Cisplatin, to a lesser extent, binds to RNA and protein, ultimately inhibiting synthesis. Other cytotoxic activities may include tumor immunogenicity and immunosuppressive, radiosensitizing, and antimicrobial properties.

DOSAGE AND ADMINISTRATION

Testicular cancer: 20–40 mg/m^2 daily for 5 d or 120 mg/m^2 as a single dose every 3–4 wk (usually in combination therapy); Ovarian cancer: 30–120 mg/m^2 as a single dose every 3–4 wk, usually in combination with doxorubicin; Bladder cancer: 50–70 mg/m^2 as a single dose every 3–4 wk, **or** 1 mg/kg once a week for 6 wk, then every 3 wk thereafter; Head and neck cancer, cervical cancer, and non–small cell lung cancer: 50–120 mg/m^2 every 3 to 6 wk; Intra-arterial dosing for regionally confined malignancies (advanced bladder cancer, malignant melanoma, osteogenic sarcoma): 75–150 mg/m^2 as a single dose every 2 to 5 wk for 1 to 4 courses; Intraperitoneal dosing for advanced ovarian carcinoma, carcinoid, mesotheliomas: 60–270 mg/m^2; Pediatric osteogenic sarcoma or neuroblastoma: 90 mg/m^2 once every 3 wk or 30 mg/m^2 once a wk; Recurrent pediatric brain tumors: 60 mg/m^2 daily for 2 d every 3–4 wk; Dosage modification: reduce dose to 75% in patients with CLcr of 10 to 50 ml/min and to 50% in patients with CLcr < 10 ml/min. Dose adjustments are controversial and may result in suboptimal therapy

SPECIAL PRECAUTIONS

Children; possibly a mutagenic and carcinogenic agent; pregnant/nursing patients; hypersensitivity reactions to platinum-containing compounds

TOXICITIES

Renal: nephrotoxicity associated with renal tubular damage (dose related—reversible in low-to-moderate doses, possibly irreversible with higher doses); **Electrolyte:** electrolyte disturbances—hypomagnesemia, hypokalemia, hypocalcemia, hypophosphatemia, hyponatremia; **GI:** immediate and delayed nausea and vomiting (severe and often intractable), anorexia (due to nausea and vomiting), and diarrhea (rare); **Otolaryngologic:** tinnitus and/or high-frequency hearing loss (31%); **Neurologic:** peripheral neuropathies—sensory (paresthesias) and motor (gait); neuronal impairment (with prolonged therapy); tonic-clonic seizures, slurred speech, loss of taste, memory loss, intention tremor; **Hematologic:** leukopenia, thrombocytopenia (mild to moderate, 25–30%); acute leukemia (rare); **Sensitivity reactions:** anaphylactoid reactions—facial edema, flushing, wheezing and respiratory difficulty, tachycardia, hypotension; **Ophthalmologic:** optic neuritis, papilledema, cerebral blindness; **Cardiovascular:** bradycardia, left bundle branch block, ST-T wave changes with congestive heart failure, postural hypotension, hypertension (all rare); **Miscellaneous:** mild and transient elevations of serum AST (SGOT) and ALT (SGPT) concentrations (rare); local phlebitis, cellulitis with fibrosis, skin necrosis after extravasation; hyperuricemia, mild alopecia, myalgia, pyrexia, gingival platinum line, aspermia, SIADH (all rare)

INDICATIONS

FDA-approved: metastatic testicular and ovarian tumors, advanced bladder cancer; **clinical studies show activity in:** head and neck cancer, cervical carcinoma, lung cancer, osteogenic sarcoma, neuroblastoma, recurrent brain tumors, advanced esophageal carcinoma, advanced prostatic carcinoma, malignant melanoma, endometrial cancer, penile carcinoma, breast carcinoma, advanced Hodgkin's, malignant lymphomas, advanced soft tissue and bone sarcomas, refractory choriocarcinoma, metastatic adrenal carcinoma, malignant thymoma, medullary carcinoma of the thyroid, gastric carcinoma

PHARMACOKINETICS

Absorption—50–100% absorbed systemically (intraperitoneal); **Distribution**—high concentrations in kidneys, liver, prostate; volume of distribution of 20–80 l, does not penetrate CNS; **Protein binding**—≥ 90%; **Elimination**—excreted unchanged in the urine; **Half-life**—73–290 hr (terminal)

DRUG INTERACTIONS

Nephrotoxic and ototoxic drugs; etoposide, bleomycin, doxorubicin, 5-FU, methotrexate, vincas, anticonvulsants

RESPONSE RATES

Testicular neoplasms—60 to 70% complete remissions with combination therapy, higher responses in less advanced cases; advanced ovarian carcinoma refractory to radiation and/or chemotherapy—objective responses of 25–33%; complete responses are rare; in combination and intraperitoneal administration—varied overall response rates of 35 to 80%; bladder cancer—partial response rates in one third of patients; metastatic squamous cell carcinoma of the head and neck—30% response rates; recurrent or advanced squamous cell carcinoma of the cervix—response rates of 25 to 50%; non–small cell lung carcinoma—objective responses of 15–20%, response rates of 25–50% with combination therapy

PATIENT MONITORING

Renal function; complete serum chemistries particularly magnesium, potassium, sodium, calcium concentrations; audiometry prior to initial and repeated doses; routine neurologic exams; CBC every 2 wk

NURSING INTERVENTIONS

Be prepared for anaphylactic reactions within minutes of administration; monitor performance; provide antiemetics; hydrate well to prevent renal toxicity; do not use aluminum-containing IV sets or needles

PATIENT INFORMATION

Call physician for unusual bruising or bleeding, fever ≥ 102°, intractable nausea and vomiting, hearing loss, numbness or tingling in extremities; avoid exposure to infection; maintain adequate fluid intake, especially with vomiting; take antiemetic for 2–3 days after cessation of therapy

FORMULATIONS

Available as Platinol®, Bristol-Myers Oncology Division, Princeton, NJ. 10- and 15-mg vials containing white, lyophilized powder. Protected from light, stored at 15–25°C. Platinol—AQ®. Aqueous solution of 1 mg/ml in 50- and 100-mg vials.

CYCLOPHOSPHAMIDE

Cyclophosphamide is a cell cycle–nonspecific alkylating agent of the nitrogen mustard class. It is metabolized in the liver to active metabolites that alkylate nucleic acids. Cyclophosphamide prevents cell division by cross-linking DNA and RNA strands, preventing cell division and leading to cell death. Cyclophosphamide has phosphorylating properties that enhance its cytotoxicity; it also possesses significant immunosuppressive activity.

DOSAGE AND ADMINISTRATION

Adults: 50–100 mg/m^2 po × 10–14d, **or** 50–1000 mg/m^2 single IV dose on days 1 and 8 or every 14–21 d
High dose therapy: 1000–4000 mg/m^2 every 21 d or 5.6 g over 3 d for 1 course; maintenance dose—1–5 mg/kg PO d, or 10–15 mg/kg IV q 7–10 d, or 3–5 mg/kg IV twice weekly
Children: 2–8 mg/kg or 60–250 mg/m^2 PO or IV qd × 6 d (divide oral doses or IV doses given once a week); maintenance dose—2–5 mg/kg or 50–150 mg/m^2 PO twice weekly

SPECIAL PRECAUTIONS

Myelosuppressed patients or patients with infection
Patients with renal impairment
Pregnant/nursing patients

TOXICITIES

Hematologic: leukopenia, bone marrow depression, thrombocytopenia, anemia
GI: nausea (increased with high doses), vomiting, diarrhea
Dermatologic: skin rash, hives, itching, increased sweating, redness swelling, pain at the injection site
Renal: uric acid nephropathy, hemorrhagic cystitis, nephrotoxicity, hyperuricemia (especially when used for leukemias and lymphomas)
Cardiac: acute myopericarditis
Pulmonary: pneumonitis, interstitial pulmonary fibrosis
Miscellaneous: hyperglycemia, alopecia, hepatitis

INDICATIONS

FDA-approved: ALL, AML, CML, CLL, acute monocytic leukemia, Hodgkin's and non-Hodgkin's, carcinoma of the ovary or breast, myeloma, mycosis fungoides, neuroblastoma, retinoblastoma; **clinical studies show activity in:** bronchogenic carcinoma, small cell lung cancer, rhabdomyosarcoma, Ewing's sarcoma, carcinomas of GI, endometrium, testes, prostate, bladder, and renal cell, Wilm's tumor, squamous cell tumors of the cervix, head, and neck

PHARMACOKINETICS

Absorption—90% absorbed from the GI tract in doses < 100 mg, > 100 mg 75% absorbed; **Distribution**— well distributed with minimal amounts found in saliva, sweat, and synovial fluid, crosses the blood–brain barrier to a limited extent, 50% bound to plasma proteins; **Metabolism**—liver; **Elimination**— primarily in urine; **Half-life**—4–6.5 hr

DRUG INTERACTIONS

Barbiturates, phenytoin, chloral hydrate; cortico-steroids, doxorubicin, probenecid, chloramphenicol, sulfinpyrazone, bone marrow depressants, radiation, cocaine, cytarabine, allopurinol (possibly)

RESPONSE RATES

Hodgkin's—objective response rate of 60% with single agent; lymphoma—complete response of 10–20% and objective response of 40–70% with single agent; in combination regimen, complete response rate of 50%; Burkitt's lymphoma—complete response rate of 90% with single agent; Myeloma—objective response rate of 30%; ALL—objective response rate of 20–40%; AML—objective response rate of 10%; neuroblastoma—objective response rate of 65%; ovarian cancer—objective response rate of 60%; breast cancer—objective response rate of 35% with single agent, up to 90% in combination

PATIENT MONITORING

CBC weekly; other serum chemistries at periodic intervals; urinary output and urine-specific gravity following high-dose IV therapy

NURSING INTERVENTIONS

Monitor performance status; encourage good oral hygiene; administer antiemetics; encourage increased fluid intake and voiding every 2 hr; educate patients regarding side effects, care of venous access devices

PATIENT INFORMATION

Avoid use of aspirin or NSAIDs during therapy; neutropenic precautions to reduce the risk of infec-tion; increase fluid intake (up to 3 l/d) and voiding; divided oral doses and taken with or after meals to lessen nausea; call physician if blood is in urine

FORMULATIONS

Available as Cytoxan®, Bristol-Myers Oncology Divi-sion, Princeton, NJ; 25 and 50-mg tablets. Available as Neosar®, Adria Laboratories, Dublin, OH.; 100-mg, 200-mg, 500-mg, 1-g, and 2-g vials of powder for reconstitution. Tablets and vials stored at < 25°C.

DACARBAZINE

Dacarbazine (DTIC) is a cell cycle phase–nonspecific alkylating agent that is a synthetic analogue of the naturally occurring purine precursor, 5-amino-1h-imidazole-4-carboxamide. It is thought to exert its cytotoxic activity by three mechanisms: formation of carbonium ions leading to inhibition of DNA and RNA synthesis by alkylation; antimetabolite activity as a false precursor for purine synthesis, and binding with sulfhydryl groups.

DOSAGE AND ADMINISTRATION

Malignant melanoma: 2–4.5 mg/kg/d × 10 d, every 28 d, or 200–250 mg/m^2 d × 5 d, every 21–28 d. Doses of 400–500 mg/m^2 on days 1 and 2 (or 1000 mg/m^2 on day 1) every 3 to 4 wk have also been used

Hodgkin's disease (in combination therapy): 150 mg/m^2 × 5 d, every 4 wk, **or** 375 mg/m^2 repeated every 15 d or 750–1500 mg/m^2 as a single dose every 3–4 wk

DOSAGE MODIFICATIONS: reduce recommended doses in patients with renal or hepatic impairment receiving repeated courses; temporarily suspend therapy if leukocyte count falls below 3000/mm^3 and platelet count falls below 100,000/mm^3

SPECIAL PRECAUTIONS

Leukocyte, erythrocyte, and platelet counts taken prior to and at regular intervals during therapy
Hypersensitivity to the drug (anaphylactic reactions possible)
Pregnant/nursing patients

TOXICITIES

Hematologic: bone marrow depression, leukopenia (dose-limiting), thrombocytopenia, and anemia; acute leukemias after therapy (rare)
GI: severe nausea and vomiting occur (90%); anorexia, stomatitis, diarrhea, intractable nausea and vomiting (rare)
Hepatic: hepatic vein thrombosis, hepatocellular necrosis
Dermatologic: phototoxicity, urticaria, alopecia
Neurologic: confusion, lethargy, blurred vision, seizures, headache
Local: pain, burning, irritation at injection site; tissue damage and severe pain if extravasated
Miscellaneous: Flu-like syndrome; numbness and flushing of face

INDICATIONS

FDA-approved: malignant melanoma and Hodgkin's lymphoma (in combination-ABVD); **clinical studies show activity in:** soft-tissue sarcomas (leiomyosarcoma, fibrosarcoma, rhabdomyosarcoma), neuroblastoma, malignant glucagonoma

PHARMACOKINETICS

Absorption—not absorbed across the GI tract; **Distribution**—localizes in body tissues, especially liver, crosses the blood–brain barrier to a limited extent; **Protein binding**—low (approximately 20%), bound to plasma; poor CSF penetration; **Metabolism:** liver; **Elimination:** urine; **Half-life:** 19 min initial phase, 5 hr terminal phase; initial phase half-life is 55 min and terminal phase half-life 7.2 hr in patients with renal or hepatic impairment

DRUG INTERACTIONS

Barbiturates, phenytoin, bacillus Calmette–Guerin, hydrocortisone sodium succinate solutions

RESPONSE RATES

Metastatic malignant melanoma—objective response of greater than 50% reduction in 20% of patients
Advanced Hodgkin's disease second-line therapy with ABVD—3-yr survival rates of approximately 60%

PATIENT MONITORING

Monitor complete blood count weekly; obtain serum chemistries at periodic intervals; monitor temperature

NURSING INTERVENTIONS

Monitor treatment tolerance, weight, nutritional status; encourage good oral hygiene; educate patients about neutropenic precautions and self-care at home; take care to avoid extravasation, if it occurs treat with hot packs; give appropriate antiemetics as needed

PATIENT INFORMATION

Patients should avoid taking aspirin and nonsteroidal anti-inflammatory agents; call physician if sore throat, fever, or unusual bruising or bleeding develops; avoid sun exposure and/or exposure to sunlamps for at least 2 days post-treatment; avoid exposure to people with infections; treat flu-like symptoms with acetaminophen; modify and supplement diet as needed

FORMULATION

Available as DTIC-Dome®, Miles Pharmaceutical Division, West Haven CT
100-mg and 200-mg vials for reconstitution (10 mg/ml). Protected from light and stored at 2–8°C.

IFOSFAMIDE

Ifosfamide is a cell cycle–nonspecific alkylating agent of the nitrogen mustard class. It is a synthetic analogue of cyclophosphamide that must be activated by hepatic microsomal enzymes to exert its antineoplastic effect. Ifosfamide is hydroxylated to 4-hydroxyifosfamide (an active metabolite) and then metabolized to 4-ketoifosfamide and to 4-carboxyifosfamide (neither of which are cytotoxic). The active metabolites interact with DNA forming cross-linking strands of DNA and RNA, inhibiting protein synthesis.

DOSAGE AND ADMINISTRATION

Non-Hodgkin's lymphoma: 700–1000 mg/m^2/d × 5 d, repeated q 3 wk
Nonseminomatous germ cell tumors: 1.2 g/m^2/d × 5 d, repeated 3 wk
Non–small cell lung cancer: 2400 mg/m^2/d × 3 d, repeated q 3 wk
Advanced lung cancer: up to 5000 mg/m^2 as a single dose should be given with mesna for prophalaxis of ifosfamide-induced hemorrhagic cystitis

DOSAGE MODIFICATIONS: patients with renal function impairment require dose adjustment

SPECIAL PRECAUTIONS

Elderly patients (particularly with renal function impairment)
Hypersensitivity to ifosfamide
Patients with WBC count < 2000/ul and/or platelet count below 50,000/ul
Pregnant/nursing patients

TOXICITIES

Hematologic: severe myelosuppression (dose-related, dose-limiting)
GI: nausea and vomiting (common); anorexia, diarrhea, constipation
Neurologic: lethargy, confusion, hallucinations, encephalopathy
Renal: hemorrhagic cystitis (frequent), dysuria, urinary frequency
Pulmonary: cough, shortness of breath
Miscellaneous: phlebitis, infection, hepatotoxicity, alopecia

INDICATIONS

FDA-approved: third-line therapy for germ-cell testicular tumors; **clinical studies show activity in:** soft tissue sarcomas, Ewing's sarcoma, Hodgkin's and non-Hodgkin's lymphoma, carcinoma of the breast, lung, pancreas, and ovaries, ALL, CLL

PHARMACOKINETICS

Absorption—not administered orally; **Distribution**—crosses the blood–brain barrier but metabolites do not; **Metabolism**—50% in liver; doses of 3.8–5 g/m^2 have biphasic decay and half-life of 15 hr; doses of 1.6–2.4 g/m^2 have monophasic decay and half-life of 7 hr; **Elimination**—70–86% renally excreted; **Half-life:** 14 hr

DRUG INTERACTIONS

Phenobarbital, phenytoin, chloral hydrate, corticosteroids, allopurinol, bone marrow depressants, radiation therapy, live virus vaccines; mesna

RESPONSE RATES

Nonseminomatous germ cell tumors (in combination with cisplatin and etoposide or vinblastine)—complete response rate of 21%; (in combination with etoposide, cisplatin, and mesna)—complete response rate of 26%; Bulky seminoma (in combination with cisplatin and vinblastine)—complete response rate of 87%; Small cell lung cancer (in combination with etoposide and radiation therapy)—complete response rate of 76% and partial response rate of 14%; Recurrent or disseminated lung cancer (with high doses)—response rate of 33%; Non–small cell lung cancer (with single agent)—response rate of 24–30%; Advanced non–small cell lung cancer: in combination with cisplatin and etoposide—response rate of 26%; in combination with cyclophosphamide—response rate of 38% with complete response rate of 7%

PATIENT MONITORING

Monitor complete blood count weekly, obtain other serum chemistries at periodic intervals; test urine for microscopic hematuria prior to each course

NURSING INTERVENTIONS

Monitor treatment tolerance, weight, nutritional status; encourage good oral hygiene; administer antiemetics as necessary; encourage fluid intake and voiding every 2 hr (once at night); educate patients regarding central venous access devices and self-care at home

PATIENT INFORMATION

Patient should avoid use of aspirin or nonsteroidal anti-inflammatory agents; ensure adequate fluid intake and frequent voiding; notify physician if blood is in urine or clinical signs of infection; modify and supplement diet to maintain adequate caloric intake

FORMULATION

Available as IFEX®, Bristol Myers Oncology Division, Princeton, NJ; 1-g and 3-g vials for reconstitution. Stored protected from light at 15–30°C.

LOMUSTINE

Lomustine is a nitrosourea derivative that has demonstrated cytotoxic activity against a wide variety of malignancies. As with other alkylating agents, lomustine is considered to be cell cycle–nonspecific. Within 1 to 6 hours after oral administration of lomustine, peak metabolite concentrations occur. These metabolites are responsible for the alkylation and carbamoylation activity that interfere with DNA, RNA, and protein synthesis. Cross-resistance between lomustine and carmustine have occurred.

Lomustine and its metabolites are widely distributed in the body. Nitrosureas as a class tend to be highly lipophilic, thus enhancing their ability to cross the blood—brain barrier and be used in the treatment of meningeal leukemias and brain tumors. The long-term use of nitrosureas has been associated with profound cumulative myelosuppression and renal failure (especially with methyl-CCNU) with lesions similar to radiation-induced nephritis.

DOSAGE AND ADMINISTRATION

Adults and children: 75–130 mg/m^2 orally every 6–8 wk. Repeated doses should not be given until WBC count is greater than 4000/mm^3 and platelet count is greater than 100,000/mm^3

DOSAGE MODIFICATIONS: reduce dose to 70% if leukocytes drop to 2000–2999 or platelets to 25,000–74,999; reduce dose by 50% if leukocytes drop to < 2000 or platelets to < 25,000

SPECIAL PRECAUTIONS

Possible prolonged myelosuppression
Hypersensitivity to the drug
Pregnant/nursing patients

TOXICITIES

Hematologic: delayed hematologic toxicity (leukopenia, thrombocytopenia); refractory anemia, acute leukemias, bone marrow dysplasias (with long-term therapy)
GI: mild-to-moderate nausea and vomiting; anorexia; stomatitis (infrequent)
Neurologic: lethargy, ataxia, dysarthria (rare)
Miscellaneous: mild hepatotoxicity (transient elevation in liver enzymes); nephrotoxicity, progressive azotemia (accumulative doses ≥ 1000 mg/m^2), pulmonary fibrosis (accumulative doses ≥ 1000 mg/m^2)

INDICATIONS

FDA-approved: palliative treatment of primary and metastatic brain tumors, disseminated Hodgkin's disease in patients refractory to established treatment regimens (in combination therapy); **clinical studies show activity in:** bronchiogenic carcinoma, non-Hodgkin's lymphoma, malignant melanoma, breast carcinoma, renal cell carcinoma, carcinoma of the GI tract

PHARMACOKINETICS

Absorption—rapidly absorbed from the GI tract; oral bioavailability of 60–90%; **Distribution**—widely distributed, rapidly crosses the blood–brain barrier; **Metabolism**—completely metabolized 1 hr after administration; **Half-life**—6 hr (initial plasma), 1–2 d (second plasma); **Elimination**—completely in the urine

DRUG INTERACTIONS

Phenobarbital, cimetidine (possibly)

RESPONSE RATES

Refractory Hodgkin's disease—not established; brain tumors—partial response rate of 40% (limited studies)

PATIENT MONITORING

Monitor complete blood cell count weekly for 6 to 8 wk after oral administration; obtain first CBC 2 to 3 wk after therapy, with weekly CBC counts thereafter; monitor renal and hepatic status until CBC counts are normal

NURSING INTERVENTIONS

Monitor treatment tolerance, weight, nutritional status; administer antiemetics if necessary; educate patients about neutropenic precautions and self-care at home

PATIENT INFORMATION

Patient should call physician immediately if vomiting occurs after taking dose or if sore throat, fever, or any unusual bruising or bleeding develops; take medication on empty stomach (2–4 hr after meals); avoid aspirin or nonsteroidal anti-inflammatory agents; avoid exposure to people with infections

FORMULATIONS

Available as CeeNU®, Bristol Myers Oncology Division, Princeton, NJ
10-mg, 40-mg, and 100-mg capsules or dose kit-containing a total of 300-mg lomustine. Stored in tightly closed containers at < 40°C.

MECHLORETHAMINE

Mechlorethamine hydrochloride (nitrogen mustard or NH_2 hydrochloride) is a nitrogen analogue of sulfur mustard. It is a bifunctional alkylating agent that interferes with DNA replication and transcription of RNA in rapidly proliferating cells, eventually resulting in disruption of nucleic acid function. Mechlorethamine also possesses weak immunosuppressive activity. The drug is cell cycle phase–nonspecific. Its cytotoxic activity is most pronounced on rapidly proliferating cells. The activity of mechlorethamine is due to the transfer of an alkyl group to cellular constituents, such as phosphate, amino, hydroxyl, sulfhydryl, carboxyl, and imidazole groups. In neutral or alkaline solution, the drug is ionized to produce a positively charged carbonium ion, which then attaches to susceptible nuclear proteins at the N-7 position of guanine, a nucleoside found in DNA. This leads to abnormal base pairing of guanine with thymine, cleaving the imidazole ring of guanine, cross-linking of DNA, and depurination of DNA. Mechlorethamine also inhibits glycolysis, respiration, and RNA-directed protein synthesis.

DOSAGE AND ADMINISTRATION
Advanced Hodgkin's disease: 0.4 mg/kg either as a single dose or 2 to 4 divided doses of 0.1–0.2 mg/kg/d or 6 mg/m² on days 1 and 8, repeated every 28 d, for 6 cycles (in combination regimen) or 6 mg/m² on days 1 and 8 repeated every other month (in combination regimen)

SPECIAL PRECAUTIONS
Highly toxic with low therapeutic index
Inhalation of dust and vapors and contact of the drug with skin or mucous membrane should be avoided
Patients with leukopenia, thrombocytopenia, or anemia caused by malignant cell infiltration of the bone marrow
CLL patients
Patients undergoing radiation therapy
Pregnant/nursing patients

TOXICITIES
Hematologic: lymphocytopenia, granulocytopenia (6–8 d after treatment, lasting for 10–21 d), agranulocytosis, thrombocytopenia, severe leukopenia, anemia, hemorrhagic diathesis
GI: nausea, vomiting, diarrhea, jaundice, anorexia
Dermatologic: maculopapular skin eruptions, alopecia, erythema multiforme, herpes zoster
Reproductive: delayed menses, oligomenorrhea, temporary or permanent amenorrhea, impaired spermatogenesis, azoospermia, total germinal aplasia
Local reactions: thrombosis, thrombophlebitis, extravasation
Miscellaneous: weakness, vertigo, tinnitus, diminished hearing, chromosomal abnormalities

INDICATIONS
FDA-approved: palliative treatment of Hodgkin's disease (Stages III and IV), lymphosarcoma, chronic myelocytic leukemia, CLL, polycythemia vera, mycosis fungoides, bronchogenic carcinoma, palliative intraperitoneal, intrapleural, and intraperizardial treatment of metastatic carcinoma; **clinical studies show activity in:** topical application for cutaneous lymphoma and mycosis fungoides

PHARMACOKINETICS
Absorption—incompletely absorbed, rapidly transformed in water or body fluids; **Metabolism**—less than 0.01% of IV dose excreted unchanged in urine; **Elimination**—apparently renal

DRUG INTERACTIONS
Uricosuric agents; blood dyscrasia-causing medications; radiation therapy; live virus vaccines

RESPONSE RATES
Previously untreated patients with advanced Hodgkin's disease—complete response of 70–80% while receiving MOPP, 60–70% disease-free at 10 yr

PATIENT MONITORING
Monitor hematocrit and hemoglobin status and platelet and total (or differential) leukocyte counts throughout course; Audiometric testing at periodic intervals (with high doses); obtain serum chemistries; x-ray examination after intracavity administration

NURSING INTERVENTIONS
If extravasated, aspirate and neutralize with isotonic sodium thiosulfate and cold compresses; monitor treatment tolerance, weight, nutritional status; administer antiemetics as necessary; educate patient regarding care of central venous access devices and self-care at home

PATIENT INFORMATION
Patients should avoid use of aspirin or nonsteroidal anti-inflammatory agents; call physician if moderate or severe adverse effects develop (nausea, fever, or signs of serious infection); modify and supplement diet. For topical solution, shower and rinse carefully before application, wear rubber or plastic gloves when applying; apply lightly to groin, inside elbow, and behind knees; avoid contact with eyes, nose, and mouth

FORMULATION
Available as Mustargen®, Merck & Co., West Point, PA
Vials containing 10 mg of mechlorethamine triturated with 100 mg of sodium chloride. Unopened vials stored protected from light at room temperature.

MELPHALAN

Melphalan (L-phenylalanine mustard, L-PAM, or L-sarcolysin) is a bifunctional alkylating agent that is a phenylalanine derivative of nitrogen mustard. It is a cell cycle–nonspecific agent. Because it is a bischloroethylamine alkylator, its antineoplastic activity occurs due to the formation of an unstable ethylene immonium ion. This unstable ion alkylates with many intracellular molecular components, including nucleic acids. The result is cross-linking of strands of DNA (at the N-7 position of guanine) and RNA and disruption of cellular division leading to cellular death. Melphalan also inhibits protein synthesis and exhibits immunosuppressant activity. It is active against both resting and rapidly dividing tumor cells.

DOSAGE AND ADMINISTRATION

Multiple myeloma: usual oral dose is 6 mg/d (adjusted based on weekly blood counts) or 10 mg/d × 7–10 d (maintenance dose of 2 mg/d when WBC > 4000 and platelets > 100,000) **or** 0.15 mg/kg/d for 7 d, rest for 3 wk, then maintenance dose of 0.05 mg/kg/d **or** 0.1–0.15 mg/kg/d × 14–21 d, rest 2–4 weeks, then maintenance dose of 2–4 mg/d **or** 7 mg/m^2 or 0.25 mg/kg/d × 5 d every 5–6 wk **or** 16 mg/m^2 IV q 2 wk × 4 doses, after recovery from toxicity, at 4-wk intervals
Ovarian carcinoma: 0.2 mg/kg/d × 5 d every 4–5 wk

DOSAGE MODIFICATIONS: in patients with BUN ≥ 30 mg/dl, reduce dosage by 50%

SPECIAL PRECAUTIONS

Patients who have had prior radiation or chemotherapy
Elderly patients (particularly with renal function impairment)
Pregnant/nursing patients

TOXICITIES

Hematologic: reversible bone marrow suppression, leukopenia, thrombocytopenia, hemolytic anemia (most common); irreversible bone marrow failure
GI: nausea, vomiting, diarrhea (primary complaints); oral ulceration (infrequent)
Dermatologic: skin hypersensitivity, allergic reaction
Pulmonary: pulmonary fibrosis, interstitial pneumonitis
Miscellaneous: vasculitis, fever, chills, cough, hoarseness, alopecia, hematuria

INDICATIONS

FDA-approved: palliative treatment of multiple myeloma and nonresectable epithelial ovarian carcinoma; **clinical studies show activity in:** carcinoma of the breast and testes

PHARMACOKINETICS

Absorption—variably and incompletely absorbed in the GI tract; **Distribution**—rapidly and widely distributed in total body water; low penetration across blood–brain barrier; **Metabolism**—process of hydrolysis, half-life—90 min; **Elimination**—chemical hydrolysis to monohydroxy-and dihydroxymelphalan, low renal clearance
Dose adjustments in organ dysfunction: patients with BUN greater than (or equal to) 30 mg/dl should be closely monitored

DRUG INTERACTIONS

Cimetidine, famotidine, nizatidine, ranitidine, cyclosporine, other bone marrow depressants, live virus vaccines

RESPONSE RATES

Multiple myeloma—not curative but possible prolonged survival; ovarian carcinoma: objective response of 30–50% (combination regimens appear more effective)

PATIENT MONITORING

Monitor complete blood count weekly during therapy; obtain BUN, serum creatinine, serum uric acid concentrations prior to therapy and monthly throughout course

NURSING INTERVENTIONS

Monitor treatment tolerance, weight, nutritional status; encourage good oral hygiene; administer antiemetics as necessary

PATIENT INFORMATION

Patients should avoid use of aspirin and nonsteroidal anti-inflammatory agents during therapy; take oral doses at one time on empty stomach; call physician if signs or symptoms of infection or bleeding develops

FORMULATION

Available as Alkeran®, Burroughs-Wellcome Co., Research Triangle Park, NC
2-mg scored tablets. Stored in a well-closed, light-resistant container at 15–30°C. Also, 50-mg vials of melphalan with 10 ml of sterile diluent. Protected from light and stored at 15–30°C.

STREPTOZOCIN

Streptozocin is an antineoplastic antibiotic produced by *Streptomyces achromogenes*. As an antibiotic, streptozocin has activity against gram-positive and gram-negative bacteria but its cytotoxicity limits its use as an antibiotic. Streptozocin exhibits alkylating action *in vivo* by decomposing into reactive methylcarbonium ions that alkylate DNA and cause interstrand cross-linking. Although streptozocin blocks progression of cells into mitosis, it also blocks other sites of the cell cycle and is considered cell cycle–nonspecific.

The presence of a D-glucopyranose moiety enhances streptozocin uptake by pancreatic islet cells. No other alkylating agent contains a sugar moiety.

DOSAGE AND ADMINISTRATION

500 mg/m^2/d for 5 d every 6 wk

DOSAGE MODIFICATIONS: in patients with creatinine clearance of 10–50 ml/min reduce dose by 75%; patients with creatinine clearance < 10 ml/min reduce dose by 50%

SPECIAL PRECAUTIONS

Possible irreversible and fatal nephrotoxicity
Pregnant/nursing patients
Children

TOXICITIES

Renal: renal toxicity (serious and dose-limiting, 25–75%); glomerular and renal tubular dysfunction (azotemia, anuria, proteinuria, hypophosphatemia, hyperchloremia, proximal renal tubular acidosis); histologic changes in kidneys possible
GI: severe nausea and vomiting (possibly dose-limiting and progressively worse), mild diarrhea
Hematologic: mild-to-moderate myelosuppression
Hepatic: transient and mild increases in serum concentrations of liver enzymes, LDH, and/or alkaline phosphatase (all of which occur in 25% of patients)
Metabolic: hypoglycemia in patients with insulinoma (possibly severe but transient)
Local reactions: severe necrosis after extravasation
Miscellaneous: confusion, lethargy, depression

INDICATIONS

FDA-approved: pancreatic islet cell carcinoma; **clinical studies show activity in:** malignant carcinoid tumors, lung cancer, squamous cell carcinoma of the oral cavity, synovial sarcoma, adenocarcinoma of the gall bladder, colorectal cancer, malignant Zollinger–Ellison tumors, Hodgkin's disease

PHARMACOKINETICS

Absorption—poor oral absorption (< 20%); **Distribution**—rapidly distributed into the liver, kidneys, intestine, pancreas, via IV and intraperitoneal administration; **Metabolism**—extensively metabolized in the liver and kidneys; **Elimination**—biphasic; **Half-life**—5 min (initial), 35–40 min (terminal); **Excretion**—urine (60–70%)

DRUG INTERACTIONS

Nephrotic drugs, phenytoin, doxorubicin

RESPONSE RATES

Pancreatic islet cell carcinoma—response rates of 35 to 60%; palliative treatment of metastatic carcinoid tumor—partial responses of short duration

PATIENT MONITORING

Assess renal function prior to and during therapy; obtain urinalyses and routine serum chemistries with attention to BUN, serum creatinine, electrolyte concentration; monitor CBC count weekly

NURSING INTERVENTIONS

Monitor treatment tolerance, weight, nutritional status; administer appropriate antiemetics; wear gloves when administering agent (irritant); test urine for protein and glucose (proteinuria); be prepared for hypoglycemia (50% dextrose)

PATIENT INFORMATION

Patient should call physician immediately if intractable nausea and vomiting, unusual bruising or bleeding, fever above 102°F occurs; avoid people with infections; increase fluid intake during therapy; diabetic patients must intensively monitor glucose

FORMULATION

Available as Zanosar®, The Upjohn Company, Kalamazoo, MI
1-g vials of powder for injection. Stored protected from light and at 2–8°C.

THIOTEPA

Thiotepa is a synthetic polyfunctional alkylating agent that also possesses some immunosuppressive activity. Thiotepa interferes with DNA replication and transcription of RNA and ultimately results in the disruption of nucleic acid function. This alkylating agent has been in clinical use for more than 30 years. It can be administered by several different routes and is primarily used as an intravesical instillation for bladder carcinoma.

Recently, several studies have investigated the value of thiotepa in high doses to treat several tumor types, such as chronic leukemias, Hodgkin's disease, non-Hodgkin's lymphoma, breast and ovarian carcinoma, and melanoma.

DOSAGE AND ADMINISTRATION

Intravesical instillation for superficial bladder tumors: 30–60 mg in 30–60 ml of sterile water instilled by catheter into the bladder and retained for 2 hr once a week ×4 wk, then once a month × 1 yr
Intratumor injection: initial doses of 0.6–0.8 mg/kg directly into tumor; maintenance dose of 0.07–0.8 mg/kg every 1 to 4 wk
Intracavitary infusions: 0.6–0.8 mg/kg every week
Intrapericardial doses: 15–30 mg
Breast, lung, and ovarian cancers, lymphomas, Hodgkin's disease: 0.2 mg/kg IV daily for 5 d repeated every 2–4 wk, **or** 0.3–0.4 mg/kg IV every 1–4 wk
High-dose therapies: 60–475 mg/m^2 with or without autologous bone marrow transplantation **or** 180–1575 mg/m^2 with autologous bone marrow transplantation
Intrathecal administration: 1 to 10 mg/m^2 once or twice a week at 1 mg/ml concentration
Ophthalmic instillation: to prevent pterygium recurrence: 0.05% solution in Ringer's injection instilled into eye every 3 hr during day for 6 to 8 wk postoperatively

DOSAGE MODIFICATIONS: discontinue therapy if WBC count falls below 3000/mm^3 and platelet count falls below 150,000/mm^3

SPECIAL PRECAUTIONS

Hypersensitivity to the drug
Pregnant/nursing patients

TOXICITIES

Hematologic: leukopenia (major adverse effect); secondary malignancies can develop
GI: nausea, vomiting, and anorexia (infrequent at usual doses, increased at high doses); mucositis, esophagitis (with high doses)
Neurologic: headache, dizziness (with IV administration—dose limiting at high doses); cognitive dysfunction; demyelination
Dermatologic: hives, rash, and pruritus (mild); novel skin toxicity (high-dose therapy), bronzing of skin, some alopecia
Miscellaneous: lower abdominal pain, vesical irritability, hematuria, and hemorrhagic chemical cystitis (rare) with intravesical administration; lower extremity weakness and pain with intrathecal route; transient elevations (less than tenfold) in liver function tests (with high dose); amenorrhea, impaired spermatogenesis

INDICATIONS

FDA-approved: superficial tumors of the bladder (transitional cell carcinoma, papilloma, carcinoma *in situ*); **clinical studies show activity in:** breast cancer, Hodgkin's disease, non-Hodgkin's lymphoma, chronic leukemias, lung cancer, ovarian cancer, malignant melanoma, pterygium

PHARMACOKINETICS

Absorption—incompletely absorbed from the GI tract; **Distribution**—lipophilic, penetrates CNS readily; extensively and rapidly distributed to all tissues, exhibiting average volume of distribution of 0.7 l/kg; **Metabolism**—extensively metabolized in the liver; metabolite may be more potent than agent itself; **Half-life**—approximately 10 min (initial), 125 min (terminal); **Excretion**—60% in urine

DRUG INTERACTIONS

Succinylcholine

RESPONSE RATES

Superficial bladder tumors—complete response rates of 38% and partial responses of 24%
Palliative treatment in breast and ovarian carcinomas—response rates of 20 to 30% and 30 to 50%, respectively

PATIENT MONITORING

Monitor complete blood cell count weekly during therapy and for 3 wk thereafter; in patients with high tumor burden, monitor uric acid concentrations and administer allopurinol; perform complete neurologic exam at start and intermittently throughout therapy

NURSING INTERVENTIONS

Monitor treatment tolerance, weight, nutritional status; administer antiemetics when appropriate (especially with high doses); evaluate cognitive function, coordination, mental status at each visit

PATIENT INFORMATION

Patient should call physician immediately if sore throat, unusual bruising or bleeding, fever above 102°F develops; avoid people with infections; abstain from fluid intake for 8 to 10 hr before bladder installation; inform physician of loss of memory or coordination

FORMULATION

Available as Thiotepa®, Immunex Corporation, Seattle, WA
15-mg vials containing 80 mg of sodium chloride and 50 mg of sodium bicarbonate. Stored at 2–8°C and protected from light.

The antitumor antibiotics comprise a heterogeneous group of chemotherapy agents, that have proven to be extremely successful in the treatment of a wide variety of tumors, both epithelial and mesenchymal. Doxorubicin, daunorubicin, their analogues epirubicin and idarubicin, respectively, and the anthracendione antibiotic mitoxantrone are successful agents in the treatment of a number of neoplastic diseases, including carcinomas of the breast, lung, thyroid, and stomach, as well as Hodgkin's disease, non-Hodgkin's lymphoma, myeloma, acute lymphocytic and myelogenous leukemia, and sarcomas of various sites. Antibiotic agents have not only proven useful clinically but also from the standpoint of the basic scientist; they have yielded a fascinating variety of structure-activity relationships that have provided insights into the mechanisms by which anticancer agents exert their effects on normal and malignant tissues.

ANTHRACYCLINES

The anthracyclines comprise a series of large multiring structures attached to a daunosamine sugar; the compounds differ in the nature of the side chain (ketone vs ketol), the stereochemistry of the attached sugar, and the presence or absence of a methoxy side group on the ring structure. The planar semiquinone ring facilitates intercalation into DNA; this is a key event, because incorporation of the anthracycline creates the local conditions critical to its cytotoxicity.

MECHANISM OF ACTION

Interference with the action of DNA topoisomerase II in regions of transcriptionally active DNA is the most widely cited and generally accepted mechanism of action for the anthracyclines (Table 1). This enzyme acts by binding to DNA and nicking one of its strands, thus allowing the supercoiled macromolecule to relax as the opposite strand passes through the break. The enzyme then reanneals the broken ends. Anthracyclines are thought to act by stabilizing the topoisomerase-DNA complex in the cleaved configuration. This event not only maintains the single-strand breaks, but also helps to create further double-strand breaks. During mitosis, topoisomerase

II levels rise rapidly and the cell becomes more vulnerable to the effects of doxorubicin, thus possibly accounting for selective effects on rapidly dividing tumors.

The ability of these drugs to generate free radicals, which are cytotoxic to both normal and malignant tissues, has attracted much attention. Doxorubicin, as well as the other anthracyclines, is highly reactive with heavy metal ions, such as Cu^2 and Al^{3+}. Following entry into the cell, free drug in the cytosol is thought to bind ferric (Fe^{3+}) iron, which then generates highly reactive hydroxyl radical species by a one-electron reduction of the hydroxyquinone structure. The drug–iron complex binds to cell membranes and causes oxidative cell damage; most tissues possess adequate defenses against this type of event (in the form of superoxide dismutase, glutathione, etc.) and are able to repair the damage. Cardiac tissue, however, is notably deficient in this respect and is thus highly vulnerable to oxidative attack. Thus, the cardiotoxicity caused by anthracyclines is not the result of a particular affinity for cardiac tissue but rather the result of a deficiency in host protective factors.

This rich and varied organometallic chemistry also carries several practical implications: the ketol side chain of doxorubicin and its analogues is highly susceptible to oxidation by iron with its resultant destruction, whereas the ketone side chain of daunorubicin and its analogues lacks this reactivity. Thus, doxorubicin is much less stable than daunorubicin when reconstituted in aqueous solution, because iron is a frequent contaminant of many buffers and glassware items. For similar reasons, contact with metal surfaces and objects (such as syringe needles or aluminum foil) should not be prolonged.

PHARMACOKINETICS

Following intravenous bolus injection, doxorubicin and the anthracyclines leave the central pharmacokinetic compartment rapidly and distribute to the peripheral tissues, except the brain, in direct proportion to the DNA content of the peripheral tissue. The anthracyclines are metabolized in the liver and excreted in the bile (Table 2). One controversial area has been whether the dose of doxorubicin should be reduced in the face of abnormal liver function. Opinion is divided on this point; however, the conservative recommendation is to adjust the drug dose downward for an elevated bilirubin level.

Table 1. Mechanisms of Action of Antineoplastic Antibiotics

Agent	Mechanisms
Doxorubicin	Topoisomerase II inhibition, free radical formation, direct membrane interactions, DNA-RNA intercalation
Daunorubicin	Topoisomerase II inhibition, free radical formation, direct membrane interactions, DNA-RNA intercalation
Idarubicin	Free radical generation
Mitoxantrone	Single/double-stranded DNA breaks, cell membrane and mitochondrial lipid peroxidation, inhibition of glutathione synthesis
Dactinomycin	DNA intercalation, DNA-directed RNA synthesis inhibition
Bleomycin	Oxygen-derived free radical generation, DNA intercalation, single/double-strand DNA breaks
Mitomycin C	Oxygen-derived free radical generation, DNA alkylation, cross-linking of DNA strands, single-strand DNA breaks
Plicamycin	DNA binding, RNA synthesis inhibition, single-strand DNA breaks

Table 2. Pharmacokinetics of Antineoplastic Antibiotics

Drug	Half-life (hr)	Total Body Clearance	Route of Excretion
Bleomycin	2–4 (IV) 3 (intrapleural) 5 (intraperitoneal)	3 l/H/m²	50–70% renal
Dactinomycin	36–48	Unknown	Possibly 15% hepatic, 20–30% renal
Daunorubicin	20	34–67 l/H/m²	40% hepatic, 10% renal
Doxorubicin	16–24	15–30 l/H/m²	40–50% hepatic, 5–10% renal
Idarubicin	10–30	30–60 l/H/m²	5% renal
Mitomycin C	1–2	30 l/H	9–20% renal
Mitoxantrone	23–47	13–34 l/H/m²	40–50% hepatic, 5–10% renal
Plicamycin	Unknown	Unknown	?50% renal

ANTIBIOTIC AGENTS

TOXICITIES

The success of ICRF-187, a cardioprotective agent, is based on protection from free radical generation. ICRF-187 is a metal chelating agent, as is ethylenediaminetetraacetic acid, which is lipid-soluble and thus able to diffuse across the cell membrane. Once inside the cell, it is hydrolyzed to form a highly active metal chelating agent that binds with iron and removes it from the cardiac myocyte, thus protecting the cell from oxidative injury.

The sugar moiety of both doxorubicin and daunorubicin binds to heparin, and concomitant administration of an anthracycline and heparin can hasten clearance of doxorubicin. Both anthracyclines are associated with a radiation recall phenomenon, in which previously irradiated tissue becomes more susceptible to anthracycline-induced toxicity than would normal tissue. In patients with Hodgkin's disease and breast and small cell lung cancer, recall becomes a significant problem because these patients are often treated with chest and/or mediastinal radiation therapy, as well as anthracycline-based chemotherapy.

The dose-limiting toxicity of the anthracyclines varies with the method of administration. When given as intermittent intravenous boluses, cardiac toxicity predominates; when given as a continuous infusion over several days' time, however, the risk of cardiac injury is lessened, and myelosuppression or mucositis becomes the major clinical problem. Anthracyclines are potent vesicants, so extravasation injury must be avoided (Table 3).

Cardiac toxicity manifests itself as both an acute pericarditis–myocarditis syndrome and chronic congestive heart failure. Generally speaking, cumulative doses of 550 mg/m^2 are associated with a 10% risk of development of congestive heart failure; treatment should not exceed this limit. This number is potentially misleading, however, because the development of heart failure appears to depend on the route of administration. Patients can be safely treated with much higher cumulative doses of doxorubicin when the drug is given by continuous infusion. Increasing age, previous mediastinal irradiation, and cardiovascular disease all appear to increase the risk of cardiac complications, and patients should be screened for the existence of these risk factors prior to beginning chemotherapy with any anthracycline. Serial radionuclide gated cardiac function studies have proven to be useful in screening for the early development of cardiotoxicity. Consideration should be given to following patients with these examinations through the course of therapy, especially if any risk factors are present. As mentioned above, ICRF-187 has proven to be a successful cardioprotective agent in clinical trials and has allowed the delivery of substantially increased amounts of doxorubicin in recent clinical trials [1].

MITOMYCIN C

MECHANISM OF ACTION

In contrast to the anthracyclines, mitomycin C is a prodrug and requires metabolic activation to realize its cytotoxic potential [2,3]. Three different chemically active sites have been identified, although the precise mechanisms by which activation occurs *in vivo* are currently unclear. The quinone structure easily forms highly reactive semiquinone intermediates by chemical reduction, which can then bind to DNA and form an alkylated DNA adduct. Alternatively, reductive activation can also form highly toxic oxygen free radical intermediates, which attack cell membranes and subcellular structures. The urethane ring and the Cl carbon can also be potentially activated to form alkylating moieties.

Mitomycin C is considered the prototypical bioreductive alkylating agent, and the predominant mode of action is thought to be alkylation of DNA at the N-6 position of adenine or at the N-2 or O-6 positions of guanine by one of the active metabolites mentioned above. The drug has been moderately successful in the treatment of breast, non–small cell lung, gastric, pancreatic, colorectal, cervical, prostate, and superficial bladder cancers.

PHARMACOKINETICS

Activation to the reactive species can occur in all tissues; thus mitomycin C is rapidly cleared from the circulation following initial intravenous injection and distributes to total body water. It demonstrates pharmacokinetic behavior consistent with a two-compartment linear model, with a beta-elimination half-life of about 1 hour. Thus, significant drug levels will remain in the body for about 4 hours following an intravenous bolus administration.

TOXICITIES

Unlike other chemotherapeutic agents, the myelosuppression associated with mitomycin C is delayed, occurring about 4 weeks after treatment, suggesting that mitomycin acts upon the hematopoietic stem cell. Thrombocytopenia is often more severe than leukopenia or anemia. Mitomycin is a potent vesicant, and precautions should be taken to avoid extravasation during administration of this drug.

Among the dose-limiting toxicities unique to mitomycin C is a vasculitis that encompasses a spectrum of disease, including

Table 3. Toxicities of Antineoplastic Antibiotics

Toxicity	Bleomycin	Dactinomycin	Daunorubicin	Doxorubicin	Idarubicin	Mitomycin C	Mitoxantrone	Plicamycin
Myelosuppression	—	X	X	X	X	X	X	X
Nausea, vomiting	—	X	X	X	X	X	X	X
Stomatitis, alopecia	X	X	X	X	X	X	X	—
Extravasation necrosis	—	X	X	X	X	X	—	X
Pulmonary	X	—	—	—	—	X	—	—
Renal	—	—	—	—	—	X	—	X
Hepatic	—	X	—	—	—	—	—	X
Skin	X	X	X	X	X	—	—	—
Hemolysis	—	—	—	—	—	—	X	X
Cardiac	—	—	X	X	X	X	X	—
Fever	X	X	—	—	—	—	—	X

hemolytic–uremic syndrome and veno-occlusive disease. Interstitial pneumonitis and cardiac failure also occur. About 200 patients treated with mitomycin C have developed a syndrome that includes renal failure and hemolysis. This development seems to be dose-related, with most cases occurring after cumulative doses of 50 mg/m^2 have been given. Although the etiology of this syndrome is unknown, an autoimmune mechanism has been postulated; the fact that red blood cell transfusions can aggravate the hemolytic process supports this notion. Treatment is mainly supportive, and consists of hemodialysis, avoidance of red cell transfusions, and the use of various immunosuppressive agents. Recently, the use of a staphylococcal protein A immunoperfusion column has been reported of benefit.

Pulmonary toxicity appears to be idiosyncratic, potentiated by exposure to vinca alkaloids. Clinically, it is similar to that produced by other antineoplastics agents and is characterized by progressive pulmonary fibrosis mediated by free radical mechanisms. When given in combination with doxorubicin, mitomycin can act synergistically to increase cardiotoxicity, a possible consequence of both agents producing free radicals. Regardless of the mechanisms by which these increased toxicities are produced, caution is indicated when administering mitomycin in combination with anthracyclines.

BLEOMYCIN

MECHANISM OF ACTION

Bleomycin is a mixture of polypeptides, all with a common structural component called bleomycinic acid. Bleomycin A$_2$ is the predominant species; currently a series of analogues based on purified forms of the various polypeptides are in development. Like the anthracyclines, bleomycin chelates iron and forms an activated complex, which then binds the guanine bases in the DNA. Once formed, the DNA-bleomycin-iron adduct catalyzes the reduction of molecular oxygen to form highly reactive free radical species that cause DNA strand scission in the linker regions between nucleosomes. Thus, bleomycin causes not only DNA strand cleavage but also actual chromosomal breaks that can be visualized microscopically.

Bleomycin is a phase-specific agent, being most active in mitosis and G$_2$ phases of the cell cycle. Further supporting the concept of schedule dependency is the *in vitro* finding that both cell death and DNA strand breaks increase proportionally with the length of drug exposure, up to a period of 6 hours. Thus, bleomycin may be better administered by continuous infusion rather than by intravenous bolus.

PHARMACOKINETICS

Following intravenous injection in patients with normal renal function, bleomycin distributes to the peripheral compartment with an alpha half-life of about 30 minutes, and then is more slowly excreted with a beta half-life of between 2 and 4 hours. In the case of patients with impaired renal function, the terminal elimination half-life is extended significantly; thus, several authorities recommend decreasing the dose of bleomycin with creatinine clearances of less than 25 ml/min/m^2.

TOXICITIES

Bleomycin is toxic to lung tissue. This toxicity can have either a diffuse or nodular radiographic pattern, follows a course of relentless pulmonary fibrosis and insufficiency, and appears to be similar to the "final common pathway" noted for a number of other pulmonary toxins. The incidence of this complication increases with cumulative doses over 250 U, reaching 10% at total doses of 450 U. Elderly patients (> 70 years), patients with underling pulmonary disease, and patients previously exposed to pulmonary or mediastinal irradiation appear to be at increased risk. Treatment is mainly supportive. In regard to the mechanism of the pulmonary toxicity, it is of interest that bleomycin is degraded by hydrolysis; the aminohydrolases responsible for this are found in low concentrations in lung tissue and in skin. These tissues are particularly susceptible to bleomycin-induced injury, and thus may be examples of injury due to a lack of host protective factors, rather than to tissue tropism of the drug itself.

Cutaneous manifestations of bleomycin appear as erythematous, hyperpigmenting, or desquamating reactions typically occurring on the pressure points and skin creases. Frank ulcerations occasionally occur. These changes affect the flexer surfaces and areas of prior exposure to radiation. A dermatographic response also occurs. Vascular changes in the form of Raynaud's phenomenon has also been reported [4]. An acute idiosyncratic reaction consisting of confusion, faintness, fever and chills, and wheezing, has been reported in patients with lymphoma receiving more than 25 U/m^2. This syndrome may progress to cardiorespiratory collapse and usually occurs after the first or second dose. Other side effects of drug administration include fever (occurring up to 48 hours after infusion) and hyperbilirubinemia.

Perioperative management of patients who have previously received bleomycin is a vexing problem, because there is evidence suggesting that high inspired fractions of oxygen can potentiate or exacerbate bleomycin-induced pulmonary toxicity [5]. The clinical picture and physical findings of dyspnea, tachypnea, dry cough, and rales should prompt the performance of baseline arterial blood gas testing and chest radiography. If results are abnormal, then pulmonary function testing with DlCO should be pursued. If these tests are abnormal, or in the presence of other pulmonary risk factors, regional anesthesia should be considered, if feasible. If general anesthesia cannot be avoided, the best guidelines call for continuous oxygen saturation analysis and intermittent arterial blood gas sampling intraoperatively. For oxygen management, a brief period of 100% oxygen should be administered immediately prior to the induction of anesthesia, with subsequent inhaled concentrations kept at the minimum level necessary. Close monitoring of the patient's volume status and gas exchange is crucial both intra- and postoperatively, and mechanical ventilation may be required postoperatively to assure adequate oxygenation [5].

DACTINOMYCIN

MECHANISM OF ACTION

Dactinomycin (or actinomycin D) one of the first chemotherapeutic agents to be introduced into general use, has a structure similar to the anthracyclines and mitomycin C in that it consists of a planar, multi-ring, phenoxazone moiety with two substituents. In this case, two identical cyclic polypeptide arms are attached to the aromatic rings. The planar nature of the phenoxazone structure allows actinomycin to intercalate itself between DNA base pairs while the polypeptide rings lie within the minor groove; the overall effect is to bind together the two complementary strands of DNA, preventing the synthesis of the corresponding RNA molecules. Interestingly, at low concentrations actinomycin mainly inhibits DNA-directed RNA synthesis, whereas at high concentrations, both RNA transcription and DNA replication are affected.

PHARMACOKINETICS

Unlike many other chemotherapeutic agents, dactinomycin freely diffuses into the cell and distributes rapidly to the peripheral tissues. It has an elimination half-life of about 36 hours, mainly due to slow release from tissue- and DNA-binding sites. The drug is not significantly metabolized and is excreted unchanged into both bile and urine.

TOXICITIES

The dose-limiting toxicity of dactinomycin is primarily myelosuppression, although nausea, vomiting, diarrhea, and mucositis also occur. It can also cause a radiation recall phenomenon by inhibiting DNA repair mechanisms. The organs most prone to this effect are the skin and the gastrointestinal tract, although late effects can be seen in the lungs and the liver.

Dactinomycin has been used extensively in the treatment of gestational trophoblastic disease, Wilms' tumor, and other pediatric malignancies.

PLICAMYCIN

Although used originally in the treatment of Paget's disease and embryonal cell carcinoma of the testis, plicamycin is now used primarily in the management of hypercalcemia due to malignancy. With the advent of newer agents such as gallium nitrate and etidronate, however, use of the drug for this indication is also declining.

The mechanism of action involves inhibition of RNA synthesis but definitive molecular pharmacology studies have not been done. Likewise, because the drug was developed and marketed in the 1960s, contemporary pharmacokinetics are not available. The dose-limiting toxicity is a diffuse hemorrhagic syndrome, which occurs with a dose-related incidence of about 5 to 10%. Other side effects of hepatotoxicity and renal toxicity are seen in high-dose regimens.

REFERENCES

1. Speyer JL, Green MD, Zeleniuch-Jacquette A, *et al.*: ICRF-187 permits longer treatment with doxorubicin in women with breast cancer. *J Clin Oncol* 1992, 10:117–127.

2. Verwij J, Pinedo HM: Mitomycin C: Mechanism of action, usefulness and limitations. *Anticancer Drugs* 1990, 1:5–13.

3. Verweij J, Pinedo HM: Mitomycin C. *Cancer Chemother Biol Resp Mod* 1991, 12:59–65.

4. Vogelzang NJ, Bosl GJ, Johnson K, *et al.*: Raynaud's phenomenon: A common toxicity after combination chemotherapy for testicular cancer. *Ann Intern Med* 1981, 95:288–292.

5. Waid-Jones MI, Coursin DB: Perioperative considerations for patients treated with bleomycin. *Chest* 1991, 99:993–999.

6. Bosl GJ, Geller NJ, Bajorin D, *et al.*: A randomized trial of etoposide + cisplatin versus vinblastine + bleomycin + cisplatin + cyclophosphamide + dactinomycin in patients with good-prognosis germ cell tumors. *J Clin Oncol* 1988, 6:1231–1238.

7. Smith MA, Ungerleider RS, Horowitz ME, *et al.*: Influence of doxorubicin dose intensity on response and outcome for patients with osteogenic sarcoma and Ewing's sarcoma. *J Nat Cancer Inst* 1991, 83:1460–1470.

8. Calero F, Rodriguez-Escudero F, Jimeno J, *et al.*: Single agent epirubicin in squamous cell cervical cancer. *Acta Oncol* 1991, 30:325–327.

9. Calero F, Asins-Codoñer, Jimeno J, *et al.*: Epirubicin in advanced endometrial adenocarcinoma: A phase II study of the Grup Ginecologico Español para el Tratamiento Oncologico (GGETO). *Eur J Cancer* 1991, 27:864–866.

10. Nielsen D, Dombernowsky P, Skovsgaard T, *et al.*: Epirubicin or epirubicin and vindesine in advanced breast cancer. A phase III study. *Ann Oncol* 1990, 1:275–280.

11. Wade JR, Kelman AW, Kerr DJ, *et al.*: Variability in the pharmacokinetics of epirubicin: a population analysis. *Cancer Chemother Pharmacol* 1992, 29:391–395.

12. Berman E, Heller G, Santorsa J, *et al.*: Results of a randomized trial comparing idarubicin and cytosine arabinoside with daunorubicin and cytosine arabinoside in adult patients with newly diagnosed acute myelogenous leukemia. *Blood* 1991, 77:1666–1674.

13. Mandelli F, Petti MC, Ardia A, *et al.*: A randomised clinical trial comparing idarubicin and cytarabine to daunorubicin and cytarabine in the treatment of acute non-lymphoid leukemia. *Eur J Cancer* 1991, 27:750–755.

14. Estape J, Grau JJ, Loobendas F, *et al.*: Mitomycin C as an adjuvant treatment to resected gastric cancer: A 10-year follow-up. *Ann Surg* 1991, 213:219–221.

15. Cowan JD, Neidhart J, McClure S, *et al.*: Randomized trial of doxorubicin, bisantrene, and mitoxantrone in advanced breast cancer. A Southwest Oncology Group study. *J Nat Cancer Inst* 1991, 83:1077–1084.

16. Nissen NI, Hansen SW: High activity of daily-schedule mitoxantrone in newly-diagnosed low-grade non-Hodgkin's lymphomas: A 5-year follow-up. *Sem Oncol* 1990, 17:10–13.

17. de Forni M, Lachau S, Huguet F, *et al.*: Phase I/II pharmacokinetic study of mitoxantrone by continuous venous infusion in patients with solid tumours and lymphoproliferative diseases. *Eur J Cancer* 1991, 27:735–739.

BLEOMYCIN

Bleomycin is a mixture of fungal polypeptides isolated from *Streptomyces verticullus*, which create DNA strand breaks. Because bleomycin is cleared mainly through the kidneys, caution is advised in using this drug in the presence of impaired renal function, although no data exist on which to base specific dosing recommendations. Most commonly, the drug is given by intravenous infusion, but it is also used frequently in the setting of intracavitary instillation for sclerosis of the pleural or peritoneal cavities. Fever may occur in the immediate peri-infusion period, and occasional instances of hypersensitivity reactions have been reported. In combination chemotherapy protocols, bleomycin is most commonly used with cisplatin and etoposide as part of the PEB regimen for testicular cancer. Recent reports, however, have shown equivalent response rates for a two-drug regimen of cisplatin and etoposide alone [6].

Raynaud's phenomenon has been described as a complication of bleomycin therapy when given as part of combination chemotherapy regimens for testicular cancer. Speculated causal mechanisms have included arterial obstruction, increased neuromuscular instability due to hypomagnesemia, and sympathetic hyper-reactivity. However, as yet no single mechanism has been proven. Fortunately, the problem remains localized to the digits and causes little life- or limb-threatening morbidity.

DOSAGE AND ADMINISTRATION

Equipment and medication necessary for treatment of a possible anaphylactic reaction should be readily available at each administration. Test dose of 1–2 U given 2–4 hr prior to therapy is frequently recommended. Some clinicians recommend premedication with acetaminophen, steroids, and diphenhydramine hydrochloride to reduce fever and risk of anaphylaxis.
Intravenous administration: 10–20 U/m^2/wk IV **or** 15 U/m^2 continuous infusion over 24 hr for 4–5 d. Maintenance dose for Hodgkin's disease: 1 U/d **or** 5 U/wk until completion of therapy; **Regional arterial infusion:** 30–60 U/d over 1–24 hr; **Intrapleural injection:** 15–120 U in 100 ml 0.9% NS injection, instilled and removed after 24 hr; **Intraperitoneal injection:** 60–120 U (base) in 100 ml 0.9% NS injection, instilled and removed after 24 hr; **Intralesional injection:** 0.2–0.8 U (base) (according to lesion size) one or more times at intervals of 2–4 wk, up to a maximum total dose of 2 U, using a solution of 15 U of bleomycin in 15 ml of 0.9% NS injection or water for injection.

DOSAGE MODIFICATIONS: Cumulative doses should not exceed 250–450 U (less in patients with risk factors mentioned above or with renal impairment, < 25 ml/min/m^2). When given intrapleurally or intraperitoneally, one half of the intracavitary dose should be counted towards this total.

SPECIAL PRECAUTIONS

Pediatric patients; patients over 70 years of age (increased risk of pulmonary toxicity and decline in renal function warrant dose reduction); patients who smoke; pregnant/nursing patients; potential for perioperative pulmonary complications.
Conditions requiring special considerations: herpes zoster, chickenpox, hepatic functional impairment, Raynaud's phenomenon, peripheral vascular disease

TOXICITIES

Degree of Severity	Frequent	Occasional	Rare
Need acute medical attention	Fever/chills, pulmonary toxicity, stomatitis	Hypersensitivity reaction	Hepatotoxicity, pleuropericarditis, renal and vascular toxicity
Medical attention if persistent/bothersome	Skin changes, vomiting, loss of appetite	Weight loss	
Less need for medical attention		Alopecia	
Medical attention if occurring after withdrawal		Shortness of breath, cough	

INDICATIONS

FDA-approved: Hodgkin's disease, non-Hodgkin's lymphoma, head and neck, laryngeal, cervical, penile, skin, and vulvar carcinoma; **clinical studies show activity in:** paralaryngeal carcinoma, osteosarcoma, malignant pleural/peritoneal effusions, germ cell and ovarian tumors, mycosis fungoides, testicular carcinoma

PHARMACOKINETICS

Distribution—45% absorbed into the systemic circulation following intrapleural or intraperitoneal administration; **Protein binding**— < 1%; **Metabolism**–unknown, although degradative pathways involve aminohydrolases. Enzyme activity is high in liver, kidneys, bone marrow, and lymph nodes, low in skin and lungs; **Half-life**—(with normal renal function) alpha, 0.25 hr; beta, 2–4 hr; increases exponentially as creatinine clearance decreases; **Excretion**—60–70% renal

DRUG INTERACTIONS

General anesthetics, cisplatin, vincristine, lomustine, digoxin, phenytoin

PATIENT MONITORING

Obtain chest radiograph, pulmonary function tests (including FVC and DL$_{CO}$), BUN, serum creatinine, hematocrit or hemoglobin, platelet count, total and/or differential leukocyte count, serum alanine aminotransferase (SGPT) concentrations, serum aspartate aminotransferase (SGOT), serum bilirubin, serum lactate dehydrogenase; check patient's mouth for ulceration and lungs for rales, decreased breath sounds, or evidence of restrictive lung disease before administration of each dose.

PATIENT INFORMATION

Patient should stop smoking due to pulmonary toxicity; continue medication despite stomach upset; careful attention and monitoring are required if surgery (including dental) or emergency treatment is needed; watch for the development of shortness of breath, cough, oral ulcerations/pain, fever, or chills

NURSING INTERVENTION

Administer acetaminophen on routine basis

FORMULATION

Available as Blenoxane®, Bristol-Myers Oncology Division, Princeton, NJ
Stored at 15–30°C and protected from light.

DACTINOMYCIN

Although it is one of the first antineoplastic agents, dactinomycin (or actinomycin D) is rarely used in current practice. Responses have been noted in patients with Wilms' tumor, Ewing's sarcoma, embryonal rhabdomyosarcoma, and gestational choriocarcinoma. Its action is via DNA intercalation, and it is rapidly distributed to tissues and DNA. Clearance is slow, however, mainly due to a slow rate of release from tissue compartments and occurs through the biliary and renal routes.

DOSAGE AND ADMINISTRATION

To avoid serious toxicity, administer in short, intermittent courses (toxicity may not appear until 2–4 d after last dose and may be maximal for 1–2 wk).
All indications: 10–15 µg (0.01–0.015 mg)/kg/d IV for maximum of 5 d, every 4–6 wk **or** 500 µg (0.5 mg)/m²/wk (maximum 2 mg/wk) IV for 3 wk
Ewing's sarcoma or sarcoma botryoids: 50 µg (0.05 mg)/kg isolation-perfusion for lower extremity or pelvis, **or** 35 µg (0.035 mg)/kg for upper extremity. Limit to 15 µg (0.015 mg)/kg **or** 400–600 µg (0.4–0.6 mg)/m²/d for 5 d (base dosage on bsa for obese/edematous patients)

SPECIAL PRECAUTIONS

Pediatric patients: increased risk of toxicity in infants (contraindicated in infants under 6 mo)
Obese patients: lower dosage based on bsa and observe daily for toxicity
Patients with previous cytotoxic drug therapy or radiation therapy (lower dose recommended)
Pregnant/nursing patients
Conditions requiring special considerations: bone marrow depression, chickenpox, herpes zoster, gout, urate renal stones, hepatic impairment, infection

TOXICITIES

Degree of Severity	Frequent	Occasional	Rare
Need acute medical attention	Anemia, leukopenia, thrombocytopenia, pharyngitis		Anaphylaxis, uric acid nephropathy, hyperuricemia, phlebitis, cellulitis
Medical attention if persistent/bothersome	Skin rash/acne, fatigue		
Less need for medical attention	Nausea/vomiting, darkening/redness of skin, alopecia		
Medical attention if occurring after withdrawal	Bone marrow depression, GI ulceration, esophagitis	Ulcerative stomatitis, hepatotoxicity	

INDICATIONS

FDA-approved: Ewing's sarcoma, sarcoma botryoides, trophoblastic tumors, endometrial carcinoma, trophoblastic tumors, testicular carcinoma, Wilm's tumor, Ewing's sarcoma, rhabdomyosarcoma; **clinical studies show activity in:** ovarian carcinoma, Kaposi's sarcoma, osteosarcoma, malignant melanoma

PHARMACOKINETICS

Distribution—does not cross the blood–brain barrier; distributes particularly to bone marrow/tumor cells, subaxillary gland, liver, and kidney; **Protein binding**—extensive, to tissues; **Half-life**—36 hr; **Excretion**—50% biliary/fecal, 10% renal (both unchanged); 30% dose in urine/feces within 1 wk

DRUG INTERACTIONS

Allopurinol, colchicine, sulfinpyrazone, bone marrow depressants, radiation therapy, blood dyscrasia-causing medications, vaccines, probenecid, doxorubicin, vitamin K

PATIENT MONITORING

Examine patient's mouth for ulceration; monitor hematocrit or hemoglobin, platelet count, total and/or differential leukocyte count, serum alanine aminotransferase (SGPT) concentrations, serum aspartate aminotransferase (SGOT), serum bilirubin, serum lactate dehydrogenase, and serum uric acid

NURSING INTERVENTIONS

Avoid contact with soft tissues; if given directly into vein, use one sterile needle for reconstituting and withdrawing dose from vial, another for administration; if extravasation occurs, stop immediately and administer remaining dose by another vein; to prevent hyperuricemia and hyperuricuria, give IV fluid therapy and allopurinol (4–5 d) during severe oral toxicity (*ie*, patient unable to drink)

PATIENT INFORMATION

Patient should take each medication at correct time and continue despite stomach upset; avoid immunization unless approved by physician; maintain ample fluid intake; call physician if unusual bleeding, bruising, or black, tarry stools, blood in urine or stools, fever, chills, cough/hoarseness, lower back/side pain painful/difficult urination, or pinpoint red spots on skin occur; call physician immediately if redness, pain, or swelling occurs at injection site; use caution with dental hygiene; avoid trauma to mucosal surfaces of eyes, nose, mouth; avoid activities or situations where bruising is likely to occur; avoid exposure to persons with bacterial infections

FORMULATION

Cosmegen®, Merck Co., Westpoint, PA
Vials of 500 µg (0.5 mg). Stored at 15–30°C and protected from light.

DAUNORUBICIN

Because it causes less mucositis than doxorubicin, daunorubicin has become the standard anthracycline for use in remission induction regimens for acute myelogenous leukemia. Furthermore, decreased mortality was seen with daunorubicin in CALGB studies than with doxorubicin.

DOSAGE AND ADMINISTRATION

Courses cannot be administered more frequently than every 21 d, to allow bone marrow to recover.

Acute lymphocytic leukemia: 45 mg/m^2 IV D 1, 2, 3 of a 32-d course in combination with vincristine, prednisone, and l-asparaginase

Acute nonlymphocytic leukemia: 45 mg/m^2 IV D 1, 2, 3 of first course and D 1, 2 of second course in combination with cytarabine

DOSAGE MODIFICATIONS: Limit total lifetime dosage to 550 mg (base)/m^2 or 450 mg (base)/m^2 in patients who have received previous chest radiation therapy. In acute leukemia, agent may be administered despite presence of thrombocytopenia and bleeding; stoppage of bleeding and increase in platelet count have occurred during treatment in some cases and platelet transfusions are useful in others.

SPECIAL PRECAUTIONS

Pediatric patients
Geriatric patients, particularly those with age-related bone marrow depression and renal impairment
Patients with inadequate bone marrow reserves
Pregnant/nursing patients
Conditions requiring special consideration: bone marrow depression, chickenpox, herpes zoster, gout, urate renal stones, heart disease, herpes/renal impairment, infection, tumor cell infiltration of the bone marrow

TOXICITIES

Degree of Severity	Frequent	Occasional	Rare
Need medical attention	Esophagitis, infection, leukopenia, thrombocytopenia	GI ulceration, uric acid nephropathy, extravasation, cellulitis, tissue necrosis, hyperuricemia, cardiotoxicity	Cardiotoxicity/pericarditis—myocarditis, allergic reaction
Medical attention if persistent/bothersome		Stomatitis	Diarrhea
Less need for acute medical attention	Nausea/vomiting, alopecia, reddish urine		Darkening/redness of skin
Medical attention if occurring after withdrawal	Irregular heartbeat, shortness of breath	Edema in lower extremities	

INDICATIONS

FDA-approved: erythroleukemia, acute lymphocytic leukemia, acute myelocytic leukemia, acute monocytic leukemia; **clinical show activity in:** neuroblastoma, non-Hodgkin's lymphomas, chronic myelocytic leukemia, Wilm's tumor, Ewing's sarcoma

PHARMACOKINETICS

Distribution—rapid, especially to major organs; does not cross blood–brain barrier; **Half-life**—45 min; **Excretion**—prolonged; 25% (active) in urine, 40% biliary

DRUG INTERACTIONS

Allopurinol, colchicine, probenecid, sulfinpyrazone, blood dyscrasia-causing medications, radiation therapy, doxorubicin, hepatotoxic medications, vaccines, bone marrow depressants

PATIENT MONITORING

Monitor with chest radiography, echocardiography, ECG, radionuclide angiography determination of ejection fraction, hematocrit or hemoglobin, platelet count, total and/or differential leukocyte count, serum alanine aminotransferase, serum aspartate aminotransferase (SGOT) concentrations, serum bilirubin, serum lactate dehydrogenase, serum uric acid

NURSING INTERVENTIONS

If extravasation occurs (local burning/stinging), stop injection and resume in an alternate vein; maintain oral hydration and (if necessary) administer allopurinol; avoid inhalation of doxorubicin or exposure to the skin (use gloves)

PATIENT INFORMATION

Patient should consume medication despite stomach upset; avoid immunization unless approved by physician; avoid exposure to those who have taken oral poliovirus vaccine; call physician immediately if unusual bleeding or bruising, black, tarry stools, blood in urine or stools, or pinpoint red spots on skin occur; use caution with dental hygiene tools; avoid trauma to mucosal surfaces of eyes, nose, mouth; call physician immediately if redness, pain, or swelling occurs at injection site; urine may turn red during the first 24–48 hr after therapy

FORMULATION

Available as Cerubidine®, Wyeth-Ayerst Laboratories, Philadelphia, PA
Vials containing 20 mg (base) (21.4 mg as HCl). Stored at 15–30°C and protected from light.

DOXORUBICIN

Doxorubicin is the standard anthracycline for use against nonhematologic tumors. A recent analysis has confirmed that the dose intensity of doxorubicin is an important determinant of favorable outcome in the treatment of osteogenic sarcomas and Ewing's sarcomas [7]. The use of the cardioprotective agent ICRF-187 appears very promising, especially in light of the data suggesting its use allows the administration of higher cumulative doses of doxorubicin to patients with advanced breast cancer [8].

DOSAGE AND ADMINISTRATION

60–75 mg/m^2 IV, repeated every 21 d; **or** 25–30 mg/m^2/d IV on 2–3 consecutive d, repeated every 3–4 wk; **or** 20 mg/m^2/wk IV.

DOSAGE MODIFICATIONS: Limit total cumulative dosage to 550 mg/m^2, and 400 mg/m^2 in patients with previous chest radiation therapy or medications increasing cardiotoxicity. In acute leukemia, doxorubicin may be administered despite the presence of thrombocytopenia and bleeding; stoppage of bleeding and an increase in platelet count have occurred during treatment in some cases and platelet transfusions are useful in others.

SPECIAL PRECAUTIONS

Pediatric patients (cardiotoxicity more frequent in those < 2 years)
Elderly patients (cardiotoxicity more frequent in those > 70 years)
Pregnant/nursing patients
Conditions requiring special considerations: bone marrow depression, heart disease, herpes zoster, hepatic function impairment, gout, tumor cell infiltration of the bone marrow, urate renal stones, chickenpox

TOXICITIES

Degree of Severity	Frequent	Occasional	Rare
Need medical attention	Esophagitis, leukopenia, infection	Uric acid nephropathy, GI ulceration, tissue necrosis, cellulitis, cardiotoxicity, postradiation erythema, recall; extravasation, hyperuricemia, thrombocytopenia, phlebosclerosis	Anaphylaxis, allergic reaction
Medical attention if persistent/bothersome	Stomatitis	Diarrhea	
Less need for acute medical attention	Nausea/vomiting, alopecia	Darkening of soles, palms, or nails; reddish urine	
Medical attention if occurring after withdrawal	Possible cardiotoxicity: fast/irregular heartbeat	Shortness of breath, peripheral edema	

INDICATIONS

FDA-approved: acute lymphocyte leukemia, acute myelocytic leukemia, neuroblastoma, ovarian carcinoma, thyroid carcinoma, Wilm's tumor, lung carcinoma, gastric carcinoma, Hodgkin's lymphomas, non-Hodgkin's lymphomas, soft tissue sarcomas, osteosarcoma; **clinical studies show activity in:** head and neck, cervical, hepatic, pancreatic, prostatic, testicular, and endometrial carcinoma, germ cell and ovarian tumors, Ewing's sarcoma, multiple myeloma

PHARMACOKINETICS

Metabolism—rapid (within 1 hr); hepatic, with one active metabolite; **Half-life**—doxorubicin: alpha phase, 0.6 hr; beta phase, 16.7 hr; metabolites: alpha phase, 3.3 hr; beta phase, 31.7 hr; **Excretion**—50% biliary (unchanged); 23% as adramycinol; < 10% renal

DRUG INTERACTIONS

Allopurinol, colchicine, probenecid, sulfinpyrazone, radiation therapy, hepatotoxic medications, streptozocin, vaccines, bone marrow depressants, daunorubicin, mitomycin C, dactinomycin, cyclophosphamide, blood dyscrasia-causing medications, digoxin, verapamil

PATIENT MONITORING

Examine patient's mouth for ulceration before each dose; monitor chest radiography, echocardiography, ECG, radionuclide angiographic determination of ejection fraction, hematocrit or hemoglobin, platelet count, total and/or differential leukocyte count, serum alanine aminotransferase (SGPT) concentrations, serum aspartate aminotransferase (SGOT), serum bilirubin, serum lactate dehydrogenase, serum uric acid

NURSING INTERVENTIONS

Maintain ample fluid intake and increase in urine output; avoid inhalation of doxorubicin or exposure to the skin (use gloves)

PATIENT INFORMATION

Patient should continue medication despite stomach upset; avoid immunization unless approved by physician; avoid exposure to those who have taken oral poliovirus vaccine; call physician immediately if unusual bleeding or bruising, black, tarry stools, blood in urine or stools, or pinpoint red spots on skin occurs; call physician immediately if redness, pain, or swelling occurs at injection site; use caution with dental hygiene; avoid trauma to mucosal surfaces of eyes, nose, mouth; urine may turn red during the first 24–48 hr after therapy

FORMULATIONS

Available as Adriamycin PFS and RDF®, Adria Laboratories, Dublin OH; Doxorubicin Hydrochloride, Astra USA, Westboro, MA and Cetus Oncology Corporation, Emeryville, CA; Rubex®, Immune Corporation, Seattle, WA
Vials of 10-, 20-, 50-, 100-, 150-, and 200-mg doxorubicin hydrochloride for injection. Stored at 15–30°C and protected from light.

EPIRUBICIN

Epirubicin is a stereoisomer of doxorubicin, differing only in the orientation of the 4'-hydroxyl group in the amino sugar. Although available commercially in Europe, it is currently available only for investigational use in the United States. It differs in its catabolic pathway from doxorubicin in that it is conjugated with glucuronic acid, and this reaction is thought to account for its shorter half-life and lessened cardiotoxicity relative to doxorubicin. Indeed, its dose-limiting toxicity is myelo-suppression, with neutropenia being most prominent.

Epirubicin has been used in phase II testing in cervical cancer [8], endometrial cancer [9], and advanced breast cancer [10], with response rates ranging from 18.5 to 26%. Population pharmacokinetic analysis shows that it follows a two-compartment model and that age and sex significantly influence the clearance rates of the drug [11].

DOSAGE AND ADMINISTRATION

75–90 mg/m^2 IV, repeated every 21 d, may be given in divided doses over 2 d. Limit cumulative dosage to 700 mg/m^2.

DOSAGE MODIFICATIONS: When given as part of combination protocols, in elderly patients or in patients with prior chemo/radiation therapy, dose should be reduced, although no guidelines are available. Reduce dose by 50% in patients with liver metastases or abnormal liver function tests.

SPECIAL PRECAUTIONS

Pediatric patients (cardiotoxicity more frequent in those < 2 years)
Elderly patients (cardiotoxicity more frequent in those > 70 years)
Patients with inadequate bone marrow reserves
Pregnant/nursing patients
Conditions requiring special considerations: bone marrow depression, heart disease, herpes zoster, hepatic function impairment, gout, tumor cell infiltration of the bone marrow, urate renal stones, chickenpox

TOXICITIES

Degree of Severity	Frequent	Occasional	Rare
Need acute medical attention	Esophagitis, leukopenia, infection	Uric acid nephropathy, GI ulceration, tissue necrosis, cellulitis, cardiotoxicity, postradiation erythema, recall; extravasation, hyperuricemia, thrombocytopenia, phlebosclerosis	Anaphylaxis, allergic reaction
Medical attention if persistent/bothersome	Stomatitis	Diarrhea	
Less need for medical attention	Nausea/vomiting, alopecia	Darkening of soles, palms, or nails; reddish urine	
Medical attention if occurring after withdrawal	Possible cardiotoxicity: fast/irregular heartbeat	Shortness of breath, peripheral edema	

INDICATIONS

Clinical studies show activity in: breast carcinoma, acute myelogenous leukemia, non-Hodgkin's lymphoma, GI tract carcinoma

PHARMACOKINETICS

Metabolism—rapid, hepatic, with one active metabolite; **Half-life**—alpha phase, 0.6 hr; beta phase, 40 hr; **Excretion**—mainly biliary

DRUG INTERACTIONS

Information not available

PATIENT MONITORING

Examine patient's mouth for ulceration before each dose; monitor chest radiography, echocardiography, ECG, radionuclide angiography determination of ejection fraction, hematocrit or hemoglobin, platelet count, total and/or differential leukocyte count, serum alanine aminotransferase (SGPT) concentrations, serum aspartate aminotransferase (SGOT), serum bilirubin, serum lactate dehydrogenase, serum uric acid

NURSING INTERVENTIONS

Maintain ample fluid intake and increase in urine output; avoid inhalation or exposure to the skin (use gloves)

PATIENT INFORMATION

Patient should continue medication despite stomach upset; avoid immunization unless approved by physician; avoid exposure to those who have taken oral poliovirus vaccine; call physician immediately if unusual bleeding or bruising; black, tarry stools, blood in urine or stools, or pinpoint red spots on skin occurs; call physician immediately if redness, pain, or swelling occurs at injection site; use caution with dental hygiene avoid trauma to mucosal surfaces of eyes, nose, mouth

AVAILABILITY

Epirubicin is not commercially available in the US at this time.

IDARUBICIN

A stereoisomer of daunorubicin, idarubicin is a less cardiotoxic substitute for daunorubicin in treatment protocols for acute myelogenous leukemia (AML). Like daunorubicin, it is metabolized to an active hydroxylated metabolite (1,3-dihydroidarubicin). A long elimination half-life (twice that of idarubicin) for idarubicinol allows for the maintenance of cytotoxic concentrations for prolonged periods of time.

Because of its similarities to daunorubicin, attempts have been made to use idarubicin in place of daunorubicin in AML protocols. One study at Memorial Sloan–Kettering Cancer Center showed a clear advantage of idarubicin over daunorubicin, with a complete response rate of 80% with idarubicin and cytosine arabinoside versus 58% in patients treated with standard-dose daunorubicin and cytosine arabinoside [12]. Furthermore, this advantage was maintained over time, with overall survival rates of 19.5 versus 13.5 months. However, another study, from the Italian Cooperative Group GIMEMA, showed no difference between patients treated with these two protocols [13].

DOSAGE AND ADMINISTRATION

12 mg/m^2/d IV for 3 d as single agent. In combination with cytosine arabinoside, 100 mg/m^2/d continuous IV infusion for 7 d or single dose of 25 mg/m^2 IV followed by 200 mg/m^2/d continuous IV infusion for 5 d. Give dose slowly (over 10–15 min) into the tubing of a freely running IV infusion of 0.9% NaCl injection USP or 5% dextrose injection USP.

SPECIAL PRECAUTIONS

Pediatric patients (cardiotoxicity more frequent in those < 2 years)
Elderly patients (cardiotoxicity more frequent in those ≥ 70 years)
Patients with inadequate bone marrow reserves
Pregnant/nursing patients
Conditions requiring special considerations: bone marrow depression, heart disease, herpes zoster, hepatic function impairment, gout, tumor cell infiltration of the bone marrow, urate renal stones, chickenpox

TOXICITIES

Degree of Severity	Frequent	Occasional	Rare
Need acute medical attention	Esophagitis, leukopenia, infection	Uric acid nephropathy, GI ulceration, tissue necrosis, cellulitis, cardiotoxicity, postradiation erythema, recall; extravasation, hyperuricemia, thrombocytopenia, phlebosclerosis	Anaphylaxis, allergic reaction
Medical attention if persistent/bothersome	Stomatitis	Diarrhea	
Less need for medical attention	Nausea/vomiting, alopecia	Darkening of soles, palms, or nails; reddish urine	
Medical attention if occurring after withdrawal	Possible cardiotoxicity: fast/irregular heartbeat	Shortness of breath, peripheral edema	

INDICATIONS

Clinical studies show activity in: acute myelogenous leukemia, acute lymphocytic leukemia, advanced breast cancer, endometrial carcinoma, non-Hodgkin's lymphoma, Hodgkin's disease, pancreatic cancer, myeloma

PHARMACOKINETICS

Metabolism—rapid, hepatic, with one active metabolite; **Protein binding**—97%, although it is concentration-dependent; **Half-life**—14–35 hr with oral dosing, 12–27 hr with IV dosing; **Excretion**—15% biliary (unchanged); 15% renal

DRUG INTERACTIONS

Allopurinol, colchicine, probenecid, sulfinpyrazone, radiation therapy, hepatotoxic medications, streptozocin, vaccines, bone marrow depressants, daunorubicin, mitomycin C, dactinomycin, cyclophosphamide, blood dyscrasia-causing medications

PATIENT MONITORING

Examine patient's mouth for ulceration before each dose; monitor chest radiography, echocardiography, ECG, radionuclide angiographic determination of ejection fraction, hematocrit or hemoglobin, platelet count, total and/or differential leukocyte count, serum alanine aminotransferase (SGPT) concentrations, serum aspartate aminotransferase (SGOT), serum bilirubin, serum lactate dehydrogenase, serum uric acid

NURSING INTERVENTIONS

Maintain ample fluid intake and increase in urine output; avoid inhalation or exposure to the skin (use gloves)

PATIENT INFORMATION

Patient should continue medication despite stomach upset; avoid immunization unless approved by physician; avoid exposure to those who have taken oral poliovirus vaccine; call physician immediately if unusual bleeding or bruising, black, tarry stools, blood in urine or stools, or pinpoint red spots on skin occur; call doctor immediately if redness, pain, or swelling occurs at injection site; use caution with dental hygiene; avoid trauma to mucosal surfaces of eyes, nose, mouth

FORMULATIONS

Available as Idamycin®, Adria Laboratories, Dublin, OH
Vials of 5- and 10-mg idarubicin hydrochloride. Stored at controlled room temperature (59–86°F).

MITOMYCIN C

Mitomycin C is a bioreductive alkylating agent, requiring *in vivo* activation to the cytotoxic species. The primary side effects are delayed myelosuppression and injury due to extravasation. Occasional cases of vasculitis with manifestations ranging from hemolytic–uremic syndrome to lethal veno-occlusive disease have been observed. Because of the potential for vascular toxicity, total cumulative doses should not exceed 50 mg/m^2. When given in combination with an anthracycline, mitomycin C can enhance the cardiotoxic effect of the anthracycline. Mitomycin C can also produce an interstitial pneumonitis.

Response rates of 16 to 30% have been noted when mitomycin C is given as a single agent for treatment of a variety of gastrointestinal tract, pancreatic, breast, genitourinary tract, and non–small cell lung cancers [1]. A recent study reported that patients receiving the agent (20 mg/m^2 IV once every 6 wk for four consecutive cycles) as adjuvant therapy following definitive surgical resection for locally advanced (T3,N0,M0) gastric cancer showed a statistically significant survival advantage over untreated control patients [14]. Recent studies have investigated the use of mitomycin C as a radiosensitizing agent; although extensive experience is lacking, this approach seems to hold promise.

DOSAGE AND ADMINISTRATION

10–20 mg/m^2 IV as a single dose, repeated every 6–8 wk

DOSAGE MODIFICATIONS: Myelosuppression usually occurs approximately 4 wk following treatment. If leukocytes are 2000–2999/mm^3 and platelets are 25,000–74,999/mm^3, reduce dose by 30%; if leukocytes are < 2000/mm^3 and platelets are < 25,000/mm^3, reduce dose by 50%. No repeat dose should be given until leukocyte count has returned to 4000/mm^3 and platelet count to 100,000/mm^3. Limit doses to 20 mg/m^3. Greater doses increase the risk of toxicity and show no increased effect. Do not administer cumulative doses of > 50 μg/m^2.

SPECIAL PRECAUTIONS

Geriatric patients (caution with those with age-related renal impairment)
Patients who have had previous cytotoxic drug or radiation therapy
Pregnant/nursing patients
Conditions requiring special consideration: bone marrow depression, chickenpox, herpes zoster, coagulation disorders, infection, renal impairment

TOXICITIES

Degree of Severity	Frequent	Occasional
Need medical attention		Numbness/tingling in extremities
Medical attention if persistent/ bothersome	Anorexia	Skin rash, fatigue
Less need for medical attention	Nausea/vomiting	Purple-colored bands on nails, alopecia
Medical attention if occurring after withdrawal	Bone marrow depression, hemolytic-uremic syndrome	

INDICATIONS

FDA-approved: gastric and pancreatic carcinoma; **clinical studies show activity in:** colorectal, breast, head and neck, bladder, biliary, lung, and cervical carcinoma, chronic myelocytic leukemia

PHARMACOKINETICS

Distribution—does not cross blood–brain barrier; particularly concentrated in kidney, tongue, muscle, heart, and lung tissue; **Metabolism**—hepatic, some in other tissues and kidney; **Half-life**—initial, 5–15 min; terminal, about 50 min; **Excretion**—renal (10% unchanged); small amounts in bile and feces

DRUG INTERACTIONS

Blood dyscrasia-causing medications, bone marrow depressants, radiation therapy, vaccines, doxorubicin

PATIENT MONITORING

Monitor blood urea nitrogen, serum creatinine, hematocrit or hemoglobin, observe for fragmented red blood cells on peripheral blood smears, platelet count, total and/or differential leukocyte count; monitor renal and hematologic function for several months after therapy (possible hemolytic–uremic syndrome)

NURSING INTERVENTIONS

If extravasation occurs, stop injection immediately and resume in alternate site (surgical excision of original area may be necessary)

PATIENT INFORMATION

Patient should continue medication despite stomach upset; avoid immunization unless approved by physician; avoid exposure to those who have taken oral poliovirus vaccine; call physician immediately if unusual bleeding or bruising, black, tarry stools, blood in urine or stools, or pinpoint red spots on skin occur; call physician immediately if redness, pain, or swelling occurs at injection site; use caution with dental hygiene; avoid trauma to mucosal surfaces of eyes, nose, mouth

FORMULATION

Available as Mutamycin®, Bristol-Myers Oncology Division, Princeton, NJ
Vials of 5, 20, and 40 mg. Stored at 15–30°C and protected from light.

MITOXANTRONE

Mitoxantrone is a substituted anthracenedione, related to a group of compounds found in nature that have been used for centuries as dyes and laxatives. It exerts a cycle-specific cytotoxic effect on cells, with most activity on cells in the G1 and G2 phases by binding to G-C-base-pair–rich regions and causing DNA strand breaks. A variety of possible mechanisms of action have been advanced, including free radical formation, steric hindrance with topoisomerase II action, and prostaglandin interference.

Mitoxantrone is primarily used as a less cardiotoxic substitute for doxorubicin, especially in advanced breast cancer protocols, where it has been shown to have a 14% response rate, with a 177-day median survival [15]. Although these response rates are not substantially different from those achieved with doxorubicin, the cardiotoxicity was notably decreased. Mitoxantrone has also been used for the treatment of non-Hodgkin's lymphomas, with complete response rates of 43% in previously untreated patients with low-grade lymphomas [16,17].

DOSAGE AND ADMINISTRATION

14 mg/m^2 IV every 21 d (introduce slowly into tubing of freely running IV infusion of 0.9% sodium chloride or 5% dextrose injection over period not less than 3 min)

DOSAGE MODIFICATIONS: *Lower initial dose (12 mg [base]/m^2) recommended in patients with inadequate bone marrow reserves. Subsequent doses only appropriate when leukocyte and platelet counts recover from previous dose. Reduce dosage if severe bone marrow depression occurs.*

SPECIAL PRECAUTIONS

Geriatric patients
Patients with inadequate bone marrow reserves
Pregnant/nursing patients
Conditions requiring special consideration: bone marrow depression, chickenpox, herpes zoster, gout, urate renal stones, heart disease, hepatic impairment, infection

TOXICITIES

Degree of Severity	Frequent	Occasional	Rare
Need acute medical attention	GI bleeding, stomach pain, cough, shortness of breath, arrhythmias, leukopenia/infection (usually asymptomatic) stomatitis/mucositis	Seizures, CHF, thrombocytopenia (usually asymptomatic), renal failure, conjuctivitis	Allergic reaction, extravasation, local irritation/plebitis
Medical attention if persistent/bothersome	Diarrhea, headache	Jaundice	
Less need for medical attention	Nausea/vomiting, alopecia, blue-green urine	Blue color in whites of eyes	

INDICATIONS

FDA-approved: acute myelocytic, acute promyelocytic, acute monocytic, and acute erythroid leukemias, **clinical studies show activity in:** breast and hepatic carcinoma, non-Hodgkin's lymphoma

PHARMACOKINETICS

Distribution—rapid and extensive; concentrated in the thyroid, liver, heart, red blood cells, pleural fluid, kidneys; **Metabolism**—hepatic; **Protein binding**—high, 78%; **Half-life**—mean, 5.8 d; range, 2.3–13.0 d; **Excretion**—25% biliary/fecal (maximum, in 5 d); 6–11% renal (unchanged); extensive tissue absorption and binding for dose (thought to be gradually released)

DRUG INTERACTIONS

Allopurinol, colchicine, probenecid, daunorubicin, doxorubicin, heparin, vaccines, sulfinpyrazone, blood dyscrasia-causing medication, radiation therapy to mediastinal area

PATIENT MONITORING

Monitor chest radiography, echocardiography, ECG, radionuclide angiographic determination of ejection fraction, hematocrit or hemoglobin, platelet count; total and/or differential leukocyte count, serum alanine aminotransferase (SGPT) concentrations, serum aspartate aminotransferase (SGOT), serum bilirubin; serum lactate dehydrogenase, serum uric acid

NURSING INTERVENTIONS

Do not administer intrathecally (paralysis has occurred); concentrate must be diluted prior to administration; administer additional course only after toxic effects of first course have subsided; alleviate volume depletion/dehydration before initiation of therapy; if extravasation occurs, discontinue infusion and resume in alternate site

PATIENT INFORMATION

Patient should call physician immediately if pregnancy is suspected; continue medication despite stomach upset; avoid both salicylate-containing medications and immunizations unless approved by physician; avoid exposure to those who have taken oral poliovirus vaccine; call physician immediately if unusual bleeding or bruising, black, tarry stools, blood in urine or stools, or pinpoint red spots on skin occur; call physician immediately if redness, pain, or swelling occurs at injection site; use caution with dental hygiene; avoid trauma to mucosal surfaces of eyes, nose, mouth

FORMULATION

Available as Novantrone®, Immunex Corporation, Seattle, WA
2 mg (base)ml. Stored at 15–30°C and protected from freezing.

PLICAMYCIN

This antibiotic, known previously as mithramycin, was originally used in the treatment of testicular cancer. It is now almost exclusively reserved for the management of hypercalcemia. Very little is known of its pharmacokinetics and tissue distribution. The side effect profile is marked by several potentially serious, and unusual, events. It can cause a diffuse hemorrhagic syndrome, probably similar to disseminated intravascular coagulation, characterized by thrombocytopenia and impaired production of factors II, V, VII, and X. As a consequence, the prothrombin time is lengthened. Death can occur from refractory gastrointestinal hemorrhage. Substantial nephro-and hepatotoxicity have also been reported, although the mechanisms of these actions are unclear.

Other side effects can include fever, myalgia, headache, and the induction of a hypercoagulable state. Plicamycin's only indication as a cytotoxic agent is testicular cancer. Much lower doses than those required for antineoplastic activity are effective in treating hypercalcemia.

DOSAGE AND ADMINISTRATION

Antineoplastic: 25–30 μg (0.025–0.03 mg)/kg/d IV infusion, over a period of 4–6 hr, for 8–10 d unless significant toxicities occur, **or** 25–50 μg (0.025–0.05 mg)/kg/d every other day for up to 8 doses or until toxicity requires discontinuation. Additional courses of therapy may be administered at 1-mo intervals.
Antihypercalcemic: Initially 15–25 μg (0.015–0.025 mg)/kg/d IV infusion, over a period of 4–6 hr for 3–4 d. Repeat at 1 wk (or more) intervals, if necessary, until desired response.

DOSAGE MODIFICATIONS: Doses > 30 μg (0.03 mg)/kg and/or duration of therapy exceeding 10 d increase risk of hemorrhagic diathesis. Alternate-day schedule has been shown to decrease toxicity potential. Delayed toxicity may occur as late as 72 hr after discontinuation with daily administration, but does not occur when alternate-day schedule is used.

SPECIAL PRECAUTIONS

Patients with previous cytotoxic drug or radiation therapy or general debilitation
Pregnant/nursing patients
Patients with renal dysfunction
Contraindications: blood dyscrasias, including thrombocytopathy and thrombocytopenia, chickenpox, herpes zoster, coagulation disorders or increased susceptibility to bleeding

TOXICITIES

Degree of Severity	Frequent	Occasional
Need acute medical attention		Pain/swelling at injection site, fever
Medical attention if persistent/bothersome	Diarrhea, irritation/soreness of mouth	Mental depression, headache, fatigue
Less need for medical attention	Nausea/vomiting, anorexia	Drowsiness
Medical attention if occurring after withdrawal	Vomiting of blood, unusual bleeding/bruising	Sore throat and fever
Symptom of toxicity	GI bleeding, thrombocytopenia, leukopenia	Petechial bleeding, toxic epidermal necrolysis, nosebleed/other bleeding

INDICATIONS

FDA-approved: testicular carcinoma, hypercalcemia (associated with neoplasms), hypercalciuria (associated with neoplasms); **clinical studies show activity in:** Paget's disease of bone (unaccepted)

PHARMACOKINETICS

Distribution—concentrated in Kupffer cells of liver, in renal tubular cells, and along formed bone surfaces; may localize in areas of active bone resorption; crosses blood–brain barrier; enters cerebrospinal fluid; **Onset of action**—reduction of plasma calcium within 24–48 hr; **Excretion**—renal

DRUG INTERACTIONS

Estrogen, heparin, thrombolytic agents, NSAIDs, aspirin, bone marrow depressants, nephrotoxic medications, hepatotoxic medications, sulfinpyrazone, anticoagulants, live vaccines, dextran, dipyridamole, valproic acid

PATIENT MONITORING

Bleeding and prothrombin time determinations, complete and differential blood count, platelet count, hepatic/renal function determinations, serum calcium, serum phosphorus, serum potassium

NURSING INTERVENTIONS

Alleviate volume depletion/dehydration before initiation of therapy; give antiemetics prior to and during treatment; avoid rapid direct infusion; if extravasation occurs, apply cold pack immediately—with swelling, apply moderate heat to aid in dispersing medication from site, with cellulitis, discontinue infusion and resume in alternate site

PATIENT INFORMATION

Patient should continue medication despite stomach upset; avoid both salicylate-containing medications and immunization unless approved by physician; avoid exposure to those who have taken oral poliovirus vaccine; call physician immediately if unusual bleeding or bruising, black, tarry stools, blood in urine or stools, or pinpoint red spots on skin occur; call physician immediately if redness, pain, or swelling occurs at injection site; use caution with dental hygiene; avoid trauma to mucosal surfaces of nose, eyes, mouth

FORMULATION

Available as Mithracin®, Miles Pharmaceutical Division, West Haven, CT
2500 μg (2.5 mg). Stored at 2–8°C protected from light.

The antimetabolites constitute a large group of anticancer drugs that interfere with metabolic processes vital to the physiology and proliferation of cancer cells. The major classes of the antimetabolites are the antifols, the purine analogues, and the pyrimidine analogues [1–4].

Antimetabolites have been used in cancer treatment since 1948, when Sidney Farber first reported that aminopterin (an antifol related to methotrexate) produced temporary remissions in children with acute lymphoblastic leukemia. The use of methotrexate in women with gestational trophoblastic neoplasia in the late 1950s demonstrated, for the first time, that chemotherapy could cure patients with metastatic cancer. The fluoropyrimidines were the first drugs found to have useful clinical activity in the treatment of gastrointestinal malignancies and continue to be important in the management of patients with several common forms of cancer. Insights gained from laboratory studies of the fluoropyrimidines have recently led to the development of new, more effective treatment regimens for advanced colorectal cancer.

Recent years have seen the discovery of important new antimetabolites, including fludarabine phosphate (a purine antimetabolite with substantial activity in lymphoid malignancies) [5] and 2-chlorodeoxyadenosine (which may cure a high percentage of patients with hairy cell leukemia with a single course of therapy) [6]. Although modern molecular biology and immunology have opened up new frontiers for cancer research, it is clear that antimetabolites will continue to play a major role in cancer treatment for the foreseeable future (Table 1).

MECHANISMS OF ACTION

Actively proliferating cancer cells must continually synthesize large quantities of nucleic acids, proteins, lipids, and other vital cellular constituents. Almost all of the antimetabolites in current clinical use inhibit the synthesis of purine or pyrimidine nucleotides (needed for DNA synthesis) and/or directly inhibit the enzymes of DNA replication. Many antimetabolites also interfere with the synthesis of ribonucleotides and RNA, and some antimetabolites (*eg*, methotrexate) may affect amino acid metabolism and protein synthesis as well. The effects of a given antimetabolite on different organs, tissues, and cell types can vary greatly due to nuances in cellular metabolism. For example, normal bone marrow is rich in purines, and these purines are actively salvaged and reutilized by normal progenitor cells in the marrow. Thus, it is not surprising that many purine antimetabolites (*eg*, thioguanine) are toxic to the bone marrow and are particularly effective against malignancies of bone marrow origin (*ie*, leukemias).

When metabolic pathways for synthesis of vital cellular constituents are blocked by antimetabolites, cancer cells may temporarily stop proliferating (enter a quiescent or noncycling state; a *cytostatic* effect of treatment). Alternatively, cancer cells that continue to proliferate, even when cellular constituents required for proliferation have been depleted by antimetabolite treatment, can be destroyed (a *cytotoxic* treatment result). Thus, by interfering with the synthesis of vital cellular constituents, antimetabolites can delay or arrest the growth of cancers.

Antimetabolites may also affect the growth of cancers by other mechanisms. For example, several antimetabolites have been shown to induce terminal differentiation in certain cancer cell lines maintained *in vitro*. In this process, actively proliferating, poorly differentiated cancer cells acquire the phenotype of mature, differentiated, nonproliferating cells. Also, antimetabolites have been shown to trigger apoptosis (or programmed cell death) in some cancer cell lines [7]. Finally, some antimetabolites are known to have effects on the immune system and may alter immune responses to cancer in treated patients.

ADVERSE EFFECTS

Many of the adverse effects of antimetabolite treatment result from suppression of cellular proliferation in mitotically active tissues, such as the bone marrow or gastrointestinal mucosa. Thus, patients treated with these agents commonly experience bone marrow suppression, stomatitis, diarrhea, and hair loss. As noted previously, however, there are significant metabolic differences among these normal tissues, and the precise pattern and severity of treatment toxicities observed can vary greatly, depending on the antimetabolite administered, the schedule of administration, and (potentially) nutritional and other factors.

In addition, many antimetabolites can produce adverse effects that appear to be unrelated to their antiproliferative effects. These effects are more commonly seen at high drug doses and may affect tissues that are not mitotically active. Examples include neurotoxicity seen with high-dose cytosine arabinoside or high-dose methotrexate treatment.

Gonadal function is usually (but not always) suppressed in patients receiving cytotoxic chemotherapy [8]. Low doses of methotrexate, as used in the treatment of psoriasis, appear to have little effect on gonadal function, but this drug is clearly embryotoxic and teratogenic. Cytosine arabinoside has been shown to produce reversible inhibition of spermatogenesis. With the advent of modern combination chemotherapy regimens, few recent data are available regarding the effects of other individual antimetabolites on gonadal function. Available laboratory and clinical data suggest, however, that the effects of other antimetabolites on gonadal function are less severe and more reversible than (for example) the effects of nitrogen mustard and certain other DNA alkylating agents.

The administration of antimetabolites in pregnant women deserves special comment. It is sometimes stated that administration of antimetabolites is contraindicated in pregnancy (primarily due to the risk of teratogenesis), whereas other anticancer medications, such as alkylating agents and anthracyclines, may be used with caution. There is, in fact, no laboratory or clinical evidence supporting the concept that antimetabolites *as a class* are more mutagenic or teratogenic than are other cytotoxic anticancer agents. The only antimetabolites known to be significant human teratogens are the antifols (methotrexate, aminopterin, and related compounds). This is consistent with the known teratogenicity of folate deficiency in pregnancy. Clearly, all cytotoxic drugs must be regarded as potentially teratogenic and embryotoxic, and administration of cytotoxic drugs should be avoided in pregnancy whenever possible (particularly in the first trimester). However, there is presently no persuasive evidence that antimetabolites other than methotrexate carry a significantly greater risk to the human fetus compared to the risks associated with other classes of cytotoxic drugs.

MECHANISMS OF RESISTANCE

Cancer cells may overcome the cytotoxic and cytostatic effects of antimetabolite chemotherapy by a variety of mechanisms, including *allosteric*, *pathophysiologic*, and *cell cycle-control mechanisms*. A comprehensive discussion of all known mechanisms of cancer cell resistance to each of the antimetabolites in clinical use is far beyond the scope of this review. Instead, important classes of resistance mechanisms are discussed, using the known mechanisms of resistance to the fluoropyrimidines as examples.

Fluorouracil, the most commonly administered fluoropyrimidine, has several antimetabolic effects on cancer cells, including 1) inhibition of the enzyme thymidylate synthase by the fluorouracil metabolite fluorodeoxyuridine monophosphate (this blocks *de novo* synthesis of thymidine nucleotides, required for DNA synthesis and repair); 2) misincorporation of fluorodeoxyuridine nucleotides into DNA, in place of thymidine nucleotides (resulting in structural damage to DNA); and 3) interference with RNA synthesis and processing. Inhibition of thymidylate synthase is currently believed to be the most important mechanism of anticancer action for fluorouracil and other fluoropyrimidines. Inhibition of this enzyme can deplete cellular levels of thymidine nucleotides, which can result in destruction of the cancer cell, in the DNA synthetic S phase of the cell cycle.

Cellular levels of vital cellular constituents, such as thymidine nucleotides, are automatically and precisely controlled by a series of

Table 1. Features of Antimetabolites in Common Clinical Use

Agent	Class	Primary Pharmacologic Action(s)	Route of Elimination	Elimination Half-life	Toxic Effects	Primary Applications
Fluorouracil (5-FU)	Pyrimidine analog	Thymidylate synthase inhibition	Metabolic	6–20 min	Mucositis, diarrhea, myelosuppression	Colorectal, breast, ENT cancers; radiosensitizer
Floxuridine (5-FUdr)	Pyrimidine deoxynucleoside analog	Thymidylate synthase inhibition	Metabolic	3–20 min IV; 70–90% first-pass clearance, hepatic artery	Chemical hepatitis, sclerosing cholangitis (hepatic artery infusion)	Liver metastases from GI cancers
Methotrexate	Antifol	Dihydrofolate reductase inhibition	Renal	Primary 2–3 hr; terminal 8–10 hr	Mucositis, diarrhea, myelosuppression	Breast, bladder, ENT carcinomas; non-Hodgkin's lymphomas; ALL; choriocarcinoma; osteosarcoma; carcinomatous or leukemic meningitis
Leucovorin	Reduced folate (vitamin)	Enhanced thymidylate synthase inhibition (with 5-FU); "rescue" from antimetabolic effects of antifols	Metabolic	Parent compound, 1 hr, active 5-methyl metabolite, 4–7 hr	Increases toxicity of 5-FU; reduces toxicity of methotrexate	With 5-FU, in colorectal cancer; "rescue" for methotrexate in osteosarcoma
Hydroxyurea	Synthetic antimetabolite	Ribonucleotide reductase inhibitor	Primarily renal	3.5–4.5 hr	Myelosuppression	CML, AML, Polycythemia vera; radiosensitizer
Thioguanine (6-TG)	Purine analog	Purine nucleotide biosynthesis inhibitor; incorporation into DNA	Metabolic	25–240 min	Myelosuppression	AML, ALL, CML
Mercaptopurine (6-MP)	Purine analog	Purine nucleotide biosynthesis inhibitor	Metabolic	90 min	Myelosuppression	AML, ALL, CML
Cytarabine	Pyrimidine deoxynucleoside analog	Incorporation into DNA; inhibition of DNA synthesis	Metabolic	7–20 min	Myelosuppression, nausea, vomiting, diarrhea, mucositis; with high doses, neurotoxicity	AML, ALL, non-Hodgkin's lymphomas, meningeal leukemia
Pentostatin	Purine deoxynucleoside analog	Adenosine deaminase inhibitor	Renal	2.5–6 hr	Nephrotoxicity, neurotoxicity, myelosuppression, immunosuppression	Hairy cell leukemia, ALL, CLL, non-Hodgkin's lymphomas
Fludarabine phosphate	Purine deoxynucleotide analog	Ribonucleotide reductase and DNA synthesis inhibitor	Primarily renal	Active metabolite, 10 hr	Myelosuppression; neurotoxicity at high doses	CLL, low-grade non-Hodgkin's lymphomas
Cladribine (2-CDA)	Purine deoxynucleoside analog	Ribonucleotide reductase and DNA synthesis inhibitor	Renal	7 hr	Myelosuppression, fever	Hairy cell leukemia, CLL, low-grade non-Hodgkin's lymphomas
Asparaginase	Enzyme	Asparagine (amino acid) depletion	Metabolic	8–30 hr	Hypersensitivity reactions	ALL; "rescue" following methotrexate

allosteric (homeostatic or feedback-control) mechanisms. Inhibition of thymidylate synthase and depletion of cellular thymidine nucleotide levels, as produced by fluorouracil treatment, lead to automatic compensatory increases in the activity of several other key enzymes of the *de novo* and salvage pathways for thymidine nucleotide synthesis. The increased activity of these other enzymes (aspartate carbamoyl-transferase, ribonucleotide reductase, thymidine kinase, and others) results in 1) production of high levels of the normal substrate for the thymidylate synthase reaction (deoxyuridine monophosphate), which can competitively overcome the inhibition of this enzyme by the fluo-rouracil metabolite fluorodeoxyuridine monophosphate, and 2) production of more thymidine nucleotides by the thymidine salvage pathway (which utilizes preformed thymidine), thus bypassing the *de novo* pathway inhibition produced by fluorouracil.

Cancer cells also exhibit pathophysiologic mechanisms of resistance to antimetabolites. For example, the gene for thymidylate synthase may be amplified in fluorouracil-resistant cancer cells. The cancer cells may thus produce higher levels of this enzyme, and it becomes much more difficult to adequately inhibit this enzyme with fluorouracil treatment. Alternatively, cancer cells may acquire a mutation in the gene for thymidylate synthase, rendering this enzyme resistant to inhibition by fluorouracil treatment.

Finally, even if thymidine nucleotide levels are successfully depleted by fluorouracil treatment, cancer cells may still evade the cytotoxic consequences of thymidine nucleotide depletion via cell cycle-control mechanisms. The progression of cells through the cell cycle is tightly regulated by cyclins and other cell-cycle regulatory elements. Cells which are thymidine nucleotide–deficient may arrest (stop cycling) at the G_1-S interface and may not proceed into the DNA synthetic S phase of the cell cycle (where thymidine nucleotide depletion is lethal) until thymidine nucleotide levels are restored.

In summary, the metabolic pathways for cellular production of vital cellular constituents are redundant and tightly controlled, and cells have a variety of mechanisms to protect against perturbations in the levels of these vital cellular constituents. Cancer cells can potentially utilize all of these normal cellular mechanisms, as well as a variety of pathophysiologic mechanisms, to evade the cytotoxic effects of antimetabolite chemotherapy. Clearly, to make further progress in the use of antimetabolites in cancer treatment, it will be important to fully understand the mechanisms of cancer cell resistance to antimetabolites and to incorporate this understanding in the design of new antimetabolite chemotherapy regimens.

BIOCHEMICAL MODULATION

Broadly defined, biochemical modulation refers to the use of antimetabolites in multidrug regimens, designed to enhance the efficacy of antimetabolites and/or overcome known mechanisms of cancer cell resistance to these agents. As noted above, laboratory studies of antimetabolites have continued to yield new insights into the mechanisms of action of these drugs and the mechanisms of cancer cell resistance [9]. These laboratory studies have further indicated that certain drug combinations could yield enhanced clinical efficacy in cancer treatment. Fluorouracil/leucovorin combination treatment regimens for advanced colorectal cancer represent the most successful clinical application of biochemical modulation research to date.

Based on studies of the mechanism of thymidylate synthase inhibition by the fluoropyrimidines, Santi *et al.* first suggested that leucovorin could enhance the efficacy of fluorouracil [10]. Their observations ultimately led to the clinical finding that fluorouracil/leucovorin combination regimens are modestly superior to fluorouracil alone in the treatment of advanced colorectal cancer [11]. The clinical success of this relatively simple biochemical modulation (which modifies only one of the many mechanisms now known to be operative in the resistance of cancer cells to fluorouracil) has stimulated a substantial resurgence in clinical and laboratory biochemical modulation research. More complex drug combination regimens, which target critical metabolic pathways at multiple points, are undergoing laboratory and clinical evaluation at a number of cancer research centers around the world. Whereas these more complex, multidrug regimens can be expected to inhibit the targeted metabolic pathways more effectively, the ultimate clinical success of these regimens will be determined by their degree of selectivity.

SELECTIVITY

Bacterial infections are usually treated easily and successfully, because normal host immune defenses efficiently recognize and clear bacteria and bacterial metabolism and human metabolism differ sufficiently to allow for use of selective antimetabolites (antibiotics), which interfere with critical bacterial metabolic pathways but do not have significant adverse effects on the patient. In contrast, cancer cells are immunologically and metabolically very similar to nonmalignant cells of the cancer patient, therefore selective destruction of cancer cells with systemic chemical or biologic treatment is much more problematic. It is clear, however, that some forms of cancer can be cured with systemic therapy. Thus, selective destruction of cancer cells can be achieved with systemic therapy, at least in some patients.

Commonly considered mechanisms for the selective destruction of cancer cells emphasize known or presumed immunologic, metabolic, and kinetic differences between cancer cells and normal cells. Biologic agents with immunomodulating properties have been shown to produce useful antitumor responses in some patients, probably by enhancing immune recognition and destruction of tumor cells (see Chapter 5). Antimetabolites are not presently known to have any therapeutically useful immunomodulatory anticancer activity, although research is continuing into possible roles for combinations of antimetabolites and biologic agents in cancer treatment.

Inherent metabolic differences between cancer and non-neoplastic cells may account for some of the selectivity observed with antimetabolites in cancer treatment. For example, useful clinical remissions can sometimes be obtained, with little clinical toxicity, in patients with colorectal cancer who are treated with prolonged continuous infusions of fluorouracil, suggesting that, in these patients, tumor cells sometimes have a greater innate sensitivity to fluorouracil than normal gastrointestinal mucosal cells (or other normal cells). The precise metabolic differences allowing for this selectivity are unclear, but they may relate to toxic effects of imbalances in deoxynucleotide levels that may follow fluorouracil treatment. Unfortunately, it appears that cancer cells usually do not have metabolic features that can be selectively targeted with antimetabolites. Rather, cancer cells commonly have (or develop) metabolic capabilities that confer *decreased* susceptibility to antimetabolites (compared to non-neoplastic cells).

Kinetic differences between cancer cells and normal cells may account for most of the clinical selectivity observed with current antimetabolite chemotherapy regimens. Antimetabolites are selectively toxic to proliferating cells and typically produce few toxic effects in nonproliferating cells and tissues. Cancers characteristically exhibit a much higher rate of proliferation than normal cells and tissues (even when compared to mitotically active tissues, such as the bone marrow and gastrointestinal mucosa) and thus are inherently more susceptible to antimetabolites. Cancers also characteristically exhibit a high rate of cell loss. Normally, cellular proliferation exceeds the rate of cell loss in a growing tumor. Periodic antimetabolite treatment may serve to alter this balance, leading to stabilization or regression of tumors (until the cancer develops resistance to the antimetabolite treatment regimen).

AREAS OF RESEARCH ACTIVITY

Many research centers are continuing to investigate the biochemical mechanisms of action and resistance of antimetabolite chemotherapy. Clinical studies are beginning to incorporate measures of *in vivo* biochemical effects of antimetabolite therapy (*eg*, determining inhibition of a targeted enzyme in a patient's tumor by post-treatment biopsy or using nuclear magnetic resonance [NMR] spectroscopy to monitor drug uptake and retention in tumors) [12]. This research will clearly enhance our understanding of the failure of current antimetabolite chemotherapy regimens to control cancer growth in many patients and may lead to more effective use of these drugs in new biochemical modulation treatment regimens.

Another area of research activity relates to circadian patterns of cellular metabolic and mitotic activity, and the possibility that these patterns may differ between malignant and normal cells. For example, if normal proliferating gastrointestinal cells enter the DNA synthetic S phase primarily in the morning hours, whereas proliferating cells of gastrointestinal malignancies enter the DNA synthetic S phase throughout the day, then it would make sense to administer S phase-selective antimetabolites to patients with these malignancies at times *other* than the morning hours [13,14]. Because most antimetabolites have narrow therapeutic indices in cancer treatment, careful attention to any details (such as the timing of administration) that may enhance the selectivity of these drugs is critical.

Finally, laboratory and clinical studies have repeatedly shown that combinations of antimetabolites with biologic agents, such as the interferons, other chemotherapeutic agents, or radiation therapy can result in synergistic anticancer activity. Research into the mechanisms of these synergistic interactions is continuing, and numerous clinical studies are further evaluating a variety of combination treatment regimens.

REFERENCES

1. Chabner BA, Collins JM (eds): *Cancer Chemotherapy: Principles and Practice.* Philadelphia: J.B. Lippincott, 1990.

2. Chen AP, Grem JL: Antimetabolites. *Curr Opin Oncol* 1992, 4:1089–1098.

3. Cheson BD: New antimetabolites in the treatment of human malignancies. *Sem Oncol* 1992, 19:695–706.

4. Clarke SJ, Jackman AL, Harrap KR: Antimetabolites in cancer chemotherapy. *Adv Exp Biol Med* 1991, 309A:7–13.

5. Keating MJ, Kantarjian H, Talpaz M, *et al.*: Fludarabine: A new agent with major activity against chronic lymphocytic leukemia. *Blood* 1989, 74:19–25.

6. Piro LD, Carrera CJ, Carson DA, *et al.*: Lasting remissions in hairy-cell leukemia induced by a single infusion of 2-chlorodeoxyadenosine. *N Engl J Med* 1990, 322:1117–1121.

7. Darry MA, Behnke CA, Eastman A: Activation of programmed cell death (apoptosis) by cisplatin, other anticancer drugs, toxins, and hyperthermia. *Biochem Pharmacol* 1990, 40:2353–2362.

8. Averette H, Boike G, Jarrell M: Effects of cancer chemotherapy on gonadal function and reproductive capacity. *CA Can J Clin* 1990, 40:199–209.

9. Grem JL, Chu E, Boarman D, *et al.*: Biochemical modulation of fluorouracil with leucovorin and interferon; Preclinical and clinical investigations. *Sem Oncol* 1992, 2(suppl 3):36–44.

10. Ullman B, Lee M, Martin DW, Santi DV: Cytotoxicity of 5-fluoro-2´-deoxyuridine: requirement for reduced folate cofactors and antagonism by methotrexate. *Proc Nat Acad Sci USA* 1978, 75:980–983.

11. Poon MA, O'Connell MJ, Wieand HS, *et al.*: Biochemical modulation of fluorouracil with leucovorin: Confirmatory evidence of improved therapeutic efficacy in advanced colorectal cancer. *J Clin Oncol* 1991, 9:1967–1972.

12. Presant C, Wolf W, Albright MJ, *et al.*: Human tumor fluorouracil trapping: Clinical correlations of *in vivo* ^{19}F nuclear magnetic resonance spectroscopy pharmacokinetics. *J Clin Oncol* 1990, 8:1868–1873.

13. Buchi KN, Moore JG, Hrushesky WJ, *et al.*: Circadian rhythm of cellular proliferation in the human rectal mucosa. *Gastroenterology* 1991, 101:410–415.

14. Von Roemeling R, Hrushesky WJ: Circadian patterning of continuous floxuridine infusion reduces toxicity and allows higher dose intensity in patients with widespread cancer. *J Clin Oncol* 1989, 7:1710–1719.

ASPARAGINASE

Asparaginase (or l-Asparaginase) is an enzyme that catalyzes the hydrolysis of asparagine (a nonessential amino acid) to aspartic acid and ammonia. While most normal cells can synthesize all asparagine required for cellular protein synthesis, some cancer cells are dependent on exogenous asparagine to support cellular protein synthesis and proliferation. Asparaginase acts to deplete plasma levels of asparagine, thus depriving susceptible cancer cells of this nutrient. Clinically, asparaginase has useful activity in the treatment of acute lymphocytic leukemia and may have some activity in treatment of lymphomas. Also, asparaginase blocks the cytotoxic effects of methotrexate and thus can be used as a rescue agent following high-dose methotrexate administration.

The clinical usefulness of asparaginase is limited due to the frequent development of hypersensitivity reactions with repeated courses of treatment. If necessary, patients hypersensitive to the commercially available formulation can be treated with an investigational one derived from *Erwinia carotovora* (available from the National Cancer Institute for treatment of acute lymphocytic leukemia).

DOSAGE AND ADMINISTRATION

Acute lymphocytic leukemia (in remission-induction combination chemotherapy only; repeated or prolonged use should be avoided):
6000 U/m^2/d (IM injection) for 10 d **or** 10,000 U/m^2/wk $\times$ 2 wk (IV infusion) **or** 12,000 U/m^2 (IM injection) on days 2, 4, 7, 9, 11, 14

SPECIAL PRECAUTIONS

Hypersensitivity reactions
Pregnant/nursing patients

TOXICITIES

Hypersensitivity: urticaria, chills, fever, rash, anaphylaxis
GI: anorexia, nausea, vomiting; elevated serum levels of hepatic enzymes, usually transient; lethal acute hepatic failure (rare); pancreatitis in 5%, with pancreatic insufficiency and hyperglycemia (rarely severe)
Neurologic: headache, lethargy, depression, confusion; obtundation, coma, seizures (rare)
Hematologic: transient myelosuppression (rare)
Miscellaneous: Decreased serum albumin levels; decreased plasma levels of fibrinogen and vitamin K–dependent clotting factors; decreased levels of antithrombin III; proteinuria; renal insufficiency, oliguric renal failure (rare)

INDICATIONS

FDA-approved: acute lymphocytic leukemia (in remission-induction therapy); **Clinical studies show activity in**: as rescue agent following administration of high-dose methotrexate

PHARMACOKINETICS

Absorption: oral bioavailability very low (administered IM or IV); **Distribution**: plasma volume, little penetration into CSF; **Elimination**—metabolic (degraded by proteolytic enzymes); **Half-life**—8–30 hr; serum levels of asparagine undetectable within minutes of injection, remain low days after treatment; **Adjustments for organ dysfunction**: probably unnecessary

DRUG INTERACTIONS

Methotrexate

RESPONSE RATES

Pediatric ALL (induction phase, combination chemotherapy)—complete remission in most patients; cure rate approximately 50%

PATIENT MONITORING

Be prepared for hypersensitivity reactions; monitor vital signs for 1 hr following administration; follow-up monitoring of symptoms, hematology, serum chemistry panel, PT, PTT

NURSING INTERVENTIONS

Monitor weight, nutritional status; encourage good oral hygiene; give antiemetics, and mouthwashes and other adjuncts as needed for stomatitis

PATIENT INFORMATION

Patient should avoid use of aspirin or nonsteroidal anti-inflammatory agents; call physician if fever or other signs of serious infection develop; maintain good nutrition

FORMULATION

Available as ELSPAR® Merck & Co., West Point, PA 10-ml vials containing 10,000 IU lyophilized *E. coli* asparaginase. Store at 2–8°C

2-CHLORODEOXYADENOSINE

2-Chlorodeoxyadenosine (2-CDA) is a synthetic analogue of the naturally occurring purine nucleoside, deoxyadenosine. Like deoxyadenosine, 2-CDA is enzymatically converted to active nucleotide metabolites by cellular kinases, and reconverted to the nucleoside parent compound by 5´-nucleotidase. Unlike deoxyadenosine, 2-CDA is resistant to inactivation by the enzyme adenosine deaminase. Substantial levels of 2-CDA nucleotides can accumulate in lymphocytes, which have a particularly high ratio of (activating) kinases to (inactivating) 5´-nucleotidase.

The active nucleotide metabolites of 2-CDA interfere with several vital cellular metabolic processes. Inhibition of ribonucleotide reductase by the triphosphate of 2-CDA results in depletion and imbalances of cellular deoxyribonucleotide pools. The triphosphate metabolite of 2-CDA is also an inhibitor of DNA polymerases and can itself be incorporated into DNA. In addition, cells exposed to 2-CDA exhibit decreased RNA synthesis and an increase in DNA double-strand breaks. Finally, cellular levels of the key cofactor nicotinamide-adenine dinucleotide (NAD) may be depleted, as NAD is consumed in the synthesis of poly (ADP-ribose), which occurs in response to DNA damage. Most of these antimetabolic effects of 2-CDA are selectively cytotoxic to proliferating cells in the DNA-synthetic S phase of the cell cycle. However, depletion of NAD is cytotoxic to resting cells as well.

In clinical studies to date, 2-CDA has demonstrated remarkable activity against hairy cell leukemia and substantial activity against certain other lymphoid malignancies.

DOSAGE AND ADMINISTRATION

Hairy cell leukemia: 0.1 mg/Kg/d × 7 d (continuous IV infusion; one course sufficient)
Chronic lymphocytic leukemia: 0.05–0.2 mg/Kg/d × 7 d (continuous IV infusion; repeat up to 4 courses)

SPECIAL PRECAUTIONS

Pregnant/nursing patients

TOXICITIES

Hematologic: lymphopenia; anemia; neutropenia and thrombocytopenia (mild at low doses; dose-limiting at high doses)
GI: occasional nausea, vomiting (mild), diarrhea, elevated serum levels of liver enzymes
Miscellaneous: fever

INDICATIONS

FDA-approved: hairy cell leukemia; **Clinical studies show activity in**: chronic lymphocytic leukemia, low-grade non-Hodgkin's lymphomas, cutaneous T-cell lymphomas

PHARMACOKINETICS

Absorption: limited data; oral bioavailability may be low and erratic (acid labile); **Distribution**—insufficient data; **Elimination**—primarily renal; **Half-life**—approximately 7 hr; **Dose adjustments for organ dysfunction**: Unknown, use cautiously in patients with renal dysfunction

RESPONSE RATES

Hairy cell leukemia—complete remission rate 75–85% (relapses are uncommon)
Chronic lymphocytic leukemia, low-grade non-Hodgkin's lymphoma, cutaneous T-cell lymphoma (previously treated)—partial remission rates 40–50%

PATIENT MONITORING

Vital signs, symptoms, examination, hematology, serum chemistry panel

NURSING INTERVENTIONS

Monitor weight, nutritional status; encourage good oral hygiene; give antiemetics, and mouthwashes and other adjuncts as needed; administer antipyretics for fever

PATIENT INFORMATION

Patient should avoid use of aspirin or nonsteroidal anti-inflammatory agents; call physician if fever or other signs of serious infection develop; maintain good nutrition

FORMULATION

Available as LEUSTATIN® (cladribine), Ortho Biotech, Raritan, NJ
10-mg vials (1 mg/ml solution). Stored at 2–8°C and protected from light.

Cytarabine (cytosine arabinoside or ara-C) acts pharmacologically as a deoxycytidine analogue and has several effects on DNA metabolism. Cellular kinases convert ara-C to active nucleotide metabolites; the triphosphate metabolite (araCTP) inhibits enzymes of DNA synthesis and repair and is incorporated into DNA. Incorporation of araCTP interferes with DNA template function and causes chain termination; this appears to be the primary mechanism of ara-C cytotoxicity. Other antimetabolic and biologic effects of ara-C described include inhibition of ribonucleotide reductase and promotion of differentiation of leukemic cells *in vitro*. Finally, several cytarabine metabolites (including araCDP-choline, araCMP, and araCTP) can inhibit metabolic pathways of glycoprotein and glycolipid synthesis and thus may affect the structure and function of cell membranes.

Deaminases convert ara-C (and its active nucleotide metabolites) to inactive uridine arabinoside (and nucleotides thereof). There is evidence that cells sensitive to the cytotoxic effects of ara-C have higher levels of activating enzymes, and/or lower levels of inactivating enzymes, than do resistant cells. Pilot studies have suggested that formation and retention of araCTP in leukemic cells may correlate with clinical response to ara-C.

DOSAGE AND ADMINISTRATION
Acute leukemia (usually with anthracycline): 100 mg/m^2/d (bolus IV injection) every 12 hr × 5–7 d **or** 100 mg/m^2/d (continuous IV infusion) × 5–7 d **or** 3 g/m^2 (IV infusion over 1 hr) every 12 hr × 4–8 doses
Leukemic meningitis: 30 mg/m^2 (intrathecal) repeated every 4 d until negative CSF cytology, then one additional dose

SPECIAL PRECAUTIONS
Patients over 50: severe neurotoxicity, GI toxicity, hepatotoxicity with high-dose ara-C
Pregnant/nursing patients

TOXICITIES
Hematologic: neutropenia, thrombocytopenia, anemia (reversible)
GI: anorexia, nausea, vomiting; oral, esophageal, GI mucositis and ulceration (possibly severe, prolonged, with gastrointestinal bleeding); abdominal pain, ileus, diarrhea (possibly severe); reversible intrahepatic cholestasis (common, mild)
Neurologic: neurotoxicity (rare)
Dermatologic: rash
Miscellaneous: fever, conjunctivitis, anaphylaxis (rare)
Intrathecal: nausea, vomiting, fever; paraparesis, paraplegia, leukoencephalopathy (rare)
Intermediate (1 g/m^2) **or high-dose** (≥3 g/m^2): cerebellar dysfunction, dementia, obtundation, coma, seizures, personality changes (usually reversible); severe GI ulceration; pneumatosis cystoides intestinalis and peritonitis; bowel necrosis; jaundice; pulmonary edema; interstitial pneumonitis; hemorrhagic conjunctivitis; severe skin rash with desquamation; alopecia totalis; cardiomyopathy; pancreatitis

INDICATIONS
FDA-approved: remission induction in acute nonlymphocytic leukemia, acute lymphocytic leukemia, blast phase of chronic myelocytic leukemia, meningeal leukemia; **Clinical studies show activity in**: non-Hodgkin's lymphomas

PHARMACOKINETICS
Absorption—oral bioavailability very low; **Distribution**—CSF concentration 20–40% of plasma concentration at steady state); **Elimination**—metabolic (deaminases); **Half-life**—7–20 min; clearance prolonged with high-dose ara-C; **Adjustments for organ dysfunction**: Use intermediate- and high-dose regimens with caution in patients with pre-existing hepatic dysfunction

DRUG INTERACTIONS
Methotrexate, thioguanine, mercaptopurine, hydroxyurea, thymidine, cisplatin, cyclophosphamide, etoposide, digoxin, gentamicin

RESPONSE RATES
Adult acute nonlymphocytic leukemia (with an anthracycline)—complete remission rate 40–75%, cure rate 5–15%

PATIENT MONITORING
Vital signs, symptoms (mucositis, abdominal pain, diarrhea), examination, hematology (weekly; daily in leukemia induction therapy), serum chemistry panel

NURSING INTERVENTIONS
Monitor weight, nutritional status; encourage good oral hygiene; give antiemetics; mouthwashes and other adjuncts; and antidiarrheals as needed; evaluate for bacterial etiology if diarrhea is severe

PATIENT INFORMATION
Patient should avoid use of aspirin or nonsteroidal anti-inflammatory agents; call physician if fever or other signs of serious infection develop; avoid excessive sun exposure; maintain good nutrition

FORMULATION
Available as Cytosar-U®, The Upjohn Company, Kalamazoo, MI
100-mg, 500-mg, 1-g, and 2-g vials of cytarabine powder. Store at 15–30°C.

FLOXURIDINE

Floxuridine (fluorodeoxyuridine or 5-FUDR) is a synthetic analogue of the naturally occurring pyrimidine nucleoside, deoxyuridine. Inhibition of thymidylate synthase (TS) by 5-fluorodeoxyuridine monophosphate (FdUMP), an active metabolite of floxuridine, is believed to be the primary mechanism of anticancer efficacy of this drug. Because 5-FUDR is a direct precursor of FdUMP, this drug may act more selectively as a thymidylate synthase inhibitor than 5-FU (fluorouracil). However, 5-FUDR can also be enzymatically hydrolyzed (to 5-FU). Depending on the precise route and schedule of administration selected, the pharmacologic effects of 5-FUDR may thus closely resemble (or differ from) those observed with fluorouracil administration. (See page on 5-FU for additional data regarding fluoropyrimidine pharmacology.)

Floxuridine is commonly administered via hepatic arterial infusion, to patients who have liver metastases from gastrointestinal malignancies. Compared to 5-FU, 5-FUDR is more water-soluble and more potent (permitting outpatient administration using small, implanted continuous infusion pumps). Also, the high first-pass hepatic metabolism of 5-FUDR results in less systemic exposure and less systemic toxicity. Randomized clinical trials have shown that hepatic arterial 5-FUDR can yield significantly higher objective response rates and a significantly delayed progression of liver metastases compared with systemic fluoropyrimidine treatment.

DOSAGE AND ADMINISTRATION

Hepatic arterial continuous infusion: 0.2–0.3 mg/kg/d × 14 d, repeat q 28 d
IV continuous infusion: 0.1–0.15 mg/kg/d × 14 d, repeat q 28 d

SPECIAL PRECAUTIONS

Arterial catheter misplacement/dislodgement/migration
Chemical hepatitis
Pregnant/nursing patients

TOXICITIES

With hepatic arterial infusions:
Hematologic: neutropenia (rare)
Hepatic: abnormal liver functions, sclerosing cholangitis, acalculous cholecystitis, biliary sclerosis in 8–21%
Other GI: anorexia (common), nausea, vomiting (mild), oral mucositis (rare), diarrhea; epigastric pain, gastritis, ulcers
Neurologic: headache, confusion, cerebellar ataxia (rare)
Dermatologic: alopecia (rare), dermatitis, pruritus, rash
Cardiovascular: myocardial ischemia (rare), angina
Catheter complications: arterial ischemia, perforation of vessel, dislodgement of catheter, catheter occlusion, thrombosis, infection

INDICATIONS

FDA-approved: hepatic arterial infusion for palliative management of hepatic metastases from gastrointestinal adenocarcinomas; **Clinical studies show activity in**: renal carcinoma and head and neck carcinomas

PHARMACOKINETICS

Absorption—oral bioavailability limited, variable; **Distribution**—no data regarding CNS or malignancy penetration; **Elimination**—metabolized 70–90% first-pass in liver; **Systemic half-life**—3–20 min; **Adjustments for hepatic or renal dysfunction**: unnecessary

DRUG INTERACTIONS

Leucovorin (increased hepatotoxicity)

RESPONSE RATES

Colorectal cancer with liver metastases—40–50%

PATIENT MONITORING

Monitor vital signs, symptoms (abdominal pain, nausea, vomiting, diarrhea—verify hepatic artery catheter placement; mucositis—interrupt treatment); examination; hematology; serum chemistry panel (significant hepatic enzyme elevations—interrupt treatment)

NURSING INTERVENTIONS

Monitor weight, nutritional status; encourage good oral hygiene; give antiemetics; mouthwashes and other adjuncts; antidiarrheals as needed; educate patients on care of vascular access devices and home infusion pumps

PATIENT INFORMATION

Patient should avoid use of aspirin or nonsteroidal anti-inflammatory agents; call physician if any moderate or severe diarrhea, fever, or other signs of serious infection develop; avoid excessive sun exposure; maintain good nutrition

FORMULATION

Available as FUDR®, Roche Laboratories, Nutley, NJ 500-mg vials containing lyophilized powder. Stored at 15– 30°C and protected from light.

FLUDARABINE PHOSPHATE

Fludarabine phosphate (2-fluoro-ara-AMP) is a synthetic analogue of the naturally occurring purine nucleotide, deoxyadenosine monophosphate, and is a fluorinated nucleotide analogue of the antiviral agent vidarabine. Compared to vidarabine, the fluorine substitution renders 2-fluoro-ara-AMP relatively resistant to inactivation by the enzyme adenosine deaminase, and the phosphate moiety enhances aqueous solubility. Following intravenous infusion, fludarabine phosphate is rapidly dephosphorylated to 2-fluoro-ara-A; intracellularly, 2-fluoro-ara-A is re-phosphorylated to the active triphosphate, 2-fluoro-ara-ATP. This triphosphate metabolite is an inhibitor of several key enzymes in deoxyribonucleotide metabolism and DNA synthesis, including ribonucleotide reductase, DNA polymerase alpha, and DNA primase. Interestingly, fludarabine phosphate has also been shown to stimulate the activity of natural killer cells in *in vitro* studies.

Fludarabine phosphate has been shown to be effective in the treatment of chronic lymphocytic leukemia and other lymphoid malignancies, but has little or no activity against solid tumors. High doses of this drug can produce profound toxicities, including a distinctive syndrome of progressive neurotoxicity, characterized by delayed onset of progressive encephalopathy with cortical blindness and eventual death. Fortunately, standard doses appear to pose little or no risk of this catastrophic syndrome, even with repeated dosing.

DOSAGE AND ADMINISTRATION

Chronic lymphocytic leukemia: 25 mg/m^2/d (30-min IV infusion) × 5 consecutive d, repeat at 28-d intervals to maximal response and for three more cycles, then discontinue

SPECIAL PRECAUTIONS

Pregnant/nursing patients

TOXICITIES

Hematologic: neutropenia, thrombocytopenia, anemia (possibly severe and cumulative)
GI: anorexia, nausea, vomiting; stomatitis, diarrhea, GI bleeding (uncommon); abnormal liver function (occasional)
Neurologic: at recommended doses—weakness, agitation, confusion, visual disturbances, coma (rare), peripheral neuropathy; at high doses—delayed dementia, cortical blindness, coma, death (onset 21–60 d after last dose)
Pulmonary: possible increased susceptibility to pneumonia; pulmonary hypersensitivity reactions (dyspnea, cough, interstitial infiltrate)
Flu-like: malaise, fatigue, fever, chills
Miscellaneous: increased frequency of serious opportunistic infections (*Pneumocystis carinii, Listeria monocytogenes,* cryptococcus); tumor lysis syndrome (with hyperuricemia, hyperphosphatemia, hypocalcemia, hyperkalemia, urate crystalluria, renal failure); edema, rash

INDICATIONS

FDA-approved: chronic lymphocytic leukemia; **Clinical studies show activity in:** low-grade non-Hodgkin's lymphomas; macroglobulinemia; mycosis fungoides, Hodgkin's disease (possibly)

PHARMACOKINETICS

Absorption—insufficient data; **Distribution**—insufficient data; **Elimination**—renal; **Half-life**—10 hr; **Adjustments for organ dysfunction:** use with caution in patients with renal insufficiency

DRUG INTERACTIONS

Pentostatin (possibly lethal), dipyridamole

RESPONSE RATES

Chronic lymphocytic leukemia—in previously treated patients, complete response rate 10–15%, overall response rate 32–57%; with no prior chemotherapy, complete response rate 33%, overall response rate 79%
Low-grade non-Hodgkin's lymphomas—overall response rate 67%

PATIENT MONITORING

Vital signs, symptoms, examination, hematology, serum chemistry panel; bone marrow examination for persistent cytopenias

NURSING INTERVENTIONS

Monitor weight, nutritional status; encourage good oral hygiene; give antiemetics, and mouthwashes and other adjuncts as needed for stomatitis; consider IV gammaglobulin to reduce frequent bacterial infections in chronic lymphocytic leukemia; give antidiarrheals as needed, evaluate for infectious etiology if diarrhea is persistent or severe

PATIENT INFORMATION

Patient should avoid use of aspirin or nonsteroidal anti-inflammatory agents; call physician if fever or other signs of serious infection develop; maintain good nutrition

FORMULATION

Available as FLUDARA®, Berlex Laboratories, Richmond, CA
50-mg vials. Stored at 2–8°C.

FLUOROURACIL

Fluorouracil (5-FU) is a synthetic analogue of the naturally occurring pyrimidine, uracil. Several active metabolites of 5-FU have pharmacologic effects on the synthesis and function of cellular DNA and RNA. Inhibition of thymidylate synthase (TS) by 5-fluorodeoxyuridine monophosphate (FdUMP) is believed to be the primary mechanism of anticancer efficacy of 5-FU. Other active metabolites include 5-fluorouridine triphosphate (FUTP) and 5-fluorodeoxyuridine triphosphate (FdUTP). FUTP is misincorporated into RNA and may affect several aspects of RNA stability and function. Similarly, FdUTP can be misincorporated into cellular DNA (in place of thymidine triphosphate); the level of this misincorporation may be enhanced by the depletion of normal thymidine nucleotides, resulting from thymidylate synthase inhibition by FdUMP. Fluorodeoxyuridine nucleotides that have been misincorporated into DNA are recognized and cleaved by a glycosylase, yielding apyrimidinic sites in the DNA double helix and leading to DNA strand breaks.

Numerous pharmacologic interactions have been observed between 5-FU and other drugs commonly administered to cancer patients. Clinically, both leucovorin and interferon alpha have been shown to significantly enhance both the toxicity and the anticancer activity of fluorouracil.

DOSAGE AND ADMINISTRATION

Solid tumors: 500 mg/m²/d (bolus IV injection) × 5 d, repeated at 4–5 wk intervals **or** 1000 mg/m²/d (continuous IV infusion) × 5 d, repeated every 4 wk **or** 500–600 mg/m² (bolus IV injection), repeated weekly × 6 wk **or** 300 mg/m²/d (continuous IV infusion) × 4 wk or longer

In combination with leucovorin: 5-FU dose usually must be reduced 25–33%.

SPECIAL PRECAUTIONS

Severe diarrhea (especially in elderly patients, and with leucovorin or interferon alpha)

Patients with dihydropyrimidine dehydrogenase deficiency

Pregnant/nursing patients

TOXICITIES

Hematologic: neutropenia, occasional thrombocytopenia (reversible)
GI: anorexia, nausea, vomiting (mild); oral, esophageal, GI mucositis and ulceration; diarrhea (sometimes severe), heartburn, taste alterations
Neurologic: cerebellar ataxia (can be irreversible), obtundation, disorientation, confusion, euphoria, nystagmus, headache; seizures (with leucovorin); acute neurotoxicity with progressive obtundation, hypotension, death (with high doses)
Dermatologic: hand-foot syndrome, rash, dry skin, fissuring, nail changes/loss, photosensitivity, alopecia, hyperpigmentation
Cardiovascular: myocardial ischemia, angina, infarction
Miscellaneous: epistaxis, conjunctivitis, generalized allergic reactions (very rare)

INDICATIONS

FDA-approved: palliative management of carcinomas of the colon, rectum, breast, stomach, and pancreas; **Clinical studies show activity in** head and neck carcinomas; as a radiosensitizer, in the adjuvant treatment of adenocarcinoma of the rectum

PHARMACOKINETICS

Absorption—oral bioavailability low, variable; **Distribution**—readily penetrates the CNS and malignant effusions, crosses the placenta; **Elimination**—metabolism (dihydropyrimidine dehydrogenase); **Half-life**—6–20 min; **Adjustments for hepatic or renal dysfunction**—unnecessary

DRUG INTERACTIONS

Leucovorin, interferon alpha, interferon gamma, methotrexate, allopurinol, PALA, uridine, thymidine, dipyridamole, hydroxyurea

RESPONSE RATES

Colorectal cancer—partial remissions 10–20%; 30–40% with leucovorin
Head and neck squamous cancers—partial remissions 10–20%
Breast cancer—partial remissions 10–20%
Gastric cancer—partial remissions 10–15%

PATIENT MONITORING

Vital signs, symptoms (mucositis, diarrhea), examination, hematology, serum chemistry panel

NURSING INTERVENTIONS

Monitor weight, nutritional status; encourage good oral hygiene; give antiemetics as necessary; mouthwashes and other adjuncts for stomatitis; antidiarrheals for mild diarrhea (inform physician); educate on care of central venous access devices and home infusion pumps

PATIENT INFORMATION

Patient should avoid use of aspirin or nonsteroidal anti-inflammatory agents. Call physician if any moderate or severe diarrhea, fever, or other signs of serious infection develop. Avoid excessive sun exposure; maintain good nutrition

FORMULATION

Available as Fluorouracil (Roche Laboratories, Nutley, NJ; Adria Laboratories, Dublin, OH; and other manufacturers)
500-mg ampules (50 mg/mL); 10-mL and 100-mL vials (50 mg/mL). Stored at 15–30°C and protected from light. Administer undiluted, or dilute with 5% dextrose in water or 0.9% sodium chloride.

HYDROXYUREA

The anticancer effects of hydroxyurea appear to be related to inhibition of ribonucleotide reductase. Clinically, it is used primarily in the treatment of chronic myelocytic leukemia and related myeloproliferative disorders. Although hydroxyurea is also approved for use in malignant melanoma and ovarian cancer, there is currently little evidence that this drug has any significant activity in solid tumors. However, potentially synergistic interactions between hydroxyurea and other drugs that affect pyrimidine nucleotide biosynthesis and DNA metabolism (such as methotrexate, the fluoropyrimidines, and cytarabine) have been identified in laboratory studies, and rationally designed combinations of hydroxyurea with other drugs continue to be the subject of numerous clinical investigations.

DOSAGE AND ADMINISTRATION

800–1200 mg/m^2/d po daily **or** 2000–3200 mg/m^2 po q 3 d (wide variations in dosing; see protocol chapters)

SPECIAL PRECAUTIONS

Pregnant/nursing patients

TOXICITIES

Hematologic: neutropenia (reversible) thrombocytopenia, anemia
GI: anorexia, nausea, vomiting (mild); oral, esophageal, GI mucositis and ulceration; constipation, diarrhea; liver function abnormalities (rarely progressing to jaundice)
Dermatologic: hyperpigmentation, erythema of face and hands, diffuse maculopapular rash, dry skin, thinning of skin, nail changes, alopecia (rare)
Neurologic: headache, drowsiness, dizziness, confusion (mild)
Miscellaneous: transient renal function abnormalities, radiation recall reactions

INDICATIONS

FDA-approved: ovarian adenocarcinoma, malignant melanoma, and chronic myelocytic leukemia; concurrently with radiation therapy for squamous carcinomas of the head and neck; **Clinical studies show activity in**: acute nonlymphocytic leukemia and essential thrombocytosis (acute control of dangerously elevated cell counts, pending initiation of standard cytarabine-based treatment regimens); polycythemia vera; as a radiosensitizer, in locally advanced cancer of the uterine cervix

PHARMACOKINETICS

Absorption—high oral availability; **Distribution**—readily penetrates the CNS and malignant effusions (excreted in significant quantities in breast milk); **Elimination**— primarily renal; **Half-life**—3.5–4.5 hr; **Adjustments for organ dysfunction**—intitial reduced doses to patients with renal dysfunction recommended

DRUG INTERACTIONS

Cytarabine, fluorouracil, methotrexate

RESPONSE RATES

Chronic myelocytic leukemia—reduction of leukocyte count in over 75% of patients

PATIENT MONITORING

Vital signs, symptoms (mucositis, diarrhea), examination, hematology (weekly), serum chemistry panel

NURSING INTERVENTIONS

Monitor weight, nutritional status; encourage good oral hygiene; give antiemetics; mouthwashes and other adjuncts for stomatitis; antidiarrheals as needed

PATIENT INFORMATION

Patient should avoid use of aspirin or nonsteroidal anti-inflammatory agents; call physician if fever or other signs of serious infection develop; avoid excessive sun exposure

FORMULATION

Hydrea® Bristol-Myers Oncology Division, Princeton, NJ
500-mg capsules. Stored at 15–30°C in tightly sealed container.

LEUCOVORIN

Leucovorin (5-formyl-tetrahydrofolate) is a reduced folate that can be readily transformed to all folates required for cellular metabolism. Thus, it serves as an effective antidote for methotrexate and other antifols and can be used to reduce the adverse effects caused by these drugs. Preliminary data indicate that leucovorin will also serve as an antidote for newer, investigational antifols (including trimetrexate, piritrexim, and edatrexate). In contrast, leucovorin increases the toxicity and enhances the efficacy of the fluoropyrimidines; the leucovorin metabolite, 5,10-methylene-tetrahydrofolate, enhances the inhibition of the enzyme thymidylate synthase produced by fluorodeoxyuridine monophosphate, an active metabolite of the fluoropyrimidines.

DOSAGE AND ADMINISTRATION

Methotrexate rescue: beginning 6–24 hr after methotrexate therapy, administer leucovorin mg 15 IV or po every 6 hr for approximately 10 doses (until methotrexate level is 0.05 μmol/L). Start rescue no later than 24 hr after high-dose methotrexate. Higher leucovorin doses and longer treatement may be required if methotrexate clearance is abnormal (see manufacturer's guidelines).
With fluorouracil (for colorectal cancer): leucovorin 20 mg/m² followed by 425 mg/m² fluorouracil **or** leucovorin 200 mg/m² followed by 370 mg/m² fluorouracil daily for 5 days. Alternate regimen: leucovorin 500 mg/m² IV infusion over 2 hr with fluorouracil injection (500–600 mg/m²) at midpoint of leucovorin infusion; repeat weekly for 6 wk.

SPECIAL PRECAUTIONS

None

TOXICITIES

Allergic: sensitization (possibly)
Neurologic: seizures (with 5-FU)

INDICATIONS

FDA-approved: antidote for overdose of methotrexate or other folic acid antagonists; osteosarcoma (adjuvant chemotherapy, with high-dose methotrexate); advanced colorectal cancer (with 5-FU); **Clinical studies show activity in:** advanced breast cancer (with 5-FU)

PHARMACOKINETICS

Absorption—high bioavailability at oral doses up to 40 mg, less at higher doses; **Distribution**—negligible CSF penetration, (approximately 1% of systemic levels); **Elimination**—metabolized and excreted renally; **Half-life**—1 hr (parent compound) and 4–7 hr (active 5-methyl-tetrahydrofolate metabolite); **Adjustments for organ dysfunction**—unnecessary

DRUG INTERACTIONS

Fluoropyrimidines, methotrexate, edatrexate, trimetrexate, piritrexim, iododeoxyuridine

RESPONSE RATES

See page on methotrexate
See chapter on lower gastrointestinal cancer

PATIENT MONITORING

None required for single-agent leucovorin (see pages on methotrexate and 5-FU for combination therapy)

NURSING INTERVENTIONS

None required for single-agent leucovorin (see pages on methotrexate and 5-FU for combination therapy)

PATIENT INFORMATION

No specific information required for single-agent leucovorin (see pages on methotrexate and 5-FU for combination therapy)

FORMULATION

Available as Leucovorin, Lederle Laboratories; (Wellcovorin®) Burroughs Wellcome Co., Research Triangle Park, NC; Elkins-Sinn, Cherry Hill, NJ; and Cetus, Oncology Corporation, Emeryville, CA 5-mg, 10-mg, 15-mg, and 25-mg tablets; 1-mL ampules containing 3-mg leucovorin; 50-mg, 100-mg, and 350-mg vials of cryodessicated powder. Stored at 15–30°C and protected from light.

METHOTREXATE

Methotrexate, a synthetic analogue of folic acid, is a potent inhibitor of dihydrofolate reductase (DHFR), a key enzyme in folate metabolism. Inhibition of DHFR results in depletion of cellular reduced folates and interferes with vital cellular enzymes that require reduced folate cofactors (including enzymes of thymidylate and purine synthesis and amino acid metabolism). Inside the cell, methotrexate is metabolized to active polyglutamate metabolites, which inhibit DHFR and several other cellular enzymes, including enzymes that catalyze formyl transfer reactions in purine biosynthesis. Active polyglutamate metabolites of methotrexate may be retained by cells for long periods of time; hence, the antimetabolic effects of this drug may persist long after circulating levels of methotrexate are undetectable.

Leucovorin can reverse most of the antimetabolic effects produced by methotrexate and rescue both normal and malignant cells from the cytotoxic effects of methotrexate. Used appropriately, leucovorin can enhance the therapeutic index of methotrexate by controlling and limiting the toxicity of higher doses of methotrexate. Pharmacologic interactions may also occur between methotrexate and many other drugs commonly administered to cancer patients. Clinically, the combination of methotrexate and fluorouracil has been extensively evaluated; available data suggest therapeutic synergy for treatment schedules in which fluorouracil administration follows methotrexate administration.

DOSAGE AND ADMINISTRATION

Solid tumors: 30–40 mg/m^2/wk (IV infusion) **or** 3–12 g/m^2 as a 4–6 hr (IV infusion) with leucovorin rescue beginning at 6–24 hr, repeated weekly × 2–3 wk
Oral regimens: 15–40 mg (total dose) po, repeated weekly (usually used for psoriasis, rheumatoid arthritis); 2.5–5 mg (total dose) po daily (used for mycosis fungoides)
Intrathecal administration: Dose according to age— <1 yr, 6 mg; 1 yr, 8 mg; 2 yr, 10 mg; 3 y or older, 12 mg. Repeat administration 1–2 times weekly, until CSF cytology has been negative for malignant cells for 1 wk; consider periodic maintenance therapy.

SPECIAL PRECAUTIONS

Patients with pleural effusions, ascites, impaired renal function (may delay clearance, increase toxicity)
Pregnant/nursing patients
Patients with poor nutritional status
Patients on high-dose regimens
Recent nitrous oxide anesthesia

TOXICITIES

Hematologic: neutropenia, thrombocytopenia (occasional, reversible)
GI: anorexia, nausea, vomiting, diarrhea; oral, esophageal, GI mucositis and ulceration; transient abnormalities in serum levels of liver enzymes; cirrhosis, hepatic failure (rare)
Neurologic: headache, drowsiness, dizziness; with high doses, acute confusion, obtundation, seizures; with intrathecal administration, chronic dementia, chemical arachnoiditis (rare, possible severe)
Dermatologic: rash, pruritus, urticaria, pigmentary changes, photosensitivity, alopecia, acne
Pulmonary: interstitial pneumonitis
Renal: acute renal failure (especially with high doses), hyperuricemia
Miscellaneous: anaphylaxis (rare), radiation recall

INDICATIONS

FDA-approved: choriocarcinoma/gestational trophoblastic disease, ALL, meningeal leukemia, breast cancer, squamous head and neck cancers, mycosis fungoides, lung cancer, non-Hodgkin's lymphomas, osteogenic sarcoma; **Clinical studies show activity in:** carcinoma of the bladder, post-transplantation immunosuppression

PHARMACOKINETICS

Absorption—good oral bioavailability (for doses up to 40 mg); **Distribution**—1–3% penetration into CSF, slow penetrating, slow release from pleural effusions or ascites; **Elimination**—80–90% renal; **Half-life**—2–3 hr (primary); 8–10 hr (terminal) **Adjustments for renal insufficiency** (creatinine clearance <40 ml/min; or, for high-dose regimens, creatinine clearance <60 ml/min)—do not administer

DRUG INTERACTIONS

Leucovorin, 5FU, ara-C, asparaginase, carboxypeptidase, thiopurines, colchicine, nitrous oxide, probenecid, aspirin, NSAID, sulfonamides, triamterene, trimethoprim, pyrimethamine

RESPONSE RATES

Choriocarcinoma/gestational trophoblastic disease— generally curative; Pediatric ALL—response to combination regimens with methotrexate 90%; cured 50%; Breast cancer—with cyclophosphamide and 5-FU, 30–50% remission; Squamous head and neck cancers—partial remissions in 30%; Mycosis fungoides—complete response rate 40–50%; Osteogenic sarcoma—cure rate of nonmetastatic disease 50–60% with adjuvant combination therapy

PATIENT MONITORING

Vital signs, symptoms, examination, hematology, serum chemistry panel; with high doses, closely monitor renal function, urine output, urine pH, serum electrolytes, serum methotrexate levels

NURSING INTERVENTIONS

Monitor weight, nutritional status; encourage good oral hygiene; give antiemetics: with high doses, monitor fluid intake and output, assess patient's oral intake and ability to take leucovorin rescue as instructed post-discharge

PATIENT INFORMATION

Patient should avoid use of aspirin or NSAIDs; call physician if moderate or severe adverse effects develop

FORMULATION

Available as Rheumatrex®, Lederle Laboratories, Wayne, NJ; Folex®, Adria Labs, Dublin, OH; Mexate®, Bristol-Myers Oncology Division, Princeton, NJ; 50- , 100- , 200- , and 250-mg vials containing 25-mg/ml preservative-free solution; 50-mg and 250-mg vials containing 25-mg/ml preservative-protected solution; 20-mg, 50-mg, and 1-g vials of freeze-dried methotrexate; 2.5-mg tablets. Stored at 15–30°C and protected from light.

MERCAPTOPURINE

Mercaptopurine (6-mercaptopurine or 6-MP) is a thiopurine that has been in clinical use as an antileukemic drug since the 1950s. Mercaptopurine is enzymatically converted to 6-thioinosine monophosphate (6-TIMP) by a purine salvage enzyme, hypoxanthine-guanine phosphoribosyltransferase (HGPRT). Although 6-TIMP is a relatively poor substrate for cellular enzymes and accumulates to significant levels in 6-MP-treated cells, 6-TIMP can be converted to a variety of other metabolites, including the corresponding ribonucleoside and deoxyribonucleoside di- and triphosphates, 6-methylmercaptopurine and its nucleotides, and 6-thioguanine nucleotides. The 6-TIMP metabolite of mercaptopurine inhibits several enzymes important in purine biosynthesis; 6-thiodeoxyguanosine triphosphate formed from 6-MP can be incorporated into DNA and can produce DNA strand breaks; and the many other metabolites of 6-MP produce additional antimetabolic effects. It is not yet clear which mechanism(s) accounts for the anticancer activity of mercaptopurine.

Relationships among the thiopurines in clinical use (mercaptopurine, thioguanine, and azathioprine) are discussed in the section on thioguanine.

DOSAGE AND ADMINISTRATION

Acute lymphoblastic leukemia: 50–75 mg/m²/d for 30–36 mo (maintenance chemotherapy, with methotrexate)
Acute nonlymphocytic leukemia: 500 mg/m²/d IV (using investigational IV formulation) × 5 d (in induction combination chemotherapy)

SPECIAL PRECAUTIONS

Pregnant/nursing patients
Patients receiving allopurinol (reduce doses at least 50%)

TOXICITIES

Hematologic: neutropenia, thrombocytopenia, anemia (reversible, dose-related)
GI: anorexia, nausea, vomiting, diarrhea, (mild); oral, esophageal, GI mucositis and ulceration; reversible cholestatic jaundice; hepatic necrosis (rare)
Dermatologic: rash, hyperpigmentation
Miscellaneous: fever, pancreatitis (rare), hematuria and crystalluria with high IV doses

INDICATIONS

FDA-approved: acute lymphocytic leukemia, acute nonlymphocytic leukemias; **Clinical studies show activity in**: chronic myelocytic leukemia

PHARMACOKINETICS

Absorption—oral bioavailability (approx 16%), erratic, extensive first-pass metabolism in intestinal mucosa and liver; **Distribution**—no CSF penetration; **Elimination**—via metabolism (xanthine oxidase, other pathways); **Half-life**—1.5 hr; **Adjustments for organ dysfunction**: insufficient data

DRUG INTERACTIONS

Allopurinol, methotrexate, tiazofurin, trimethoprim-sulfamethoxazole, coumadin

RESPONSE RATES

Not applicable (used in maintenance phase treatment following complete remission of pediatric ALL; overall cure rate 50%)

PATIENT MONITORING

Vital signs, symptoms (mucositis, diarrhea), examination, hematology (weekly), serum chemistry panel

NURSING INTERVENTIONS

Monitor weight, nutritional status; encourage good oral hygiene; given antiemetics; mouthwashes and other adjuncts for somatitis; antidiarrheals as needed

PATIENT INFORMATION

Patient should avoid use of aspirin or nonsteroidal anti-inflammatory agents; call physician if fever or other signs of serious infection develop; avoid excessive sun exposure; maintain good nutrition

FORMULATION

Available as Purinethol®, Burroughs Wellcome Co., Research Triangle Park, NC
50-mg tablets. Stored at 15–25°C in a dry place.
Investigators with NCI-approved research protocols can obtain investigational tablet (10 mg) and IV formulations from the Pharmaceutical Resources Branch, National Cancer Institute
50-mL vials containing 500-mg mercaptopurine (sodium salt), lyophilized powder. Store unopened vials at room temperature (22–25°C).

PENTOSTATIN

Pentostatin (2′-deoxycoformycin or DCF) is a purine deoxynucleoside analogue isolated from fermentation cultures of *Streptomyces antibioticus*. Pentostatin is a potent inhibitor of the enzyme adenosine deaminase, which hydrolyzes adenosine to inosine. The pharmacologic actions of pentostatin are believed to be mediated by the accumulation of adenine nucleotides, which can occur when adenosine hydrolysis is blocked. High intracellular levels of deoxyadenosine triphosphate can inhibit the activity of the enzyme ribonucleotide reductase, resulting in depletion of levels of other cellular deoxyribonucleotides. High levels of deoxyadenosine nucleotides can also inhibit the enzyme S-adenosylhomocysteine hydrolase, thus interfering with cellular methylation pathways and causing accumulation of S-adenosylhomocysteine (a toxic metabolite). Cells (such as lymphocytes) that have low levels of the nucleotide-cleaving enzyme 5′-nucleotidase may be particularly sensitive to these antimetabolic effects of pentostatin. Other known antimetabolic effects of pentostatin include inhibition of RNA synthesis and misincorporation of the triphosphate metabolite of pentostatin into cellular DNA.

In initial phase I studies using high doses of pentostatin, toxicities were frequently observed, with limited evidence of clinical efficacy. However, subsequent research has shown that this agent is highly active against hairy cell leukemia (a B-cell lymphoid neoplasm), has activity in other lymphoid malignancies as well, and can be used safely and effectively at lower doses. Pentostatin is not active in the treatment of solid tumors, and significant immunosuppression occurs as an adverse effect even at low doses of pentostatin.

DOSAGE AND ADMINISTRATION

Hairy cell leukemia: pretreat with allopurinol (300 mg/d) × 7 d. Then pentostatin (4 mg/m²) once every 2 wk until complete response, followed by two additional doses, or to maximum of 12 mo. If no partial response by 6 mo, change to alternate treatment. Adjust dose if creatinine clearance is less than 60 ml/min.

SPECIAL PRECAUTIONS

Opportunistic (eg, *Pneumocystis carinii*) and severe infections
Pregnant/nursing patients

TOXICITIES

Hematologic: lymphopenia (particularly T cells), neutropenia, thrombocytopenia, immunosuppression (possibly severe and prolonged); infectious complications (common), including opportunistic infections
Neurologic: anxiety, depression, confusion, lethargy, obtundation, coma, seizures
Renal: azotemia, acute renal failure, long-term residual impairment (possible)
Dermatologic: rash (possibly severe and increased with continued treatment)
GI: anorexia, nausea, vomiting (not severe), stomatitis, elevations in liver function tests (reversible)
Miscellaneous: fever, pneumonitis, myalgias, arthralgias, pleuritis, peritonitis, pericarditis, keratoconjunctivitis

INDICATIONS

FDA-approved: interferon alpha–refractory hairy cell leukemia; **Clinical studies show activity in:** T- and B-cell lymphomas, acute lymphoblastic leukemia, chronic lymphocytic leukemia, mycosis fungoides, Sézary syndrome, Waldenstrom's macroglobulinemia; **Possible activity:** multiple myeloma, Hodgkin's lymphomas

PHARMACOKINETICS

Absorption—insufficient data; **Distribution**— insufficient data on CNS penetration; **Elimination**—renal; **Half-life**—2.5–6 hr; **Adjustments for organ dysfunction:** delayed elimination of pentostatin with renal dysfunction; patients should have a creatinine clearance ≥60 mL/min

DRUG INTERACTIONS

Fludarabine phosphate, vidarabine

RESPONSE RATES

Hairy cell leukemia (refractory to interferon-alpha)—50–60% complete response in blood and bone marrow (durable, at least some cured); plus 20–30% partial response

PATIENT MONITORING

Vital signs, symptoms, examination, hematology, serum chemistry panel; creatinine clearance pretreatment and during treatment; bone marrow examination for persistent cytopenias

NURSING INTERVENTIONS

Monitor weight, nutritional status; encourage good oral hygiene; give antiemetics as necessary; give mouthwashes and other adjuncts as needed for stomatitis; give antidiarrheals as needed; evaluate for infectious etiology if diarrhea is persistent or severe

PATIENT INFORMATION

Patient should avoid use of aspirin or nonsteroidal anti-inflammatory agents; call physician if fever or other signs of serious infection develop; maintain good nutrition

FORMULATION

Available as NIPENT® Parke-Davis, Morris Plains, NJ
10-mg vials of lyophilized powder. Stored at 2–8°C.

THIOGUANINE

Thioguanine (6-thioguanine or 6-TG) a purine analogue, has been in clinical use as an antileukemic drug since the 1950s. Thioguanine is activated to 6-thioguanosine monophosphate by a purine salvage enzyme, hypoxanthine-guanine phosphoribosyltransferase (HGPRT). This ribonucleotide can be further phosphorylated by cellular kinases to generate thioguanosine di- and triphosphates or reduced (via the action of the enzyme ribonucleotide reductase) to generate thioguanine deoxyribonucleotides. Thioguanine and its metabolites produce numerous antimetabolic effects in cells, and it is not clear which mechanism(s) accounts for the anticancer activity of this drug.

The thiopurines are active agents in the treatment of acute and chronic leukemias and may have modest activity in the treatment of non-Hodgkin's lymphomas, but they have demonstrated no significant clinical activity against solid tumors. For historic reasons, azathioprine is used as an immunosuppressive, 6-thioguanine is used primarily in treatment of nonlymphocyctic leukemias, and 6-mercaptopurine is used primarily in treatment of lymphocytic leukemias. Although clinical comparative studies have not been performed, it is likely that any of these drugs could be used for any of these indications, with comparable results. The only clinically significant pharmacologic difference among these three drugs is that the metabolic elimination of thioguanine is *not* significantly affected by allopurinol; hence, thioguanine doses need not be adjusted in patients receiving allopurinol.

DOSAGE AND ADMINISTRATION

Acute leukemia (in combination chemotherapy): 75–200 mg/m^2/d × 5 to 7 d in one or two divided oral doses

SPECIAL PRECAUTIONS

Pregnancy/nursing patients
Hepatic impairment

TOXICITIES

Hematologic: neutropenia, thrombocytopenia, anemia (reversible, dose-related)
GI: anorexia, nausea, vomiting (mild), diarrhea; oral, esophageal, GI mucositis and ulceration; cholestatic jaundice
Dermatologic: rash, hyperpigmentation

INDICATIONS

FDA-approved: acute nonlymphocyctic leukemias; chronic myelocyctic leukemia (alternative to busulfan); **Clinical studies show activity in:** acute lymphocyctic leukmeia

PHARMACOKINETICS

Absorption—limited oral bioavailability (approx 30%), highly variable (food intake reduces bioavailability); **Distribution**—does not penetrate CNS; **Elimination**— metabolism (methylation); **Half-life**—25–240 min; **Adjustments for organ dysfunction**—insufficient data, use with caution in hepatic impairment

DRUG INTERACTIONS

Methotrexate, other antifols, tiazofurin

RESPONSE RATES

Adult acute nonlymphocytic leukemia (with cytosine arabinoside and daunorubicin or doxorubicin)—complete remission rate 40–75%; cure rate 5–10%

PATIENT MONITORING

Vital signs, symptoms (mucositis, diarrhea), examination, hematology (weekly, daily in leukemia induction therapy), serum chemistry panel

NURSING INTERVENTIONS

Monitor weight, nutritional status; encourage good oral hygiene; give antiemetics; mouthwashes and other adjuncts for stomatitis; antidiarrheals as needed

PATIENT INFORMATION

Patient should avoid use of aspirin or nonsteroidal anti-inflammatory agents; call physician if fever or other signs of serious infection develop; avoid excessive sun exposure; maintain good nutrition

FORMULATIONS

Available as Tabloid® from Burroughs Wellcome Co., Triangle Research Park, NC
40-mg tablets. Stored at 15–25°C in a dry place.
Investigators with NCI-approved research protocols can obtain the investigational IV formulation from the Pharmaceutical Resources Branch, National Cancer Institute.
Investigational IV formulation, 10-ml vials containing 75-mg thioguanine (base), lyophilized powder. Unopened vials are refrigerated (2–8°C), but are also stable at room temperature (22–25°C).

The conventional treatment of cancer includes chemotherapy, radiation therapy, or surgery used singly or in combination. A fourth modality, biologic therapy, utilizes biologic reagents to elicit tumor regression. The biotherapeutic pharmacopeia includes recombinant cytokines, some of which possess profound immunomodulatory and antitumor activity. These include interleukin 2 (aldesleukin) and interferon alpha. Other recombinant cytokines, termed *colony-stimulating factors* (CSF), exert profound effects on hematopoiesis and immune function. This group of agents includes erythropoietin (epoietin-alpha), granulocyte-CSF (filgrastim), and granulocyte-macrophage–CSF (sargramostim). Although they do not have antitumor activity, these recombinant proteins have been shown to blunt chemotherapy-induced myelopoietic toxicity, and they have become useful adjuvants to bone marrow transplantation.

Other immunomodulating reagents with demonstrated antitumor activity include bacillus Calmette–Guérin and levamisole. Although the latter is not a biologic reagent *per se*, both of these agents purportedly mediate their antitumor effects through immune modulation. Octreotide is a long-acting octapeptide that mimics the effects of the naturally occurring hormone somatostatin. Its plieotropic effects include antiproliferative activity against several diverse types of tumor. Additional anticancer biologic reagents, including interleukin 1 (IL-1), IL-4, IL-6, IL-7, and IL-12, as well as adoptively transferred lymphoid cells, are currently being evaluated for clinical efficacy and are not discussed herein because of their experimental nature.

ALDESLEUKIN

Aldesleukin or interleukin 2 (IL-2) is a T-cell growth factor that is central to T-cell mediated immune responses [1,2]. It is a hydrophobic, 15kD, 133 amino acid glycoprotein that is elaborated primarily by activated CD4+ T lymphocytes. Its production is regulated at the transcriptional level by signals transduced across the plasma cell membrane when a mature T cell encounters its cognate antigen in concert with secondary signals provided by accessory cells. Aldesleukin is the recombinant protein elaborated by *Escherichia coli* that contains the human IL-2 gene. The cysteine residue at position 125 is substituted in the recombinant product by similar space-occupying amino acids in order to avoid aggregation and disulfide exchange, leading to the accumulation of less active forms.

IL-2 has been approved for the treatment of patients with metastatic renal cell carcinoma, in whom response rates between 20 and 30% have been observed. Complete responses are generally durable and may persist for several years. IL-2 also has demonstrated activity against metastatic melanoma. Treatment of these patients is associated with a response rate approaching 20%.

MECHANISM OF ACTION

IL-2 plays a central role in T-cell activation. It is requisite for cell cycle progression from G_1 to S phase and the subsequent T-cell proliferation that is the *sine qua non* of cell-mediated immune responses. These effects of IL-2 are mediated through a heterotrimeric receptor (IL-2R) that may take many cell surface forms based on which of its three subunits are expressed. The IL-2 receptor a chain (IL-2Rα, also referred to as p55, CD25, or Tac) has low affinity for IL-2 ($K_d \sim 10^{-8}$ M) and is not constitutively expressed. The beta chain of the IL-2R (or p75) is a 70- to 75-Kd,

525 amino acid molecule with intermediate affinity for IL-2 ($K_d \sim 10^{-9}$ M). IL-2Rβ is constitutively expressed by monocytes, some mature CD4+ and CD8+ T cells, and large granular lymphocytes. It is also constitutively expressed in concert with IL-2R α on a subset of CD16- natural killer (NK) cells. In the presence of large concentrations of IL-2, the IL-2Rβ chain is capable of signal transduction. The high-affinity IL-2R ($K_d \sim 10^{-11}$ M) is a noncovalently linked heterotrimer comprised of the alpha, beta, and recently described gamma subunits.

Ligation of either the high- or intermediate-affinity IL-2R with IL-2 leads to internalization of the complex and a subsequent cascade of genetic events that serves to activate a cell. Large granular lymphocytes proliferate and develop lymphokine-activated killer activity. The cytotoxic activity of monocytes and CD8+ T cells is stimulated as well. Activated B cells are induced to proliferate and elaborate secretory rather than membranous IgM. T cells that express the high-affinity IL-2R will undergo cell division upon exposure to IL-2. The ability of IL-2-stimulated mononuclear cells to elaborate IFN-γ, tumor necrosis factor-alpha (TNF-α), IL-6, and IL-1 accounts for additional pleiotropic effects. Although IL-2 has been shown to downregulate the help provided by CD4+ T cells to humoral effector cells in certain models, the net effect on immune function is generally stimulatory.

The selective antitumor effects seen in some patients treated with aldesleukin are thought to be the result of a cell-mediated immune response that discriminates between self and nonself. This intimates that antigenic differences exist between some cancers and normal cells. There is compelling evidence derived from both murine models and clinical trials that this immune response is primarily T-cell mediated.

MECHANISMS OF RESISTANCE

At least 70% of patients with renal cell carcinoma who are treated with IL-2 have no measurable clinical response to therapy. The majority of patients who manifest treatment-related tumor regression eventually develop progressive disease, despite retreatment. Although responses have also been reported in patients with metastatic melanoma, colorectal carcinoma, ovarian cancer, lymphoma, and lung cancer, these responses have generally been transient or infrequent. The mechanisms that underlie this apparent escape from immune-mediated tumor regression have not been elucidated. Antigenic heterogeneity within a tumor may allow for the outgrowth of antigenically distinct clones that are not recognized by the immune system. Alternatively, defects in cell trafficking or tumor cell susceptibility to lysis may develop that lead to unchecked tumor progression. Definition of the mechanisms of resistance must await a better understanding of the mechanisms of response.

ADVERSE EFFECTS

The supraphysiologic doses of IL-2 that have been used for therapy are associated with a myriad of side effects, which are most likely mediated by other cytokines. Hematologic toxicity, including anemia requiring transfusion and thrombocytopenia with platelet counts less than 20,000, have been observed in 60% and about 15% of treatment courses, respectively. Effects on the kidney include oliguria and decreased fractional excretion of sodium associated with rising serum creatinine and blood urea nitrogen in most patients. These can be successfully managed in the majority of patients with the intravenous administration of volume expanders and dopamine infusions (2–3 µg/kg/min). Renal toxicity resolves in nearly all instances within several days. Cardiovascular toxicity includes increased heart rate and myocardial depression manifest by decreased ejection fraction. Elevations of adrenocorticotropic hormone, endorphins, growth hormone, prolactin, and glucocorticoids have been observed in treated patients. Some patients develop clinically overt hypothyroidism that requires long-term thyroid hormone replacement therapy. Nearly all patients develop a vascular leak syndrome that is associated with egress of intravascular fluid into the soft tissues where it remains sequestered until therapy ends. This redistribution of fluid probably contributes to the hypotension observed in most treated patients and can be effectively managed with vigorous fluid resuscitation using plasma-volume expanders. The volume of administered fluid is limited in some patients by noncardiogenic pulmonary edema secondary to capillary leak. In these patients, phenylephrine can be used to support the blood pressure in lieu of volume expansion.

INTERFERONS

The interferons include more than 20 antigenically discrete but related immunomodulatory proteins [2,3]. They differ in their physicochemical properties but manifest similar effects on the immune system, albeit to different degrees and with some exceptions. Despite the profound immunomodulatory and antiproliferative effects manifest by the interferons, their use as single agents has ostensibly had limited impact on the treatment of solid tumors [4].

Interferon alpha (also referred to as type I, leukocyte interferon, or IFN α) includes more than 23 related subtypes with overlapping activities. These are primarily elaborated by macrophages, large granular lymphocytes, and B cells upon exposure to viruses, double-stranded RNA, tumor necrosis factor-alpha (TNF-α), and IL-1. Most of the naturally occurring IFN α subtypes are composed of 166 amino acids and have molecular weights between 18,000 and 20,000. Their structure is that of an alpha-helix that is stabilized by disulfide bonds between cysteine residues at positions 1, 29, 99, and 139. The IFN α gene, located on chromosome 9, is constitutively transcribed in some cell types and may confer a degree of protection against viral infection.

Natural IFN α (IFN α-n3) is prepared from pooled human leukocytes that have been induced by infection with the avian Sendai virus. The specific composition of this preparation has not been elucidated. The two recombinant IFN α formulations available in the United States differ from natural IFN α in that amino acid 44 has been deleted and amino acid 23 has been replaced by lysine (IFN α-2a) or arginine (IFN α-2b). The half-lives of IFN α-2a and IFN α-2b differ slightly after intravenous administration and are 5 hours (3.7 to 8.5) and 2 to 3 (0.5 to 3) hours, respectively.

Interferon-β (type I, fibroblast interferon, or IFN β) is a 166 amino acid glycoprotein that shares 30% homology with IFN α. The predominant sources of IFN β *in vivo* are fibroblasts and epithelial cells. Its production is upregulated by the same stimuli that induce the production of IFN α. Both IFN α and IFN β share a common cell surface receptor. Unlike most naturally occurring IFN α subtypes, IFN β is N-glycosylated, its functional unit is a dimer, its alpha-helical content is less than 50%, and there is only one molecular species that is encoded by a gene located on chromosome 9. Recombinant IFN β is a nonglycosylated analogue in which cysteine has been replaced by serine at position 17 to maintain stability. Its

activity is similar to that of the naturally occurring protein. It has not been approved for clinical use.

Interferon γ (type II, immune interferon, or IFN γ) is a 143 amino acid glycoprotein that shares little homology to the type I interferons alpha and beta. It is encoded by a gene on chromosome 12 and is made predominantly by CD4+ and CD8+ T cells, NK cells, and macrophages upon exposure to antigen, mitogen, or IL-2. The dimeric molecule interacts with a unique, high-affinity, cell surface receptor that is specific for IFN γ. There are an estimated 1000 receptors per cell, with perhaps higher numbers on some tumor cells. IFN γ has been approved by the FDA for the treatment of chronic granulomatous disease. In addition to natural IFN γ, several recombinant products are available in the United States. Differences in the N-terminal sequences and the number of amino acids account for variable pharmacokinetics and bioavailability between the commercial products.

IFN α has demonstrated activity against many solid and hematologic malignancies. The latter appear to be particularly sensitive. An 80 to 90% response rate has been observed among patients with hairy cell leukemia treated with IFN α. Complete response in the bone marrow is rare, however, and most patients eventually relapse with the median time to clinically significant hematologic deterioration being 18 to 24 months. Benefits of therapy include a decrease in the incidence of serious infection and a reduced requirement for blood products. Survival appears to be prolonged compared to historical controls.

The hematologic response among patients with chronic myelogenous leukemia who are treated within 1 year of diagnosis is 50 to 70%. Despite an associated 20% complete cytogenetic response rate that appears to be durable, a survival benefit has not been demonstrated. The role of interferon in the treatment of other hematologic malignancies appears to be limited with the exception of essential thrombocythemia in which response rates approaching 80% have been observed.

Kaposi's sarcoma is the only solid tumor for which treatment with IFN α has been approved by the FDA. The use of high doses (> 20 × 10^6 U/m^2/day) administered intramuscularly or subcutaneously is associated with a response rate of 30% among treated patients without B symptoms, without prior opportunistic infection, and with CD4+ lymphocyte counts greater than 200. Half of these responses are complete and durable. Several other solid tumors manifest some degree of sensitivity to interferons. These include renal cell carcinoma, malignant melanoma, carcinoid tumor, malignant endocrine pancreatic tumors, basal cell carcinoma, and superficial bladder cancer.

MECHANISM OF ACTION

The interferons have been intensely investigated as anticancer agents because of their pleiotropic effects on immune reactivity, cell differentiation, and rate of cell proliferation. These effects are mediated through the ligation of cell surface receptors that are specific for the interferons. About 1000 high-affinity receptors, encoded by a gene on chromosome 21, are present on most cells and interact with both IFN α and IFN β. Interferon interacts with a different receptor. Following receptor binding, incompletely understood cytoplasmic events ensue that lead to alterations in gene transcription and, as a result, the generation of regulatory enzymes and oncogenes that underlie the disparate biologic effects of interferon.

Interferons retard proliferation of both normal and malignant cells by prolonging all stages of the cell cycle. Some cellular proto-oncogenes including c-myc, c-fos, c-ras, and c-src are downregulated, suggesting that this effect is mediated in part at the transcriptional level. The action of growth factors, including platelet-derived growth factor, epidermal growth factor, fibroblast growth factor, insulin, and macrophage colony-stimulating factor, is also antagonized. 2',5'-Oligoadenylate synthetase, protein kinase, and indoleamine 2,3-dioxygenase are three interferon-induced enzymes that could also account for the observed antiproliferative effects.

Interferons modulate immune reactivity by enhancing target cell immunogenicity and activating immune effector cells. Major histocompatibility complex (MHC) class I antigen expression is upregulated by all three classes of IFN. The expression of some tumor-associated antigens, such as carcinoembryonic antigen and TAG-72, is also enhanced. These alterations in cell-surface antigen expression are thought to render tumors more susceptible to immune recognition. Direct effects on immune reactivity include enhanced cytotoxic T-cell activity, macrophage and NK-cell activation, induction of B-cell immunoglobulin production, and enhanced NK-cell–mediated, antibody-dependent cellular cytotoxicity. Effects on cellular differentiation and angiogenesis may also contribute indirectly.

MECHANISMS OF RESISTANCE

The clinical responses associated with the use of IFN α, which are dramatic in some hematologic malignancies, suggest that some neoplastic cells are much more sensitive to IFN than are normal cells. This could be accounted for by antigenic differences that exist between some cancers and normal cells or differences in cell-cycle kinetics. Resistance to IFN is poorly understood. At the cellular level, freshly isolated tumor cells demonstrate a range of sensitivity to interferon that does not correlate with tumor cell type. Resistance *in vitro* is not necessarily accompanied by changes in the number of cell surface receptors. A better understanding of resistance must await elucidation of the mechanisms underlying tumor regression.

ADVERSE EFFECTS

Therapy with IFN α is usually well tolerated. Fewer than 10% of patients discontinue treatment as a result of severe toxicity. The most common adverse effect is a flu-like syndrome occurring in as many as 98% of treated patients and consisting of fever (40–98%), chills (40–65%), myalgias (30–75%), headache (20–70%), malaise (50–95%), and arthralgias (5–24%). Fever may be as high as 40° C and occurs within 6 hours of a dose. Chills may be severe. Pretreatment with acetaminophen or nonsteroidal anti-inflammatory drugs can attenuate these toxicities, which become less severe with continued therapy. Adverse hematologic effects are mild and include neutropenia, anemia, and thrombocytopenia. Some patients manifest elevated serum concentrations of aspartate aminotransferase (AST) and alanine aminotransferase (ALT). Other gastrointestinal side effects include nausea, vomiting, diarrhea, and a metallic taste. Dyspnea, alopecia, rashes, proteinuria, thyroid dysfunction, and edema have also been reported.

BIOCHEMICAL MODULATION

Synergistic interactions between IFN and other anticancer agents have been well documented [5]. Antiproliferative synergy against transformed cell lines has been demonstrated for IFN α and IFN γ. Their immune-potentiating effects on NK cells are also enhanced in combination. Synergistic effects are seen with combinations of IFN α and IL-2 as well. The mechanisms underlying the observed synergy between IFN α and other cytokines have not been well-defined. Their interaction with two distinct sets of cell surface receptors, each with different but complimentary effects on immune effectors and tumor targets, may play a role.

IFN α has been observed to enhance the efficacy of many cancer chemotherapeutic agents including 5-FU, cisplatinum, cyclophosphamide, and doxorubicin. This may be a result of altered pharmacokinetics. IFN α-mediated inhibition of the cytochrome P450 system may delay the metabolism of doxorubicin and cyclophosphamide. The clearance of 5-FU is also inhibited by unknown mechanisms. It is also possible that the antitumor immune response generated by IFN may complement the pharmacologic tumor debulking characteristic of chemotherapy by eradicating microscopic residual disease.

BACILLUS CALMETTE–GUÉRIN

The history of immunotherapy is replete with examples of attempts to treat cancer using agents that were casually observed to augment immunoreactivity. The panoply of agents has included lectins, viable or nonviable bacteria, and bacterial products. No well-executed trial has demonstrated any clinical advantage to the use of these agents until recently.

Bacillus Calmette–Guérin (BCG) is a live, attenuated strain of *Mycobacterium bovis* with nonspecific, immunostimulating properties [2]. Intradermal administration of BCG in some animal models has been demonstrated to restore immunocompetence and to protect against infection and malignancy. The mechanisms responsible for these systemic effects are unknown although the effects have been attributed to reticuloendothelial cell activation, decreased suppressor cell activity, and macrophage and lymphocyte activation.

A number of trials have now demonstrated prolonged disease-free survival, prolonged survival, delayed tumor progression, and eradication of carcinoma *in situ* of the urinary bladder in patients treated with intravesical BCG after transurethral resection compared with patients treated with resection alone [6]. Papillary carcinoma and carcinoma *in situ* of the bladder seem particularly well suited for local therapy with BCG because of the minimal tumor burden remaining after transurethral resection, the ease of exposing all at-risk surfaces to treatment, the immunocompetence of most patients, and the ease of follow-up evaluation. A BCG-based, autologous tumor vaccine was recently evaluated as adjuvant therapy for patients at high risk of recurrence after resection of colon carcinoma (Gunderson–Sosin stages B_2, B_3, C_{1-3}). A randomized, prospective trial has not yet confirmed earlier, uncontrolled observations suggesting that vaccination was associated with prolonged disease-free survival.

MECHANISM OF ACTION

BCG is a nonspecific immunostimulant that is thought to exert its antitumor effect through the induction of a delayed-type hypersensitivity–like response. According to this paradigm, tumor cells are destroyed as innocent bystanders, either directly by activated macrophages and lymphoid cells or indirectly by the local secretion of cytokines. These nonspecific immune effectors are thought to represent a reaction to components of the bacillus cell wall. Rare regional responses, which are characterized by regression of some uninjected tumors, suggest that specific antitumor immunity is induced in some treated patients. This, however, has been difficult to prove.

MECHANISMS OF RESISTANCE

Clinical experience has defined criteria that are associated with a low likelihood of response to therapy with BCG. These relate primarily to tumor size and patient immunocompetence. Large tumors are unlikely to regress. The reason for this observed inverse relationship between tumor size and response to therapy is not known; however, tumor vasculature is thought to play a role. This observation has led to the use of intravesical BCG as an adjuvant to transurethral resection of tumors rather than as a primary mode of therapy. For the same reason, it is also applied to the treatment of carcinoma *in situ*.

ADVERSE EFFECTS

The risk of developing toxicity from BCG depends in large measure on the integrity of intravesical and systemic immunity. Impairment of either one of these can lead to dissemination of viable organisms and overwhelming mycobacterial infection. Patients who are receiving systemic steroids, bone marrow depressants, or radiation therapy or who have compromised immune systems for other reasons should not be treated. Local factors that predispose patients to disseminated infection include ongoing urinary tract infection and healing bladder mucosal injury secondary to instrumentation. Other adverse manifestations of therapy include local effects on the bladder and systemic symptoms.

Patients who are immunocompromised at the time of therapy are also unlikely to respond. This is not surprising, even in light of our limited understanding of the mechanism of response, which probably involves immune effectors that have been nonspecifically activated by BCG. Commonly encountered causes of immunosuppression in these patients include previous chemotherapy and radiation therapy, use of corticosteroids, poor nutrition, or advanced disease.

LEVAMISOLE

Levamisole is an immunomodulatory drug initially developed as an anthelminthic agent and introduced for that purpose in 1965 [7]. The anthelminthic effect has been shown to be mediated by inhibition of a unique succinate dehydrogenase-fumarate system that serves as a terminal electron acceptor in the generation of ATP. This effectively paralyzes treated worms.

The immunologic effects of levamisole *in vitro* are protean and include enhancement of polymorphonuclear and mononuclear phagocytosis and chemotaxis. Lymphocyte proliferation in response to mitogens and cytotoxic activity are also enhanced. B-cell and NK-cell function appear to be unaffected. A direct antitumor effect has not been demonstrated [8].

The results of studies designed to evaluate the immunologic effects of levamisole in animals and humans are conflicting and have provided little insight into the design of future clinical trials. In 1989, the North Central Cancer Treatment Group (NCCTG) reported that adjuvant therapy of colorectal cancer with levamisole and 5-FU may be of benefit. This combination was based on the presumption that enhanced immunoreactivity engendered by levamisole would contribute to the minimal effects of 5-FU in eliminating microscopic disease. A subsequent intergroup trial conducted by the Eastern Cooperative Oncology Group, the NCCTG, the Southwest Oncology Group, and the Mayo Clinic corroborated these findings [9]. There was a statistically significant prolongation of disease-free and overall survival among patients with Stage III disease who were treated with the combination of levamisole, 50 mg every 8 hours, and 5-FU, 450 mg/m2/d both for 1 year. The observed toxicity was generally that expected with 5-FU. These results have been questioned on the basis of the experimental design, which did not include a 5-FU control arm. This issue may be rendered clinically irrelevant as the results of ongoing trials evaluating the more efficacious combination of 5-FU and leucovorin in the adjuvant setting become available.

MECHANISM OF ACTION

It is not known whether levamisole mediates a salutary effect by reversing the immunosuppression associated with 5-FU or whether it biochemically modulates the anticancer activity of 5-FU [10]. Levamisole is a heterocyclic compound that is purported to exert immunomodulatory effects through either its imidazole or thiazol rings. The cytoplasmic or cell wall targets for this molecule are not known, nor are the mechanisms by which subsequent biochemical events within the cell are effected. One theory holds that the sulfhydryl group leads to glutathione repletion. Others have suggested that cholinergic-like effects of the imidazole ring underlie the observed enhancement of IL-2–induced T-cell proliferation. It is known that levamisole increases the level of cytoplasmic cyclic GMP and reciprocally decreases levels of cyclic AMP in treated lymphocytes. It may also increase the intracellular calcium concentration. Decreased cell membrane adenylate cyclase activity has also been observed. Whether or not these findings are relevant to the observed immunomodulatory effects is not known.

MECHANISMS OF RESISTANCE

Evasion of a levamisole-induced immune response is one theoretical mechanism by which cancer cells may overcome the effects of levamisole and 5-FU. Clinically exploitable antigenic differences between colon cancer and normal cells have yet to be demonstrated, however. Resistance may also arise through modulation of the levels of certain vital intracellular constituents. For example, gene duplication or a compensatory increase in the activity of certain enzymes may lead to elevated levels of thymidylate synthetase. This could partially overcome the detrimental effect that 5-FU exerts upon DNA and RNA synthesis and repair.

ADVERSE EFFECTS

Adverse reactions to levamisole are generally mild. Agranulocytosis, which is usually reversible following discontinuation of treatment, has rarely been reported. This may be accompanied by a flu-like syndrome. Neutropenia, thrombocytopenia, and anemia occur frequently in patients treated with levamisole and 5-FU in combination. Almost all patients treated with levamisole and 5-FU experience toxicity that is otherwise associated with 5-FU alone.

COLONY-STIMULATING FACTORS

Colony-stimulating factors (CSF) are cytokines that control hematopoiesis and possess intrinsic immunomodulatory activity.

These glycoproteins are elaborated by a variety of cell types, including T cells, B cells, NK cells, granulocytes, macrophages, vascular endothelial cells, smooth muscle cells, and fibroblasts. Some are produced constitutively and probably maintain steady-state levels of circulating cells. Their elaboration can also be induced by a variety of physiologic stimuli including mononuclear cell-derived cytokines, bacterial endotoxin, and hypoxemia.

CSFs exert their effects at several stages of blood cell development [11]. Multi-CSF (IL-3) and steel factor (c-kit ligand) act on the pluripotent stem cell as well as more differentiated cells in multiple lineages. Granulocyte-macrophage–CSF (GM-CSF) acts slightly later in blood cell development, probably in concert with IL-3 and steel factor. Monocyte-CSF (M-CSF), granulocyte-CSF (G-CSF), and erythropoietin act on more differentiated cells, and are more lineage specific, as their names imply. The picture that has emerged is one characterized by multiple regulatory proteins with overlapping functions that interact with one another within the stromal microenvironment of the bone marrow. Their effects are mediated either directly, through cell surface receptors, or indirectly, through the induction of other cytokines. The outcome is hematopoietic homeostasis that gives way to adaptive increases in the levels of circulating mature and immature cells during periods of stress.

Three CSF species have been approved for clinical use. Erythropoietin (epoietin-α) is a 166 amino acid glycoprotein that serves as an obligate growth factor for red blood cell progenitors [12–15]. It is made primarily by peritubular cells within the kidney in response to an oxygen-sensing heme protein. The liver contributes a fraction to the total amount of circulating protein as well. Under normal conditions the serum level of erythropoietin ranges from 4 to 24 mU/ml. There is an inverse correlation between serum erythropoietin level and hemoglobin concentration below 10.5 g%. Levels may rise as high as 10,000 mU/ml in response to profound anemia. A normal response to a specific degree of anemia is difficult to define due to large variations from the mean that have been observed.

Patients with cancer often suffer concomitant anemia, the causes of which may be manifold. Effective management of hemorrhage, infection, nutritional deficiency, and immune-mediated hemolysis often leads to its resolution. Patients undergoing chemotherapy or radiation therapy or whose bone marrow is replaced by tumor may develop anemia that is more difficult to manage. Some of these patients have lower erythropoietin levels than patients with comparable degrees of iron-deficiency anemia, and the inverse correlation between serum hemoglobin concentration and erythropoietin may be attenuated. The administration of epoietin-α, 1500 U/kg subcutaneously twice a week between courses of chemotherapy, has been observed to reduce the transfusion requirement of some patients, including those with solid tumors, lymphoma, and multiple myeloma. Patients whose pretreatment erythropoietin level is greater than 500 mU/ml are unlikely to respond to epoietin-α.

Granulocyte-CSF is a 174 amino acid glycoprotein produced by mononuclear phagocytes, endothelial cells, fibroblasts, and neutrophils [16,17]. G-CSF is central to the control of circulating blood neutrophil numbers, during both times of health and of infection. G-CSF also has profound effects on mature granulocyte function. Phase III studies have evaluated the efficacy of recombinant G-CSF (filgrastim) in patients with solid tumors who are treated with myelosuppressive chemotherapy. Patients treated with filgrastim have manifested less profound and less persistent neutropenia, decreased incidence of neutropenic fever, and fewer culture-positive infections. This has translated to a decreased use of antibiotics and shorter hospital stays.

Granulocyte-macrophage–CSF is a 127 amino acid protein with a molecular weight ranging from 18 to 22 Kd due to variable glycosylation [18]. GM-CSF stimulates the growth and differentiation of cells committed to the neutrophil and macrophage lineages. It also synergizes with other CSFs to stimulate multipotential progenitor cells. Randomized, placebo-controlled trials of recombinant GM-CSF (sargramostim) after bone marrow transplantation have revealed shorter periods of neutropenia and fewer infectious complications among treated patients resulting in shorter hospital stays.

The availability of reagents that augment the *in vivo* production of erythrocytes and granulocytes may have profound implications for the palliation and treatment of cancer [19,20]. Anemia associated with malignancy and chemotherapy may be debilitating. Red blood cell transfusion is associated with a small risk of serious infection, as well as a variety of immune-mediated transfusion reactions. Many chemotherapeutics also cause life-threatening bone marrow toxicity manifest as granulocytopenia or thrombocytopenia. The risk of infection and bleeding associated with these dose-limiting toxicities is significant and the impact on treatment efficacy may be substantial.

MECHANISM OF ACTION

Each CSF mediates its effects by binding to specific cell surface receptors that share structural characteristics with those of other CSFs and interleukins. High-affinity receptors unique for each growth factor have been identified. Together they comprise the cytokine receptor family that includes the receptors for erythropoietin, G-CSF, GM-CSF, IL-2β, IL-3, IL-4, IL-5, IL-6, IL-7, prolactin, and growth hormone. All share amino acid sequences that may be functionally important.

Receptor activation leads to the modulation of second messengers, which then initiate a cascade of cytoplasmic events culminating in increased gene transcription. This is probably mediated by nuclear proteins that release cytokine promoters from inhibition. CSF-specific signal transduction pathways remain to be completely defined, but protein kinase C and elevated levels of intracellular calcium are thought to be involved.

The cellular distribution of receptors determines the effect of each CSF. The receptors for GM-CSF are found on pluripotent progenitors, as well as on more differentiated cells of the macrophage and granulocyte lineages. This accounts for its effects on many mature lineages, including neutrophils, eosinophils, basophils, macrophages, and Langerhans cells, as well as its effects on most blast-forming and colony-forming unit precursors. Receptors for erythropoietin and G-CSF are generally distributed on more mature cells in a lineage-restricted fashion, which accounts for their effects being confined mainly to red blood cells and neutrophils, respectively. Receptors for G-CSF and GM-CSF are also present on endothelial cells. The pleiotropic effects of GM-CSF may also be due, in part, to the release of other cytokines.

Effects of filgrastim include decreased transit time of granulocytes from the mitotic to the postmitotic compartment, with more rapid release of mature granulocytes from the bone marrow. Mature granulocytes are primed to produce superoxide and their migration is enhanced. Antibody-dependent cellular cytotoxic activity, immunoglobulin A-mediated phagocytosis, and release of inflammatory mediators are also augmented. The net effect is to increase the number of mature, circulating granulocytes and to enhance their function.

Sargramostim shares many of these properties with filgrastim. It also enhances the cytotoxic activity of mature eosinophils and macrophages. The latter develop tumoricidal activity as well. The circulating half-life of neutrophils is prolonged. A role for GM-CSF in wound healing is suggested by its augmentation of vascular endothelial cell migration.

ADVERSE EFFECTS

Therapy with filgrastim is rarely associated with clinical toxicity. Mild bone marrow discomfort, which responds to treatment with acetaminophen, occurs in 20% of treated patients. Exacerbation of pre-existing cutaneous inflammatory disorders, including eczema and vasculitis, have been observed and resolves with discontinuation of filgrastim. Prolonged therapy has been associated with splenomegaly in small numbers of patients. This is a result of extramedullary hematopoiesis. Serum uric acid and LDH may also become elevated, reflecting increased cell turnover.

Sargramostim produces dose-dependent toxicities, some of which may be mediated through the release of other cytokines. Side effects seen in patients treated with high doses ($1000 \mu g/m^2$) include thrombosis, pleural or pericardial effusion, peripheral edema, headache, and a flu-like syndrome. Lower, clinically effective doses are better tolerated but may cause flu-like symptoms. A first-pass effect characterized by respiratory distress has been seen in some patients coincident with the first dose of sargramostim. This may require treatment with steroids if severe, and cases that go unrecognized may ultimately require mechanical ventilation. Induction of cell surface adhesion molecules on circulating granulocytes by sargramostim or release of cytokines from alveolar macrophages may underlie this toxicity.

OCTREOTIDE

Octreotide (SMS 201-995) is a long-acting, synthetic octapeptide with pharmacologic actions that mimic those of the naturally occurring, 14 amino acid hormone somatostatin (SMS 14) [21,22]. Other naturally occurring analogues have been identified including prosomatostatin (SMS 28) and preprosomatostatin (SMS 128). This family of peptides generally exerts inhibitory effects on a variety of organ systems. It downregulates the release of growth hormone, prolactin, and all gastrointestinal hormones. It inhibits gastric acid secretion, gastrointestinal motility, intestinal absorption, pancreatic secretion, and portal blood flow. The secretion of gastroenteropancreatic peptides, including insulin, vasoactive intestinal peptide, gastrin, and glucagon is also reduced. Interest in octreotide as an anticancer agent has been stimulated by its documented antiproliferative activity against many tumor cell lines. The mechanism underlying this effect has not been fully elucidated, however.

The half-life of the naturally occurring hormone somatostatin is so ephemeral ($t_{1/2}$ = 3 min) that it is of no clinical utility. The D amino acid substitutions of octreotide and other synthetic analogues such as the octapeptide Somatuline (Ipsen International, Paris, France) confer resistance to serum peptidases, prolonging their half-lives. The half-life of octreotide is about 60 minutes after intravenous administration and 2 hours after subcutaneous injection. Although a formulation for oral use has been developed, its use is limited by very poor bioavailability.

Octreotide acetate has been approved for use as an agent to palliate patients who suffer from diarrhea as a result of carcinoid syndrome or VIPoma. It has demonstrated clinical efficacy in the treatment of other hypersecretory disorders, including insulinoma, glucagonoma, Zollinger–Ellison syndrome, acromegaly, and pancreatic ascites. It has also proven to be a useful adjunct in the management of enterocutaneous and pancreaticocutaneous fistulae. Its use as an anticancer agent remains investigational.

MECHANISM OF ACTION

Octreotide exerts its pleiotropic effects through cell surface receptors that vary in their affinity for different somatostatin analogues. They are widely distributed throughout the body and have been demonstrated on cells that comprise the central nervous system, gastrointestinal tract, exocrine glands, and kidneys. These receptors have also been detected in human meningioma, breast carcinoma, and carcinoid tumors.

Its antiproliferative effects are thought to be mediated in several ways. Octreotide inhibits and reduces the levels of several growth factors that have been associated with tumor growth, including epidermal growth factor, platelet-derived growth factor, fibroblast growth factor, transforming growth factor-α, and bombesin. Octreotide also possesses direct antiproliferative effects that are poorly understood. Receptor binding may also be associated with dephosphorylation of cell membrane proteins that are necessary for proliferation. Stimulation of the reticuloendothelial system may be responsible, in part, for the antitumor effects of octreotide that have been observed in murine models.

ADVERSE EFFECTS

The therapeutic index for octreotide is very wide and serious toxicity is unusual. Nausea, diarrhea, and abdominal discomfort have been observed in about 5 to 10% of treated patients. Less common side effects (less than 2%) include headache, dizziness, flushing, fatigue, hypoglycemia, and hyperglycemia.

RETINOIDS

Retinoids are a family of structurally and functionally related molecules that exercise a profound effect upon cell growth and differentiation [23,24]. This class of compounds includes all-trans-retinol (vitamin A), which is obtained primarily through the conversion of dietary precursors, including retinyl palmitate and beta-carotene. This occurs within the intestinal lumen and in enterocytes, respectively. The conversion of carotenoids to retinol is tightly regulated so that ingestion of excessive amounts of beta-carotene does not produce hypervitaminosis A. Retinol is transported in chylomicrons via intestinal lymph. It is taken up by hepatocytes and transferred to stellate cells within the liver. These cells contain about 80% of the body's store of vitamin A and maintain plasma levels at about $2 \mu m$.

Retinol, secreted by stellate cells complexed with a binding protein, is further reversibly bound to transthyretin, a protein that protects vitamin A from loss through glomerular filtration. The mechanism by which target tissues take up retinol remains an enigma. Many of its effects are thought to be mediated by its intracellular conversion to all-trans-retinoic acid (tretinoin). Another metabolite of vitamin A with therapeutic potential is 13-cis-retinoic acid (isotretinoin).

Retinoids are essential to embryonic development, epithelial cell differentiation, and growth. They may also be requisite for immunologic integrity because they have been shown to enhance certain cell-mediated immune responses, augment IL-2-induced LAK-cell generation, and upregulate macrophage phagocytic activity. Vitamin A also plays an important role in vision, reproduction, and hematopoiesis.

Retinoids possess antineoplastic activity and may have some clinical value in the treatment of a variety of malignancies. Transient complete remissions are associated with the use of single agent tretinoin in most patients with acute promyelocytic leukemia. The role of concomitant chemotherapy remains to be defined. Isotretinoin has induced complete clinical responses in about 50% of patients with basal cell and squamous cell carcinoma of the skin. Tumor regression has been seen less frequently among treated patients with mycosis fungoides. These responses are also ephemeral.

Retinoids prevent the development of tumors in a variety of animal models. This has led to several chemoprevention trials in patients at high risk for malignancy. Isotretinoin has been associated with a decreased tumor frequency among treated patients with xeroderma pigmentosum. This effect lasted only as long as treatment was continued. Among patients with treated head and neck cancer, isotretinoin is associated with a lower frequency of secondary aerodigestive malignancy. Unfortunately, the incidence of tumor recurrence appears to be unaffected and as many as 33% of patients required discontinuation of therapy due to intolerable toxicity.

MECHANISM OF ACTION

Retinol and retinoic acid are bound within the cell cytoplasm by proteins whose function is unclear. Retinoic acid is then transported to the nucleus where it forms a complex with any of three receptors. These share substantial homology and are members of the steroid–thyroid superfamily of nuclear receptors. Retinoic acid receptor alpha (RAR-α) is widely distributed throughout the body. The distribution of RAR-beta is more limited, and RAR-γ is expressed in high levels almost exclusively by epithelial cells of the skin and oral mucosa.

Retinoic acid mediates many of its effects through the induction of gene expression. The RA-RAR complexes bind to specific DNA sequences termed *retinoic acid response elements*. Some of these sequences encode DNA-binding proteins that regulate the transcription of genes, encoding proteins that are necessary for cell growth and differentiation.

Antitumor activity may be mediated by any of several proposed mechanisms. Retinoic acid has been shown to induce cell differentiation. This is evident for some human acute myeloid leukemia, melanoma, neuroblastoma, and teratocarcinoma tumor cell lines. These effects are enhanced by some cytokines including interferon alpha, tumor necrosis factor-alpha, and granulocyte colony-stimulating factor. Retinoic acid also reverses squamous metaplasia in vitamin A–deficient animals. These observations have served as the basis for chemoprevention trials.

A number of tumor cell lines respond to retinoic acid with growth inhibition. This may be mediated by a direct effect of retinoic acid on the cells or in a paracrine fashion through the induction of transforming growth factor–beta expression. The latter may also be responsible for the induction of apoptosis, which has been associated with the use of retinoic acid. Growth inhibitory effects of retinoic acid are enhanced by IFN α and IFN γ.

MECHANISMS OF RESISTANCE

Resistance to the antitumor effects of retinoids is not understood. Some observations suggest that this has a pharmacokinetic basis. Specifically, plasma levels of tretinoin decline during prolonged therapy. This may be a result of homeostatic mechanisms that regulate retinoid metabolism because it is not reversed by dose escalation.

ADVERSE EFFECTS

The spectrum of toxicity differs somewhat between tretinoin and isotretinoin. Both are teratogenic and their use in women who are or may become pregnant is contraindicated. It is recommended that these drugs not be used in women of childbearing age unless they understand the risks and are capable of following mandatory contraceptive measures. These include the use of effective contraception for 1 month before, during, and 1 month after therapy.

The most frequent complication associated with both drugs is cheilitis, which occurs in 90% of treated patients. Xerosis is seen in about 50% of patients, possibly complicated by conjunctivitis, epistaxis, and pruritus. Rash, thinning hair, photosensitivity, and nail changes are seen less frequently. Gastrointestinal morbidity includes nausea and vomiting, which is seen in 20 to 30% of patients. The onset of inflammatory bowel disease has been temporally associated with the use of retinoids, although a cause-and-effect relationship has not been established. Headache is frequently associated with the use of tretinoin but is uncommon among patients treated with isotretinoin. Other neurologic toxicities are rare and include fatigue, depression, and pseudotumor cerebri. Moderate musculoskeletal symptoms are seen in about 15% of treated patients.

An unusual and potentially fatal complication of therapy with tretinoin has been seen among patients who have acute promyelocytic leukemia. This syndrome includes respiratory distress, fever, pulmonary infiltrates, pleural and pericardial effusions, edema, and myocardial depression. This is almost invariably associated with hyperleukocytosis. Resolution of this syndrome has been associated with the use of dexamethasone, 10 mg intravenously twice daily. Metabolic effects include hypertriglyceridemia, hepatic transaminasemia, hyperglycemia, hyperuricemia, hypercholesterolemia, and decreased high-density lipoproteins. These effects are reversible upon discontinuation of therapy.

The information here is provided as guidance only. Prescribers should always consult the manufacturer's current prescribing information.

54

REFERENCES

1. Rubin JT: Interleukin-2: Its biology and clinical application in patients with cancer. *Cancer Invest* 1993, 11:460–472.

2. DeVita VT, Hellman S, Rosenberg SA (eds): *The Biologic Therapy of Cancer*. Philadelphia: JB Lippincott, 1991.

3. Itri LM: The interferons. *Cancer* 1992, 70:940–945.

4. Wadler S: The role of interferons in the treatment of solid tumors. *Cancer* 1992, 70:949–958.

5. Wadler S, Schwartz EL: Principles in the biomodulation of cytotoxic drugs by interferons. *Sem Oncol* 1992, 19(suppl 3):45–48.

6. Lamm DL, Blumenstein BA, Crawford ED, *et al.*: A randomized trial of intravesical doxorubicin and immunotherapy with bacille calmette–guerin for transitional cell carcinoma of the bladder. *N Engl J Med* 1991, 325:1205–1210.

7. Janssen PAJ: Levamisole as an adjuvant in cancer treatment. *J Clin Pharmacol* 1991, 31:396–400.

8. Stevenson HC, Green I, Hamilton JM, *et al.*: Levamisole: Known effects on the immune system, clinical results, and future applications to the treatment of cancer. *J Clin Oncol* 1991, 9:2052–2066.

9. Moertel CG, Fleming TR, MacDonald JS, *et al.*: Levamisole and fluorouracil for adjuvant therapy of resected colon carcinoma. *N Engl J Med* 1990, 322:352–358.

10. Schiller JH, Witt PL: Levamisole: Clinical and biological effects. *Biol Ther Cancer Up* 1992, 2:1–14.

11. Crosier PS, Clark SC: Basic biology of the hematopoietic growth factors. *Sem Oncol* 1992, 19:349–361.

12. Brugger W, Rosenthal FM, Kanz L, *et al.*: Clinical role of colony stimulating factors. *Acta Haematol* 1991, 86:138–147.

13. St Onge J, Jacobson RJ: The role of hematopoietic growth factors in the treatment of neoplastic diseases. *Sem Hematol* 1992, 29(suppl 2):53–63.

14. Spivak JL: The application of recombinant erythropoietin in anemic patients with cancer. *Sem Oncol* 1992, 19(suppl 8):25–28.

15. Erslev AJ: The therapeutic role of recombinant erythropoietin in anemic patients with intact endogenous production of erythropoietin. *Sem Oncol* 1992, 19(suppl 8):14–18.

16. Glaspy JA, Golde DW: Granulocyte colony-stimulating factor (G-CSF): Preclinical and clinical studies. *Sem Oncol* 1992, 19:386–394.

17. Gabrilove JL: Granulocyte colony-stimulating factor and granulocyte-macrophage colony-stimulating factor in chemotherapy. *Biol Ther Cancer Upd* 1992, 2:1–11.

18. Demetri GD, Antman KHS: Granulocyte-macrophage colony-stimulating factor (GM-CSF): Preclinical and clinical investigations. *Sem Oncol* 1992, 19:362–385.

19. Neidhart JA: Hematopoietic colony-stimulating factors. uses in combination with standard chemotherapeutic regimens and in support of dose intensification. *Cancer* 1992, 70:913–920.

20. Quesenberry PJ: Biomodulation of chemotherapy-induced myelosuppression. *Sem Oncol* 1992, 19(suppl 8):8–13.

21. Evers MB, Parekh D, Townsend CM, *et al.*: Somatostatin and analogues in the treatment of cancer. *Ann Surg* 1991, 213:190–198.

22. Parmar H, Bogden A, Mollard M, *et al.*: Somatostatin and somatostatin analogues in oncology. *Cancer Treat Rev* 1989, 16:95–115.

23. Smith MA, Parkinson DR, Cheson BD, *et al.*: Retinoids in cancer therapy. *J Clin Oncol* 1992, 10:839–864.

24. Hofmann SL: Retinoids—differentiation agents for cancer treatment and prevention. *Am J Med Sci* 1992, 304:202–213.

25. Olin BR (ed): *Facts and Comparisons Drug Information*, Philadelphia: JB Lippincott, 1993.

ALDESLEUKIN

Aldesleukin (interleukin-2 or IL-2) is a highly purified lymphokine produced by genetically engineered *Escherichia coli*. It differs from native IL-2 in that it is not glycosylated, it does not have an N-terminal alanine, and cysteine 125 has been replaced by serine. Aldesleukin possesses the same immunoregulatory capacity as natural IL-2. Some of its effects include T-cell and NK-cell activation, the generation of lymphokine activated killer (LAK) activity, and induction of interferon gamma production by macrophages.

The systemic administration of IL-2 to patients with selected malignancies has been associated with tumor regression in variable numbers of patients. IL-2 is potentially active against renal cell carcinoma and metastatic melanoma, with response rates of 30 and 20%, respectively. Its use with adoptively transferred lymphocytes, chemotherapeutics, as well as other cytokines is an area of ongoing investigation.

DOSAGE AND ADMINISTRATION

Renal cell cancer: 600,000 IU/kg (0.037 mg/kg) administered IV over 15 min every 8 hr for 2 cycles (neither exceeding 14 doses) and administered 7 to 10 days apart.

Decision to withhold doses or terminate a cycle is based on patient status. Median number of doses is 20 out of 28. Evidence of tumor regression 2 months after treatment indicates retreatment if there are no contraindications.

SPECIAL PRECAUTIONS

Patients with significant cardiac, pulmonary, hepatic, or renal dysfunction
Patients with untreated brain metastases with edema
Patients with GI or GU tract bleeding (risk of thrombocytopenia)
Patients whose tumors encroaching on the spinal canal
Patients with pre-existing infection except when adequately treated prior to therapy
Patients with angina or MI
Transplant recipients (risk of allograft rejection)

TOXICITIES

Cardiovascular: ventricular and supraventricular dysrhythmias, myocardial infarction (2% of patients), myocarditis, hypotension (due to capillary leak syndrome)
Pulmonary: frequent noncardiogenic pulmonary edema (secondary to capillary leak syndrome) with dyspnea (50%) and rarely reversible respiratory failure; ascites and pleural effusions with attendant shortness of breath (possibly due to capillary leak)
Renal: frequent reversible oliguria accompanied by elevations of BUN and creatinine (1% of patients require dialysis)
Neurologic: mental status changes infrequent; impaired cognitive function may precede more profound central nervous system (CNS) impairment, rarely leading to coma
Dermatologic: pruritus (50%), exfoliative dermatitis, dry skin, hair loss
GI: nausea, vomiting, diarrhea; stomatitis (less frequently); life-threatening intestinal perforation (rare)
Musculoskeletal: reversible arthralgia, myalgia (< 50%)
Hematologic: anemia, thrombocytopenia, leukopenia, and eosinophilia are common; rebound lymphocytosis after cessation; impaired neutrophil function associated with central venous catheter-associated *S. aureus* infection
Capillary leak syndrome: very common and responsible for hypotension, decreased organ profusion, and development of noncardiogenic pulmonary edema, ascites, pleural effusions, and anasarca
Miscellaneous: fever and rigors 1 to 2 hr after dose; hypothyroidism (10%); hypophosphatemia, hypomagnesemia, metabolic acidosis, hepatic transaminasemia, hyperbilirubinemia

INDICATIONS

FDA-approved: metastatic renal cell carcinoma; **Clinical studies show activity in:** metastatic melanoma, non-Hodgkin's lymphoma, colorectal carcinoma

PHARMACOKINETICS

Distribution—with IV infusion, rapid penetration of extravascular space with preferential uptake by liver, kidneys, and lungs; little penetration of CNS; **Half-life**—85 minutes; **Elimination**—glomerular filtration and peritubular extraction

DRUG INTERACTIONS

Drugs metabolized by hepatic or renal routes, or causing nephrotoxic and hepatotoxic effects, may require dosage modification during combination therapy; steroids

RESPONSE RATES

Patients with metastatic renal cell carcinoma—partial or complete response of 20–30%; patients with metastatic melanoma—10–20% response

PATIENT MONITORING

In-hospital administration, monitor vital signs immediately before each dose and every 4 hr after; urine output, oxygen saturation (if hypoxemia develops), frequent physical exams, daily CBC, biochemical evaluation of thyroid function (if hypothyroidism is suspected)

NURSING INTERVENTIONS

Evaluate for nausea, vomiting, diarrhea, stomatitis; encourage use of bicarbonate mouthwash; give doses of antiemetics and antidiarrheals as needed; evaluate for rigors (provide blankets and IV meperidine); evaluate mental status; monitor central venous catheter site for evidence of infection; control pruritus with diphenhydramine or hydroxyzine

PATIENT INFORMATION

Avoid direct sunlight; refrain from driving until fully recovered; report symptoms of hypothyroidism; use emollients to manage dry skin

FORMULATIONS

Available as Proleukin®, distributed by Cetus Oncology Corporation, Emoryville, CA
22×10^6 IU (1.3 mg) of lyophilized IL-2 in vial with a dodecyl sulfate. Vials stored at 2–8°C.

BACILLUS CALMETTE–GUÉRIN

Bacillus Calmette–Guérin (BCG) is a live, attenuated strain of *Mycobacterium bovis* that has demonstrated efficacy in the treatment of primary or recurrent *in situ* carcinoma of the urinary bladder. The mechanism of this therapeutic effect is unknown, but it is thought to be immunologic.

DOSAGE AND ADMINISTRATION

Carcinoma of the urinary bladder: Start therapy 7 to 14 days after bladder biopsy or transurethral resection;

Thera-Cys—3 vials (27 mg) reconstituted with the diluent provided and further diluted with 50 ml of sterile, preservative-free saline (53 ml total) are administered by bladder catheter. Dose is repeated at 3, 6, 12, 18, and 24 mo **or** TICE BCG—1 ampule (50 mg) suspended in 50 ml of sterile, preservative-free saline instilled weekly for 6 wk, then monthly for 6 to 12 mo [25]

SPECIAL PRECAUTIONS

Immunosuppressed patients
Patients with urinary tract infection
Patients with small bladder capacity
Pregnant/nursing patients

TOXICITIES

GU: dysuria, urinary frequency, hematuria, and urinary urgency (40% of patients); bladder toxicity occurs after third installation, begins within 2 to 4 hr, persists 1 to 3 d; side effects are bladder cramps, nocturia, passage of urinary debris, and urethritis (less frequent)
GI: nausea, vomiting, diarrhea, anorexia, mild abdominal pain (infrequent)
Systemic: fever, malaise, chills (resolve within 3 d)
Miscellaneous: anemia, neutropenia, allergic reactions, systemic infection, hepatitis and hepatic granuloma (infrequent)

INDICATIONS

FDA-approved: primary and relapsed carcinoma *in situ* of the urinary bladder

DRUG INTERACTIONS

Immunosuppressive or myelosuppressive drugs, radiation therapy

RESPONSE RATES

Cancer of the urinary bladder—complete response rate of 75%; median time to failure 48 mo and median time to death 2 yr

PATIENT MONITORING

Monitor for systemic infection, including fever, severe malaise, and cough (may also represent hypersensitivity reactions—give antihistamines); monitor bladder for inflammation (manage with phenazopyridine, propantheline, or oxybutynin); rule out urinary tract infection

NURSING INTERVENTIONS

BCG contains a viable, attenuated mycobacteria and therefore should be handled as infectious accordingly; monitor patients for bladder irritation, urinary tract infection, and systemic infection

PATIENT INFORMATION

Report signs or symptoms of systemic infection and bladder irritation; avoid pregnancy during treatment; disinfect all urine voided within 6 hr of treatment

FORMULATIONS

TICE® BCG, Oclassen Pharmaceuticals, San Rafael, CA (distributed by Organon, West Orange, NJ); TheraCys® Connaught Laboratories, Swift Water, PA
TICE BCG—2 ml ampules with BCG 50 mg ($1–8 \times 10^8$ CFU).
TheraCys—3 vials of 27 mg ($3.4 \pm 3 \times 10^8$ CFU).
All stored at 2–8°C and protected from light.

ERYTHROPOIETIN

Erythropoietin (epoietin-alpha, EPO) is a 166 amino acid glycoprotein and an obligatory growth factor for erythroid progenitors. It is produced predominantly by the kidney in response to decreased tissue oxygen tension as sensed by a heme-like protein in the renal tubules. The recombinant product is made by gene-modified mammalian cells that contain the human gene.

The anemia associated with cancer is thought to be due in part to a blunted response to erythropoietin. This can be overcome to some extent by administering epoietin-alpha, although it is unclear whether transfusion requirements or quality of life is significantly affected.

DOSAGE AND ADMINISTRATION

Cancer or chemotherapy-associated anemia: 100 U/kg SC 3 x wk for 8 wk; hematocrit should be assessed regularly and dose adjusted based on this value
Preoperatively for autologous transfusion: 600 U/kg IV 2 x wk for 3 wk; surgery is performed 1 month after phlebotomy

LAB MONITORING: Serum iron studies should be assessed prior to starting treatment and deficits should be corrected with oral iron preparations. Determine endogenous erythropoietin level; data suggest that patients whose levels are > 500 mU/ml are unlikely to respond to therapy.

DOSAGE MODIFICATION: Assess hematocrits 2 x wk— decrease dosage by 25 U/kg; if hematocrit > 36%, withhold dose until value is in range of 30–33%; resume at dose 25 U/kg less than the preceding dose. If the response to 100 U/kg is not satisfactory within 8 wk, increase dose by 50 U/kg to 100 U/kg administered 3 x wk. Patients who do not respond to this therapy over 8 wk are unlikely to respond to higher doses; evaluate for other causes of anemia.

SPECIAL PRECAUTIONS

Patients with uncontrolled hypertension
Patients with pre-existing vascular disease
Patients with pre-existing porphyria
Pregnant/nursing patients

TOXICITIES

Epoietin-alpha is well tolerated even at high doses
Cardiovascular: exacerbation of pre-existing hypertension
Musculoskeletal: mild arthralgias
Miscellaneous: increased incidence of thrombosis of venous access devices

INDICATIONS

FDA-approved: treatment of anemia associated with chronic renal failure; used with AZT in HIV-infected patients; **clinical studies show activity in:** cancer and chemotherapy-associated anemia; increase volume of donated blood for autologous transfusion

PHARMACOKINETICS

Half-life about 3–10 hr; **Plasma levels**—detectable for at least 24 hr; **Peak serum levels**—between 5 and 24 hr after SC dose

DRUG INTERACTIONS

None known

PATIENT MONITORING

Evaluate blood pressure regularly; prior to therapy, assess transferrin saturation, serum iron, total iron binding capacity, and serum ferritin; initiate oral iron therapy if iron stores are low

NURSING INTERVENTIONS

Flush central venous catheters well to reduce risk of thrombosis; evaluate perfusion of lower legs in patients with significant peripheral vascular disease; treat arthralgia with acetaminophen

PATIENT INFORMATION

Patient taking iron concomitantly should be instructed about the possible side effects of erythropoietin; advise to treat associated arthralgias with acetaminophen

FORMULATIONS

Available as Epogen®, Amgen, Inc., Thousand Oaks, CA; Procrit®, Ortho Biotech, Raritan, NJ
1-ml vials of 2000, 3000, 4000, and 10,000 U. Stored at 2–8°C; do not shake.

FILGRASTIM

Filgrastim (granulocyte colony-stimulating factor or G-CSF) is a 174 amino acid glycoprotein that serves as an obligate factor in maintaining adequate numbers of circulating polymorphonuclear leukocytes (PMN). It targets granulocyte precursors, which are induced to proliferate when G-CSF binds to its cell surface receptor. PMN leukocyte chemotaxis, phagocytosis, and intracellular killing through enhanced generation of reactive oxygen intermediates are also augmented.

Filgrastim is the recombinant glycoprotein that has been expressed in *Escherichia coli* containing the human gene. It is well tolerated and has been shown to be of benefit in the setting of chemotherapy-induced neutropenia. Its use after myelosuppressive chemotherapy has been associated with decreased duration of neutropenia, decreased frequency of infection, decreased incidence of neutropenic fever, and decreased use of antibiotics. Because receptors for G-CSF have been found on small cell lung carcinoma lines, there is a theoretic risk that filgrastim may serve as a growth factor for this and other solid tumors. No clinically evident tumor progression has been noted, however.

DOSAGE AND ADMINISTRATION

5 μg/kg/day SC or IV [25] (the former route may be more effective). Do not administer within 24 hr of chemotherapy. Doses may be increased incrementally by 5 μg/kg each cycle, depending on response to previous cycle. Continue treatment until WBC count reaches 10,000/mm^3 after the chemotherapy-induced nadir. Avoid premature termination of treatment based on initial increase in WBC count that is due to the release of WBC stores.

SPECIAL PRECAUTIONS

Patients with atherosclerotic cardiovascular disease
Patients with sepsis
Pregnant/nursing patients
Filgrastim could serve as growth factor for some myeloid malignancies and possibly other tumors

TOXICITIES

Hematologic: small risk of excessive leukocytosis (WBC count > 100,000/mm^3)
Cardiovascular: transient decreases in blood pressure (rare)
Dermatologic: exacerbation of pre-existing inflammatory conditions
Musculoskeletal: mild-to-moderate medullary bone pain
Reticuloendothelial: splenomegaly (3% of patients)
Miscellaneous: reversible, mild elevations of lactic dehydrogenase (LDH) and alkaline phosphatase

INDICATIONS

FDA-approved: treatment of patients with nonmyeloid malignancies who have severe neutropenia as a consequence of myelosuppressive anticancer drugs

PHARMACOKINETICS

Peak plasma levels—2–8 hr after SC injection;
Half-life—3.5 hr (both SC or IV)

DRUG INTERACTIONS

May sensitize myeloid progenitors to the toxic effects of chemotherapy

PATIENT MONITORING

Evaluate WBC counts 2 x wk to avoid leukocytosis and assess response; monitor platelet counts

NURSING INTERVENTIONS

Train patients in self-administration if treated at home, including safe disposal of needles, drug vials, syringes after doses

PATIENT INFORMATION

Mild bone pain can be managed with acetaminophen but aspirin and nonsteroidal anti-inflammatory drugs must be avoided; discard unused drug, used needles, syringes after dose is administered

FORMULATIONS

Available as Neupogen®, Amgen, Thousand Oaks, CA
300 μg/ml in 1-ml and 1.6-ml single-dose vials. Stored at 2–8°C and warmed to room temperature for no more than 6 hr prior to use.

INTERFERON ALPHA-2

Interferons (IFN) are a group of naturally occurring proteins and glycoproteins subdivided according to differences in antigenic, biologic, and chemical properties, designated as IFN α, IFN β, and IFN γ. Human leukocyte IFN α is made up of a complex mixture of more than 14 glycoprotein subspecies each of approximately 165 amino acids encoded by chromosome 9. The development of techniques for large-scale production and purification of lymphoblastoid-cell IFN α and the advent of recombinant IFNs has allowed extensive clinical trials. The recombinant IFNs available for use include IFN α-2a, IFN α-2b, and IFN α-2c.

DOSAGE AND ADMINISTRATION

Hematologic neoplasms: (hairy cell leukemia, chronic myelogenous leukemia): dosage of $0.5-3 \times 10^6$ U/m^2, as tolerated, SC, 3 x wk
Solid tumors: escalation of dosage up to 10×10^6 U/m^2 as tolerated, IV, IM, SC, daily, 3 x wk. Administration before bedtime may reduce toxicity.

SPECIAL PRECAUTIONS

Patients with cardiac rhythm disturbance (ventricular or supraventricular)
Patients with congestive heart failure
Patients with cardiotoxicity following prior anthracycline
Elderly, or patients with organic brain syndrome, or the elderly
Pregnent/nursing patients

TOXICITIES

GI: nausea (mild, after 1 wk), diarrhea (mild), vomiting (rare), anorexia, taste alterations, xerostomia
Neurologic: mild confusion, somnolence, irritability, poor concentration, seizures, transient aphasia, hallucinations, paranoia, psychosis
Cardiopulmonary: tachycardia, pallor, cyanosis, tachypnea, nonspecific ECG changes, myocardial infarction (rare), orthostatic hypotension
Renal/hepatic: increased BUN, creatinine, proteinuria, elevated transaminase (dose-related, usually asymptomatic, occasional interstital nephritis); elevations of bilirubin (less frequent and of greater concern)
Hematologic: neutropenia (reversible, dose-related), thrombocytopenia (reversible, dose-related)
Flu-like: fever, chills (onset 30–90 min after dosing), fatigue, malaise, myalgia

INDICATIONS

FDA-approved: hairy cell leukemia, AIDS-related Kaposi's sarcoma and condyloma; **Clinical studies show activity in:** multiple myeloma, renal cell carcinoma, T-cell lymphomas (nodular and cutaneous), chronic myeloid leukemia, melanoma, superficial bladder cancer

PHARMACOKINETICS

Excretion—renal; **Metabolism**—renal; Blood terminal half-life—4–6 hr

DRUG INTERACTIONS

Aspirin, prostaglandin synthetase inhibitors, antihistamines, other immunomodulators, NSAIDs

RESPONSE RATES

Hairy cell leukemia—60 to 80%; cutaneous T-cell lymphoma and Kaposi's sarcoma—50%; metastic melanoma and renal cell carcinoma—18 to 20%

PATIENT MONITORING

Symptoms, hematologic values, bilirubin, vital signs, hepatic enzyme profile

NURSING INTERVENTIONS

Give acetaminophen for flu-like symptoms prior to treatment and every 4 hr as needed after IFN; assess patient performance and mental status; monitor weight; encourage adequate fluid, caloric, and protein intake; give antiemetics, food supplements as necessary; describe the number, volume, and consistency of stool.

PATIENT INFORMATION

Patient may experience flu-like symptoms: fever, chills, nausea; fatigue likely; arrange most activities in morning and allow for frequent rest periods

FORMULATIONS

IFN α-2a is available as Roferon-A®, Roche Laboratories, Nutley, NJ; Interferon A®, Schering Corporation, Kenilworth, NJ
Roferon —18-MU vial—3 m (6 MU/ml), 3-MU vial—1 ml (3 MU/ml) lyophilized powder or solution. Intron A—3-, 5-, 10-, 25-MU vials lyophilized powder. All stored at 4°C.

LEVAMISOLE

Levamisole was originally developed as an anthelminthic agent. The anthelminthic effect is mediated by its inhibition of a helminth-specific electron transport system. Levamisole exerts anticholinergic and immunomodulatory activity in humans. Effects on the immune system include enhanced T-cell activation and proliferation, augmented macrophage activity, increased neutrophil chemotaxis, and enhanced antibody formation. Two clinical trials have demonstrated a statistically significant prolongation of disease-free and overall survival among patients who were treated with adjuvant levamisole and 5-FU following resection of Duke's C colon carcinoma. The mechanism of this effect is unknown and the results of these studies have been questioned due to the omission of a 5-FU control group.

DOSAGE AND ADMINISTRATION

Colon cancer: begin therapy within 7–30 d of surgery [25]. Levamisole, 50 mg orally every 8 hr for 3 d, repeated every 14 d. Start 5-FU concomitantly with a cycle of levamisole 21–35 d postoperatively. 5-FU, 450 mg/m^2/d rapid IV bolus daily for 5 d. This should be followed after 28 d by weekly doses of 5-FU, 450 mg/m^2/wk. Continue therapy for 1 yr.

DOSAGE MODIFICATION: Hold 5-FU if mild stomatitis or diarrhea develop; if symptoms are moderate to severe, reduce dose of 5-FU by 20% when it is resumed; WBC count is 2500–3500/mm^3, hold 5-FU until WBC count ≥ 3500/mm^3; WBC ≤ 2500/mm^3, hold 5-FU until WBC count ≥ 3500/mm^3, resume at 80% of dose; WBC count ≤ 2500/mm^3 for 10 or more days, discontinue levamisole; platelet count ≤ 100,000, hold both drugs.

SPECIAL PRECAUTIONS

Epileptics must have phenytoin levels closely monitored
Pregnant/nursing patients

TOXICITIES

Hematologic: reversible agranulocytosis (rare); neutropenia, thrombocytopenia, anemia (frequent with levamisole and 5-FU combination)
Dermatologic: rashes (2% of treated patients)
Musculoskeletal: myalgia and arthralgia (2% of treated patients)
GU: renal failure (rare)
Neurologic: confusion, convulsions, hallucinations, impaired concentration, and encaphalopathic syndrome (rare)
Miscellaneous: flu-like: fevers, chills, fatigue (accompanying agranulocytosis)

INDICATIONS

FDA-approved: adjuvant treatment of Duke's C colon cancer following surgical resection (in combination with 5-FU)

PHARMACOKINETICS

Distribution—rapidly absorbed after oral administration; **Metabolism**—extensively metabolized in the liver; **Half-life**—is 3–4 hr; **Elimination**—mainly through kidneys

DRUG INTERACTIONS

Alcoholic beverages, 5-FU, phenytoin

RESPONSE RATES

Patients with Duke's C colon cancer (adjuvant levamisole and 5-FU)—about a 30% reduction in recurrence and death rates

PATIENT MONITORING

Perform baseline CBC with differential and platelet counts, serum electrolytes, and liver function tests; take weekly CBC with differential and platelet counts prior to each 5-FU dose; monitor electrolytes and liver function studies monthly; monitor for mucositis and diarrhea (modify 5-FU accordingly); evaluate phenytoin levels regularly

NURSING INTERVENTIONS

Monitor treatment tolerance, weight, nutrition; instruct patients on oral hygiene; manage stomatitis with combinations of benadryl, Maalox and viscous lidocaine (rule out oral candidiasis); treat diarrhea aggressively, particularly in the aged

PATIENT INFORMATION

Patients should report flu-like symptoms to physician immediately; avoid alcohol; avoid pregnancy and nursing during treatment

FORMULATION

Available as Ergamisol® by Janssen Pharmaceutica, Titusville, NJ
50-mg tablets. Stored at room temperature.

OCTREOTIDE

Octreotide is a long-acting somatostatin analogue (SMS 201-995), the effects of which are pleiotropic and generally inhibitory. Its activity is mediated through binding to widely distributed cell surface receptors. These have been identified on the cells of some tumor types, suggesting that they may be susceptible to the inhibitory effects of octreotide. Antitumor efficacy is also suggested by its ability to downregulate the activity of myriad growth factors, its direct antiproliferative effects on some tumor cell lines, and its stimulation of reticuloendothelial activity.

The therapeutic index of octreotide is broad. It has demonstrated activity against some symptoms associated with hypersecretory neuroendocrine tumors. Its inhibitory effects on gastrointestinal function are useful in the management of enterocutaneous fistulae. Its use in the treatment of cancer, however, remains investigational.

DOSAGE AND ADMINISTRATION

50 µg once or twice daily, with gradual dosage adjustment thereafter to achieve control of symptoms [25].
Carcinoid syndrome or VIPoma: 200–300 µg daily given in 2 to 4 divided doses during initial 2 weeks of therapy

SPECIAL PRECAUTIONS

Patients with renal dysfunction who require dialysis
Diabetic patients (possible dosage modification of insulin or sulfonylureas required)
Transplant recipients taking cyclosporin
Pregnant/nursing patients

TOXICITIES

GI: nausea, diarrhea, abdominal discomfort (5–10% of patients); cholelithiasis (< 1%)
Endocrine: hyperglycemia or hypoglycemia (2% of patients)
Miscellaneous: pain at injection site (5% of patients)

INDICATIONS

FDA-approved: symptomatic treatment of patients with carcinoid syndrome or VIPoma with diarrhea, electrolyte abnormalities, and flushing; **clinical studies show activity in:** metastic colon cancer

PHARMACOKINETICS

Distribution—rapid and complete absorption after SC injection; **Protein binding**—lipoprotein and albumin in a concentration-independent manner; **Half-life**—about 100 min; **Elimination**—30% unchanged in the urine

DRUG INTERACTIONS

Insulin, sulfonylureas, cyclosporin, TPN

PATIENT MONITORING

Monitor for hyper- or hypoglycemia (particularly in diabetics) and thyroid function; evaluate some patients with 72 h fecal fat and serum carotene determinations periodically; take periodic ultrasound examinations of the gall bladder and biliary tree in patients undergoing prolonged therapy; antitumor effects may be monitored by measurements of serum serotonin, substance P and urinary 5-hydroxyindole acetic acid (5-HIAA) in patients with carcinoid syndrome; measurement of serum vasoactive intestinal peptide in patients with VIPoma

NURSING INTERVENTIONS

Assess for signs and symptoms of hyperglycemia, hypoglycemia, hypothyroidism; teach self-administration to patients treated at home; instruct in safe disposal of needles, drug vials, syringes; avoid multiple injection sites; do not use drug if discoloration or particulates develop

PATIENT INFORMATION

Diabetic patients should monitor their blood glucose closely; patients should report episodes of upper abdominal pain to physician

FORMULATION

Available as Sandostatin® by Sandoz Pharmaceuticals, East Hanover, NJ
1-ml ampules of 0.05, 0.1, or 0.5 mg octreotide. Stored at room temperature for the day of use; otherwise, refrigerated at 2–8°C.

RETINOIDS

Retinoids are a family of structurally and functionally related molecules that exercise a profound effect on cell growth and differentiation. This class of compounds includes all-trans-retinol (vitamin A), its metabolites all-trans-retinoic acid (tretinoin) and 13-cis-retinoic acid (isotretinoin), and beta-carotene. Retinoids possess antineoplastic activity and may have some clinical value in the treatment of acute promyelocytic leukemia, basal cell and squamous cell carcinoma of the skin, and mycosis fungoides. The efficacy of retinoic acid in the treatment of these and other malignancies is being intensely investigated.

Retinoids prevent the development of tumors in a variety of animal models. This has led to several chemoprevention trials in patients at high risk for malignancy. Isotretinoin has been associated with a lower frequency of secondary aerodigestive tumors among patients with surgically treated squamous cell carcinoma of the head and neck. Applications in lung cancer, cervical cancer, and melanoma are under investigation.

DOSAGE AND ADMINISTRATION

Acute promyelocytic leukemia: tretinoin, 45 mg/m^2/d orally, with food
Solid tumors: isotretinoin, 1–3 mg/kg/d orally, with food (use is investigational, and optimal doses have not been defined)

SPECIAL PRECAUTIONS

Patients of childbearing age must use effective contraceptive for 1 month before and after therapy and during the course of therapy
Patients at risk for hypertriglyceridemia, including those with diabetes mellitus, obesity, increased alcohol intake, and a positive family history
Diabetic patients (possible adjustment of hypoglycemic medications required)
Patients allergic to parabens
Pregnant/nursing patients

TOXICITIES

Dermatologic: frequent chelitis and xerosis, possibly leading to pruritus, conjunctivitis, blepharitis, and epistaxis; hair thinning, brittle nails
GI: dry mouth, nausea, vomiting (common); inflammatory bowel disease
Ophthalmic: conjunctivitis (40% of patients); optic neuritis, corneal opacities, photophobia (rare)
Neurologic: fatigue and headache are frequent with tretinoin but uncommon with isotretinoin; pseudotumor cerebri
Musculoskeletal: moderate symptoms (15% of patients)
Metabolic: reversible hypertriglyceridemia, hyperglycemia, hyperuricemia, hypercholesterolemia: elevations of AST, ALT, and LDH (10% of patients)

INDICATIONS

Clinical studies show activity in: acute promyelocytic leukemia and solid tumors

PHARMACOKINETICS

Peak plasma levels (isotretinoin)—3 hr after dose; **Metabolism**—tretinoin and isotretinoin metabolized by cytochrome P-450-dependent hydroxylation and undergo conjugation with glucuronide; **Excretion**—about 70% of an oral dose in urine and feces in equal portions

DRUG INTERACTIONS

Minocycline, tetracycline, vitamin A, topical dermatologics (benzoyl peroxide, sulfur), ethanol

PATIENT MONITORING

Negative serum pregnancy test within 2 weeks of beginning therapy in women of childbearing age, monthly pregnancy testing thereafter; monitor for development of headache, nausea, vomiting, or visual disturbances—if present, evaluate for papilledema or ophthalmalogic disorders; obtain baseline lipid profile (repeated once or twice weekly until lipid response to therapy has been determined, usually 8 wk); follow other blood tests (glucose, liver function studies, uric acid, cholesterol, CBC, and platelet counts)

NURSING INTERVENTIONS

Frequent counseling about contraception (two methods of contraception used simultaneously is recommended unless abstinence is practiced); monitor for signs and symptoms of inflammatory bowel disease

PATIENT INFORMATION

Decreased night vision requires precautions; avoid exposure to sun; do not donate blood for 30 days after treatment ends; if diabetic, insulin medication may require adjustment; take medications with meals and avoid crushing capsules; avoid vitamin A supplements and benzoyl peroxide; minimize intake of ethanol

FORMULATIONS

Isotretinoin is available as Accutane® by Roche Dermatologies, Nutley, NJ
Capsules containing 10, 20, or 30 mg of drug as a suspension in soybean oil. Stored at 15–30°C protected from light.
Tretinoin is also manufactured by Roche but is not commercially available.

SARGRAMOSTIM

Sargramostim (granulocyte-macrophage–colony-stimulating factor, GM-CSF) is a 127 amino acid recombinant, human GM-CSF that is produced in a yeast expression system. It differs from the natural glycoprotein by the substitution of leucine at amino acid position 23. The carbohydrate moiety may also differ. Sargramostim affects progenitors of multiple lineages, including granulocytes, monocytes, eosinophils, megakaryocytes, and erythrocytes. Its effect on these immature cells requires other CSFs, including erythropoietin. Sargramostim's greatest effect is on lineage-committed granulocyte and monocyte precursors. In addition to increasing the number of circulating PMN and monocytes, it enhances their function.

DOSAGE AND ADMINISTRATION

Myeloid reconstitution after autologous bone marrow transplantation:
250 μg/m²/d, 2-hr IV infusion daily for 21 d. Begin treatment 2–4 hr after marrow infusion [25]

Bone marrow transplant failure or engraftment delay: 250 μg/m²/d, 2-hr IV infusion daily for 14 d, repeat after 7 d if engraftment has not occurred. A third 14-d course, 500 μg/m², can be given after 7 d if engraftment has not occurred. Further therapy is not useful.

DOSAGE MODIFICATIONS: In both instances, discontinue drug if blast cells appear or disease progresses. If severe drug reactions occur, the dose may be decreased or delayed until reactions abate.

SPECIAL PRECAUTIONS

Patients with a history of cardiac disease
Patients with pre-existing hypoxemic lung disease
Patients with pre-existing pericardial effusion, plural effusion, or congestive heart failure
Patients with pre-existing hepatic or renal dysfunction
Pregnant/nursing patients
Patients with acute myelocytic leukemia and myelodysplastic syndrome
Patients who have been treated previously with intensive chemotherapy or radiation therapy and who require myeloid reconstitution after bone marrow transplantation may have less responses.
Patients with excessive myeloid blasts in the bone marrow or peripheral blood (> 10%)
Do not administer within 24 hr of or during chemotherapy or within 12 hr of or during radiation therapy

TOXICITIES

Cardiovascular: development of transient supraventricular tachydysrhythmias (in patients with pre-existing heart disease); exacerbation of congestive heart failure and pericardial effusion due to fluid retention; hypotension, flushing, and syncope associated with first dose
Respiratory: dyspnea; exacerbation of pre-existing lung disease
Immunologic: neutralizing antibodies to sargramostim (3% of patients)
Renal: exacerbation of pre-existing renal disease
Hepatic: exacerbation of pre-existing liver disease
Hematologic: reversible thrombocytosis and leucocytosis
Musculoskeletal: mild-to-moderate medullary bone pain
GI: diarrhea
Miscellaneous: flu-like syndrome

INDICATIONS

FDA-approved: myeloid reconstitution after autologous bone marrow transplantation, bone marrow transplantation failure, delay of bone marrow transplant engraftment; **clinical studies show activity in:** patients with myelodysplastic syndrome and HIV-positive patients treated with zidovudine (increase WBC count), patients with leukopenia secondary to chemotherapy, preleukemic patients with myelosuppression, patients with aplastic anemia, recipients of organ transplants with neutropenia

PHARMACOKINETICS

Serum concentration—23,000 pg/ml after a dose of 250 μg/m² given by 2-hr IV infusion;
Distribution—good absorption with SC administration; **Peak serum levels**—2 hr after injection;
Half-life—15 min (alpha), 2 hr (beta)

DRUG INTERACTIONS

Lithium, corticosteroids

PATIENT MONITORING

Perform CBC twice weekly; evaluate renal and hepatic function twice weekly in patients with pre-existing renal or hepatic dysfunction as well

NURSING INTERVENTIONS

To reduce flu-like symptoms to tolerable levels administer drug in evening and give acetaminophen concomitantly; monitor patients for flushing, dyspnea, hypotension

PATIENT INFORMATION

Patients should report signs of fluid retention, including weight gain and edema, particularly those with heart or lung disease

FORMULATION

Available as Leukine®, Immunex Corporation, Seattle, WA; Prokine®, Hoechst–Roussel Pharmaceuticals, Somerville, NJ
Vials of 250 or 500 mg of lyophilized recombinant GM-CSF. Stored at 2–8°C.

The fundamental role of ovarian hormones in the growth of some breast cancers has been known since 1896 when Sir George Beatson first described the control of advanced disease following oophorectomy. However, by 1900 it was clear that not all women with breast cancer would respond to oophorectomy; only one third of the patient population received palliation. The question of who would respond to the procedure remained unresolved for more than half a century until Dr. Elwood Jensen proposed that the presence of estrogen receptors (ER) in tumor tissue could be a predictor of response to endocrine manipulation. Simply stated, the hypothesis was that if no ERs were present, the tumor was hormone-dependent but the ER should be present for the tumor to be dependent upon estrogen for growth.

The ER test is now performed on all patients with breast cancers (Table 1). For advanced disease only 10% of patients will respond to endocrine therapy if ER is absent, but 60% of patients will respond if the tumor is ER positive. The reasons all ER-positive tumors do not respond to endocrine therapy are twofold: 1) the tumor may be a heterogeneous mix of ER-positive and ER-negative cells and 2) there are ERs made by the cell that are no longer involved in cell growth. To determine the hormonal responsiveness of the patient more accurately, it is now possible to use immunocytochemistry on frozen section using monoclonal antibodies to ER so that the distribution of positive cells can be estimated. It is also possible to estimate the functionality of the ER by determining the progesterone receptor (PgR). The PgR is only made as a result of estrogen action through functional ER; if no PgR is present, the possibility that the patient will respond to endocrine therapy is reduced. However if a patient with advanced disease is both ER and PgR positive, there is an 80% chance of a response to endocrine therapy (Table 2).

It is usual for breast tumors to be classified with both ER and PgR values at the time of surgery. This information can then be used to establish a strategy for adjuvant therapy.

The incidence of prostate cancer, like breast cancer, increase with advancing age. Prostate cancer maintains hormonal characteristics similar to breast cancer. Gonadectomy will control a majority of metastatic prostate cancers by denying the tumor androgens that are necessary for growth. This surgical approach has been employed for more than half a century, but with our increased understanding of reproductive endocrinology, it has been possible to use therapeutic measures to control the growth of both breast and prostate cancer (Tables 3 and 4).

PRINCIPLES OF ENDOCRINE PHARMACOLOGY

Since estrogen and androgen are necessary to maintain the growth of some breast and prostate tumors, respectively, the therapeutic strategies rely on either reduction of the source of steroids or blockade of steroid action in the tumor itself (Figs. 1 and 2). Naturally the simplest way to reduce circulating sex steroids is to remove either the ovaries or testes. This is standard practice. High-dose estrogen (diethylstilbestrol) is used as an alternative to castration in men but the side effects to the drug are significant. However, a range of pharmacologic agents is now available to control or block hormone action. An alternative approach to gonadectomy or estrogen therapy in men is the use of luteinizing hormone-releasing hormone (LHRH) superagonists to desensitize the pituitary gland and prevent the release of gonadotropins. Two LHRH preparations are routinely used to treat prostate cancer: goserelin and leuprolide. Although the use of LHRH agonists can reduce circulating androgens, this strategy is not absolute. The adrenal gland is a rich source of secreted androgens that can maintain prostate tumor growth. For this reason the LHRH agonists may be given with an antiandrogen, usually flutamide, to block the androgen receptor. The strategy is therefore dual in men with prostate cancer: reduction of gonadal steroid secretion by stopping gonadotrophin release and blocking of adrenal androgen action with a pure antiandrogen (Fig. 3) [1].

A similar treatment strategy is used in postmenopausal women with breast cancer who no longer have active ovarian steroid synthesis; an antiestrogen, tamoxifen, is given to block low levels of endogenous estrogen from binding to ER in the tumor. The estrogen, usually estrone and estradiol, is produced by peripheral aromatization of androstenedione of adrenal origin. Progestins can be used as second-line therapy if tamoxifen or aminoglutethimide/ hydrocortisone combinations have failed to prevent steroidogenesis. There is little endocrine responsiveness after aminoglutethimide treatment failure. Compared with tamoxifen, halotestin alone offers little advantage as an endocrine therapy, as response rates are low and side effects are significant. High-dose estrogen therapy (diethylstilbestrol) is equally as effective as tamoxifen in the postmenopausal patient, but the side effects are greater. Premenopausal patients with breast cancer can benefit from tamoxifen, but large clinical studies have not been performed to compare efficacy with oophorectomy. Premenopausal patients who initially respond and then fail with tamoxifen treatment can benefit from subsequent oophorectomy.

Table 1. Prediction of Hormone Response

Estrogen receptor content
  Biochemical assay
  Immunocytochemistry
Proggesterone receptor content

Table 2. Response Rates to Endocrine Therapy

Advanced breast cancer		Advanced prostate cancer	
All	30%	All	70%
ER+	60%		
ER, PR+	80%		

Table 3. Role of Endocrine Therapy: Hormonally Responsive Tumors

Advanced	Adjuvant
Breast carcinoma	Breast carcinoma
Prostate carcinoma	
Ovarian (epithelial) cancer	
Endometrial cancer	

Table 4. Tumors Not Classically Hormone Responsive

As single agents
  Medroxyprogesterone acetate—renal cell carcinoma
As combined modality
  Tamoxifen—to alter drug resistance with a variety of cytotoxic drugs

Detailed descriptions of the pharmacologic agents available to treat breast and prostate cancers can be found elsewhere [2] but a brief overview is given below.

ENDOCRINE THERAPY FOR ADVANCED BREAST CANCER

A majority of metastatic prostate cancer responds to endocrine manipulation. Androgen receptor determinations are not of clinical significance. In contrast only about one third of advanced breast cancer is responsive. The majority of advanced breast cancer is noted in postmenopausal women, but when it is found in premenopausal women either oophorectomy or tamoxifen can be used to treat the ER-positive patient.

ADJUVANT THERAPY FOR BREAST CANCER

Breast cancer that does not have any clinically detectable distant metastases can, at the time of surgery, be classified as axillary node positive or negative. Women with axillary nodes that are determined positive for tumor by a pathologist have a shorter time to recurrence than do node-negative women. Indeed, clinical experience demonstrates that the greater the number of nodes involved, the sooner the disease will recur. By contrast, approximately 70% of node-negative women will be cured of their breast cancer.

Adjuvant therapy with tamoxifen is used following breast surgery to control the growth of micrometastases. In general, 2 to 5 years of adjuvant tamoxifen therapy is the treatment of choice for either postmenopausal woman with node-positive breast cancer, irrespective of ER/PgR status, or postmenopausal woman with node-negative ER-positive disease. Tamoxifen produces both an increase in disease-free survival and overall survival even 10 years after mastectomy [3]. Tamoxifen is also an available option to treat the premenopausal woman with node-negative ER-positive disease, largely because side effects are minor compared with those from combination chemotherapy. The latter regimen is standard treatment for premenopausal women with node-positive disease; a survival advantage is to be expected.

A 40% decrease in the occurrence of primary cancers in the contralateral breast has been noted with the use of tamoxifen. This finding is an important basis for the trial on breast cancer prevention, which is testing the value of tamoxifen in normal and high-risk women.

TAMOXIFEN

NSABP/NCI Prevention Trial

Tamoxifen is not available for the treatment of women who do not have a diagnosis of breast cancer. However, it is being studied in a clinical trial with normal women. Sixteen thousand women are being currently recruited in the United States and Canada to be randomized in a double-blind, placebo-controlled clinical study to determine whether 5 years of tamoxifen (20 mg daily) will reduce the risk of breast cancer.

Any woman over the age of 60 is eligible for recruitment, but women over the age of 35 must have accumulative risk factors, determined by the NSABP, equivalent to the risk experienced by a woman of 60 years. Risk factors that are important are first-degree relatives with breast cancer, no children, children after the age of 25, multiple breast biopsies, breast hyperplasia, menarche before the age of 12, and lobular carcinoma *in situ*.

This study will also assess the effects of tamoxifen on bones and lipids to establish its action on associated physiologic functions of estrogen. The principal aim of the study is not only to reduce deaths from breast cancer but also to improve the rate of long-term health in women. Similar prevention trials are being conducted by groups in Great Britain and Italy.

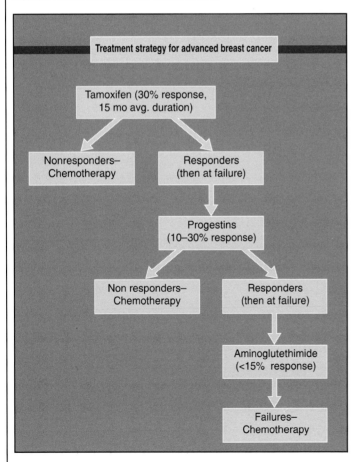

FIGURE 1

Therapy for women with advanced breast cancer is to block the action of estrogen.

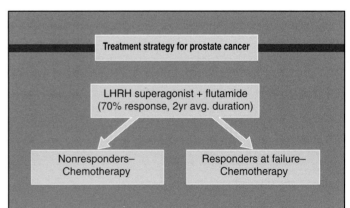

FIGURE 2

The strategy for controlling prostate cancer is similar to that for controlling breast cancer—blocking the action of hormone.

Advantages

Estrogen is essential to maintain bone density in women and protects them from coronary heart disease. It is possible that the administration of tamoxifen could predispose women to both osteoporosis and coronary heart disease. However tamoxifen is a weak estrogen agonist and expresses a variety of estrogen-like effects in the postmenopausal woman. Tamoxifen maintains bone density in the lumbar spine [4] and lowers circulating levels of cholesterol [5]. At present, it is possible that tamoxifen may prevent osteoporosis and reduce the incidence of coronary heart disease [6–8].

Disadvantages

The estrogen-like effects of tamoxifen are responsible for a modest increase in thromboembolic disorders and endometrial carcinoma during long-term therapy. Each of these side effects is serious and should be treated accordingly. However, women undergoing tamoxifen therapy should not be treated with coumadin anticoagulants. Although tamoxifen can, like estrogen, promote liver carcinogenesis in laboratory rats, there are only two reported instances of hepatocellular carcinomas in the 4.5 million women-years of experience.

Special attention should be paid to eye examinations during tamoxifen therapy. Most experience is anecdotal but there is concern about the possibility of retinopathies and changes in visual acuity. Women with macular degeneration may have deterioration of vision from tamoxifen. In premenopausal women tamoxifen causes an increase in circulating estrogen, but at present it is not thought that this will be detrimental to patient care. Tamoxifen should not be given to the pregnant patient. The endocrine effects of tamoxifen [9,10] in pre- and postmenopausal women are illustrated in Figure 4.

FIGURE 3

Potential targets for the treatment of prostate cancer. Luteinizing hormone-releasing hormone (LHRH) agonists are standard with or without the antiandrogen flutamide. The inhibitor of adrenal steroidogenesis, aminoglutethimide, is only used experimentally and has little clinical application.

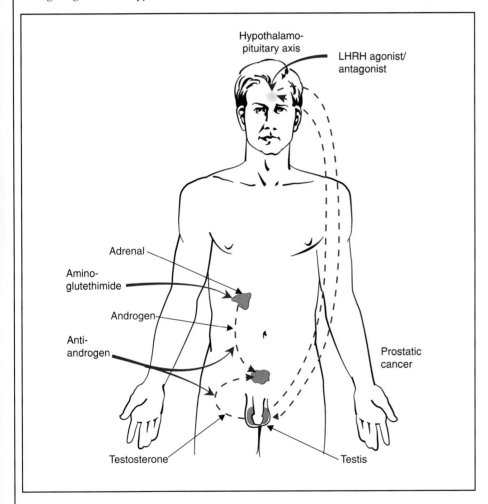

The information here is provided as guidance only. Prescribers should always consult the manufacturer's current prescribing information.

67

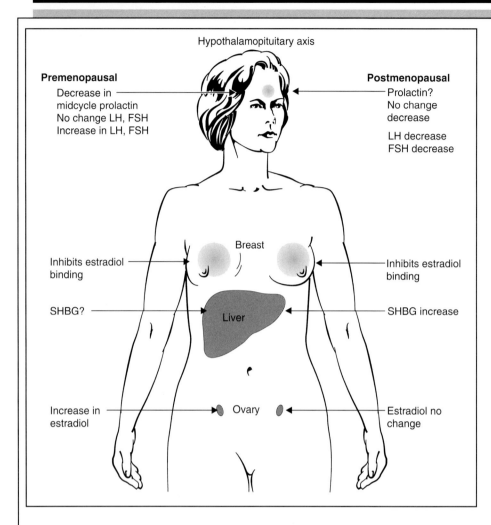

Hypothalamopituitary axis

Premenopausal

Decrease in midcycle prolactin
No change LH, FSH
Increase in LH, FSH

Inhibits estradiol binding

SHBG?

Increase in estradiol

Postmenopausal

Prolactin?
No change decrease

LH decrease
FSH decrease

Inhibits estradiol binding

SHBG increase

Estradiol no change

Breast

Liver

Ovary

FIGURE 4

The endocrine effects of tamoxifen in pre- and postmenopausal patients. FSH—follicle-stimulating hormone; LH—luteinizing hormone, SHBG—sex hormone-binding globulin.

REFERENCES

1. Geller S, Albert S, Vik A: Advantages of total androgen blockade in the treatment of advanced prostate cancer. *Sem Oncol* 1988, 15:53.

2. Robinson SP, Jordan VC: Metabolism of steroid-modifying anticancer agents. *Pharmacol Ther* 1988, 36:41–97.

3. Early Breast Cancer Trialists Collaborative Group: Systemic treatment of early breast cancer by hormonal, cytotoxic or immune therapy. *Lancet* 1992, 339:1–15.

4. Love RR, Mazess RB, Barden HS, *et al.*: Effects of tamoxifen on bone mineral density in postmenopausal women with breast cancer. *N Engl J Med* 1992, 26:852–856.

5. Love RR, Weibe DA, Newcomb PA, *et al.*: Effects of tamoxifen on cardiovascular risk factors in postmenopausal women. *Ann Intern Med* 1991, 115:860–864.

6. McDonald CC, Stewart HJ: Fatal myocardial infarction in the Scottish adjuvant tamoxifen trial. The Scottish Breast Cancer Committee. *Br Med J* 1991, 303:435–437.

7. Rutqvist LE, Mattsson A: Cardiac and thromboembolic morbidity among postmenopausal women with early stage breast cancer in a randomized trial of adjuvant tamoxifen. *J Natl Cancer Inst* 1993, 85:1398–1406.

8. Jordan VC: Can all postmenopausal women with a diagnosis of breast cancer benefit from tamoxifen treatment? *Rev Endo Cancer* 1993, 43:23–31.

9. Wolf DM, Jordan VC: Gynecological complications associated with long-term tamoxifen therapy for breast cancer. *Gynecol Oncol* 1992, 45:118–128.

10. Jordan VC: A current review of tamoxifen for the treatment and prevention of breast cancer. *Br J Pharmacol* 1993, 110:507–517.

AMINOGLUTETHIMIDE

Aminoglutethimide inhibits the conversion of cholesterol to Δ^5 pregnenolone in the adrenals and the aromatization of androstenedione to estrone in peripheral tissues. Hydrocortisone must be administered simultaneously because the decrease in glucocorticoids produced by aminoglutethimide causes an increase in adrenocorticotropic hormone (ACTH) that will reverse the agent's action in the adrenals. The drug combinations can be used as a second-line treatment for ER-positive breast cancer after the failure of tamoxifen. Side effects with this drug are more troublesome than those with tamoxifen.

DOSAGE AND ADMINISTRATION: 250 mg four times a day at 6 hr intervals. As cortisol decreases, dose increases by 250 mg daily at 1–2-wk intervals to a total daily dose of 2 g. Hydrocortisone, 20–30 mg orally each morning, to replace glucocorticoid insufficiency

SPECIAL PRECAUTIONS: Patients with hypersensitivity to glutethimide and aminoglutethimide; Pregnant patients; Elderly patients; Diminishes effects of warfarin and coumadin

TOXICITIES: Neurologic: drowsiness, dizziness, headache; **Dermatologic:** morbilliform skin rash, pruritus ;**GI:** nausea, vomiting; **Endocrine:** hypothyroidism; **Hematologic:** various conditions; **Cardiopulmonary:** hypotension; **Flu-like:** fever, myalgia

INDICATIONS: FDA-approved: selected patients with Cushing's syndrome; clinical studies show activity in experimental treatment of advanced breast cancer as second-line therapy

PHARMACOKINETICS: Distribution—ubiquitous; **Absorption**—rapid/complete; **Biotransformation/Metabolism**—50%; **Onset of action**—rapid; **Peak concentration**—5.9 µg/ml 1.5 hrs after 500-mg dose; **Half-life**—12.5 hr; **Elimination**—urine

DRUG INTERACTIONS: Coumadin; warfarin; rapid metabolism of dexamethasone

RESPONSE RATES: 10–15% after tamoxifen failure

PATIENT MONITORING: Check for rashes (5–8 days or severe), glucocorticoids, hematologic values, thyroid

NURSING INTERVENTION: Careful monitoring and documentation of signs and symptoms

PATIENT INFORMATION: Patient may experience drowiness, dizziness, rashes, nausea

FORMULATION: Available as Cytadren®, CIBA Pharmacauticals, Woodbridge, NJ; 250-mg tablets scored into quarters; Protect from light in tight, light-resistant container.

DIETHYLSTILBESTROL

Diethylstilbestrol is a synthetic estrogen used for the palliative treatment of advanced breast cancer in postmenopausal women or advanced prostate cancer in men. In prostate cancer, diethylstilbestrol lowers circulating testosterone by reducing gonadotropins. In breast cancer, the mechanism of action is unknown. The high doses of diethylstilbestrol used produces beneficial effects in ER-positive breast cancer and may desensitize the receptor system to estrogen stimulation.

DOSAGE AND ADMINISTRATION: Breast cancer: 15 mg daily; **Prostate cancer:** 1–3 mg daily, reduced to 1 mg daily

SPECIAL PRECAUTIONS: Pregnant/nursing patients; Depressed patients; Patients with renal insufficiency; Patients with hypercalcemia; Patients with endometrial problems; Patients with poor liver function; Patients with fluid retention; Patients with gallbladder disease; Patients with thromboembolic disease

TOXICITIES: GU: breakthrough bleeding, vaginal candidiasis, cystitis-like symptoms; **Breasts:** tender, discharge; **GI:** cholestatic jaundice, nausea, vomiting; **Neurologic:** depression, headaches; **Dermatologic:** chloasma, melasma, erythema multiforme, loss of scalp hair; **Ophthalmologic:** contact lens intolerance

INDICATIONS: FDA-approved: advanced prostate cancer, advanced breast cancer in postmenopausal women

PHARMACOKINETICS: Absorption—2–4 hr ; **Protein binding**—40–50%; **Biotransformation/Metabolism**— extensive; **Onset of action**—physiologically 1 d, anticancer action 2–3 d; **Half-life**—2 hr; **Elimination**—biliary excretion

DRUG INTERACTIONS: None

RESPONSE RATES: 10–70% in advanced breast cancer based on hormone receptor status; 70% in advanced prostate cancer

PATIENT MONITORING: Monitor symptoms, calcium, blood pressure, uterine malignancy, gallbladder disease, liver function

NURSING INTERVENTIONS: Careful monitoring and documentation of signs and symptoms

PATIENT INFORMATION: Patient may experience nausea, cystitis-like symptoms, vaginal candidiasis, tender breasts, changes in libido, increase/decrease in weight

FORMULATIONS: Available as Diethystilbestrol, Eli Lilly and Company, Indianapolis, IN; Enseals: 1 mg and 5 mg; Tablets: 1 mg and 5 mg; Protect contents from light.

FLUOXYMESTERONE

A synthetic androgenic hormone with a steroidal structure used to treat postmenopausal women with hormone-responsive breast cancer. The high incidence of androgeneric side effects make this compound a second-line agent. The patients that have ER-positive breast tumors respond better than those with ER-negative tumors. The mechanism of action is unknown but probably involves blocking the stimulating effect of estrogen.

DOSAGE AND ADMINISTRATION: 10–40 mg total daily

SPECIAL PRECAUTIONS: Hypercalcemic patients

TOXICITIES: Dermatologic: hirsuitism, male pattern baldness, acne **Renal/hepatic:** alterations of liver function, electrolyte disturbances, cholestatic hepatitis and jaundice, fluid retention **Hematologic:** suppression of clotting factors

INDICATIONS: FDA-approved: advanced ER-positive breast cancer in postmenopausal women

PHARMACOKINETICS: Distribution—ubiquitous; **Absorption**—rapid/oral administration; **Biotransformation/ metabolism**—conjugated in liver; **Onset of action**—within 24 hr; breast cancer treatment up to 8 wk; **Peak concentration**—**Half-life**—9.2 hr; **Elimination**—bile, urine

DRUG INTERACTIONS: Oral anticoagulants

RESPONSE RATES: 30% as first-line therapy in advanced breast cancer 10–20% as second-line therapy after tamoxifen failure

PATIENT MONITORING: Monitor anticoagulants; insulin—drug lowers blood glucose; Hypercalcemia—discontinue drug

NURSING INTERVENTIONS: Careful monitoring and documentation of signs and symptoms

PATIENT INFORMATION: Patient may experience hirsuitism, deepening of the voice, changes in skin color, ankle swelling, nausea, vomiting

FORMULATION: Available as Halotestin®, The Upjohn Company, Kalamazoo, MI; 2-, 5-, 10-mg tablets of fluoxymesterone

FLUTAMIDE

Flutamide is an orally active antiandrogen used with LHRH agonist to treat men with prostate cancer. The drug blocks androgen binding to the receptor. Flutamide is considered a prodrug. The active metabolite hydroxyflutamide is the pharmacologically active agent.

DOSAGE AND ADMINISTRATION: Two 125-mg capsules 3 times daily

SPECIAL PRECAUTIONS: Hepatic injury

TOXICITIES: Cardiovascular: hypertension (1% of patients); **CNS:** drowsiness; **GI:** nausea and vomiting (6% of patients); **Hematopoietic:** anemia, leukopenia, hepatitis, jaundice

INDICATIONS: FDA-approved: with leuprolide for prostatic cancer

PHARMACOKINETICS: Absorption—within 2–6 hr; completely absorbed, steady state after third dose; **Protein binding**—96%; **Biotransformation/metabolism**—metabolically activated to hydroxy compound; **Peak concentration**—parent 24–78 ng/mL, metabolite 1556–2284 ng/mL; **Half-life**—active metabolite 6 hr; **Elimination**—urine

DRUG INTERACTIONS: None, although close monitoring of prothrombin time is recommended in patients on warfarin

RESPONSE RATES: 70% when given with leuprodide

PATIENT MONITORING: Monitor symptoms, take periodic liver function tests

NURSING INTERVENTIONS: Careful monitoring and documentation of signs and symptoms

PATIENT INFORMATION: Patient should not interrupt dosing

FORMULATION: Available as Eulexin®, Schering Corporation, Kenilworth, NJ; 125-mg capsules; Protect from moisture and store between 2 and 30°C

GOSERELIN ACETATE

Goserelin acetate contains a potent synthetic decapeptide analogue of luteinizing hormone releasing hormone (LHRH). The depot preparation is designed for subcutaneous injection for a 28-day release to desensitize the pituitary gland and reduce the release of gonadotrophins. The drug is used to treat prostate cancer in men.

DOSAGE AND ADMINISTRATION: 3.6 mg in sustained-release preparation. The skin may be anesthetized and the hypodermic needle of the applicator inserted into the subcutaneous fat on the upper abdominal wall.

SPECIAL PRECAUTIONS: Patients with metastatic vertebral lesions Patients with urethral obstructions

TOXICITIES: Exacerbation of signs and symptoms; **Cardiovascular:** angina, cardiac arrhythmias; **GI:** anorexia, diarrhea; **Endocrine:** gynecomastia, decreased libido; **GU:** dysuria, urgency, hematuria, testicular pain; **Neurologic:** paresthesia, insomnia

INDICATIONS: FDA-approved: metastatic prostate cancer; clinical studies show activity in advanced breast cancer in premenopausal women

PHARMACOKINETICS: Distribution—plasma compartment; **Absorption**—slow for the first 8 d and continues up to 28 d; **Protein binding**—40%; **Onset of action**—24 hr to stimulate gonadotrophins, 10 days to inhibit gonadotrophins; **Peak concentration**—2.5 ng/mL within 12–15 d; **Half-life**—4.2 hr; **Elimination**—not reported, possibly liver

DRUG INTERACTIONS: None reported

RESPONSE RATES: 70–80% of men with advanced prostate cancer

PATIENT MONITORING: Monitor symptoms, urine flow; watch for spinal metastasis

NURSING INTERVENTIONS: Careful monitoring and documentation of signs and symptoms

PATIENT INFORMATION: Patient may experience hot flashes, sexual dysfunction, decreased erections

FORMULATION: Zoladex® with 16-gauge needle and disposable syringe device, Zeneca Pharmaceuticals, Wilmington, DE; Supplied as sterile and totally biodegradable DL lactic and glycolic acids copolymer impregnated with goserlin acetate equivalent to 3.6-mg goserelin; Store at room temperature (do not exceed 25° C).

KETOCONAZOLE

Ketoconazole is a synthetic broad-spectrum antifungal agent. High doses will significantly lower serum testosterone. Experimental studies have demonstrated its value in treating prostate carcinoma in men. Ketoconzole can be used when orchiectomy is contraindicated or cannot be performed immediately.

DOSAGE AND ADMINISTRATION: 1200 mg daily

SPECIAL PRECAUTIONS: Hypersensitivity to the drug; Hepatotoxicity

TOXICITIES: Sudden death within 2 weeks of therapy; Anaphylaxis Neuropsychiatric disorders

INDICATIONS: Clinical studies show activity in patients with prostate cancer

PHARMACOKINETICS: Absorption—rapid 1–2 hr; **Protein binding**—99%; **Biotransformation/metabolism**—extensive oxidation; **Onset of action**—rapid, <48 hr; **Peak concentration**—3.5 μg/mL after 200-mg dose; **Half-life**—biphasic 2 hr, thereafter 8 hr; **Elimination**—bile (major), urine (13%)

DRUG INTERACTIONS: Terfenadine (Seldane)—ventricular dysrhythmia

PATIENT MONITORING: Monitor testosterone (long-term therapy is slowly reversed); adrenal function (may cause sudden death)

NURSING INTERVENTIONS: Management of overdosage—gastric lavage with sodium bicarbonate

PATIENT INFORMATION: Patient may experience fatigue, nausea, anorexia, jaundice, pale stool, dark urine

FORMULATION: Available as Nizoral®, Janssen Pharmaceutica, Titusville, NJ; 200-mg tablet; Store at room temperature.

The information here is provided as guidance only. Prescribers should always consult the manufacturer's current prescribing information.

LEUPROLIDE ACETATE

Leuprolide acetate is a synthetic nonapeptide analogue of naturally occurring gonadotropin-releasing hormone (LHRH). It is a superagonist. The depot preparation provides sustained release of the product, causing desensitization of the pituitary gland. The decrease in gonadotropin causes a drop in steroidogenesis (testes in males, ovaries in females). This decrease in sex steroids can be used to produce a medical castration.

DOSAGE AND ADMINISTRATION: 7.5-mg depot in single monthly IM injection administered under the supervision of a physician

SPECIAL PRECAUTIONS: Patients with metastatic vertebral lesions; Patients with urinary tract obstruction

TOXICITIES: Exacerbation of signs and symptoms; **Cardiovascular:** angina, cardiac arrhythmias; **GI:** anorexia, diarrhea; **Endocrine:** gynecomastia, decreased libido; **GU:** dysuria, urgency, hematuria, testicular pain; **Neurologic:** paresthesia, insomnia

INDICATIONS: FDA-approved: advanced prostate cancer; clinical studies show activity in endometriosis

PHARMOCOKINETICS: Distribution—unknown; **Absorption**—rapid max at 4 hr; **Protein binding**—50%; **Biotransformation/metabolism**—not determined in man; **Onset of action**—24 hr (stimulation of gonadotrophins), in 2 wk (suppression of gonadotrophins); **Peak concentration**—20 ng/mL at 4 hr; **Half-life**—4 hr; **Elimination**—unknown

DRUG INTERACTIONS: None reported

RESPONSE RATES: 70% in advanced prostate cancer

PATIENT MONITORING: Monitor cardiovascular symptoms

NURSING INTERVENTIONS: Careful monitoring and documentation of signs and symptoms

PATIENT INFORMATION: Patient may experience increase/decrease of libido, diarrhea, anorexia, insomnia, paresthesias

FORMULATION: Available as Lupron Depot®, TAP Pharmaceuticals, Deerfield, IL; Lupron depot 7.5 mg as lyophized microspheres single-dose vial; Store at room temperature; Do not freeze

MEDROXYPROGESTERONE ACETATE

Medroxyprogesterone acetate is a synthetic progestin used for the treatment of endometrial and advanced breast cancer in women. High-dose therapy is effective in breast cancer as a second-line treatment after tamoxifen failure in postmenopausal patients. The drug acts to prevent the stimulating actions of estrogen but the precise mechanism of action is unknown.

DOSAGE AND ADMINISTRATION: Effective at doses of 1 g daily

SPECIAL PRECAUTIONS: Patients with existing thrombophlebitis Patients with liver dysfunction

TOXICITIES: Hematologic: thromboembolic disorders; breakthrough bleeding; **GI:** weight changes, cholestatic jaundice; **Neurologic:** depression; **Dermatologic:** rashes

INDICATIONS: FDA-approved: bleeding associated with endometrial carcinoma; clinical studies show activity in: high-dose therapy may provide benefit for advanced breast cancer patients as a second-line agent. Depoprovera is approved for endometrial and renal cancer

PHARMACOKINETICS: Not available

DRUG INTERACTIONS: Aminoglutethimide—reduces bioavailability

RESPONSE RATES: In advanced disease with *high*-dose regimen—20–40%; 10–20% response rates as second-line therapy after tamoxifen failure

PATIENT MONITORING: Monitor any signs of thromboembolic disorders, watch for early signs of failed liver functions

NURSING INTERVENTIONS: Careful monitoring and documentation of signs and symptoms

PATIENT INFORMATION: Patient should immediately report any side effects to physician

FORMULATION: Available as Depo-Provera® (injection) and Provera® (tablets), The Upjohn Company, Kalamazoo, MI; Injection—400-mg/mL, 2.5-mL vial, 100-mg/mL, 5-mL vial; Tablets—10-mg

MEGESTROL ACETATE

Megestrol acetate is a synthetic steroid with progestational and anti-neoplastic activity used as a second-line agent after tamoxifen for the treatment of advanced breast cancer in postmenopausal women. High doses reduce adrenal steroidogenesis and block action of estrogen in women with breast tumors through an unknown mechanism.

DOSAGE AND ADMINISTRATION: 40 mg four times daily

SPECIAL PRECAUTIONS: Thrombophlebitis

TOXICITIES: GI: weight gain, nausea, vomiting; **Hematologic:** hypercalcemia, breakthrough bleeding, hyperglycemia, thrombophlebitis and pulmonary embolism; **Cardiovascular:** hypertension

INDICATIONS: FDA-approved: palliative treatment of ER-positive advanced breast cancer in postmenopausal women; inoperable endometrial carcinoma

PHARMACOKINETICS: Distribution—ubiquitous; **Absorption**—variable; **Biotransformation/metabolism**—negligible (5%); **Peak concentration**—30 ng/mL; **Half-life**—24 hr; **Elimination**—urine (major), biliary (minor)

DRUG INTERACTIONS: None

RESPONSE RATES: Unselected patients with breast cancer as a first-line therapy—response rate of 30–40%, higher rates in ER-positive patients; Second-line therapy after tamoxifen failure—10–30%

PATIENT MONITORING: No special tests

NURSING INTERVENTIONS: Careful monitoring and documentation of signs and symptoms

PATIENT INFORMATION: Patient should tell physician of any adverse reactions

FORMULATION: Available as Megace®, Bristol-Myers Oncology Division, Princeton, NJ; 20- and 40-mg tablets; Store at room temperature, not above 40°C.

TAMOXIFEN

Tamoxifen is a nonsteroidal antiestrogen used for the treatment of all stages of breast cancer. The agent blocks estrogen binding to ER in tumors. The compound also has estrogen-like activity, which can produce beneficial effects on bone density and decrease circulating cholesterol.

DOSAGE AND ADMINISTRATION: One or two 10-mg tablets twice a day

SPECIAL PRECAUTIONS: Patients with existing leukopenia or thrombocytopenia; Pregnant patients; Patients with existing hyperlipidemia

TOXICITIES: GI: nausea, vomiting; **Ophthalmologic:** visual disturbances, corneal changes, cataracts, retinopathy, macular degeneration; **GYN:** increased incidence of endometrial carcinoma; **Vascular:** increase in thrombophlebitis

INDICATIONS: FDA-approved: advanced breast cancer (post-menopausal), ER-positive advanced breast cancer (premenopausal), adjuvant therapy with chemotherapy, adjuvant therapy for node-positive disease, ER-positive adjuvant therapy for pre- and post-menopausal node-negative disease; clinical studies show activity in: melanoma, endometrial carcinoma, male breast cancer

PHARMACOKINETICS: Distribution—ubiquitous; steady state achieved in 4 wk; **Absorption**—4–6 hr after dosing; **Protein binding**—98%; **Biotransformation/ metabolism**—30% parent drug; **Onset of action**—3–4 d; **Peak concentration**—100–150 ng/mL at steady state; **Half-life**—initial 7–14 hr, at steady state 7 d; **Elimination**—biliary

DRUG INTERACTIONS: Coumadin-type anticoagulants; CMF chemotherapy (increased thromboembolic events)

RESPONSE RATES: 10–70% related to hormone receptors in advanced disease, adjuvant therapy related to receptor status, only single agent that produces survival advantage

PATIENT MONITORING: Periodic platelet counts, abnormal vaginal bleeding, periodic plasma triglycerides

NURSING INTERVENTIONS: Careful monitoring and documentation of signs and symptoms

PATIENT INFORMATION: Patient may experience amenorrhea, hot flashes, altered menses, some nausea

FORMULATION: Available as Nolvadex®, Zenaca Pharmaceutica, Wilmington, DE; 10-mg tablets; Protect from heat and light.

CHAPTER 6: PLANT-DERIVED AGENTS
Sanjiv S. Agarwala

Plants have been the source for agents used to treat cancer since the nineteenth century. The oldest known plant-derived (or alkaloid) chemotherapeutic agent is colchicine, which was shown to bind to the mitotic spindle and lead to mitotic arrest. The traditional plant alkaloids, vincristine and vinblastine, are derived from the pink periwinkle and are the most widely used plant-derived agents in chemotherapy. Vindesine (desacetyl vinblastine) is another vinca alkaloid, derived from vinblastine and displaying similar activity. Although vindesine has shown efficacy in a number of malignancies, particularly non–small cell lung cancer, its use is not yet approved in the United States. Vinzolidine and navelbine are two newer derivatives of vinblastine that have aroused considerable interest, particularly due to their availability in both oral and parenteral forms. These two agents are currently being tested in clinical trials.

Paclitaxel is the prototype of a new class of agents, the taxanes, currently garnering significant attention as potentially effective chemotherapeutic agents. The epipodophyllotoxins, etoposide and teniposide, are semisynthetic compounds derived from podophyllotoxin, a plant product. A brief overview of these classes and the key individual agents within them is presented in this chapter (Table 1).

SOURCE

Although extracts of the common periwinkle plant (*Vinca rosea lynn*) were initially tested for their potential hypoglycemic properties, they were found instead to cause bone marrow suppression in rats. This finding led to the systematic extraction of vincristine and vinblastine for use as cancer chemotherapeutic agents. Podophyllotoxin is a substance extracted from the May apple or mandrake plant *Podophyllum peltatum*, a tree that holds a well-established place in American Indian folklore. Paclitaxel, originally isolated in 1971, is obtained from the Western yew known as *Taxus brevofolia*.

MECHANISMS OF ACTION

Unlike most chemotherapeutic agents, the vinca alkaloids and paclitaxel do not target DNA. Vincristine, vinblastine, and their related agents cause mitotic arrest of the cell in metaphase by reversibly binding to tubulin. Tubulins are structural proteins that are an integral part of eukaryotic cells and are the major component of the mitotic spindle. Microtubules of the mitotic spindle are responsible for mitotic separation of the chromosomes during mitosis. The tubulins possess several distinct sites that bind to the vinca alkaloids. Separate binding sites have been isolated for colchicine, the vinca alkaloids, and paclitaxel. The vinca alkaloids exert their antineoplastic effect by binding to tubulin and inhibiting microtubule assembly.

The vinca alkaloids may also alter the structure and function of lipid membranes, leading to cellular disruption by virtue of their hydrophobic properties. Paclitaxel, on the other hand, alters the dynamics of microtubule assembly and disassembly and stabilizes the microtubule, "freezing" the cell in the $G_2 + M$ phase of the cell cycle [1].

Although podophyllotoxin itself acts on microtubules to inhibit their polymerization, its two clinically useful derivatives etoposide and teniposide act on DNA. Their target is the nuclear enzyme DNA topoisomerase II, the enzyme responsible for catalyzing the separation of daughter DNA strands prior to miosis [2]. By inhibiting this enzyme, these drugs lead to permanent cross-linking of DNA strands and, consequently, to cell death.

MECHANISMS OF RESISTANCE

Of particular relevance to this drug class is the phenomenon of cross-resistance, whereby resistance to one of these drugs is often associated with resistance to many of the naturally derived chemotherapeutic drugs. Included in this group of cross-resistant agents are the podophyllotoxins and the DNA intercalators duanorubicin, doxorubicin, and mitoxantrone but not the antimetabolic or alkylating agents. The most widely studied mechanistic component of this multi-drug–resistant phenotype is the membrane protein p-glycoprotein, which is found in high concentration in drug-resistant cells. This protein is encoded by the *mdr1* gene and is thought to function as a membrane efflux pump that actively extrudes chemotherapeutic drugs from the interior of the cell by an energy ATP-dependent

Table 1. Properties of Plant-derived Chemotherapeutic Agents

Agent	Class	Mechanism of Action	Metabolism	Elimination Half-life (hr)	Major Toxicity	Major Clinical Application
Vincristine	Vinca alkaloid	Binds to tubulin arresting mitotic cells	Hepatic	28–30	Peripheral neuropathy	ALL, lymphoma, childhood tumors
Vinblastine	Vinca alkaloid	Binds to tubulin arresting mitotic cells	Hepatic	24–26	Myelosuppression (leukopenia)	Hodgkin's disease, testicular cancer
Etoposide	Epipodophyllotoxin	Inactivation of topoisomerase II alters DNA synthesis	Unknown (30–40% excreted unchanged in urine, 2% in bile)	4–8	Leukopenia	Testicular cancer, small cell lung cancer
Teniposide	Epipodophyllotoxin	Inactivation of topoisomerase II alters DNA synthesis	Unknown (15–20% excreted unchanged in urine)	6–48	Leukopenia	Refractory ALL, AML
Paclitaxel	Taxane	Promotes microtubule assembly	Uncertain (possibly hepatic)	1.3–8.6	Neutropenia, cardiotoxicity, allergic reaction	Refractory ovarian carcinoma, breast cancer

mechanism, leading to decreased intracellular drug concentration. P-glycoprotein is present in small quantities in drug-sensitive cells; amplification of the *mdr1* gene is the basis for increasing the expression of this protein. The degree of resistance to the agents correlates with the p-glycoprotein content of the cell. Cells resistant to chemotherapy due to increased p-glycoprotein show homogeneously staining chromosomal regions or double-minute chromosomes on cytogenetic analysis.

P-glycoprotein is significantly homologous to a number of ATP-binding proteins in bacteria, suggesting that it functions as a general transport protein. This thought is further borne out by the fact that significant amounts of p-glycoprotein are found in various epithelial tissues, such as colonic mucosa and renal tubular epithelium.

The *mdr1* gene has been found to be overexpressed in many tumor types that are traditionally resistant to chemotherapy. Certain classes of drugs, particularly the calcium channel blockers (*eg*, verapamil, quinidine), actively compete to bind with p-glycoprotein. This phenomenon has led to efforts to modulate or circumvent this resistance by combining these agents with chemotherapeutic agents [3].

Another less well-explored mechanism for resistance to the vinca alkaloids is the genetically mediated mutations of the alpha and beta subunits of tubulin. As a consequence of these mutations, binding of the alkaloid to the tubulin substrate is decreased [4]. This mechanism may also underlie the potential resistance to paclitaxel, which has been noted in a rodent cell line.

PHARMACOKINETICS

The pharmacokinetics of the vinca alkaloids depend upon the route of administration. When the agents are given by traditional intravenous bolus, they exhibit a triphasic pattern of plasma clearance with a terminal half-life of approximately 24 hours [5]. Vinblastine and vincristine are rapidly taken up by various tissues, including platelets, which may account for the initial rapid clearance from circulation; the drug is then slowly released from these sites, leading to the prolonged terminal phase. Both of these alkaloids are actively metabolized in the liver, which is the primary mode of excretion. Dosage reductions of 50% are therefore recommended in patients with a serum bilirubin > 3 mg/dl. The administration of these drugs by continuous intravenous infusion is thought to lead to higher steady-state concentrations than those achieved by bolus therapy [6].

Etoposide can be given both orally and intravenously. The oral bioavailability is approximately 50%, with peak concentrations occurring about 1 hour after administration. Absorption is not affected by food. Intravenous injection leads to peak plasma concentrations of 30 µg/ml, with biphasic clearance and a terminal half-life of about 8 hours that is independent of both dose and mode of administration (bolus or continuous infusion). Teniposide exhibits bi- or triphasic plasma clearance, with a terminal half-life of about 40 hours. Both etoposide and teniposide are highly protein bound. Etoposide is metabolized in the liver. About 40% of etoposide is excreted unchanged in the urine, which necessitates dosage reduction in patients with renal insufficiency. Teniposide is metabolized to inactive metabolites before it is excreted in the urine, therefore dosage reduction is unnecessary in the setting of renal insufficiency. Neither agent penetrates the cerebrospinal fluid to any significant degree.

Based upon results of various phase I studies, paclitaxel is usually given by 24-hour intravenous infusion. It is extensively bound to plasma proteins and displays a biphasic pattern of elimination [7]. Its site of metabolism and mode of excretion are as yet undefined.

TOXICITIES

Although the vinca alkaloids are similar in structure, vincristine and vinblastine display markedly different spectrums of clinical toxicity. Much of the toxicity induced by vincristine is derived from its action on microtubules. Microtubules are ubiquitous structures found in diverse, dividing and nondividing cell types. For example, microtubules are involved in neuronal transport; neurotoxicity, dose-limiting for vincristine, may result as a direct consequence of this inhibition of neuronal function. Disruption of the microtubular structure of platelet membranes may lead to altered platelet function. The dose-limiting toxicity of vinblastine is myelosuppression. Vindesine causes leukopenia without thrombocytopenia; it also produces neurotoxicity similar to that of vincristine. Paclitaxel causes dose-limiting neutropenia with relative sparing of the other hematopoietic cell lines. Type I hypersensitivity reactions have largely been prevented by the prophylactic administration of dexamethasone.

The major toxicity of the epipodophyllotoxins is hematologic in character (neutropenia and thrombocytopenia). Other side effects include transient hepatic enzyme abnormalities, alopecia, allergic reactions, and peripheral neuropathy.

EFFICACY AND USE

The vinca alkaloids have been widely incorporated into several combination chemotherapy protocols. Such application is based upon their distinct mechanism of action, and because their toxic properties differ considerably from the alkylators, antimetabolites, and other agents. For instance, because of its dose-limiting neurologic toxicity, vincristine is an attractive candidate for incorporation into regimens using myelosuppressive drugs. Vincristine is used in the therapy of the leukemias, Hodgkin's disease, non-Hodgkin's lymphoma, and the childhood tumors neuroblastoma, rhabdomyosarcoma, and Wilms' tumor. Vinblastine is used effectively against the lymphomas, testicular cancer, renal cell carcinoma, mycosis fungoides, and Kaposi's sarcoma [8].

Paclitaxel has undergone intensive investigation in a number of phase I and II trials and has demonstrated activity against ovarian carcinoma, including disease refractory to other agents, breast carcinoma, non–small cell lung carcinoma, and melanoma. Etoposide is active against a wide range of neoplasms, of which small cell lung cancer, testicular cancer, and non–small cell lung cancer are the most responsive. It has also shown promise in various hematologic malignancies, including acute myeloid leukemia. Teniposide is an investigational agent that has demonstrated activity in combination with cytarabine in acute myeloid leukemia and other pediatric hematologic malignancies. Other tumors against which this agent is active include non-Hodgkin's lymphoma, bladder cancer, and small cell lung cancer.

ACKNOWLEDGMENT

I wish to gratefully acknowledge the generous help of Dr. Jack Yalovich, PhD in the preparation of this chapter.

REFERENCES

1. Schiff PB, Fant J, Horwitz SB: Promotion of microtubule assembly in vitro by taxol. Nature 1979, 277:665–667.
2. Wozniak AJ, Ross WE: DNA damage as a basis for 4'-demethylepipodophyllotoxin-9-(4,6-O-ethylidene-beta-D-glucopyranoside) (etoposide) cytotoxicity. *Cancer Res* 1983, 43:120–124.
3. Beck WT: Multidrug resistance and its circumvention. *Eur J Cancer* 1990, 26:513–515.
4. Cabral FR, Brady RC, Schibler MJ:A mechanism of cellular resistance to drugs that interfere with microtubule assembly. *Ann NY Acad Sci* 1986, 466:745–756.
5. Nelson RL: The comparative clinical pharmacology and pharmacokinetics of vindesine, vincristine, and vinblastine in human patients with cancer. *Med Ped Oncol* 1982, 10:115–127.
6. Wiernik PH, Schwartz EL, Strauman JJ, *et al.*: Phase 1 clinical and pharmacokinetic study of taxol. *Cancer Res* 1987, 47:2486–2493.
7. Clark PI, Slevin ML: The clinical pharmacology of etoposide and teniposide. *Clin Pharmacokinet* 1987, 12:223–252.
8. Rowinsky EK, Donehower RC: The clinical pharmacology and use of antimicrotubule agents in cancer chemotherapeutics. *Pharmacol Ther* 1991, 52:35–84.
9. Greco FA, Johnson DH, Hainsworth JD: Chronic daily administration of oral etoposide. *Sem Oncol* 1990, 17(suppl 2):71–74.
10. Cavalli F, Sonntag RW, Jungi F, *et al.*: VP-16-213 monotherapy for remission induction of small cell lung cancer: A randomized trial using three dosage schedules (abstract). *Cancer Treat Rep* 1978, 62:473–475.
11. Slevin ML, Clark PI, Joel SP, *et al.*: A randomized trial to evaluate the effect of schedule on the activity of etoposide in small-cell lung cancer (abstract). *J Clin Oncol* 1989, 7:1333–1340.
12. O'Dwyer PJ, LaCreta FP, Daugherty JP, *et al.*: Phase I pharmacokinetic study of intraperitoneal etoposide (abstract). *Cancer Res* 1991, 51:2041–2046.
13. Porter LL III, Johnson DH, Hainsworth JD, *et al.*: Cisplatin and etoposide combination chemotherapy for refractory small cell carcinoma of the lung. *Cancer Treat Rep* 1985, 69:479–481.
14. Greco FA, Johnson DH, Hainsworth JD: Etoposide/cisplatin-based chemotherapy for patients with metastatic poorly differential carcinoma of unknown primary site (abstract). *Sem Oncol* 1992, 19(suppl 13):14–18.
15. Lasser EC, Walters A, Reuter SR, Lang J: Histamine release by contrast media. *Radiology* 1971, 100:683–686.
16. Rowinsky EK, Eisenhauer EA, Chaudhry V, *et al.*: Clinical toxicities encountered with paclitaxel (Taxol). *Sem Oncol* 1993, 20(suppl 3):1–15.
17. Swenerton K, Eisenhauer E, ten Bokkel Huinink W, *et al.*: Taxol in relapsed ovarian cancer: High vs low dose and short vs long infusion (abstract). *Proc ASCO* 1993, 12:256.
18. Rowinsky EK, Gilbert MR, McGuire WP, *et al.*: Sequences of taxol and cisplatin: A phase I and pharmacologic study. *J Clin Oncol* 1991, 9:1692–1703.
19. Madoc-Jones H, Mauro F: Interphase action of vinblastine and vincristine: Differences in their lethal action through the mitotic cycle of cultured mammalian cells. *J Cell Physiol* 1968, 72:185–196.
20. Jackson DV, Bender RA: Cytotoxic thresholds of vincristine in a murine and human leukemia cell line *in vitro*. *Cancer Res* 1979, 39:4346–4349.

ETOPOSIDE

Etoposide is a derivative of podophyllotoxin, an ancient substance used in the nineteenth century as a topical agent for the treatment of skin cancers. Chemically, etoposide is a β-glycoside of podophyllotoxin, with a molecular weight of 588 and with reduced toxicity and greater therapeutic efficacy than the parent compound.

It was originally thought that etoposide and teniposide exerted their neoplastic activity through mitotic inhibition, similar to podophyllotoxin. However, their major mechanism of action is now known to be interference of DNA synthesis by interaction with the enzyme topoisomerase II. Topoisomerase II is responsible for "untangling" daughter chromosomes during mitosis. During this process it causes transient breaks in DNA strands. These breaks are then resealed by this same enzyme. This resealing is inhibited by the podophyllotoxin derivatives, leading to permanent breaks in DNA strands. Maximal cytotoxic effect occurs on cells in the G2–S phase; this may be due to the decreased topoisomerase content of resting cells. Another postulated mechanism of action is the formation of toxic-free radicals with consequent cytotoxicity. Prolonged low-dose exposure to etoposide may be more important than intermittent bolus doses; therefore there has been an increased interest in chronic, low-dose oral administration of etoposide [9].

DOSAGE AND ADMINISTRATION

Testicular cancer: 50–100 mg/m^2 IV for 3–5 d [10,11] employed in combination with other agents
Small cell lung carcinoma: 35–50 mg/m^2/d IV for 3–5 d **or** 400–800 mg/m^2/d IV, with or without autologous bone marrow support
Kaposi's sarcoma: 150 mg/m^2/d IV for 3 d every 4 wk
Peritoneal metastases: max dose of 700 mg/m^2 by intraperitoneal infusion [12]

DOSAGE MODIFICATIONS: hold treatment if absolute neutrophil count < 500/mm^3 or platelets < 500,000/mm^3.

SPECIAL PRECAUTIONS

Anaphylaxis and anaphylactoid reactions (slow rate of infusion is preferred)
Close monitoring of hematologic function agent
Patients with impaired renal function (dosage reductions may be indicated)

TOXICITIES

Hematologic: leukopenia (dose-limiting and possibly severe); thrombocytopenia and anemia (less common)
GI: moderately severe nausea and vomiting (30–40% of patients); diarrhea and stomatitis (10%, particularly at high doses and may be dose-limiting)
Anaphylaxis: following IV administration (reduce rate of infusion)
Cardiovascular: transient hypotension (more common in the elderly)
Dermatologic: reversible alopecia (70% of patients); pruritus, hyperpigmentation, radiation recall dermatitis (uncommon)
Neurologic: mixed (sensorimotor) neuropathy (1–2%, greater frequency with combination of vincristine or other agents)
Miscellaneous: dystonic reactions, radiation recall, phlebitis

INDICATIONS

FDA-approved: testicular cancer, small cell lung cancer; **clinical studies show activity in:** Kaposi's sarcoma, peritoneal metastases

PHARMACOKINETICS

With IV infusion: Distribution highly bound to plasma proteins with a steady-state volume of distribution of 7–20 l/m^2; **Absorption**—CSF penetration is poor (< 5%) unless given at high doses; **Half-life**—90 min and 3–12 hr (terminal); **Elimination**—30–40% excreted unchanged in the urine, 2% in bile; **Dose adjustment**—possibly indicated in patients with compromised renal function
With oral administration: Distribution—oral bioavailability is about 50%; **Absorption**—not affected by food; **Peak plasma concentrations**—1–4 hr after oral administration

DRUG INTERACTIONS

Cisplatin [13], cyclophosphamide, vincristine, cytosine arabinoside, and 5-fluorouracil

RESPONSE RATES

Nonseminomatous testicular germ cell cancer (as single agent)—response rates of 35% in patients, both *de novo* and in those with refractory disease; in combination regimen—61% complete response rate; Stage II seminoma (in cisplatin-based regimens)—complete response rate of 61%; small cell lung cancer (as single agent)—response rates of 30–35%; in combination with cisplatin—response rates of approximately 50% in previously treated patients; non–small cell lung cancer (with cisplatin)—response rates of up to 40%; non-Hodgkin's and Hodgkin's disease—objective response rates of 30–40% in previously treated non-Hodgkin's lymphoma of unfavorable histology; metastatic carcinoma of unknown primary site (with cisplatin)—73% response rate in 78 evaluable patients (31% were complete [14])

PATIENT MONITORING

Observe closely for anaphylactoid reactions (discontinue if hypotension occurs); monitor hematologic function before and frequently during therapy; monitor CBC and platelet counts twice weekly

NURSING INTERVENTIONS

Administer by slow IV infusion; avoid extravasation of drug (a vesicant), wear protective gloves during handling

PATIENT INFORMATION

Patients should notify physician at first signs of infection while on treatment

FORMULATION

Available as VePesid®, Bristol-Myers Oncology Division, Princeton, NJ
Multiple-use vials of 20 mg/ml. Stored at room temperature. 50-mg capsules. Stored at 2–8°C.

PACLITAXEL

Paclitaxel is the prototype of the taxanes, a new and important group of antineoplastic agents. It was originally derived from the bark of the Pacific or Western yew, a comparatively rare and ancient inhabitant of the Pacific Northwest forests. Ongoing efforts to produce synthetic analogues have resulted in the development of taxotere, an analogue with promising potential.

As a promoter of microtubule assembly, paclitaxel is distinct from the vinca alkaloids and other tubulin-interacting drugs. All aspects of tubulin polymerization are enhanced at concentrations as low as 50 nM. By stabilizing the microtubule and preventing its disassembly, paclitaxel causes tubulin-microtubule disequilibrium, which eventually leads to cell death. Aggregates, or bundles, of microtubules are induced by paclitaxel to interact with other cellular organelles, including myosin, the Golgi apparatus, and smooth and rough endoplasmic reticulum. Due to the widespread presence of microtubules in various cell types, paclitaxel affects multiple cellular functions, including fibroblast activity, leukocyte migration, and sperm motility. The clinical significance of these observations is unknown.

DOSAGE AND ADMINISTRATION

Three hour infusion: The FDA has recently approved the following: for ovarian cancer: 135 mg/m^2 or 175 mg/m^2. IV over 3 hr every 3 wk; for breast cancer: 175 mg/m^2 over 3 hr every 3 wk. The 3-hr infusion may be associated with a lower incidence of neutropenia [17].

SPECIAL PRECAUTIONS

Hypersensitivity and hypotensive reactions (premedicate with H$_1$ and H$_2$ blockers and steroids [15] and use longer infusion rates)
Patients with pre-existing cardiac disease

TOXICITIES

Myelosuppression: neutropenia (frequently severe and dose-limiting) [16]; anemia and thrombocytopenia (much less common)
Cardiac: arrhythmias, transient bradycardia (up to 30% of patients); hemodynamically significant progressive atrioventricular or bundle branch block (about 5% of patients treated in phase II trials)
Hypersensitivity: possibly severe reactions, manifesting as hypotension, bronchospasm, urticaria
Neurologic: sensory neuropathy presenting as glove-and-stocking anesthesia; motor neuropathy (less common)
GI: anorexia, nausea, vomiting (uncommon and not severe); mucositis (at high doses)
Dermatologic: alopecia (universal at doses above 130 mg/m^2) reversible, but involves all hair sites

INDICATIONS

FDA-approved: relapsed metastatic ovarian cancer; metastatic breast cancer that has failed an anthracycline-based regimen.

PHARMACOKINETICS

Peak plasma concentrations–range from 0.6–13 umol/l, with higher peaks following shorter infusion times; **Distribution**—mean volume of distribution about 87 l/m^2; **Half-life**—biphasic; 1.3–8.6 hr (terminal); **Absorption**—detected in ascitic fluid but not in cerebrospinal fluid; **Elimination**—site of metabolism uncertain (possibly liver); 5% recovered unchanged in the urine

DRUG INTERACTIONS

Cisplatin [18]

RESPONSE RATES

Non–small cell lung cancer—responses of 21–24% in two phase II studies of previously untreated patients; response rate of 34% in patients with advanced small cell lung cancer; Ovarian cancer—20–35% response rate in patients refractory to other agents including platinum (phase II studies); Breast cancer—objective responses of 56–62% in previously treated patients

PATIENT MONITORING

Monitor carefully for neutropenia; reduce dose if infections develop; observe for hypersensitivity reaction

NURSING INTERVENTIONS

Watch for hypersensitivity; avoid extravasation (can lead to local pain, erythema, swelling); prepare infusions in glass bottles and infuse through polyethylene-lined sets with in-line filter

PATIENT INFORMATION

Patient should be aware of possibility of hypersensitivity reaction and neutropenia

FORMULATION

Available as Taxol®, Bristol-Myers Oncology Division, Princeton, NJ
30 mg/5 cc single dose.

TENIPOSIDE

Teniposide shares a common source and mechanism of action with etoposide. Although the synthesis of this agent preceded that of etoposide, it is not approved for use in this country except as a second-line agent in the treatment of acute lymphoblastic leukemia (ALL) in children. It has been widely tested and extensively used in Europe.

DOSAGE AND ADMINISTRATION

Acute lymphoblastic leukemia in children: 165—250 mg/m^2 slow IV infusion (30–60 min) to avoid reactions or hypotension
Bladder carcinoma: 50 mg/30–50 ml of sterile water or 0.9% sodium chloride instilled directly into bladder

SPECIAL PRECAUTIONS

Patients with hepatic and renal impairment
Patients who have been heavily pretreated with myelosuppressive agents or radiation therapy

TOXICITIES

Hematologic: leukopenia (dose-limiting)
GI: moderate nausea and vomiting, stomatitis, diarrhea, mucositis
Cardiovascular: hypotension with rapid infusion (probably due to Cremaphor® diluent), decreased with slower infusion rates (> 30 min)

INDICATIONS

FDA-approved: second-line agent for ALL in children

PHARMACOKINETICS

Distribution—8–30 l/m^2 volume; **Absorption**—limited penetration into CSF; **Half-life**—bi- or triphasic plasma clearance, 6–48 hr terminal half-life; **Protein binding**—more than etoposide and more completely metabolized; **Metabolism**—uncertain; **Elimination**—10–20% unchanged in the urine

DRUG INTERACTIONS

Cytosine arabinoside (combination used to treat myeloid leukemia)

RESPONSE RATES

ALL in children refractory to other agents—effective in combination with cytosine arabinoside; Hodgkin's and non-Hodgkin's lymphoma—response rates of about 30%; Other responsive malignancies—acute myeloid leukemia (AML), small cell lung cancer, carcinoma of the bladder, neuroblastoma

PATIENT MONITORING

Observe closely for anaphylactoid reactions (discontinue if hypotension occurs); monitor hematologic function before and frequently during therapy; monitor CBC and platelet counts twice weekly.

NURSING INTERVENTIONS

Administer by slow IV infusion; avoid extravasation; wear protective gloves during handling

PATIENT INFORMATION

Patient should be aware of possibility of anaphylactic reaction

FORMULATION

Available as Vumon®, Bristol-Myers Oncology Division, Princeton, NJ
Vials of 10 mg/ml concentration for injection. Stored at room temperature.

VINBLASTINE

Vinblastine is formulated as vinblastine sulfate, an alkaloid also isolated from *Vinca rosea lynn*. It differs from vincristine by one alkyl group. Its mechanism of action is similar to that of vincristine, that is, it arrests cells as they enter metaphase by binding to tubulin.

DOSAGE AND ADMINISTRATION

3.7 mg/m^2 (5 mg in adult) by continuous 24-hr infusion, gradually increasing to 18.5 mg/m^2; most patients are unable to tolerate more than 10–12 mg/wk. Give drug at weekly intervals. (When used as part of the ABVD [doxorubicin, bleomycin, vinblastine, dacarbazine] regimen for Hodgkin's disease, the dose is 6 mg/m^2.)

DOSE MODIFICATIONS: *hold drug if WBC count < 4000/mm^3; reduce dose by 50% if serum bilirubin ≥ 3 mg/dl.*

SPECIAL PRECAUTIONS

Elderly, cachectic patients
Patients who have had prior chemotherapy or radiation (risk of leukopenia)
Patients with elevated liver enzymes or serum bilirubin
Extreme irritant to tissues: free-flowing IV line only; precautions against extravasation; corneal ulceration possible upon eye contact

TOXICITIES

Hematologic: myelosuppression (dose-limiting) with leukopenia (common), thrombocytopenia and anemia (less frequent)
GI: nausea and vomiting (common), abdominal pain, constipation, ileus (possibly due to neurotoxicity); mucositis of the oral and pharyngeal membranes (frequent)
Dermatologic: alopecia (partial and reversible)
Neurologic: sensorimotor neuropathy (less severe and less frequent than with vincristine, only occurring at high doses); autonomic neuropathy (see **GI** toxicity above)
Cardiovascular: hypertension more commonly than hypotension, Raynaud's phenomenon (possible late and prolonged side effect, usually with combination chemotherapy)
Endocrine: syndrome of inappropriate antidiuretic hormone secretion

INDICATIONS

FDA-approved: Hodgkin's disease, testicular cancer, choriocarcinoma, non–small cell lung cancer, bladder carcinoma, head and neck and cervical cancer; **palliative therapy** for choriocarcinoma, breast cancer, Kaposi's sarcoma, mycosis fungoides

PHARMACOKINETICS

Absorption: not administered orally, erratic absorption through GI tract, does not penetrate into CSF; **Distribution**—rapidly taken up by tissues; **Protein binding**—80%; **Half-life**—25 hr; **Metabolism**—primarily in liver; **Elimination**— <20% excreted in urine; **Dose adjustment**—indicated in patients with liver dysfunction

DRUG INTERACTIONS

L-Asparaginase, methotrexate, digoxin, phenytoin

RESPONSE RATES

Hodgkin's disease (with ABVD regimen)—response rates of 50–80%, complete responses of 10–30%; advanced nonseminomatous germ cell tumors of the testis (with PBV [cisplatin, bleomycin, vinblastine] regimen)—produced dramatic cures in patients (largely replaced now by BEP [bleomycin, etoposide, platinum] regimen)

PATIENT MONITORING

Monitor WBC count before treatment and weekly thereafter, check liver function at initiation of treatment

NURSING INTERVENTIONS

Give antiemetics; avoid extravasation of drugs (aspirate venous blood into syringe before and after administration to assure line placement); if extravasation occurs aspirate residual drug, apply heat to effected area, inject 150 mg of hyaluronidase SC around injection site

PATIENT INFORMATION

Patient should notify physician at first signs of infection while on treatment

FORMULATIONS

Available as Vinblastine Sulfate Injection, Lyphomed, Deefield, IL;
Velban®, Eli Lilly and Company, Indianapolis, IN;
Velsar®, Adria Laboratories, Dublin, OH;
Vinblastine Sulfate Sterile, Cetus Oncology Corporation, Emeryville, CA
Vials of 10 mg of vinblastine lyophilized powder. Stored at room temperature and protected from light.

VINCRISTINE

Vincristine is an alkaloid derived from **Vinca rosea lynn**, the common periwinkle. It is a dimeric compound formed from two multiringed units, vindoline and catharanthine, that are joined by a carbon–carbon bridge. It is available as vincristine sulfate. Its major mechanism of action appears to be the arrest of cells as they enter metaphase, by binding to tubulin.

DOSAGE AND ADMINISTRATION

IV bolus (in combination chemotherapy regimens): 1.4 mg/m^2 at weekly intervals (adult dose).
IV continuous infusion: low, sustained concentrations inhibit the formation of microtubules *in vitro* [19] and clinically [20]. The superiority of this method of administration remains to be confirmed in the clinical setting.

DOSE MODIFICATION: reduce by 50% when serum bilirubin ≥ 3 mg/dl.

SPECIAL PRECAUTIONS

Patients with liver disease, particularly those with obstructive jaundice
In elderly patients, neurotoxicity may manifest as constipation
Extreme irritant: give only through free-flowing IV line

TOXICITIES

Neurologic: dose-limiting sensorimotor neuropathy, manifesting first as numbness and paresthesias in the toes and fingers and loss of ankle jerk reflex (do not mandate dose reduction); painful paresthesias, muscle cramps, and ataxia (dose reduction or discontinuation is recommended); foot and wrist drop are late manifestations and are irreversible; autonomic neuropathy—unexplained abdominal pain, severe constipation, and ileus (particularly in elderly); possible urinary retention and incontinence; cranial nerve involvement leading to hoarseness, diplopia, and facial weakness; occasionally headache and jaw pain; depression, confusion, and other alterations in mental status
Dermatologic: reversible alopecia (20% of patients), skin rashes (rare)
Endocrine: syndrome of inappropriate antidiuretic hormone excretion (rare)
Hematologic: much less pronounced effects on bone marrow than with vinblastine; occasional leukopenia and/or thrombocytopenia; possible increase in platelet count by stimulation of endoreduplication of megakaryocytes
Cardiovascular: occasional hypo- or hypertension

INDICATIONS

FDA-approved: acute lymphoblastic leukemia in children and adults, lymphoma (Hodgkin's and non-Hodgkin's), childhood tumors (Wilms', Ewing's sarcoma, and rhabdomyosarcoma); **clinical studies show activity in:** small cell lung cancer, multiple myeloma, breast cancer

PHARMACOKINETICS

Absorption: not given orally due to poor oral bioavailability; **Distribution**—limited penetration into CSF, triphasic serum clearance when given by bolus IV injection, rapidly taken up by plasma tissues and slowly released; **Peak plasma concentrations**—about 500 nM and steady-state concentrations between 1–2 nM; **Half-life**—longer than that of other vinca alkaloids; **Metabolism**—in liver; **Elimination:** excretion in the bile—70% in feces, 15% unchanged in urine

DRUG INTERACTIONS

L-Asparaginase, methotrexate, digoxin

RESPONSE RATES

ALL—in combination regimens complete remission rate of 90%; Hodgkin's disease (in MOPP [mechlorethamine, vincristine, procarbazine, prednisone] regimen)— complete remission rate in 70–80% of patients (about two thirds are disease-free for 10 yr and presumed cured); Childhood tumors (with cyclophosphamide)—responses in up to 100% of children with neuroblastoma; response rates of 80—90% in rhabdomyosarcoma and Wilms' tumor (in combination with other drugs)

PATIENT MONITORING

Assess for neurotoxicity (loss of Achilles tendon reflex, note further signs of peripheral neuropathy); monitor liver functions closely, especially if abnormal at start

NURSING INTERVENTIONS

Avoid extravasation during administration; if extravasation occurs, apply moderate heat together with hyaluronidase at site

PATIENT INFORMATION

Patient should be aware of potential neurotoxicity; if foot drop occurs, special caution while driving

FORMULATIONS

Available as Oncovin®, Eli Lilly and Company, Indianapolis, IN;
Vincasar PFS® (preservative free), Adria Laboratories, Dublin, OH;
Vincristine Sulfate Injection, Lymphomed, Deerfield, IL
Vials containing 1 mg/ml of drug. Stored at 2–8°C and protected from light.

ETIOLOGY AND RISK FACTORS

The incidence of breast cancer in the United States has been rising steadily during the past few decades. Early detection through patient screening and self-examination accounts for only part of this trend. The death rate and incidence of advanced breast cancer have remained stable, while the number of early stage, particularly node-negative, and *in situ* lesions has increased. This trend may be due in part to earlier detection, improvement in surgical and radiation therapy techniques, and the increasing use of systemic adjuvant therapy. Approximately 185,000 new cases and 45,000 deaths from breast cancer are projected in 1993. Risk factors for the development of breast cancer include older age, immediate family history of breast cancer at a young age or bilateral breast cancer, early menarche, late menopause, nulliparity, the use of prolonged, high doses of conjugated estrogens, exposure to ionizing radiation at a young age, and a past history of atypical hyperplasia on breast biopsy. Dietary risks from high-fat or low-fiber diets, however, have been hard to demonstrate.

Table 1. Staging of Breast Cancer

Primary tumor	Criteria
Tx	Primary tumor size cannot be assessed
Tis	Carcinoma in situ
T1	
T1a	<0.5 cm
T1b	0.5–1.0 cm
T1c	>1.0–2.0 cm
T2	>2–5 cm
T3	>5 cm
T4	Tumor of any size fixed to the chest wall or skin
T4a	Fixation to chest wall only
T4b	Edema (peau d'orange), ulceration of skin, satellite skin nodules
T4c	Both T4a and T4b
T4d	Inflammatory changes
Nodes	
Nx	Regional lymph nodes cannot be assessed
N0	No regional lymph node metastases
N1	Involved, movable ipsilateral axillary lymph nodes
N2	Involved, fixed ipsilateral axillary lymph nodes
N3	Involved, ipsilateral internal mammary lymph nodes
Metastases	
Mx	Metastases cannot be assessed
M0	No metastases
M1	Distant metastases present, including nonregional (ie, ipsilateral supraclavicular) lymph nodes
Stage	**TNM Staging**
I	T1N0
IIA	T2N0, T0N1, T1N1, T2N0
IIB	T2N1, T3N0
IIIA	T0–3N2, T3N1
IIIB	T4N0–3M0, T0–4N3M0
IV	Any M1

From Beahrs et al. [17]; with permission.

STAGING AND PROGNOSIS

Patients presenting with a palpable breast lesion, new breast asymmetry, or mammographic abnormalities (including microcalcifications, dominant mass, significant architectural distortion or asymmetric density) should undergo a biopsy. Fine-needle aspiration performed and interpreted by an experienced pathologist has a positive predictive value of close to 100%, although negative predictive values ranging from 87 to 99% may warrant examination of additional tissue based on the situation [1]. Excisional biopsy, or needle localization for nonpalpable mammographic abnormalities, can also be carried out, with suitable tissue preparation for histopathologic examination and measurement of hormone receptor content.

Apart from the measurement of hormone receptor content, no clear consensus exists on how to base clinical decisions on other tumor parameters such as ploidy, S-phase percent, cathepsin D, epidermal growth factor receptor, or HER2/*neu* oncogene expression; therefore, these determinations need not be performed outside of the investigative setting. Full surgical TNM staging should be determined for all invasive tumors after partial or complete mastectomy and axillary lymph node dissection (Table 1). Testing for preoperative staging should include a complete blood count, serum measurements of liver function, and a chest radiograph. Radionuclide bone scintigraphy and liver scan are of low yield in asymptomatic Stage I disease, but may be considered in more advanced stages.

THERAPY FOR PRIMARY DISEASE

Primary local therapy for patients with clinical Stage I and II disease can be accomplished with either a modified radical mastectomy or partial mastectomy followed by external beam irradiation. Local and distant recurrence rates are equal with either approach if negative margins are accomplished with breast-conserving surgery [2]. Axillary lymph node dissection is necessary for staging as such information is needed to choose the appropriate adjuvant therapy, although there is conflicting evidence as to whether or not lymph node dissection reduces on distant recurrences or improves survival time. Locally advanced (Stage III) disease is generally treated with initial induction chemotherapy, followed by mastectomy, radiotherapy, or both. Primary therapy, including mastectomy or radiotherapy for metastatic disease, can improve local control but does not effect survival. This approach may be suitable for patients with large primary lesions who have a good functional status; it is sometimes facilitated after an initial response to hormonal therapy or chemotherapy.

ADJUVANT THERAPY FOR REGIONAL DISEASE

The single most powerful predictor of relapse in operable breast cancer (Stages I and II) is the presence of axillary nodal involvement. Multiple randomized trials have demonstrated the benefit of cytotoxic and hormonal therapy in delaying the recurrence of breast cancer and improving 5- and 10-year overall survival in certain subsets of patients. An overview analysis, including data from 133 such trials, has recently been published [3]. Relative reductions in annual rates of recurrence and death of 25 and 17%, respectively, were seen with tamoxifen treatment compared to similar treatment without tamoxifen. Treatment with polychemotherapy compared to similar treatment without polychemotherapy yielded relative reductions of 28 and 17%.

Node-positive Patients

Outcome among node-positive patients in the overview analysis has confirmed the findings of many individual trials. A significant reduction in mortality was seen with tamoxifen treatment among women aged over 50 years with node-positive disease; the benefit was nearly doubled for patients with tumors classified as estrogen receptor (ER) rich (≥10 fmol/mg) compared to ER poor. Indirect comparisons suggested that 2 to 5 years of tamoxifen therapy was superior to 1 year. The addition of chemotherapy to tamoxifen in older women reduced the odds of recurrence, but not the mortality rate. Only one study has demonstrated a survival benefit from the addition of chemotherapy to tamoxifen [4], and further trials are under way to address this controversial issue. For women aged under 50 years, the analysis found a significant reduction in mortality rates with chemotherapy. In the chemotherapy trials, results with combination chemotherapy regimens were superior to those with single agents, but there was no advantage to long-term administration (≥12 months) over short-term administration (≤6 months). The CMF combination regimen was the most represented in the analysis. No benefit was seen with the addition of tamoxifen to chemotherapy among women aged under 50.

There is as of yet no firm evidence that adjuvant chemotherapy regimens other than standard CMF provide a greater advantage for node-positive patients. Although doxorubicin-containing regimens produce superior response rates in metastatic breast cancer, few trials have directly assessed anthracycline content in the adjuvant setting. A comparison of CMF to CAF has not demonstrated a difference in outcome [5]. Alternatively, doxorubicin-based regimens have been examined in order to shorten the duration of chemotherapy without compromising effectiveness. Short, intensive doxorubicin and cyclophosphamide (AC) was found to be equally effective as standard oral CMF [6]. AC treatment required less than half the total time of treatment and one third the number of health professional visits as standard CMF, but it was accompanied by more vomiting and greater hair loss.

The roles of total dose and dose intensity (defined as the amount of drug administered per unit of time) beyond conventional ranges are currently being studied. Preliminary results from one such trial that randomized patients to low-, moderate-, and high-dose CAF revealed a significant survival difference between low and moderate or high doses, but no difference between moderate and high doses [7]. However, since the low doses used in this study are lower than conventional CAF, this difference may be more indicative of a threshhold effect, signifying a minimal effective dose necessary to delay recurrence. A true dose intensity effect might be shown if future follow-up reveals an outcome difference between moderate- and high-dose arms that contain equal total doses but a dose intensity ratio of about 2.

In summary, adjuvant chemotherapy is indicated in women aged under 50 with positive axillary lymph nodes. Standard oral CMF for 6 months remains the standard regimen, while shorter, more intensive AC for 4 cycles is an alternative for patients who prefer shorter treatment times and fewer clinic visits, at the cost of greater toxicities [6]. The use of more intense doxorubicin-containing regimens, dose intensification, multiagent sequential therapy, or chemohormonal therapy remains investigational. Therefore, current recommendations for adjuvant therapy for node-positive patients include tamoxifen administration for 2 to 5 years for women aged over 50 and CMF polychemotherapy for 6 months for women aged under 50. Additionally, the use of tamoxifen in patients under age 50 and chemotherapy in older women remain experimental and are being evaluated in ongoing trials.

Node-negative Patients

Due to the comparatively low 10-year recurrence rate of about 30% among node-negative patients, large numbers of patients must be studied to detect significant outcome differences. It has therefore been difficult to demonstrate a benefit of systemic adjuvant therapy from earlier trials within this subset of patients. In 1990, a National Institutes of Health Consensus Conference recommended the consideration of adjuvant hormonal or cytotoxic therapy for some patients with node-negative breast cancer, although no criteria were provided on whom to treat. This was based on the findings of four trials limited to node-negative patients that differed considerably in design yet all demonstrated small but significant improvements in relapse-free (but not overall) survival among treated patients compared to those receiving no treatment. The Intergroup Study included ER-negative patients with tumors of any size and ER-positive patients with tumors greater than 3 cm; the treatment group received CMF plus prednisone [8]. In the Ludwig V Study, the treated group received a single cycle of perioperative intravenous CMF and leucovorin [9], whereas the National Surgical Adjuvant Bowel and Breast Project Group treated ER-positive patients with tamoxifen (10 mg twice a day) and ER-negative patients with sequential methotrexate and 5-fluorouracil for 12 cycles [10,11].

Although it is plausible that certain node-negative patients may benefit from tamoxifen treatment if their tumor is ER positive or from chemotherapy if their tumor is ER negative or greater than 3 cm, results from the overview analysis suggest that absolute survival benefits from adjuvant therapy are discernable but very small; those due to chemotherapy do not reach statistical significance [3]. A new generation of studies is now ongoing to assess the independent values of cytotoxic and hormonal therapy, as well as the relative merits of alkylating and doxorubicin-based regimens. Considerable variability in outcome exists within node-negative patients, and a greater absolute benefit of therapy may be derived from high-risk patients, whereas the the potential long-term risks of hormonal and cytotoxic therapy must be weighed against the smaller benefit in low-risk patients [12]. Further risk stratification based on tumor size, hormone receptor content, and other indices, including DNA ploidy, S-phase percent, and HER2/*neu* expression, may help select appropriate candidates for treatment [13]. However, such approaches need to be validated prospectively before they can be incorporated into standard clinical practice [14].

THERAPY FOR ADVANCED DISEASE

Locally Advanced Breast Cancer

Locally advanced breast cancer generally encompasses Stage III disease, defined by the presence of a large primary tumor (>5 cm) or bulky ipsilateral axillary or internal mammary nodes (N2 or N3). Surgery alone results in low long-term survival rates, whereas the addition of radiation therapy appears to lower the incidence of local, but not distant recurrence. The advent of preoperative induction chemotherapy followed by definitive local therapy (mastectomy, radiation therapy, or both) has resulted in improved disease-free and overall survival times compared to historical controls, although few randomized, comparative trials have been performed. The largest such trial reported improvement in local recurrence, but not distant recurrence or survival, with endocrine and/or cytotoxic therapies added to radiation therapy compared to radiation therapy alone [15]. When combined with chemotherapy, the local control modalities of mastectomy versus radiation therapy have resulted in equal relapse-free and overall survival rates in a randomized trial [16]. Recently published series using doxorubicin-containing induction regimens, such as FAC (due to this agent's superior response rate in metastatic breast cancer), followed by either radiation therapy, mastectomy, or both, followed by additional chemotherapy, have yielded complete response rates (at the time of surgery) of 58 to 100%, 3- to 5-year relapse-free survival rates of 20 to 73% and local recurrence rates of 13 to 38%.

Inflammatory breast cancer is identified by the clinical appearance of a diffuse erythema, peau d'orange (edema), and ridging in the skin overlying the tumor or by histopathologic evidence of tumor emboli within dermal lymphatics [17]. Strategies similar to those used for locally advanced breast cancer have yielded similar or slightly lower response and survival rates [18]. Due to the small number of patients that present with locally advanced or inflammatory breast cancer, the optimal treatment has not been defined by a series of controlled, randomized studies. A reasonable approach includes initial hormonal treatment (in ER-positive, older patients) or combination chemotherapy such as CMF or CAF (in ER-negative, younger patients) for two to four cycles or until a plateau in the response is reached, followed by modified radical mastectomy and/or radiation therapy, and then additional chemotherapy. The role of dose intensification (with or without bone marrow support), optimal agents, duration of use, and sequence of modalities remains undetermined.

Metastatic Breast Cancer

Of the approximately 45,000 deaths in the United States due to breast cancer, virtually all are associated with progressive metastatic disease. Although metastatic breast cancer is not curable with any current modality, the length and quality of life of patients with relapsed or newly diagnosed disseminated breast cancer upon presentation vary greatly. The median survival rate from time of presentation of 2 to 3.5 years has been reported, with 25 to 35% of patients living beyond 5 years and up to 10% living beyond 10 years [19]. Factors associated with a more favorable prognosis include longer interval from initial diagnosis to recurrence, older age, lower number of involved sites, sites limited to bone or soft tissue, ER-positive disease, and low histologic grade. The effect of any therapy on survival is modest at best. Therefore, the timing of therapy and the selection of agents should reflect therapeutic goals whose benefits outweigh the toxicity of treatment. In general, palliation of organ-specific symptoms related to tumor or a rapid clinical course suggestive of impending multiorgan involvement would be a greater impetus for systemic therapy, whereas local therapy such as radiation of an isolated symptomatic boney lesion or close observation of asymptomatic patients with few sites of involvement may be more appropriate.

Endocrine Therapy

Approximately one third of unselected patients with metastatic breast cancer (and two thirds of those with ER-positive tumors) will respond to endocrine manipulation [20]. Endocrine agents are best used as initial therapy in patients with ER-positive tumors in older patients, and in those exhibiting low-burden, predominantly nonvisceral disease. These modalities yield equivalent results, with the possible exception of androgens and corticosteroids alone resulting in slightly lower response rates (Table 2). For premenopausal patients, oophorectomy or tamoxifen treatment may be considered first, followed by progestin or androgen treatment in the event of progression.

First-line endocrine therapy for postmenopausal patients generally consists of tamoxifen, followed by a progestin, an estrogen, an aromatase inhibitor, or androgen upon progression. Ablative thera-

pies, such as adrenalectomy and hypophysectomy, are not used today due to surgical risks and complications. There is no evidence that doses higher than those listed in Table 2 for tamoxifen, megestrol acetate, fluoxymesterone, or aminoglutethimide are more effective. Only a few studies have demonstrated superior response rates when using combinations of these agents, and generally there has not been an improvement in median survival rates [19]. The median duration of response to any of these endocrine therapies is between 1 and 2 years. Response rates and durations of response are less with retreatment with a second or third agent upon progression. There is no evidence that combination hormonal treatment results in greater response rates. Although chemohormonal treatment may lead to higher response rates compared to hormonal treatment alone, a survival benefit has not been demonstrated [19]. Furthermore, in ER-positive patients with metastatic breast cancer, response rates to hormonal therapy and chemotherapy are equal. The roles of newer antiestrogens, aromatase inhibitors, luteinizing hormone-releasing hormone analogues, antiprogestins, and somatostatin analogues are under investigation (see Chapter 5 for further discussion).

Chemotherapy

About two thirds of all patients with metastatic breast cancer will have a response to some form of chemotherapy, although complete response rates in the range of 5 to 25% have been reported in most trials. The median duration of response to chemotherapy is 6 to 12 months [19]. Previous phase II trials have demonstrated single-agent response rates of 27 to 33% for the four drugs considered to be the most active in patients with metastatic breast cancer: doxorubicin, cyclophosphamide, methotrexate, and 5-fluorouracil [19]. Combination chemotherapy can achieve higher response rates, albeit at the cost of greater toxicity. Therefore, the most widely used combinations in the treatment of metastatic breast cancer are CMF and CAF. Doxorubicin, taken as a single agent, is a less toxic alternative, especially in patients previously exposed to CMF, to which no cross resistance exists. Although doxorubicin-containing regimens such as CAF appear to result in superior response rates compared to doxorubicin alone, the difference in survival time is modest and it is accompanied by higher toxicity. In the responding patients, the duration of therapy for optimal palliation and survival is not clear. Comparative studies that have examined regi-

Table 2. Endocrine Therapy for Metastatic Breast Cancer

Endocrine Maneuver	Setting	Dose
Ablative oophorectomy	Premenopausal	
Competitive antiestrogen Tamoxifen	Premenopausal (esp ER-positive) Postmenopausal	20 mg/d
Progestin Megestrol acetate	Any age	40 mg qid
Estrogen Diethylstilbesterol Ethinyl estradiol Conjugated estrogen	Postmenopausal	5 mg tid 1 mg tid 2.5 mg tid
Aromatase inhibitor Aminoglutethimide	Postmenopausal	250 or 500 mg bid
Androgen Fluoxymesterone	Any age	10 mg bid

mens of increasing dose intensity have failed to show a benefit, except in those trials in which the lower doses were less intensive than standard CMF or CAF [21]. Two studies that randomized patients to receive intermittent chemotherapy (3 to 6 cycles) and retreatment at time of progression versus continuous or longer term (18 cycles) therapy demonstrated increased response rates and better quality of life, but no or only marginal improvement in survival rates [22, 23].

It should be emphasized that cumulative doses of doxorubicin exceeding 450 mg/m^2 are associated with significant cardiotoxicity [24]; therefore, doxorubicin should not be given beyond this total dose, avoided entirely in patients with clinical evidence of congestive cardiomyopathy, and used with caution (perhaps accompanied by frequent measurement of ejection fraction [EF] and withheld for EF <40% or a fall of >10–20% from baseline) in patients at risk for cardiac disease or those approaching toxic cumulative doses. Likewise, systemic side effects need to be monitored, with therapy modified or adjusted accordingly (see protocol).

Salvage chemotherapy for refractory patients generally results in lower response rates and durations of response compared to those for front-line therapy. There are few comparative trials to guide the clinician in the most appropriate regimen. Patients who have not previously received doxorubicin are best treated with either doxorubicin as a single agent or in combination with other drugs such as vinblastine and thiotepa. Alternatively, single agents, including mitomycin C and vinblastine, yield response rates of 25 to 30% [19]. Although many small uncontrolled trials have examined combinations including these and other drugs, the latter are associated with increased toxicity and direct comparative studies are lacking. There are no definitive data on the merit of combination or sequential chemohormonal regimens. The roles of other active agents (including taxanes, platinum, etoposide, mitoxantrone, and 5-fluorouracil with leucovorin modulation, as well myeloablative regimens with peripheral stem cell or bone marrow support and subablative therapy with recombinant hematopoietic growth factors) are under active investigation.

REFERENCES

1. Harris JR, Lippmann ME, Veronesi U, et al.: Breast cancer. N Engl J Med 1992, 327:319–328.

2. Fisher B, Redmond C, Poisson R, et al.: Eight year results of a randomized clinical trial comparing total mastectomy and lumpectomy with or without irradiation in the treatment of breast cancer. N Engl J Med 1989, 320:822–828.

3. Early Breast Cancer Trialists' Collaborative Group: Systemic treatment of early breast cancer by hormonal, cytotoxic, or immune therapy. Lancet 1992, 339:1–15, 71–85.

4. Fisher B, Redmond C, Legault-Poisson S, et al.: Postoperative chemotherapy and tamoxifen compared with tamoxifen alone in the treatment of positive-node breast cancer patients aged 50 years or older with tumors resposive to tamoxifen: Results from NSABP B-16. J Clin Oncol 1990, 8:1005–1018.

5. Carpenter JT, Velez-Garcia E, Aron BS, et al.: Prospective, randomized comparison of cyclophosphamide, doxorubicin (Adriamycin) and fluorouracil (CAF) vs. cyclophosphamide, methotrexate and fluorouracil (CMF) for breast cancer with positive axillary nodes: A Southeastern Cancer Study Group Study. Proc ASCO 1991, 10:45.

6. Fisher B, Brown AM, Dimitrov NV, et al.: Two months of doxorubicin-cyclophosphamide with and without interval reinduction therapy compared with 6 months of cyclophosphamide, methotrexate and fluorouracil in positive-node breast cancer patients with tamoxifen-nonresponsive tumors: Results from the National Surgical Adjuvant Breast and Bowel Project B-15. J Clin Oncol 1990, 8:1483–1496.

7. Budman DR, Wood W, Henderson IC, et al.: Initial findings of CALGB 8541: A dose and dose intensity trial of cyclophosphamide, doxorubicin, and 5-fluorouracil as adjuvant treatment of stage II, node +, female breast cancer. Proc ASCO 1992, 11:51.

8. Mansour EG, Gray R, Shatila AH, et al.: Efficacy of adjuvant chemotherapy in high-risk node-negative breast cancer. N Engl J Med 1989, 320:485–490.

9. The Ludwig Breast Cancer Study Group: Prolonged disease-free survival after one course of perioperative adjuvant chemotherapy for node-negative breast cancer. N Engl J Med 1989, 320:491–496.

10. Fisher B, Constantino J, Redmond C, et al.: A randomized clinical trial evaluating tamoxifen in the treatment of patients with node-negative breast cancer who have estrogen-receptor-positive tumors. N Engl J Med 1989, 320:479–484.

11. Fisher B, Redmond C, Dimitrov NV, et al.: A randomized clinical trial evaluating sequential methotrexate and fluorouracil in the treatment of patients with node-negative breast cancer who have estrogen-receptor-negative tumors. N Engl J Med 1989, 320:473–478.

12. Curtis RE, John MA, Boice JD, et al.: Risk of leukemia after chemotherapy and radiation treatment for breast cancer. N Engl J Med 1992, 326:1745–1751.

13. McGuire WL, Clark GM: Prognostic factors and treatment decisions in axillary node-negative breast cancer. N Engl J Med 1992, 326:1756–1761.

14. Henderson IC: Breast cancer therapy—The price for success. New Engl J Med 1992, 326:1774–1775.

15. Rubens RD, Bartelink H, Engelsman E, et al.: The contribution of cytotoxic and endocrine treatment to radiotherapy. An EORTC Breast Cancer Co-operative trial (10792). Eur J Cancer Clin Oncol 1989, 25:667–678.

16. Perloff M, Lesnick GJ, Korzun A, et al.: Combination chemotherapy with mastectomy or radiation for stage III breast carcinoma: A Cancer and Leukemia Group B study. J Clin Oncol 1988, 6:261–269.

17. Beahrs OH, Henson DE, Hutter RVP, et al.: Manual for Staging of Cancer, 4th ed. 1992, Philadelphia: JB Lippincott, pp 149–154.

18. Jaiyesimi IA, Buzdar AU, Hortobagyi G: Inflammatory breast cancer: A review. J Clin Oncol 1992, 10:1014–1024.

19. Henderson IC, Harris JR: Principles in the management of metastatic disease. In Harris JR, Hellman S, Henderson IC, et al. (eds): Breast Diseases. 1991, Philadelphia: JB Lippincott, pp 547–679.

20. Glauber JG, Kiang DT: The changing role of hormonal therapy in advanced breast cancer. Sem Oncol 1992, 19:308–316.

21. Sledge GW, Antman KH: Progress in chemotherapy for metastatic breast cancer. Sem Oncol 1992, 19:317–332.

22. Coates A, Gebski V, Bishop JF, et al.: Improving the quality of life during chemotherapy for advanced breast cancer. A comparison of intermittent and continuous treatment strategies. N Engl J Med 1987, 317:1490–1495.

23. Ejlerten B, Pfeiffer P, Pederson D, et al.: Diminished efficacy by reducing duration of CEF from 18 to 6 months in the treatment of metastatic breast cancer. Proc ASCO 1990, 9:23.

24. Von Hoff DD, Layard MW, Basa P, et al.: Risk factors for doxorubicin-induced congestive heart failure. Ann Intern Med 1979, 91:710–717.

25. Bonadonna G, Valagussa P, Rossi A, et al.: Ten-year results with CMF-based adjuvant chemotherapy in resectable breast cancer. Breast Cancer Res Treat 1985, 5:95–115.

26. Umsawasdi T, Valdivieso M, Booser DJ, et al.: Weekly doxorubicin vs doxorubicin every 3 weeks in cyclophosphamide, doxorubicin and cisplatinum chemotherapy for non-small cell lung cancer. Cancer 1989, 64:1995–2000.

27. Shapiro J, Gotfried M, Lishner M, et al.: Reduced cardiotoxocity of doxorubicin by a 6-hour infusion regimen: A prospective randomized evaluation. Cancer 1990, 65:870–873.

CMF
Cyclophosphamide, Methotrexate, and 5-Fluorouracil

Cyclophosphamide is an alkylating agent that inhibits DNA replication and is therefore toxic to dividing cells. Methotrexate is an antimetabolite that inhibits dihydrofolate reductase and the subsequent generation of thymidine necessary for DNA synthesis. 5-Fluorouracil is likewise an antimetabolite that blocks the methylation of deoxyuridylate to thymidylate, inhibiting the synthesis of RNA and DNA. This combination of agents is used because the agents possess different modes of action and are noncross-resistant and can therefore eradicate resistant clones.

DOSAGE AND SCHEDULING

Cyclophosphamide 100 mg/m^2 po daily d 1-14	████████████████████													
MTX 40 mg/m^2 iv, d1,8	■							■						
5-FU 600 mg/m^2 iv, d1,8	■							■						
CBC, lytes, Cr, LFT	☐							☐						
Day	1	2	3	4	5	6	7	8	9	10	11	12	13	14

6 cycles for adjuvant therapy

DOSAGE MODIFICATIONS: *50% of cyclophosphamide, MTX, or 5-FU for WBC<3.5k, platelet 75-100k; hold therapy for WBC<2.5k, platelet<75k. Use 75% MTX for creatinine clearance <50 mL/min, 50% if <25 mL/min.*

RECENT EXPERIENCES AND RESPONSE RATES

Study	Evaluable patients, n	Dosage/schedule	Response (%) for metastatic dis.
Valagussa et al, Proc Am Soc Clin Oncol 1983, 2:111	53	C 100 mg/m^2 po d 1–14 M 40 mg/m^2 iv d 1, 8 F 600 mg/m^2 iv d 1, 8	53
Canellos et al, Cancer 1976, 38: 1882-1886	93	C 100 mg/m^2 po d 1–14 M 60 mg/m^2 iv d 1, 8 F 600 mg/m^2 iv d 1,8	53
Muss et al, Arch Int Med 1977, 137: 1711-1714	38	C 10 mg/kg iv d 1, 5 mg/kg iv d 15 then q 7 d M 0.2 mg/kg iv d 1, 0.1 mg/kg iv d 15 then q 7 d F 12 mg/kg iv d 1, 10 mg/kg d 15 then q 7 d	34
Aisner et al, J Clin Oncol 1987, 5: 1523-1533	99	C 100 mg/m^2 po d 1–14 M 40 mg/m^2 iv d 1, 8 F 500 mg/m^2 iv d 1, 8	37
Creech et al, Cancer 1975 35:1101-1107	46	C 50 mg/m^2 po d 1–14 M 25 mg/m^2 iv d 1, 8 F 500 mg/m^2 iv d 1, 8	46

CANDIDATES FOR TREATMENT

Adjuvant treatment of premenopausal node-positive and selected node-negative patients, metastatic disease in patients with aggressive visceral disease or failed initial hormonal therapy

SPECIAL PRECAUTIONS

Enhanced leukopenia and skin toxicity with concomitant radiation therapy

ALTERNATIVE THERAPIES

CAF or AC combination chemotherapy for adjuvant therapy; CAF or single-agent doxorubicin for metastatic disease

TOXICITIES

Cyclophosphamide: nausea, vomiting, anorexia, fatigue, cystitis, leukopenia, anemia, thrombocytopenia, alopecia, pigment changes in skin and nails; pulmonary fibrosis, hepatitis, renal tubular necrosis (rare); **Methotrexate:** nausea, vomiting, mouth sores, fatigue, dermatitis, leukopenia, hepatitis; interstitial pneumonitis, renal tubular damage (rare); **5-FU:** nausea, vomiting, anorexia, diarrhea, abdominal cramps, mouth sores, dermatitis, hyperpigmentation, photosensitivity, phlebitis, increased tearing of eyes, leukopenia, anemia; vascular complications including heart attack and stroke (rare)

DRUG INTERACTIONS

Cyclophosphamide: phenobarbital; **methotrexate:** nonsteroidal anti-inflammatory agents, sulfa drugs, nonabsorbable antibiotics; **5-FU:** interferon, leucovorin

NURSING INTERVENTIONS

Give antiemetic (usually prochlorperazine and/or lorazapam) and evaluate blood counts and sometimes renal and hepatic function prior to administration.

PATIENT INFORMATION

Patient should immediately report severe mucositis, chest pain, shortness of breath, signs of infection (fever, chills, dysuria), diarrhea, and abdominal cramps. High fluid intake is necessary while taking cyclophosphamide.

CAF
Cyclophosphamide, Doxorubicin, and 5-Fluorouracil

Doxorubicin is an anthacycline whose mode of action is inhibition of mitosis by intercalation of DNA. Although there is no clear evidence that this combination of drugs is superior to CMF in the adjuvant setting, it is clear that it is more toxic. In metastatic breast cancer, CAF is associated with a higher rate and duration of response, but no difference in the overall survival rate. Due to doxorubicin's superior single-agent activity in metastatic breast cancer, this regimen is commonly used in high-risk Stage II and in Stage III and IV breast cancers (see discussion on CMF).

DOSAGE AND SCHEDULING

ORAL CYCLOPHOSPHAMIDE REGIMEN

Cyclophosphamide 100 mg/m² po daily days 1-14	■													
Doxo 30 mg/m² iv, d 1,8	■							■						
5-FU 500 mg/m² iv, d 1,8	■							■						
CBC, lytes, Cr, LFT	□							□						
Day	1	2	3	4	5	6	7	8	9	10	11	12	13	14

IV CYCLOPHOSPHAMIDE REGIMEN

Cyclo 500 mg/m² iv	■							
Doxo 50 mg/m² iv	■							
5-FU 500 mg/m² iv, d 1,8	■							■
CBC, lytes, Cr, LFT	□							□
Day	1	2	3	4	5	6	7	8

DOSAGE MODIFICATIONS: *Use 50% of cyclophosphamide, 5-FU, or doxorubicin for WBC<3.5k, platelet 75-100k; hold therapy for WBC<3.5k platelet<75k. Use 50% doxorubicin for bilirubin 1.5-3.0 mg/dl, 25% dose for >30 mg/dl.*

RECENT EXPERIENCES AND RESPONSE RATES

Study	Evaluable patients, n	Dosage/schedule	Response (%) for metastatic dis.
Kardinal, *et al*, Breast Cancer Res Treat 1983 3:365-372	116	C 100mg/m² po d 1-14 A 25 mg/m² iv d 1,8 F 500 mg/m² iv d 1,8 q 4 wk	51
Tranum, *et al*, Cancer 1978, 41:2078-2083	105	C 400 mg/m² iv d 1 A 40 mg/m² iv d 1 F 400 mg/m² iv d 1,8 q 3 wk	49
Smalley, *et al*, Cancer 1977, 40:625-632	59	C 500 mg/m² iv d 1 A 50 mg/m² iv d 1 F 500 mg/m² iv d 1 q 3 wk	64
Tormey, *et al*, Cancer Clin Trials 1979, 2:247-256	46	C 100 mg/m² po d 1-14 A 30 mg/m² iv d 1,8 F 500 mg/m² iv d 1,8 q 4 wk	52
Vogel, *et al*, J Clin Oncol 1984, 2:643-651	66	C 500 mg/m² iv d 1 A 50 mg/m² iv d 1 F 500 mg/m² iv d 1 q 3 wk	29
Bull, et al, *Cancer* 1978, 41:1649-1657	38	C 100 mg/m² po d 1-14 A 30 mg/m² iv d 1,8 F 500 mg/m² iv d 1,8 q 4 wk	82

CANDIDATES FOR TREATMENT
Adjuvant treatment of premenopausal, node-positive patients and patients with locally advanced disease; metastatic disease in patients with aggressive visceral disease or failed initial hormonal therapy

SPECIAL PRECAUTIONS
Patients undergoing radiotherapy; cardiotoxicity with cumulative doxorubicin >450 mg/m², further enhanced with concommitant radiotherapy; extravasation of doxorubicin, a vesicant, may lead to tissue necrosis; it should be administered by experienced personnel through large peripheral or central vein.

ALTERNATIVE THERAPIES
CMF or AC combination chemotherapy for adjuvant therapy; CMF or single-agent doxorubicin for metastatic disease

TOXICITIES
Cyclophosphamide: nausea, vomiting, anorexia, fatigue, cystitis, leukopenia, anemia, thrombocytopenia, alopecia, pigment changes in skin and nails; pulmonary fibrosis, hepatitis, renal tubular necrosis (rare); **Doxorubicin:** nausea, vomiting, anorexia, mucositis, alopecia, onycholysis, extravasation reaction, anaphylaxis (rare); congestive cardiomyopathy (with high doses); **5-FU:** nausea, vomiting, anorexia, diarrhea, abdominal cramps, mouth sores, dermatitis, hyperpigmentation, photosensitivity, phlebitis, increased tearing of eyes, leukopenia, anemia; vascular complications including myocardial infarction and stroke (rare)

DRUG INTERACTIONS
Cyclophosphamide: phenobarbital; **Doxorubicin:** cyclophosphamide, 6-mercaptopurine; **5-FU:** interferon, leucovorin

NURSING INTERVENTIONS
Give antiemetic and evaluate blood counts and renal and hepatic function prior to administration.

PATIENT INFORMATION
Patient should report severe mucositis, chest pain, shortness of breath, diarrhea and abdominal cramps, signs of infection, skin redness, or pain at infusion site immediately. High fluid intake is necessary while taking cyclophosphamide.

AC
Doxorubicin and Cyclophosphamide

In the NSABP B-15, the AC regimen was used in the adjuvant setting for node-positive women. The rates for relapse-free and overall survival were equivalent to those with standard CMF. However, the AC regimen was delivered in half the total time with one third the office visits, but at the expense of more vomiting and alopecia. (See discussions on CMF and CAF.)

DOSAGE AND SCHEDULING

Cyclo 600 mg/m² iv	■							
Doxo 60 mg/m² iv	■							
CBC, lytes, Cr, LFT	☐							
Day		1	2	3	4	5	6	7

Cycle q 3 wk × 4 cycles

DOSAGE MODIFICATIONS: *Dose is withheld if granulocytes are <1000 and platelets <100,000. If fever accompanies neutropenia, reduce subsequent AC dose by 25% or consider full doses with recombinant G-CSF. Use 50% doxorubicin for bilirubin 1.5–3.0 mg/dl, 25% dose for 30 mg/dl.*

RECENT EXPERIENCE AND RESPONSE RATES

Study	Evaluable patients, *n*	Dosage/schedule	3-Yr Disease-free survival (%)
Fisher *et al*, J Clin Oncol 1990 8:1483-1496	535	Doxo 60 mg/m² iv q 3 wk x 4 cycles	68
		Cyclo 600 mg/m² iv q 3 wk x 4 cycles	

CANDIDATES FOR TREATMENT
Adjuvant treatment of node-positive patients

SPECIAL PRECAUTIONS
Enhanced toxicity with radiotherapy. Cardiotoxicity with cumulative doxorubicin >450 mg/m², further enhanced with concommitant radiotherapy. Extravasation of doxorubicin, a vesicant, may lead to tissue necrosis; it should be administered by experienced personnel through large peripheral or central vein.

ALTERNATIVE THERAPIES
CMF or CAF combination chemotherapy

TOXICITIES
Cyclophosphamide: nausea, vomiting, anorexia, fatigue, cystitis, leukopenia, anemia, thrombocytopenia, alopecia, pigment changes in skin and nails; pulmonary fibrosis, hepatitis, renal tubular necrosis (rare); **Doxorubicin:** nausea, vomiting, anorexia, mucositis, alopecia, onycholysis, extravasation reaction, anaphylaxis (rare)

DRUG INTERACTIONS
Cyclophosphamide: phenobarbital; **Doxorubicin:** cyclophosphamide, 6-mercaptopurine

NURSING INTERVENTIONS
Give antiemetic and evaluate blood counts and renal and hepatic function prior to administration.

PATIENT INFORMATION
Patient should report severe mucositis, chest pain, shortness of breath, diarrhea and abdominal cramps, skin redness, signs of infection, or pain at infusion site immediately. High fluid intake is necessary while taking cyclophosphamide.

VATH
Vinblastine, Doxorubicin, Thiotepa, and Fluoxymesterone

VATH is a doxorubicin-based combination commonly used as second-line chemotherapy for metastatic breast cancer, especially if the patient has not had prior exposure to doxorubicin. Single-agent regimens are preferable, since no randomized comparative trials have been performed to compare this to other less-toxic single-agent regimens.

DOSAGE AND SCHEDULING

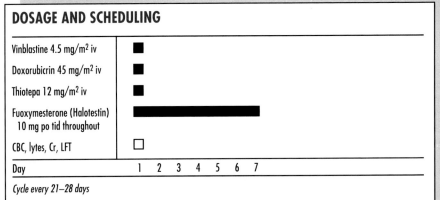

	Day	1	2	3	4	5	6	7

Vinblastine 4.5 mg/m² iv

Doxorubicrin 45 mg/m² iv

Thiotepa 12 mg/m² iv

Fuoxymesterone (Halotestin) 10 mg po tid throughout

CBC, lytes, Cr, LFT

Cycle every 21–28 days

DOSAGE MODIFICATIONS: *Delay vinblastine if neutrophil count <2000, platelet count <120,000; 50% doxorubicin or vinblastine if total bilirubin 1.5–3.0 mg/dL; 25%, >3.0 mg/dL.*

RECENT EXPERIENCE AND RESPONSE RATES

Study	Evaluable patients, *n*	Dosage/schedule	Response (%) for metastatic disease*
Perloff, *et al*, Cancer 1978, 42:2534-2537	19	V 2.25 mg/m² iv d 1,5 A 11.25 mg/m² iv d 1,5 T 6 mg/m² iv d 1 H 30 mg po q d continuous q 4 wk	52
Hart, *et al*, Cancer 1981, 48:1522-1527	29	V 4.5 mg/m² iv d 1 A 45 mg/m² iv d 1 T 12 mg/m² iv d 1 H 20 mg po q d continuous q 3 wk	45
Skeel *et al*, Cancer 1989, 64:1393-1399	84	V 4.5 mg/m² iv d 1 A 45 mg/m² iv d 1 T 12 mg/m² iv d 1 H 20 mg po q d continuous q 3 wk	38

No patients had received doxorubicin prior to therapy

CANDIDATES FOR TREATMENT
Recurrent or metastatic breast cancer in those patients who have failed first- or second-line therapy and have no prior exposure to doxorubicin

SPECIAL PRECAUTIONS
Administer through large or central vein. Enhanced marrow suppression with concommitant radiotherapy

ALTERNATIVE THERAPIES
Single-agent doxorubicin, vinblastine or mitomycin C

TOXICITIES
Drug combination: nausea, vomiting, anorexia, mucositis, alopecia, onycholysis, extravasation reaction, anaphylaxis (rare), myalgias, parathesias, neutropenia, anemia, thrombocytopenia.
Fluoxymesterone: hirsutism and cholestatic jaundice

DRUG INTERACTIONS
Cyclophosphamide, 6-mercaptopurine (doxorubicin)

NURSING INTERVENTIONS
Give antiemetic and evaluate blood counts and renal and hepatic function prior to administration.

PATIENT INFORMATION
Patient should report any redness or pain at infusion site. Severe headaches, confusion, nausea, vomiting, fever, and signs of infection should be reported immediately.

MITOMYCIN C AND VINBLASTINE

The combination of mitomycin C and vinblastine is used as second-line therapy for metastatic breast cancer. No comparative trials assessing this regimen over either single agent have been reported. It is possible that this combination is associated with a higher response rate at the cost of greater toxicity, particularly myelosuppression, given the known single-agent toxicities.

DOSAGE AND SCHEDULING

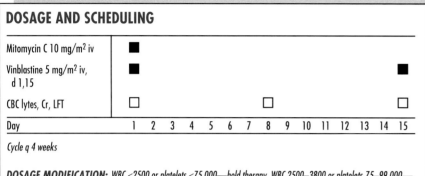

	1	2	3	4	5	6	7	8	9	10	11	12	13	14	15
Mitomycin C 10 mg/m² iv	■														
Vinblastine 5 mg/m² iv, d 1,15	■														■
CBC lytes, Cr, LFT	☐							☐							☐
Day	1	2	3	4	5	6	7	8	9	10	11	12	13	14	15

Cycle q 4 weeks

DOSAGE MODIFICATION: *WBC <2500 or platelets <75,000—hold therapy. WBC 2500–3800 or platelets 75–99,000— decrease all drugs by 25%.*

RECENT EXPERIENCES AND RESPONSE RATES

Study	Evaluable patients, n	Dosage/schedule	Response (%) for metastatic disease
Denefrio, *et al*, Cancer Treat Rep 1978, 62:2113–2115	14	M 6 mg/m² iv d 1 V 5 mg/m² iv d 1 q 2 wk	7
Konits, *et al*, Cancer 1981,48:1295–1298	303	M 20 mg/m² iv d 1 V 0.15 mg/mg iv d 1 q 3 wk	40
Garewal, *et al*, J Clin Oncol 1983, 1:772–775	22	M 10 mgm² iv d 1* V 5 mg/m² iv d 1 q 2 wk	32

CANDIDATES FOR TREATMENT

Recurrent or metastatic breast cancer in patients who have failed doxorubicin or other first- or second-line therapy containing doxorubicin

SPECIAL PRECAUTIONS

Patients with hepatic insufficiency; extravasation of vinblastine, a vesicant, may lead to tissue necrosis

ALTERNATIVE THERAPIES

Doxorubicin or VATH in patients not previously exposed to doxorubicin; single-agent mitomycin C or vinblastine

TOXICITIES

Drug combination: fevers, nausea, vomiting, anorexia, anemia, prolonged leukopenia, thrombocytopenia, hemolytic uremic syndrome, rare pulmonary fibrosis, renal toxicity, peripheral paresthesias, neuropathy, constipation and rare ileus

DRUG INTERACTIONS

None known

NURSING INTERVENTIONS

Give antiemetic and evaluate blood counts and renal and hepatic function prior to administration.

PATIENT INFORMATION

Patient should report any redness or pain at infusion site. Severe headaches, confusion, nausea, vomiting, fever, and signs of infection should be reported immediately.

Malignancies of the upper gastrointestinal tract pose substantial challenges for therapy. In most cases, surgery remains the mainstay of therapy and is the only known curative therapeutic modality for this group of diseases. However, the 5-year survival rates remain low and range from 3% for pancreatic adenocarcinoma to 15% for gastric cancer. These statistics have stimulated interest in alternate forms of management for these malignancies. Experience with chemotherapy and radiation therapy often as combined modality treatment with or without surgery is growing. In this chapter, a variety of chemotherapeutic approaches within each disease group are discussed and compared, and selected chemotherapeutic regimens that are in common use or that have unique applications in upper gastrointestinal tract cancer are highlighted. Risk factors and guidelines for the prevention of these cancers are presented in Tables 1 and 2.

ESOPHAGEAL CANCER

In 1993, 11,300 new cases of epidermoid and adenocarcinoma of the esophagus are expected in the United States and men have a more than twofold increase in risk compared with women. The overall 5-year survival rate is 9% for Caucasians and only 6% for African-Americans. Locoregional or systemic spread of disease is often attributed to the lack of anatomic barriers to dissemination. The esophagus does not have a serosa to provide a natural barrier for local invasion and this organ is rich in submucosal lymphatics, which may facilitate longitudinal spread from the primary site. Autopsy findings from patients who have recently undergone surgery for squamous cell carcinoma of the esophagus have demonstrated a high incidence of unsuspected early metastatic disease. TNM classification and staging criteria for esophageal cancer are provided in Table 3.

THERAPY FOR ADVANCED DISEASE

Historically, the use of single agent or combination chemotherapeutic regimens was restricted to patients with widespread metastatic disease, and the value of therapy was the subject of debate. Agents that have undergone adequate testing as single agents include bleomycin, mitomycin C, doxorubicin, cisplatin, carboplatin, plant alkaloids, various antimetabolites, lomustine, ifosfamide, and mitoguazone. Among the noninvestigational drugs, the most active agents appear to be cisplatin, mitomycin C, methotrexate, and 5-fluorouracil (5-FU) with or without leucovorin. The majority of regimens involving combination chemotherapy for metastatic disease

Table 1. Risk Factors for Cancers of the Upper Gastrointestinal Tract

Pancreas	Stomach
Cigarette smoking	*Helicobacter pylori* infection
Exposure to beta-napthylamine, benzidine	Achlorhydria
Chronic pancreatitis	Previous gastrectomy, Billroth II procedures
Liver	Esophagus
Hepatitis B carrier state	Exposure to nitrosamines
Chronic liver disease (chronic active	Cigarette smoking
hepatitis, cirrhosis)	Excessive alcohol use
Exposure to mycotoxin, ionizing	Lye ingestion
radiation, steroid hormones, arsenic	Achalasia
Bile ducts	Barrett's mucosa
Sclerosing cholangitis	Tylosis
Parasitic infections	
Use of steroid hormones	

Table 2. General Guidelines for Prevention and Early Detection of Cancers of the Upper Gastrointestinal Tract

Prevention	Early Detection*
Avoid cigarette smoking	Esophagus
Use alcohol in moderation	Annual upper gastrointestinal endoscopy
Eat a low-fat diet rich in fresh fruit and	in patients with known Barrett's mucosa,
vegetables	tylosis, or history of caustic esophageal
Avoid exposure to occupational toxins	injury
Immunize against infectious hepatitis	Hepatoma
Avoid unnecessary use of steroid	Periodic alpha-fetoprotein measurement
hormones	and liver ultrasound for patients with
	chronic liver disease

*Applicable only in certain high-risk conditions.

Table 3. TNM Staging Criteria for Esophageal Cancer

Staging	Criteria
T1	Tumor limited to lamina propria or submucosa
T2	Tumor involving muscularis propria
T3	Involvement of adventitia but no extraesophageal structures
T4	Extension to extraesophageal structures
Thoracic esophagus	
N0	No nodal involvement
N1	Regional* nodes involved
Cervical esophagus	
N0	No nodal involvement
N1	Regional† nodes involved
N2	(No longer defined)
N3	(No longer defined)
(Both)	
M0	No distant metastases
M1	Distant metastases present
Stage	TNM
I	T1, N0, M0
II	
IIA	T2-3, N0, M0
IIB	T1-2, N1, M0
III	T3, N1, M0
	T4, any N, M0
IV	Any T, any N, M1

Adapted from Hermanek and Sobin [1]; with permission.
*Mediastinal, perigastric (excluding celiac).
†Cervical, supraclavicular.

have built on this single-agent experience, and cisplatin has become the anchor in most combination regimens. Many of these trials have combined cisplatin with 5-FU, methotrexate, or bleomycin and occasionally have included a variety of agents with marginal single-agent activity. To date, there have been no prospective randomized trials comparing any combination regimen to single-agent therapy. However, the response rates for combination therapy appear to be higher than those achieved with single agents. For example, the objective response rate with cisplatin and 5-FU may be as high as 42% [2]. The response rates achieved with various other permutations of this regimen or regimens involving cisplatin and methotrexate or bleomycin range from 26 to 76% [32]. Recently, a phase II trial was reported in which the novel combination of interferon alpha-2a and 5-FU was tested in patients with advanced esophageal cancer [4]. A response rate of 27% (complete and partial responses) was reported in this trial. Further investigation with this regimen is expected in the future.

THERAPY FOR LOCALLY UNRESECTABLE DISEASE

Perhaps the most vigorously tested role of combination chemotherapy in esophageal cancer has been in the multimodality management of patients with local or regional involvement. In the past, radiation therapy has been the mainstay of therapy for patients who were believed to have disease that could not be resected with chance for cure. The definition of unresectable disease is somewhat debatable; however, it is commonly held that presenting lesions greater than 5 cm in length or with circumferential involvement or apparent local extension or evidence for lymph node involvement on a computed tomographic (CT) scan are less likely to be resectable for cure. The palliative effect of radiation to relieve dysphagia in these patients is excellent, with reported palliative responses of up to 80%. However, it is now well established that even a small change in tumor size can lead to a marked functional improvement resulting from a decrease in the resistance to flow (based on the law of LaPlace). This phenomenon may explain why the high palliative rate observed with radiation therapy alone has not resulted in significant changes in median survival. A variety of studies have assessed the safety, feasibility, and regression rates of combination chemotherapy and radiation for patients with locally unresectable disease. The mainstay of drug therapy in this setting has been 5-FU (which may have a radiation-enhancing effect) combined with a radiation-sensitizing drug such as cisplatin or mitomycin C. Pilot study experiences with this approach have shown encouragingly high 2-year survival rates. In some cases, durable complete responses have been observed [5]. An additional intriguing report of this approach in the treatment of patients with adenocarcinoma of the esophagus and gastroesophageal junction involved a combination of 5-FU and mitomycin C in addition to radiation therapy as definitive treatment. Complete responses in eight of nine patients with T1 and T2 disease and a median relapse-free survival of 10 months was observed [6]. Studies such as these led the Radiation Therapy Oncology Group (RTOG), the Southwest Oncology Group (SWOG), and the North Central Cancer Treatment Group (NCCTG) to conduct a randomized trial comparing a combination of 5-fluorouracil (1000 mg/m² by continuous infusion daily for 4 days) and cisplatin (75 mg/m² on day 1) plus 5000 cGy of radiation therapy with 6400 cGy of radiation therapy alone in patients with epidermoid carcinoma or adenocarcinoma of the thoracic esophagus [7]. As might be expected, the incidence of severe and life-threatening side effects (predominantly mucositis and myelosuppression) were

more frequently seen in patients treated with combined-modality therapy. One patient in the combined-modality group died from complications of renal and bone marrow failure. However, the group undergoing combination therapy experienced a prolonged median survival with a survival rate at 24 months of 38% in the combined-modality arm and 10% in the group treated with radiation alone. Control of both local and distant metastases was also superior in the combined-modality group. Both physicians and patients will have to weigh the benefits and side effects of these forms of therapy in electing treatment for unresectable esophageal cancer.

NEOADJUVANT THERAPY

An increasing amount of experience is also developing with combination chemotherapy with or without radiation prior to surgery. This neoadjuvant approach with combined radiation and chemotherapy, while encouraging, carries with it many caveats concerning additive and potentially life-threatening toxicities. As with regimens used in advanced disease, cisplatin is a common denominator and the reported response rates to preoperative therapy are remarkably similar; a recent report by Ajani et al. [8] suggests that a preoperative response rate of 49% can be achieved. Preliminary data are available from two randomized trials comparing preoperative chemotherapy with either immediate surgery [9] or with radiation therapy prior to surgery [10]. In both of these trials, major objective responses (47 and 53%, respectively) were reported for preoperative chemotherapy. However, median survival rates did not differ significantly in the trial that compared preoperative chemotherapy with immediate surgery. Because of a crossover design in the study comparing preoperative chemotherapy with preoperative radiation therapy, it is difficult to analyze the effect of therapy on disease-free or overall survival.

Experience with the combined use of chemotherapy and radiation therapy prior to esophagectomy is growing. Most of these studies use 5-FU as a common denominator in the induction chemotherapy as a single agent [11] in combination with cisplatin [12], or mitomycin C [13], or as a multiagent regimen [14]. Although all of these trials vary in their study populations with respect to the proportion of epidermoid carcinomas and adenocarcinomas and for presenting stages of disease, these reports are notable for the documentation of both complete and pathologic responses in all instances. Naunheim et al. [15] have reported an overall median survival of 23 months; in the report by Forastiere et al. [14], the median survival time had not been reached at a median follow-up of 26 months. These results appear to be better than those achieved historically. In both of the studies, the complete response rate assessed pathologically was more than 20%. Because the natural history of the disease in patients with complete pathologic response to therapy is not well understood and because durable complete responses have been reported in patients who were treated with chemotherapy and radiation therapy but not with esophagectomy [5], one question raised is whether esophagectomy is necessary for all responding patients. Confirmation of the value of this multimodality treatment, then, awaits testing in randomized trials comparing this approach to standard management for both resectable and unresectable disease.

STOMACH CANCER

Cancer of the stomach represents the only gastrointestinal malignancy that appears to be decreasing in incidence. The explanation for this perplexing change in incidence is not known; however, some have attributed this decrease to the common practice of adding ascorbic acid as a food preservative, which decreases the gastric pH and limits endogenous nitrosoamine production by bacteria in the upper gastrointestinal tract. A new link between gastric cancer and *Helicobacter pylori* infection as a risk factor has now been described [16]. In 1993, approximately 24,000 new cases of stomach cancer are expected and the overall 5-year survival rate for affected patients remains low, at approximately 16%. Because the presenting symptoms of stomach cancer tend to be extremely vague, the majority of patients are diagnosed with extensive local involvement or regional lymph node metastases and this tendency undoubtedly explains in part the poor 5-year survival rate following surgery. TNM classification and staging criteria for stomach cancer are provided in Table 4.

THERAPY FOR ADVANCED DISEASE

Both single-agent and combination chemotherapy have been widely tested in advanced metastatic gastric cancer. Among the most active agents are 5-FU, trimetrexate, mitomycin C, hydroxyurea, epirubicin, and carmustine (BCNU), which demonstrate partial response rates of 18 to 30% [17]. Combination chemotherapy with these and other marginally active agents appears to produce higher objective response rates than those observed with single agents and single institution trials have reported objective response rates of as high as

53% [18]. Unfortunately, these higher objective response rates have not always held up in phase III trials and, to date, no single combination chemotherapy program tested in prospective randomized trials has shown a statistically significant improvement in median survival compared with other regimens. One notable trial compared 5-FU, doxorubicin (Adriamycin), and mitomycin C (FAM) with 5-FU and doxorubicin or 5-FU alone and showed no improvement in median survival with combination chemotherapy [19]. The FAM regimen was one of the first described active combination regimens with a partial response rate of 42% [20]. More recent modifications of this regimen have included the addition of high-dose leucovorin as a biochemical modulator of 5-FU [21]. When using this approach, an objective response rate of 38% and an encouraging overall median survival of 11.5 months have been reported. Another novel combination of etoposide, doxorubicin, and cisplatin (EAP) was first reported in 1989 and an objective response rate of 64% with a complete response rate of 21% was observed in patients with advanced metastatic disease [22]. Unfortunately, severe myelosuppression was experienced in this trial and other investigators failed to confirm these early encouraging results [23]. Another notable combination chemotherapy regimen includes high-dose methotrexate, 5-FU, doxorubicin, and leucovorin rescue (FAMTX). This regimen was initially shown to have an objective response rate in the range of 33 to 50% with a 10% complete response rate [24]. A phase III trial of this regimen compared with FAM chemotherapy showed a superior objective response rate (41 vs 9%) and a significant improvement in median survival (10.5 vs 7.2 months) [25]. Finally, the combination of etoposide, leucovorin, and 5-FU, initially chosen for expected better tolerance in elderly patients or patients with cardiac disease, has proved to be an active regimen with an objective response rate of 52% and a median survival time of 11.5 months [26]. Thus, a variety of multiagent regimens are available with established activity in gastric cancer. Unfortunately, it is not yet clear whether any specific regimen can improve median survival compared with the best single or other combination regimens, and further phase III trials are needed to clarify the role of combination chemotherapy in patients with advanced metastatic gastric cancer.

ADJUVANT THERAPY

The higher objective response rates observed with combination chemotherapy have stimulated interest in adjuvant therapy for gastric cancer. Older studies focused primarily on postoperative chemotherapy. The majority of these studies used the FAM regimen or 5-FU either in combination with radiation therapy or with methyl-CCNU [2]. An initial encouraging report evaluating 5-FU and methyl-CCNU therapy from the Gastrointestinal Tumor Study Group (GITSG) [27] was not confirmed in an identical study performed by the Eastern Cooperative Oncology Group (ECOG) [28]. A small trial evaluating the role of postoperative mitomycin C suggested an improved median survival time, and confirmation of this finding awaits testing [29]. More recently, the NCCTG has evaluated intensive 5-FU plus doxorubicin and has reported no evidence of therapeutic benefit [30].

The disappointing results with postoperative adjuvant chemotherapy have spawned attempts at improving surgical outcome with preoperative chemotherapy. Two studies are noteworthy in this regard. EAP was tested preoperatively in patients with advanced locoregional disease (positive lymph nodes, T3 or T4 primary lesions) [31]. EAP therapy was continued until patients achieved a maximum response to therapy and resection was then attempted. The objective response rate

Table 4. TNM Staging Criteria for Gastric Cancer

Staging	Criteria
Tis	Limited to mucosa, does not penetrate basement membrane
T1	Limited to mucosa or submucose
T2	To or into but not through serosa
T3	Through serosa without invasion of adjacent tissue
T4a	Involves immediately adjacent structures (lesser omentum, perigastric fat, regional ligaments, greater omentum, transverse colon, spleen) or extends intraluminally into esophagus or duodenum
T4b	Direct extension to liver, diaphragm, pancreas, abdominal wall, adrenals, kidney, retroperitoneum, or small bowel or extension extraluminally to esophagus or duodenum
N0	No nodes involved
N1	Perigastric nodes along lesser or greater curvature, within 3 cm of tumor
N2	Other regional nodes, resectable
N3	Other intra-abdominal nodes
M0	No distant metastasis
M1	Distant metastasis present

Stage	TNM
0	Tis, N0, M0
I	T1, N0, M0
II	T2-3, N0, M0
III	T1-3, N1-2, M0
	T4a, N0-2
IV	T1-4a, N3, M0
	T4b, any N, M0
	Any T, any N, M1

From Ahlgren and Macdonald [18]; with permission.

to preoperative EAP was 70% including a 21% complete response rate. Twenty patients subsequently underwent surgery and, at the time of initial publication, the median follow-up was 20 months, with a relapse rate of 60% and a median survival time of 18 months. A more recently reported study evaluated the preoperative response rate and resectability following etoposide, 5-FU, and cisplatin therapy [32]. In this study, 24% of the patients had major preoperative responses to chemotherapy, including two complete responses. The resection rate was 72% and, with a median follow-up of 25 months, the median survival time was 15 months. In both of these trials, additional postoperative chemotherapy was given for patients who demonstrated an initial response to treatment. These early promising reports will require confirmation in larger trials before this approach can be accepted as standard management for gastric cancer.

PANCREATIC CANCER

ADENOCARCINOMA

Adenocarcinoma of the pancreas represents the fourth most common cause of cancer-related death in American males. Approximately 27,700 cases are expected to occur in 1993. The incidence of this disease approximately equals the age-adjusted mortality rate, underscoring the aggressive nature of this malignancy. TNM classification and staging criteria for pancreatic cancer are presented in Table 5. In large studies, only 5 to 22% of presenting patients have resectable tumors. Unfortunately, even successful resection is associated with a low survival rate, ranging from 3.5 to 19%. Patients with unresectable adenocarcinomas of the pancreas confined to the pancreas often undergo palliative surgery or biliary stent placement for relief of jaundice in addition to prophylactic duodenal bypass procedures to prevent obstruction (observed in 10% of patients).

Therapy for Locoregional Disease

The role of chemotherapy in the management of pancreatic carcinoma is best understood in the context of combined modality treatment as adjuvant therapy for pancreatic carcinoma after resection or in the management of locally unresectable lesions. The Gastrointestinal Tumor Study Group (GITSG) has reported a better than twofold increase in the 2-year actuarial survival rate (46 and 43% vs 18%) for patients treated with a combination of 5-FU and split-course radiation therapy after resection, compared with observation [33]. In addition, the GITSG has also demonstrated an almost twofold increase in median survival in patients with unresectable disease treated with 5-FU plus splitcourse radiation therapy compared with high-dose radiation therapy alone [34]. 5-FU has also been studied in combination with intraoperative radiation therapy and with brachytherapy, although randomized trials are not available to determine the role of 5-FU in this clinical setting.

Therapy for Advanced Disease

The use of chemotherapy for patients with widespread metastatic disease has been extremely disappointing. There appear to be no highly active single agents and virtually all approved chemotherapeutic drugs have now been tested. In the past, 5-FU was believed to have activity as a single agent; however, a recent well-designed phase II trial that used 5-FU and more optimal biochemical modulation with leucovorin did not show acceptable clinical activity [35].

Combination chemotherapy regimens have, in some cases, demonstrated improved objective response rates. However, randomized trials with popular regimens such as FAM and streptozocin, mitomycin C, and 5-FU (SMF) have failed to demonstrate any prolongation in median survival time compared with the use of 5-FU alone [19,36]. A pilot study exploring a novel regimen involving the use of cisplatin, cytosine arabinoside, and caffeine has been reported to produce an objective response rate of 39%; however, this early study awaits confirmation in a larger trial [37].

It seems clear that either new drugs or novel therapeutic approaches for pancreatic adenocarcinoma are desperately needed. Currently, an active area of investigation is the use of preoperative chemotherapy and radiation therapy to improve the opportunities for complete resection. It is unclear, however, whether these approaches will alter the pattern of disseminated disease recurrence. Pilot trials are in progress to address these concerns.

ISLET CELL CARCINOMA

Another important subgroup of pancreatic tumors includes islet cell tumors. These tumors include malignant insulinoma, gastronoma, VIPoma, glucogonoma, and somatostatinoma. It is important to recognize these lesions histologically because the natural history and management of these pancreatic tumors is very different.

Many of the islet cell tumors produce fascinating and distinctive syndromes related to secretory hormones produced. Although it is beyond the scope of this chapter to discuss these syndromes in detail, it is worth noting that the management of these tumors is often directed at palliation of the associated symptoms. Treatment may include surgical reduction of tumor bulk, up to and including total orthotopic liver transplantation, hepatic artery occlusion for symptomatic metastatic disease, and specific end organ blockade of the hormonal syndrome. Examples of the latter would include the use of omeprezole for the treatment of gastronoma, or the somatostatin analogue, octreotide, for vasoactive intestinal peptide syndrome.

In the past, chemotherapy was reserved for patients with these indolent tumors as a last resort. Active drugs have included streptozocin, doxorubicin, chlorozotocin, and dacarbazine. Recently, a

Table 5. TNM Staging Criteria for Pancreatic Cancer

Staging	Criteria
T1	No direct extension beyond pancreas
T2	Limited extension to duodenum, bile duct, or stomach
T3	Advanced local extension, incompatible with resection
N0	Regional nodes uninvolved
N1	Regional nodes involved
M0	No known distant metastases
M1	Distant metastases present

Stage	TNM
I	T1-2, N0, M0
II	T3, N0, M0
III	T1-3, N1, M0
IV	T1-3, N0-1, M1

From Ahlgren and Macdonald [18]; with permission.

randomized trial was conducted that showed the superiority of streptozocin and doxorubicin over streptozocin plus 5-FU or single-agent chlorozotocin [38]. In this trial, the combination of streptozocin and doxorubicin produced an improved response rate over the other two arms (69 vs 45 and 30%) and a significant survival advantage (median survival, 2.2 vs 1.4 and 1.4 years). These results may justify the use of this therapy as an initial approach in some patients.

HEPATOBILIARY CANCER

THERAPY FOR LOCOREGIONAL DISEASE

Hepatoma and biliary tract cancer account for approximately 15,000 new cancer cases annually. Worldwide, the most common risk factor for hepatoma is hepatitis B infection. In the United States, other causes of chronic liver disease, such as alcoholic cirrhosis, may be more important predisposing factors. Regardless of the etiology, the only known curative modality for hepatoma is surgical resection. Patients whose cancers are not resectable because of severe underlying liver disease, anatomic location of tumor, or the presence of distant metastases have

an extremely poor prognosis. Tables 6 and 7 list staging criteria and TNM classification for biliary cancer and hepatocellular carcinoma.

Carcinoma of the gall bladder is often found incidentally at surgery. Nonetheless, advanced local and regional disease is usually present and the overall 5-year survival rate is less than 5%. The prognosis for patients with carcinoma of the distal bile duct is more optimistic, with an average 5-year survival rate after radical pancreaticoduodenectomy of approximately 40%. However, proximal bile duct carcinomas and hilar cholangiocarcinomas are much more difficult to treat surgically. In some cases, palliation and disease control can be achieved with brachytherapy by using iridium 192 placed through a biliary drainage catheter. Localized but otherwise unresectable hepatobiliary tumors are sometimes managed with the orthotopic liver transplant; however, the role of liver transplantation in malignancy remains undefined. Aggressive neoadjuvant chemotherapy protocols have been designed with the hope of improving outcome with transplantation.

THERAPY FOR ADVANCED DISEASE

The use of systemic chemotherapy in the management of unresectable or metastatic hepatoma has been extremely disappointing. Although doxorubicin is often considered to be an active single agent

Table 6. TNM Staging for Biliary Cancer

Staging	Criteria
T1	Invades mucosa or muscle layer
T1a	Invades mucosa
T1b	Invades muscle layer
T2	(Gallbladder): invades perimuscular connective tissue; no extension beyond serosa or into liver
	(Extrahepatic ducts): invades perimuscular connective tissue
T3	(Gallbladder): beyond serosa and/or into one adjacent organ, ≤ 2 cm into liver
	(Extrahepatic ducts): invades adjacent structures
T4	(Gallbladder only): > 2 cm liver extension, or more than one adjacent organ involved
N0	No nodal metastases
N1	Regional node metastasis
N1a	Involvement of cystic duct nodes, pericholedochal nodes, and/or hilar nodes
N1b	Peripancreatic (head only), periduodenal, periportal, celiac, and/or superior mesenteric nodes involved
M0	No distant metastatic sites
M1	Distant metastases present

Group staging criteria

Stage	Gallbladder	Extrahepatic ducts
I	T1, N0, M0	T1, N0, M0
II	T2, N0, M0	T2, N0, M0
III	T1-2, N1, M0	T1-2, N1, M0
	T3, any N, M0	
IV	T4, any N, M0	
	Any T/N, M1	
IVA		T3, any N, M0
IVB		Any T/N, M1

From Ahlgren and Macdonald [18]; with permission.

Table 7. TNM Staging Criteria for Hepatocellular Carcinoma

Staging	Criteria
T1	Solitary tumor ≤ 2 cm, without vascular invasion
T2	Solitary tumor ≤ 2 cm, with vascular invasion or
	Multiple tumors, in one lobe only, ≤ 2 cm, without vascular invasion or
	Solitary tumor > 2 cm, without vascular invasion,
T3	Solitary tumor > 2 cm, with vascular invasion, or
	Multiple tumors, in one lobe only, ≤ 2 cm, with vascular invasion, or
	Multiple tumors, in one lobe only, > 2 cm, with or without vascular invasion
T4	Multiple tumors involving more than one lobe, or
	Involvement of a major branch of portal or hepatic vein
N0	No nodal involvement
N1	Regional nodes involved
M0	No distant metastases
M1	Metastases present

Stage	TNM
I	T1, N0, M0
II	T2, N0, M0
III	T1-2, N1, M0
	T3, N0-1, M0
IVA	T4, any N, M0
IVB	Any T, any N, M1

From Ahlgren and Macdonald [18]; with permission.

in hepatoma, the objective response rate to this agent is very low and therapy with doxorubicin probably does not influence group survival when compared with no antitumor therapy [39]. Possible promising experimental approaches for hepatoma confined to the liver include chemoembolization [40], hepatic artery infusion chemotherapy [41], and percutaneous ethanol injection [42].

The role of systemic chemotherapy in unresectable metastatic biliary tract cancers also has not been well defined. Because of the low incidence of these diseases, associated medical complications, and poor performance status of affected patients, few patients are referred for clinical trials. A recent review of the use of chemotherapy in the treatment of bile duct cancer suggests that possible active agents include 5-FU and mitomycin C either as single agents or in combination therapy with doxorubicin (FAM) [43]. In addition, hepatic artery infusion chemotherapy with agents such as 5-FU, FUDR, and doxorubicin have been studied in small patient populations, and objective partial responses have been reported [43]. Clearly, a concerted effort to define the role of chemotherapy in biliary tract cancer is needed.

REFERENCES

1. Hermanek P, Sobin LH (eds): *VICC: TNM Classification of Malignant Tumors*. 1987, Berlin: Springer-Verlag, 40–42.

2. Kies MS, Rosen St, Tasang TK, *et al.*: Cisplatin and 5-fluorouracil in the primary management of squamous esophageal cancer. *Cancer* 1987, 60:2156–2160.

3. Kelsen D, Omar AT: Therapy of upper gastrointestinal cancer. *Cancer* 1991, 15:253–285.

4. Kelsen D, Lovett D, Wong J, *et al.*: Interferon alpha-2a and fluorouracil in the treatment of patients with advanced esophageal cancer. *J Clin Oncol* 1992, 10:269–274.

5. Leichman L, Herskovic A, Leichman CG, *et al.*: Nonoperative therapy for squamous cell cancer of the esophagus. *J Clin Oncol* 1987, 5:365–370.

6. Coia LR, Paul AR, Engstrom PF: Combined radiation and chemotherapy as primary management of adenocarcinoma of the esophagus and gastro-esophageal junction. *Cancer* 1988, 61:643–649.

7. Herskovic A, Martz K, Al-Sarraf M, *et al.*: Combined chemotherapy and radiotherapy compared with radiotherapy alone in patients with cancer of the esophagus. *N Engl J Med* 1992, 326:1593–1598.

8. Ajani J, Roth JA, Ryan B, *et al.*: Evaluation of pre- and post-operative chemotherapy for resectable adenocarcinoma of the esophagus or the gastro-esophageal junction. *J Clin Oncol* 1990, 8:1231–1238.

9. Roth JA, Pass HI, Flanagan MM, *et al.*: Randomized clinical trial of pre-operative and post-operative adjuvant chemotherapy with cisplatin, vindisine, and bleomycin for carcinoma of the esophagus. *J Thorac Cardiovasc Surg* 1988, 96:242–248.

10. Kelsen D, Bains M, Burt M, *et al.*: Randomized comparison of pre-operative (Pre-OP) chemotherapy (CT) versus radiation (RT) in epidermoid esophageal cancer (EEC). *Proc ASCO* 1988, 7:98.

11. Urba SJ, Orringer MB, Perez-Tamayo C, *et al.*: Concurrent preoperative chemotherapy and radiation therapy in localized esophageal adenocarcinoma. *Cancer* 1992, 69:285–291.

12. Lackey VL, Reagan MT, Smith RA, Anderson WJ: Neoadjuvant therapy of squamous cell of the esophagus: Role of resection and benefit in partial responders. *Ann Thorac Surg* 1989, 48:218–221.

13. Parker EF, Reed CE, Marks RD, *et al.*: Chemotherapy, radiation therapy and resection for carcinoma of the esophagus. *J Thorac Cardiovasc Surg* 1989, 98:1037–1044.

14. Forastiere AA, Orringer MB, Perez-Tamayo C, *et al.*: Concurrent chemotherapy and radiation therapy followed by transhiatal esophagectomy for local-regional cancer of the esophagus. *J Clin Oncol* 1990, 8:119–127.

15. Naunheim KS, Petruska PJ, Roy TS, *et al.*: Preoperative chemotherapy and radiotherapy for esophageal carcinoma. *J Thorac Cardiovasc Surg* 1992, 103:87–95.

16. Parsonnet J, Friedman GD, Vandersteen DP, *et al.*: Helicobacter pylori infection and the risk of gastric carcinoma. *N Engl J Med* 1991, 325:1127–1131.

17. Macdonald JS, Steele G Jr, Gunderson LL: Cancer of the stomach. In Devita VT, Hellman S, Rosenberg SA (eds): *Cancer Principles and Practice of Oncology*, 3rd ed. Philadelphia: JB Lippincott, 1989, 765–799.

18. Ahlgren J, Macdonald J, eds: *Gastrointestinal Oncology*. 1992, Philadelphia: JB Lippincott.

19. Cullinan SA, Moertel CG, Fleming TR, *et al.*: A comparison of three chemotherapeutic regimens in the treatment of advanced pancreatic and gastric carcinoma. *JAMA* 1985, 253:2061–2067.

20. Macdonald J, Schein P, Wooley P, *et al.*: 5-Fluorouracil, doxorubicin, and mitomycin (FAM) combination chemotherapy for advanced gastric cancer. *Ann Intern Med* 1980, 93:533–536.

21. Arbuck SG, Silk Y, Douglass HO, *et al.*: A phase II trial of 5-fluorouracil, doxorubicin, mitomycin-C, and leucovorin in advanced gastric carcinoma. *Cancer* 1990, 65:2442–2445.

22. Preusser P, Wilke H, Achterrath W, *et al.*: Phase II study with the combination etoposide, doxorubicin, and cisplatin in advanced measurable gastric cancer. *J Clin Oncol* 1989, 7:1310–1317.

23. Kelsen D, Atiq OT, Saltz L, *et al.*: FAMTX vs. etoposide, doxorubicin, and cisplatin: A random assignment trial in gastric cancer. *J Clin Oncol* 1992, 10:541–542.

24. Wils J, Bleiber GH, Dalesio O, *et al.*: An EROTC gastrointestinal group evaluation of the combination sequential methotrexate and 5-fluorouracil combined with Adriamycin (FAMTX) in advanced measurable gastric cancer. *J Clin Oncol* 1986, 4:1799–1803.

25. Wils J, Klein H, Wagener DJ, *et al.*: Sequential high-dose methotrexate and fluorouracil combined with doxorubicin: A step ahead in the treatment of advanced gastric cancer: A trial of the European Organization of Research and Treatment of Cancer. Gastrointestinal Tract Cooperative Group. *J Clin Oncol* 1991, 9:827–831.

26. Wilke H, Preusser P, Fink U, *et al.*: High dose folinic acid/etoposide/5-fluorouracil in advanced gastric cancer: A phase II study in elderly patients or patients with cardiac arrest. *Invest New Drugs* 1990, 8:65–70.

27. Gastrointestinal Tumor Study Group: Control trial of adjuvant chemotherapy following curative resection for gastric cancer. *Cancer* 1982, 49:1116–1122.

28. Engstrom P, Lavin P, Douglas H, Brunner K: Post-operative adjuvant 5-fluorouracil plus methyl-CCNU therapy for gastric cancer patients. *Cancer* 1985, 55:1868–1873.

29. Estape J, Grau J, Lcobendas F, *et al.*: Mitomycin-C as an adjuvant treatment to resected gastric cancer: A 10 year follow up. *Ann Surg* 1991, 213:219–222.

30. Crook JE, O'Connell MJ, Wieand HS, *et al.*: A perspective, randomized evaluation of intensive-course 5-fluorouracil plus doxorubicin: A surgical adjuvant chemotherapy for resected gastric cancer. *Cancer* 1991, 67:2454–2458.

31. Wilke H, Preusser P, Fink U, *et al.*: Preoperative chemotherapy in locally advanced and nonresectable gastric cancer: A phase II study

with etoposide, doxorubicin and cisplatin. *J Clin Oncol* 1989, 7:1318–1326.

32. Ajani JA, Ota DM, Jessup JM, *et al.*: Resectable gastric carcinoma. An evaluation of preoperative and post operative chemotherapy. *Cancer* 1991, 68:1501–1506.

33. Gastrointestinal Tumor Study Group: Further evidence of effective adjuvant combined radiation and chemotherapy following curative resection of pancreatic cancer. *Cancer* 1987, 59:2006–2010.

34. Moertel CG, Fryta KS, Hahn RG, *et al.*: Therapy of locally unresectable pancreatic carcinoma: A randomized comparison of high dose (6,000 rads) radiation alone, moderate dose radiation (4,000 rads + 5 fluorouracil), antidose radiation + 5 fluorouracil: The Gastrointestinal Tumor Study Group. *Cancer* 1991, 48:1705–1710.

35. DeCaprio JA, Mayer RJ, Gonin R, Arbuck SG: Fluorouracil and high dose leucovorin in previously untreated patients with advanced adenocarcinoma of the pancreas: Results of a phase 2 trial. *J Clin Oncol* 1991, 9:2128–2130.

36. Bukowski RM, Balcerzak SP, O'Bryan RM, *et al.*: Randomized trial 5 fluorouracil and mitomycin C with or without streptozocin for advanced pancreatic cancer. *Cancer* 1983, 52:1577–1582.

37. Dougherty JB, Kelsen D, Kemeny N, *et al.*: Advanced pancreatic cancer: A phase II trial of cisplatin, high dose cytarabine, and caffeine. *J Nat Cancer Inst* 1989, 81:1735–1738.

38. Moertel CG, Lefkopoulo M, Lipsitz S, *et al.*: Streptozocin-doxorubicin, streptozocin-fluorouracil, or chlorozotocin in the treatment of advanced islet cell carcinoma. *N Engl J Med* 1992, 326:519–523.

39. Lai CL, Wu PC, Chan GC, *et al.*: Doxorubicin vs. no antitumor therapy in an inoperable hepatocellular carcinoma: A prospective randomized trial. *Cancer* 1988, 62:479–483.

40. Venook AP, Stagg RJ, Lewis BJ, *et al.*: Chemoembolization for hepatocellular carcinoma. *J Clin Oncol* 1990, 8:1108–1114.

41. Patt Y, Mavligit GM: Arterial chemotherapy in the management of colorectal cancer: An overview. *Sem Oncol* 1991, 18:478–490.

42. Livraghi T, Bolondi L, Lazzaroni S, *et al.*: Percutaneous ethanol injection in the treatment of hepatocellular carcinoma and cirrhosis: A study on 207 patients. *Cancer* 1992, 69:925–929.

43. Oberfield RA, Rossi RL: The role of chemotherapy in the treatment of bile duct cancer. *World J Surg* 1988, 12:105–108.

STREPTOZOCIN AND DOXORUBICIN

Streptozocin is a methyl nitrosourea produced by the fermentation of *Streptomyces archromogenes*. It decomposes spontaneously to generate alkylating and carbamoylating moieties, with alkylation thought to be its principal mechanism of antitumor activity. Streptozocin is capable of transferring methyl groups to DNA but cannot form cross-links.

Doxorubicin is an antitumor antibiotic agent with an extremely wide spectrum of activity. It does not have a single mechanism of cytotoxicity but can produce cellular dysfunction and death by multiple means. Two of its most important mechanisms of cytotoxicity include intercalation among DNA base pairs and generation of toxic intracellular free radicals. These actions can cause single- and double-stranded DNA breaks, which in turn lead to inhibition of RNA and protein synthesis and defective mitoses.

DOSAGE AND SCHEDULING

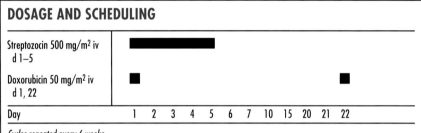

Streptozocin 500 mg/m² iv d 1–5												
Doxorubicin 50 mg/m² iv d 1, 22												
Day	1	2	3	4	5	6	7	10	15	20	21	22

Cycles repeated every 6 weeks.

PRIOR TO THERAPY: *CBC and platelets, liver chemistry, BUN, creatinine. Baseline estimates of cardiac ejection fraction using a gated pool scan may be useful in some patients.*

RECENT EXPERIENCE AND RESPONSE RATES

Study	Evaluable patients, n	Dosage and scheduling	Any regression/ complete regression (%)	Median duration of regression (mo)
Moertel *et al.*, N Engl J Med 1992, 326:519–523	36	Streptozocin 500 mg/m²/d × 5 Doxorubicin 50 mg/m²/d; days 1 and 22	69/14	22
	33	Chlorozotocin, 150 mg/m² q 7 wk	30/6	21
	33	Streptozocin 500 mg/m²/d × 5 5-FU 400 mg/m²/d × 5 (repeat q 6 wk)	45/4	13

CANDIDATES FOR TREATMENT
Patients with metastatic islet cell tumors

SPECIAL PRECAUTIONS
Patients with pre-existing renal or heart disease

ALTERNATIVE THERAPY
Chlorozotocin, dacarbazine

TOXICITIES
Streptozocin: renal toxicity (azotemia, anuria, hypophosphatemia, glycosuria, renal tubular acidosis), severe nausea and vomiting possible; mild-to-moderate abnormalities of glucose tolerance (hypoglycemia); hepatic toxicity and myelosuppression possible (usually mild); **Doxorubicin:** bone marrow suppression, anorexia, nausea and vomiting, alopecia, possible cardiotoxicity

DRUG INTERACTIONS
Streptozocin—none known; **doxorubicin**—digoxin (suspected)

NURSING INTERVENTIONS
Monitor blood counts, liver function, pulmonary function, cardiac function; administer appropriate antiemetics to avoid severe nausea and vomiting; avoid extravasation—can cause severe necrosis

PATIENT INFORMATION
Myelosuppression may occur—call physician if signs and symptoms of infection develop; call physician if injection site becomes painful, red, or swollen; possible red-colored urine for 1 to 2 days after treatment; nausea and vomiting may occur; hair loss likely

EAP
Etoposide, Doxorubicin, and Cisplatin

Etoposide is a semisynthetic derivative of podophyllotoxin. Its mechanism of cytotoxic action involves the inhibition of the nuclear enzyme topoisomerase II. This enzyme has the ability to disentangle topologically intertwined DNA helices, cleave double-stranded DNA, and then covalently bond to DNA to form DNA–topoisomerase II complexes. The cleaved DNA is then reunited after a second duplex DNA has passed through. Etoposide is believed to stabilize the DNA–topoisomerase II complex and prevent rejoining of the double-stranded DNA.

Doxorubicin is an antitumor antibiotic agent with an extremely wide spectrum of activity. It does not have a single mechanism of cytotoxicity but can produce cellular dysfunction and death by multiple means. Two of its most important mechanisms of cytotoxicity include intercalation among DNA base pairs and generation of toxic intracellular free radicals. These actions can cause single- and double-stranded DNA breaks, which in turn lead to inhibition of RNA and protein synthesis and defective mitoses.

Cisplatin is activated intracellularly to generate a positively charged aquated complex. This complex functions similarly to a bifunctional alkylating agent by interacting with the nucleophilic sites on DNA, RNA, and protein, producing intrastrand links and cross-links. These reactions alter the DNA template and inhibit DNA synthesis. Cisplatin lacks cell-cycle specificity.

Combination therapy with these drugs is based on *in vitro* and *in vivo* experimental data that have suggested synergistic cytotoxicity.

CANDIDATES FOR TREATMENT
Patients with advanced locoregional or metastatic gastric cancer prior to surgery

SPECIAL PRECAUTIONS
Patients with cardiac dysfunction
Patients with renal dysfunction

ALTERNATIVE THERAPIES
ELF or 5-FU, cisplatin, and etoposide for neoadjuvant therapy; FAM, FAMTX, or ELF for metastatic disease

TOXICITIES
Drug combination: severe myelosuppression (leukopenia, anemia, thrombocytopenia); **cisplatin:** renal toxicity, alopecia

DRUG INTERACTIONS
Etoposide: synergistic *in vitro* with cytarabine, cyclophosphamide, carmustine, vincristine, cisplatin, hydroxyurea, 5-fluorouracil, methotrexate, verapamil; **Doxorubicin:** digoxin (suspected)

NURSING INTERVENTIONS
Monitor blood counts, liver function, cardiac function, renal function, electrolytes; administer doxorubicin with caution—an extravasant; give adequate antiemetics and maintain adequate hydration; hypotension may occur with rapid administration of etoposide

PATIENT INFORMATION
Myelosuppression common—call physician if signs and symptoms of infection develop; call physician if injection site becomes painful, red, or swollen; possible red-colored urine for 1 to 2 days after treatment; nausea and vomiting may occur; hair loss likely

DOSAGE AND SCHEDULING

	Day	1	2	3	4	5	6	7	8	9	10
Etoposide 120 mg/m² iv d 4,5,6					■	■	■				
Doxorubicin 20 mg/m² iv d 1,7		■						■			
Cisplatin 40 mg/m² iv d 2,8			■						■		

Cycles repeated q 3–4 weeks

PRIOR TO THERAPY: *CBC and platelets, liver chemistries, BUN, creatinine, electrolytes. Baseline estimates of cardiac ejection fraction using a gated pool scan may be useful in some patients.*

RECENT EXPERIENCES AND RESPONSE RATES

Study	Evaluable patients, *n*	Dosage and scheduling	CR/PR (%)	Median duration of survival (mo)
Lerner *et al.*, J Clin Oncol 1992, 10:536–540	36	Etoposide 120 mg/m²/d days 4,5,6 Doxorubicin 20 mg/m²/d days 1,7 Cisplatin 40 mg/m²/d days 2,8	3/9 (33)	7.5
Kelsen *et al.*, J Clin Oncol 1992, 10:541–548	30	Etoposide 120 mg/m²/d days 4,5,6 Doxorubicin 20 mg/m²/d days 1,7 Cisplatin 40 mg/m²/d days 2,8	0/6 (20)	6.1
Preusser *et al.*, J Clin Oncol 1989, 7:1310–1317	67	Etoposide 120 mg/m²/d days 4,5,6 Doxorubicin 20 mg/m²/d days 1,7 Cisplatin 40 mg/m²/d days 2,8	14/29 (64)	9
Wilke *et al.*, Sem Oncol 1990, 17:61–70	145	Etoposide 120 mg/m²/d days 4,5,6 Doxorubicin 20 mg/m²/d days 1,7 Cisplatin 40 mg/m²/d days 2,8	22/61 (57)	

FAMTX
5-Fluorouracil, Doxorubicin, Methotrexate, and Leucovorin

5-Fluorouracil (5-FU) is a fluorinated uracil analogue that is metabolized intracellularly to its active forms, fluorouridine triphosphate (FUTP) and fluorodeoxyuridine monophosphate (FdUMP). FdUMP inhibits the enzyme, thymidylate synthetase, which is necessary for DNA synthesis. Another mechanism of cytotoxicity involves the false incorporation of 5-FUTP into RNA, causing transcription errors.

Doxorubicin is an antitumor antibiotic agent with an extremely wide spectrum of activity. It does not have a single mechanism of cytotoxicity, but can produce cellular dysfunction and death by multiple means. Two of its most important mechanisms of cytotoxicity include intercalation among DNA base pairs and generation of toxic intra-cellular free radicals. These actions can cause single- and double-stranded DNA breaks, which in turn lead to inhibition of RNA and protein synthesis and defective mitoses.

Methotrexate is an antifolate antimetabolite that exerts its primary cytotoxic effect during the S phase. Methotrexate is actively transported across the cell membrane where it binds to its target enzyme, dihydrofolate reductase (DHFR). This enzyme is essential for regenerating the oxidized folates produced during thymidine synthesis to their active forms. In the absence of unbound DHFR, thymidylate and purine biosynthesis can no longer occur.

Leucovorin, also known as folinic acid, is the active, chemically reduced derivative of folic acid, which is involved as a cofactor for one-carbon transfer reactions in the biosynthesis of purines and pyrimidines. It is a potent antidote for the hematopoietic and reticuloendothelial effects of folic acid antagonists because it is easily converted to tetrahydrofolic acid derivatives. Leucovorin also acts as a biochemical modulator of 5-fluorouracil by enhancing the ability of 5-fluorouracil to bind and then block the action of thymidylate synthetase.

DOSAGE AND SCHEDULING

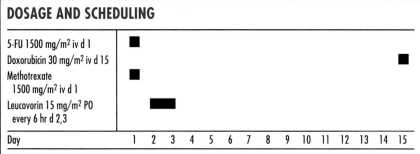

5-FU 1500 mg/m² iv d 1
Doxorubicin 30 mg/m² iv d 15
Methotrexate 1500 mg/m² iv d 1
Leucovorin 15 mg/m² PO every 6 hr d 2,3

Day   1 2 3 4 5 6 7 8 9 10 11 12 13 14 15

Cycles repeated q 4 weeks.

PRIOR TO THERAPY: *CBC and platelets, liver chemistries, BUN, creatinine. Baseline estimates of cardiac ejection fraction using a gated pool scan may be useful in some patients.*

RECENT EXPERIENCES AND RESPONSE RATES

Study	Evaluable patients, *n*	Dosage and Scheduling	CR/PR (%)	Median duration of survival (mo)
Kelsen *et al.,* J Clin Oncol 1992, 10:541–548	30	5-FU 1.5 g/m²/d day 1 Doxorubicin 30 mg/m²/d day 15 Methotrexate 1.5 g/m²/d day 1 Leucovorin 15 mg/m² PO q 6 hr × 3 days starting day 2	3/7 (33)	7.3
Wils *et al.,* J Clin Oncol 1991, 9:827–831	81	5-FU 1.5 g/m²/d day 1 Doxorubicin 30 mg/m²/d day 15 Methotrexate 1.5 g/m²/d day 1 Leucovorin 15 mg/m² PO q 6 hr × 48 hr starting day 2	5/28 (41)	10.5
Wils *et al.,* J Clin Oncol 1986, 4:1799–1803	67	5-FU 1.5 g/m²/d day 1 Doxorubicin 30 mg/m²/d day 15 Methotrexate 1.5 g/m²/d day 1 Leucovorin 15 mg/m² PO q 6 hr × 48 hr starting day 2	9/13 (33)	6

CANDIDATES FOR TREATMENT
Patients with metastatic gastric cancer

SPECIAL PRECAUTIONS
Patients with cardiac dysfunction, renal dysfunction, any third-space fluid collection or ascites, pleural effusion, seroma

ALTERNATIVE THERAPIES
EAP, FAM, ELF, 5-FU (with or without leucovorin)

TOXICITIES
Drug combination: myelosuppression, mucositis, alopecia, **5-FU:** diarrhea; **methotrexate:** renal toxicity, pulmonary fibrosis

DRUG INTERACTIONS
5-Fluorouracil: leucovorin, methotrexate, interferon alpha, dipyridamole, allopurinol, thymidine; **Doxorubicin:** digoxin (suspected); **Methotrexate:** salicylates, sulfonamides, tetracycline, phenylbuta-zone, chloramphenicol, phenytoin, probenecid, NSAIDs, L-asparaginase, vincristine, etoposide, 5-FU

NURSING INTERVENTIONS
Monitor blood counts, renal function; patient must have normal renal function, adequate hydration, and urine alkalinization prior to high-dose methotrexate administration; monitor use of all NSAIDs (can enhance methotrexate toxicity); investigate/report pulmonary symptoms (such as dry nonproductive cough); monitor for ascites or other third-space fluid collection (can enhance methotrexate toxicity); give antiemetics as necessary; monitor hepatic function; administer doxorubicin with caution—an extravasant; monitor methotrexate levels.

PATIENT INFORMATION
Myelosuppression can occur—call physician if signs and symptoms of infection develop (fever, chills, flu-like symptoms); oral mucositis and diarrhea possible; hair loss likely; call physician if injection site becomes painful, red, or swollen; possible red-colored urine for 1 to 2 days after treatment; maintain adequate hydration

ELF
Etoposide, Leucovorin, and 5-Fluorouracil

Etoposide is a semisynthetic derivative of podophyllotoxin. Its mechanism of cytotoxic action involves the inhibition of the nuclear enzyme topoisomerase II. This enzyme has the ability to disentangle topologically intertwined DNA helices, cleave double-stranded DNA, and then covalently bond to DNA to form DNA–topoisomerase II complexes. The cleaved DNA is then reunited after a second duplex DNA has passed through. Etoposide is believed to stabilize the DNA–topoisomerase II complex and prevent rejoining of the double-stranded DNA.

Leucovorin, also known as folinic acid, is an active, chemically reduced derivative of folic acid. Reduction by the enzyme dihydrofolate reductase is not required for leucovorin to participate in reactions that use folates as a source of one-carbon moieties. Leucovorin also acts as a biochemical modulator of 5-fluorouracil by enhancing the ability of 5-fluorouracil to bind and then block the action of thymidylate synthetase.

5-Fluorouracil (5-FU) is a fluorinated uracil analogue that is metabolized intracellularly to its active forms, fluorouridine triphosphate (FUTP) and fluorodeoxyuridine monophosphate (FdUMP). FdUMP inhibits the enzyme, thymidylate synthetase, which is necessary for DNA synthesis. Another mechanism of cytotoxicity involves the false incorporation of 5-FUTP into RNA, causing transcription errors.

Etoposide and 5-fluorouracil are both active agents in gastric carcinoma. In combination, they act synergistically and are not cross-resistant *in vitro* or *in vivo*.

Leucovorin contributes to the synergism of this regimen by enhancing the cytotoxicity of 5-FU by increasing its ability to bind and then block the action of thymidylate synthetase.

CANDIDATES FOR TREATMENT
Patients with metastatic or advanced locoregional gastric cancer, especially for elderly or high-risk patients

SPECIAL PRECAUTIONS
None noteworthy

ALTERNATIVE THERAPIES
EAP, FAMTX, FAM, 5-FU (with or without leucovorin)

TOXICITIES
Myelosuppression, possible mucositis, diarrhea

DRUG INTERACTIONS:
Etoposide: synergistic *in vitro* with cytarabine, cyclophosphamide, carmustine, vincristine, cisplatin, hydroxyurea, 5-fluorouracil, methotrexate, verapamil; **Leucovorin:** 5-fluorouracil; **5-Fluorouracil:** leucovorin, methotrexate, interferon alpha, dipyridamole, allopurinol, thymidine

NURSING INTERVENTIONS
Monitor blood counts; administer etoposide slowly over 45 to 60 minutes or longer (hypotension can occur if given too rapidly)

PATIENT INFORMATION
Oral mucositis may occur; skin reactions possible; call physician if diarrhea develops

DOSAGE AND SCHEDULING

	Day
Etoposide 120 mg/m² iv d 1,2,3	
Leucovorin 300 mg/m² iv d 1,2,3	
5-FU 500 mg/m² iv d 1,2,3	
Day	1 2 3 4 5 6 7 8 9 10 11 12 13 14 15

PRIOR TO THERAPY: CBC and platelets

RECENT EXPERIENCES AND RESPONSE RATES

Study	Evaluable patients, n	Dosage and Scheduling	CR/PR (%)	Median duration of survival (mo)
Preusser et al., Sem Oncol 1990, 17:61–70	51	Etoposide 120 mg/m²/d days 1,2,3 Leucovorin 300 mg/m²/d days 1,2,3 5-FU 500 mg/m²/d days 1,2,3	8/16 (53)	11
Wilke et al., Invest New Drugs 1990, 8:65–70	33	Etoposide 120 mg/m²/d days 1,2,3 Leucovorin 300 mg/m²/d days 1,2,3 5-FU 500 mg/m²/d days 1,2,3	4/12 (48)	10.5

FAM

5-Fluorouracil, Doxorubicin, and Mitomycin C

5-Fluorouracil (5-FU) is a fluorinated uracil analogue that is metabolized intracellularly to its active forms, fluorouridine triphosphate (FUTP) and fluorodeoxyuridine monophosphate (FdUMP). FdUMP inhibits the enzyme, thymidylate synthetase, which is necessary for DNA synthesis. Another mechanism of cytotoxicity involves the false incorporation of 5-FUTP into RNA, causing transcription errors.

Doxorubicin is an antitumor antibiotic agent with an extremely wide spectrum of activity. It does not have a single mechanism of cytotoxicity but can produce cellular dysfunction and death by multiple means. Its two most important mechanisms of cytotoxicity include intercalation among DNA base pairs and generation of toxic intracellular free radicals. These actions can cause single- and double-stranded DNA breaks, which in turn lead to inhibition of RNA and protein synthesis and defective mitoses.

Mitomycin C contains both quinoline and aziridine ring structures, allowing it to exert antitumor activity by two different mechanisms. Reduction of the quinoline ring by one electron transfer allows for free radical reactions similar to those seen with the anthracyclines. The aziridine ring functions as an alkylator producing DNA cross-links.

CANDIDATES FOR TREATMENT

Patients with metastatic gastric cancer

SPECIAL PRECAUTIONS

Patients with pre-existing heart disease or pulmonary dysfunction

ALTERNATIVE THERAPIES

EAP, FAMTX, ELF, 5-FU (with or without leucovorin)

TOXICITIES

Drug combination: cumulative bone marrow suppression, including enhanced leukopenia and thrombocytopenia, alopecia, anorexia, nausea and vomiting; **Doxorubicin:** congestive cardiomyopathy, **Mitomycin C:** hemolytic anemia-like syndrome, pulmonary fibrosis

DRUG INTERACTIONS

5-FU: leucovorin, methotrexate, interferon alpha, dipyridamole, allopurinol, thymidine; **Doxorubicin:** digoxin (suspected); **Mitomycin C:** none

NURSING INTERVENTIONS

Monitor blood counts, liver function, pulmonary function, cardiac function; administer doxorubicin and mitomycin C with great caution—extravasation injury can be extremely severe.

PATIENT INFORMATION

Myelosuppression common—call physician if signs and symptoms of infection develop; call physician if area around site of injection becomes painful, red, or swollen; oral mucositis and diarrhea may occur—call physician if diarrhea persists; skin reactions possible; possible red-colored urine for 1 to 2 days after treatment

DOSAGE AND SCHEDULING

	Week
5-FU 600 mg/m² iv d 1 of wk 1,2,5,6	■ ■ ■ ■
Doxorubicin 30 mg/m² d 1 of wk 1,5	■ ■
Mitomycin C 10 mg/m² iv d 1 of wk 1	■
Week	1 2 3 4 5 6 7 8 9 10 11 12 13 14

Cycles repeated every 6 weeks.

PRIOR TO THERAPY: *CBC, platelets, liver chemistries. Baseline estimates of cardiac ejection fraction using a gated pool scan may be useful in some patients. Pulmonary function tests may be useful in selected patients.*

RECENT EXPERIENCES AND RESPONSE RATES

Study	Evaluable patients, *n*	Dosage and Scheduling	CR/PR (%)	Median duration of response (mo)
MacDonald *et al.*, Ann Intern Med 1980, 93:533–536	62	5-FU 600 mg/m²/d days 1,8,29,36 Doxorubicin 30 mg/m²/d days 1,29 Mitomycin C 10 mg/m²/d day 1	0/26 (42)	9
Brian *et al.*, Oncology 1989, 46:83–87	43	5-FU 600 mg/m²/d days 1,8,29,36 Doxorubicin 30 mg/m²/d days 1,29 Mitomycin C 10 mg/m²/d day 1	0/18 (42)	7
Arbuck *et al.*, Cancer 1990, 65:2442–2445	26	Leucovorin 500 mg/m²/d IV over 2 hr days 1,8,29,36 5-FU 600 mg/m²/d IVP 1 hr after leucovorin, days 1,8,29,36 Doxorubicin 30 mg/m²/d day 1,29 Mitomycin C 10 mg/m²/d day 1	1/9 (38)	6

5-FLUOROURACIL AND RADIATION THERAPY

5-Fluorouracil (5-FU) is a fluorinated uracil analogue that is metabolized intracellularly to its active forms, fluorouridine triphosphate (FUTP) and fluorodeoxyuridine monophosphate (FdUMP). FdUMP inhibits the enzyme, thymidylate synthetase, which is necessary for DNA synthesis. Another mechanism of cytotoxicity involves the false incorporation of 5-FUTP into RNA, causing transcription errors.

When 5-FU is combined with radiation, enhancement of radiation effects is observed. It is known that 5-FU can significantly affect the slope of the radiation therapy survival curve when present in cytotoxic concentrations. The mechanism of this effect is unknown but may involve incorporation into DNA or RNA and cell-cycle effects. Inhibition of sublethal damage repair does not seem to play a role.

DOSAGE AND SCHEDULING

5-FU—500 mg/m^2/d × 3 d every 2 wk × 2, then 500 mg/m^2/q wk for a total of 2 years of therapy—weekly doses begin 1 mo after radiation therapy is complete.
Radiation—2000 cGy over 5 days × 2 courses; 2-wk separation between doses

RECENT EXPERIENCES AND RESPONSE RATES

Study	Evaluable patients, n	Dosage and Scheduling	Median duration of survival (mo)	2-yr actuarial survival (%)
GI Tumor Study Group, Arch Surg 1985, 120:899–903	21	5-FU 500 mg/m^2/d x 3 days q 2 wk x 2; then 500 mg/m^2/wk starting 1 month after radiation therapy complete Plus Radiation 2000 rads/5 d x 2 (2 wk separation between doses)	21	43
	22	No treatment—control group	10.9	18
GI Tumor Study Group, Cancer 1987, 59:2006–2010	30	5-FU 500 mg/m^2/d x 3 days q 2 wk x 2; then 500 mg/m^2/wk starting 1 month after radiation therapy complete Plus Radiation 2000 rads/5 d x 2 (2 wk separation between doses)	18	46

Chemotherapy was continued on a weekly schedule for 2 years of therapy.

CANDIDATES FOR TREATMENT
Patients with locally unresectable pancreatic cancer or with pancreatic cancer causing severe back pain from retroperitoneal extension of disease

SPECIAL PRECAUTIONS
None noteworthy

ALTERNATIVE THERAPIES
Radiation therapy alone, chemotherapy

TOXICITIES
Mucositis, diarrhea, myelosuppression, anorexia, nausea, vomiting, diarrhea, skin irritation

DRUG INTERACTIONS
5-FU: leucovorin, methotrexate, interferon alpha, dipyridamole, allopurinol, thymidine

NURSING INTERVENTIONS
Monitor blood counts; inform patients of possible skin reactions, diarrhea, mucositis

PATIENT INFORMATION
Possible nausea, vomiting, anorexia, oral mucositis, skin reactions, diarrhea

CISPLATIN, 5-FLUOROURACIL, AND RADIATION THERAPY

Cisplatin is activated intracellularly to generate a positively charged aquated complex. This complex functions similarly to a bifunctional alkylating agent by interacting with the nucleophilic sites on DNA, RNA, and protein, producing intrastrand links and cross-links. These reactions alter the DNA template and inhibit DNA synthesis. Cisplatin lacks cell-cycle specificity.

5-Fluorouracil (5-FU) is a fluorinated uracil analogue that is metabolized intracellularly to its active forms, fluorouridine triphosphate (FUTP) and fluorode-oxyuridine monophosphate (FdUMP). FdUMP inhibits the enzyme, thymidylate synthetase, which is necessary for DNA synthesis. Another mechanism of cytotoxicity involves the false incorporation of 5-FUTP into RNA, causing transcription errors.

Both cisplatin and 5-FU, as single agents, are moderately active against esophageal carcinoma. When used in combination with radiation therapy, a radiation-enhancing effect is seen. Ideally, this multimodality approach would enhance the effects of radiation on local tumors and the systemic drug therapy would reduce the chance of distant micrometastases.

DOSAGE AND SCHEDULING

5-FU 1000 mg/m^2/d by continuous infusion every day × 5 d,
Cisplatin 70 to 100 mg/m^2 d 1 only

PRIOR TO THERAPY: *CBC, platelets, electrolytes, BUN, creatinine*

RECENT EXPERIENCES AND RESPONSE RATES

Patients with Localized Disease

Study	Evaluable patients, n	Dosage and Scheduling	Median duration of survival (mo)	Survival rates, (%) 12 mos	24 mos
Herskovic *et al.*, N Engl J Med 1992, 326:1593–1598	121	5-FU 1000 mg/m^2/d x 4 days continuous infusion Cisplatin 75 mg/m^2 day 1 only Radiation 5000 cGy/5 wk	12.5	50	38
		Radiation alone, 6400 cGy/6.4 wk	8.9	33	10
Seitz *et al.*, Cancer 1990, 66:214–219		5-FU 1000 mg/m^2/d x 5 days continuous infusion Cisplatin 70 mg/m^2/d day 2 only Radiation 20 Gy/5 d	17	—	41

Patients with Metastatic Disease and Control of Primary Tumor

Study	Evaluable patients, n	Dosage and Scheduling	CR/PR	Response rate (%)
Debesi *et al.*, Cancer Treat Rep 1986, 70:909–910	37	5-FU 1000 mg/m^2/d x 5 days continuous infusion Cisplatin 100 mg/m^2 day 1 only Allopurinol 600 mg daily day -2 to +5	3/10	35
Kies *et al.*, Cancer 1987, 60:2156–2160	26	5-FU 1000 mg/m^2/d x 5 days continuous infusion Cisplatin 100 mg/m^2/d day 1 only	3/8	42

CANDIDATES FOR TREATMENT
Patients with esophageal carcinoma

SPECIAL PRECAUTIONS
Patients with renal dysfunction

ALTERNATIVE THERAPIES
Preoperative: 5-FU and mitomycin C; 5-FU, vinblastine, and cisplatin plus radiation; cisplatin and bleomycin with or without vindesine; cisplatin and 5-FU; etoposide, cisplatin, and 5-FU; etoposide, doxorubicin, and cisplatin; **Inoperable or metastatic disease:** cisplatin and bleomycin with or without vindesine; cisplatin, methotrexate, and bleomycin

TOXICITIES:
Cisplatin: myelosuppression, nausea, vomiting, renal dysfunction, possible ototoxicity, possible neurotoxicity; **5-FU:** myelosuppression, mucositis, diarrhea; **Chemotherapy plus radiation therapy:** enhanced myelosuppression, severe esophagitis or stomatitis, nausea, vomiting, anorexia, diarrhea, possible ototoxicity, possible neurotoxicity

DRUG INTERACTIONS
5-FU: leucovorin, methotrexate, interferon alpha, dipyridamole, allopurinol, thymidine; **Cisplatin:** none

NURSING INTERVENTIONS
Monitor blood counts, renal function, electrolytes; inform patients of possible skin reactions; give adequate amounts of antiemetics before and after cisplatin therapy; maintain adequate hydration; use diuretics as indicated

PATIENT INFORMATION
Oral mucositis and severe esophagitis may occur; myelosuppression is likely—call physician if signs of infection or diarrhea develop; call physician if hearing loss occurs; nausea and vomiting possible (possibly protracted); skin reactions possible, taste changes (metallic) possible

COLORECTAL CANCER

Cancers of the large bowel are common and increasing in incidence. In the United States, the number of cases of colorectal carcinoma diagnosed annually exceeds 155,000. Cancer deaths from colorectal malignancies number approximately 55,000 each year. The incidence increases by 2 to 3% each year as the general population ages, but the number of deaths has remained fairly constant over the past 10 to 20 years. As a result, the overall death rate has declined from more than 50% of all cases to less than 40%. Earlier diagnosis and advancements in surgical and supportive care most likely account for the major portion of this improved survival rate. Advances in adjuvant therapy and progress in treatment of metastatic disease have only recently been shown to influence survival.

Three fourths of new cases originate in the colon, that is, the segment of the large bowel proximal to the peritoneal reflection. The remaining new cases arise in the rectum. Adenocarcinomas account for more than 90% of large bowel cancers. Carcinoid tumors account for most of the rest of malignant neoplasms arising in the colorectum. Rarely, primary lymphomas, melanomas, and sarcomas are reported.

ETIOLOGY AND RISK FACTORS

The average age of disease onset is 60 to 64 years, but the incidence per 100,000 patients at risk increases linearly with age: from 8 per 100,000 at 40 years, to 150 per 100,000 at 60 years, to 500 per 100,000 at 80 years. An individual's lifetime risk for developing colorectal cancer is about 1 in 10. This risk increases about threefold if a first-degree relative develops a large bowel carcinoma. Several inherited syndromes are associated with an increased risk for colorectal cancer, including ulcerative colitis, Crohn's disease, familial polyposis, and hereditary nonpolyposis colon cancers, such as Lynch syndromes I and II (Table 1). Cancer screening with colonoscopy or double-contrast barium enema in such settings should begin at an early age (as early as age 20, not later than age 35) and occur regularly. Other individuals at increased risk include those with a personal history of adenomas of the large bowel or a family history of breast, endometrial, or ovarian cancer. In asymptomatic individuals at normal risk, recommendations for screening are 1) annual digital examination of the rectum beginning at age 40 and 2) yearly fecal occult blood testing, with sigmoidoscopy every 3 to 5 years, beginning at age 50.

Progression of adenomatous polyps to large bowel adenocarcinoma is clearly documented. The risk for malignant conversion of polyps is related to polyp size, number, and histology. Polyps less than 1 cm in size have about a 1% chance of containing a malignant focus. Risk increases from 5–10% chance for polyps 1 to 2 cm in diameter and 20–50% for those greater than 2 cm. In addition to the additive risk of multiple polyps (each of which has an independent chance of neoplastic transformation), a colonic epithelium in which multiple polyps develop tends to show increasing tendency for neoplasia with increasing numbers of polyps. Whether this tendency is due to increased exposure to environmental factors, an intrinsic genetic susceptibility, or both is unclear. The most frequently encountered adenomatous polyps (75%) are tubular adenomas. Less than 5% of these will contain foci of cancer. Tubulovillous (15% of all adenomas) or villous adenomas (10% of adenomas) show malignant features in 20 and 40% of polyps, respectively.

SURGICAL CONSIDERATIONS

All polyps should be removed when detected. Even if a malignant focus is found, local removal may be curative if there is no invasion beyond the mucosa. Surgery remains the primary means for curative therapy for colorectal cancer as well. Perioperative adjuvant chemotherapy or chemoradiation therapy further decreases the risk for recurrence and improves survival rates in node-positive (Stage III or Dukes' C) patients with colon or rectal primaries. A beneficial role for adjuvant therapy has also been shown for patients with rectal cancer and bowel wall penetration by tumor (Stage II or Dukes' B2). There are insufficient data to confirm a benefit for similar patients with colonic (ie, nonrectal) primaries. Among patients with Stage II colon cancers, a poorer prognostic group that has a higher potential to benefit from adjuvant treatment can be identified by such characteristics as bowel obstruction or perforation by tumor, direct extension of tumor to adjacent structure (T3 or Dukes' B3), or aneuploid DNA content [1].

STAGING AND PROGNOSIS

The most reproducible prognostic indicator for large bowel cancers is operative staging in one of the variations of the Dukes' system or the tumor-node metastasis (TNM) system. TNM staging is preferable to Dukes' stagings because it has been standardized by the Union Internationale Contre Cancer (UICC) and the American Joint Commission on Cancer (AJCC) and is recognized internationally. Details of this staging may be found elsewhere [2] (Table 2). In brief, Stage I tumors demonstrate partial bowel invasion with exten-

Table 1. Risk Factors of Colorectal Cancer	
Risk Factor	**Lifetime Risk* (%)**
Individual (no predisposing history)	1–3
Individual (with one first-degree relative with colorectal cancer)	5–10
Ulcerative colitis	15–30
Crohn's disease	15
Nonpolyposis hereditary colorectal cancer (Lynch I or II)	15–20
Familial polyposis	30–100

*Risk depends on the severity and treatment of underlying disease.

Table 2. Staging and Prognosis of Colorectal Cancer

AJCC/UICC TNM Staging				Dukes'-MAC Staging	5-yr Survival (%)
Stage 0	Tis	N0	M0	—	< 95
Stage I	T1	N0	M0	A	85–90
	T2	N0	M0	B1	
Stage II	T3	N0	M0	B2	65–70
	T4	N0	M0	B3	
Stage III	Any T	N1,2,3	M0	C1–3	45–55
Stage IV	Any T	Any N	M1	D	< 5

sion to the muscularis propria and no lymph node involvement or distant metastatic disease. Stage II tumors invade through the thickness of the bowel wall and may extend to adjacent structures, but show no further tumor involvement. Lymph node involvement without metastatic disease defines Stage III. The presence of distant metastases is described as Stage IV.

The approximate distribution of patients at the time of diagnosis will be 15% with Stage I tumor, 20 to 30% Stage II, 30 to 40% Stage III, and 20 to 25% Stage IV. Excluding the Stage IV patients, who rarely can be cured, the remaining three quarters of individuals will have a tumor that may be approached with curative intent resection. Based on 5-year survival rates of all stages of patients with colon and rectal primaries, only about 50% of patients are cured by surgery. Patients with Stage I colorectal cancer have an 85 to 90% survival rate after surgery alone. This percentage is nearly identical to that of an age-matched cohort of the general population. Sixty-five to 75% of Stage II patients may be alive at 5 years postdiagnosis. For Stage III, the average 5-year survival rate is 55% for patients with colon cancer and 45% for those with rectal cancer. Patients with advanced disease (Stage IV) rarely are alive five years after diagnosis (< 5%); median survival in this group ranges from 6 to 12 months (Table 2).

TREATMENT STRATEGY

Follow-up after curative intent surgery with or without adjuvant therapy includes history and physical examination, liver function tests, and chest radiograph every 3 to 4 months for the first 2 years, at 6-month intervals for the next 3 years, and annually thereafter. Serum CEA and abdominal•pelvic CT scans are often obtained at these same intervals and/or when symptoms indicate a possible recurrence. Colonoscopy is usually performed annually, especially if the initial diagnosis of cancer was preceded or accompanied by the discovery of colonic polyps. The cost and intensity of follow-up must be guided by the patient's ability and willingness to undertake aggressive treatment of any recurrent disease. Anastomotic or locoregional recurrences may be completely resected and a small (5–20%) but real cure rate can be associated with resection of isolated metastases in the liver or other sites [3].

Consideration for preoperative radiation therapy may be given to patients with resectable tumors. Proponents for this approach point out that preoperatively, tumor tissue is well vascularized (and, therefore, more radiosensitive) and surgical adhesions that may retain normal loops of bowel in a radiation port have not formed. Detractors observe that without full surgical staging, 15 to 25% of patients may receive radiation therapy inappropriately for Stage I or IV disease, the full extent of tumor may be best defined and marked for radiation planning at surgery, and surgical techniques for excluding the small bowel from a radiation port are effective. Definitive comparisons of pre- versus postoperative adjuvant irradiation are planned, but convincing data for superiority of either approach do not exist at this time. Preoperative irradiation of local regionally unresectable tumors is more generally accepted. Locally advanced tumors that cannot be resected with tumor-free margins may be reduced in size and possibly approached with curative attempt after radiation therapy, but dosing and the inclusion of chemotherapy remain variable.

ADJUVANT THERAPY

Standards for therapy are more clearly established for adjuvant therapy than for treatment of advanced disease. For Stage III colon cancer primaries, 5-fluorouracil (5-FU) in combination

with levamisole has reduced recurrence rates by 39% [4] and death rates at 5 years by 31%. Mature figures from the largest clinical trial that evaluated this therapy showed overall recurrence-free rates of 47% for surgery alone and 63% for patients receiving adjuvant 5-FU and levamisole [5]. The corresponding overall survival rates were 52 and 64%. A benefit from this therapy has as yet not been demonstrated for patients with Stage II colon cancer.

For rectal cancer, studies have demonstrated an important role for 5-FU-based adjuvant chemotherapy, especially in combination with pelvic irradiation. Such therapy has reduced pelvic recurrences by 46%, systemic relapse by 37%, and has lowered death rates by 29% [6,7]. Ongoing clinical trials are testing the efficacy of various 5-FU regimens in conjunction with radiation therapy for rectal cancer, as well as comparing adjuvant 5-FU and leucovorin to standard 5-FU and levamisole or to 5-FU, leucovorin, and interferon (Table 3). Radiation therapy may be incorporated into a multimodality, adjuvant regimen for T4 and/or N+ tumors arising from anatomically fixed areas of the colon outside the rectum (ie, the cecum, splenic, and hepatic flexures). As in the rectum, radiation with chemotherapy to these areas may reduce risk for local relapse.

Table 3. Current and Planned Cooperative Group Adjuvant Trials for Treatment of Colorectal Cancer

Group	Regimens (Randomized)
Colon	
NSABP C-05	A. 5-FU/leucovorin
Stages II/III	B. 5-FU/leucovorin/interferon
NCCTG	A. 5-FU/leucovorin/stnd-dose levamisole
Stages II/III	B. 5-FU/leucovorin/high-dose levamisole
INT-0089	A. 5-FU/levamisole
Stages II/III	B. 5-FU/leucovorin weekly
	C. 5-FU/leucovorin monthly
	D. 5-FU/leucovorin/levamisole
EST 5283/1290	A. Surgery only
Stage II	B. Autologous tumor vaccine
Stage III	A. 5-FU/levamisole
	B. Autologous vaccine + 5-FU/levamisole
INT-0130	A. 5-FU/levamisole
Locally advanced	B. 5-FU/levamisole + radiation/5-FU
Intergroup	A. 7-day periop 5-FU infusion + 5-FU/levamisole
Stages II/III (perioperative)	B. 5-FU/levamisole
Intergroup	A. 5-FU/leucovorin/levamisole
Stages II/III (postoperative)	B. Prolonged-infusion 5-FU/levamisole
Rectal	
INT-0114	A. 5-FU + RT/5-FU
Stages II/III	B. 5-FU/levamisole + RT/5-FU
	C. 5-FU/leucovorin monthly + RT/5-FU
	D. 5-FU/leucovorin/levamisole + RT/5-FU
Intergroup	A. 5-FU bolus + RT/5-FU
Stages II/III (postoperative)	B. Prolonged-infusion 5-FU + RT/5-FU
NSABP R-03	A. Preop 5-FU/leucovorin/RT
	B. Postop 5-FU/leucovorin/RT

THERAPY FOR ADVANCED DISEASE

For advanced disease, 5-FU combined with leucovorin (folinic acid) has approximately twice the response rate than that seen with 5-FU alone. A meta-analysis of randomized clinical trials comparing 5-FU with or without leucovorin revealed a collective response rate of 11% for 5-FU alone and 23% for 5-FU and leucovorin [8]. Less than 25% of the number of responses from either regimen achieved complete remission. No difference in survival of all randomized patients was seen for the two treatments, possibly because the impact of even the "best available therapy" on advanced colorectal cancer is so limited.

Several doses and schedules of 5-FU and leucovorin have been used and none is clearly superior to the others [9]. The two most widely used schedules are a 5-day bolus regimen repeated every 29 days and a weekly regimen administered for 6-week cycles separated by 2-week rests [10]. Stomatitis and myelosuppression are more commonly associated with the former schedule and profound diarrhea with the latter. A prolonged continuous infusion schedule of 5-FU also has achieved a higher response rate than that obtained with bolus therapy (30 vs. 7%, respectively), but no survival difference was realized [11].

Further modulation of the effect of 5-FU with other agents, including interferon, PALA, dipyridamole, uridine, thymidine, and various combinations of these agents with or without leucovorin is the subject of ongoing clinical and preclinical research. Although reports can be found that cite provocative response rates, these combinations still should be regarded as experimental even when they employ commercially available agents. Similarly, although high response rates have been achieved with regional therapy for liver metastases [12], this approach has not produced improved survival rates and is associated with additional cost and toxicities, such as biliary sclerosis. Hepatic perfusion is an important area of clinical research, but remains experimental (Table 4).

Measures may be taken to reduce oral toxicity and to treat the diarrhea associated with 5-FU therapy. Because the half-life of 5-FU is short (8–12 min), stomatitis may be markedly reduced in severity with oral cryotherapy, that is, holding ice chips on or an iced slurry in the mouth before, during, and for about 30 minutes after bolus infusion [13]. This approach, however, is impractical with prolonged infusion schedules.

Routine antidiarrheal preparations, such as diphenoxylate hydrochloride with atropine sulfate or loperamide hydrochloride, are usually adequate to control drug-induced diarrhea. With a weekly bolus regimen of 5-FU with leucovorin, diarrhea may be cholera-like

in intensity and life-threatening. Patients receiving this regimen must be questioned carefully about any change in stool frequency or consistency before the administration of each week's dose, and the dose must be withheld if, compared to baseline, stools are loose or increase in number. Management of severe or greater diarrhea includes early, vigorous parenteral replacement of fluids and electrolytes. In addition, subcutaneous injections of octreotide, 50 to 150 µg twice a day, may reduce or completely ablate the diarrhea within 24 to 72 hours [14].

ANAL CANCER

Anal cancer is quite distinct from carcinomas of the colon and rectum. It is an uncommon tumor and one that is undergoing a demographic shift due to an association with sexually transmitted disease. The predominant squamous and transitional cell histologies differ from carcinoma of the large bowel, where adenocarcinomas predominate. Most of the tumor morbidity and mortality are associated with uncontrolled locoregional disease. Nodal and distant patterns of spread tend to be systemic (beginning with inguinal nodes) rather than intra-abdominal and intrahepatic metastases, as seen with colorectal cancers. Radical surgery, which remains a mainstay of curative therapy of colorectal cancers, has largely been replaced in anal cancers with radiation or chemoradiation therapy and limited, sphincter-sparing resections.

ETIOLOGY AND RISK FACTORS

In the United States 1500 to 3000 cases of anal cancer are reported annually. The average age at diagnosis is above 60 years. Cancers of the anal canal (from the anal verge proximal to the pectinate line) tend to occur more commonly in older females, and cancers of the anal margin (within 5 cm distal or caudal from the anal verge) more commonly in young men. Anal intercourse in men (but not in women) is a strong risk factor [15]. Sexually transmitted papilloma virus, development of condylomata acuminata, and other sexually transmitted diseases are probable causative agents. Immunosuppression related to organ transplant has been associated with increased incidence [16], and AIDS may have a etiologic role independent of any coexisting sexually transmitted conditions. Chronic anal fistulas, fissures, and other benign conditions have been associated with anal carcinomas, particularly adenocarcinoma.

STAGING AND PROGNOSIS

Staging based on the TNM system is provided in Table 5 [2]. Early stage lesions (Stages 0–II) have 5-year survival rates of 80% or greater. The presence of any nodal metastases, even with small

Table 4. Standard Therapy by Stages of Colorectal Cancer

Stage	Options
I—Colon and rectum	Observation after curative intent resection
II—Colon	Postop observation or postop adjuvant chemotherapy with 5- FU and levamisole or 5-FU and leucovorin
II—Rectum	Postop radiation + 5-FU (with or without leucovorin)
III—Colon	Postop adjuvant chemotherapy with 5-FU and levamisole or 5- FU and leucovorin
III—Rectum	Postop radiation + 5-FU (with or without leucovorin)
IV—Colon and rectum	Palliative chemotherapy with 5-FU and leucovorin or prolonged-infusion 5-FU (with local radiation if needed)

Table 5. Staging of Anal Cancer

AJCC/UICC TNM Staging		Criteria
Stage 0	Tis, N0	Carcinoma *in situ*
Stage I	T1, N0	Tumor < 2 cm
Stage II	T2–3, N0	Tumor 2–5 cm
Stage III	T2–4, N1	Tumor any size; node involvement
Stage IV		Distant metastasis

tumors, confers approximately a 50% or worse 5-year survival rate. Locally invasive tumors, distant metastatic disease, and recurrent cancers are associated with a 7- to 12-month median survival. The major prognostic indicators are tumor size (< 2 cm versus all others), degree of differentiation, (well vs. poorly differentiated), and site of origin (anal canal vs. anal margin).

TREATMENT STRATEGY

Initial diagnostic evaluation includes anorectal digital examination and palpation of inguinal nodes, as well as direct visualization with anoscopy and proctoscopy. Suspicious lesions and enlarged lymph nodes should be biopsied, but an inguinal node dissection is not useful. Concurrent benign anal pathology such as fissures or fistulas are commonly present. These may mask the malignant process; after a 2-week trial of appropriate analgesics and topical therapy, a malignant cause for persistent symptoms should be pursued. It is essential in the primary diagnosis and management of perianal complaints to re-evaluate after no more than 2 to 4 weeks. If a presumed benign condition has not responded markedly to treatment by that time, it must be biopsied and/or evaluated under anesthesia.

Follow-up after treatment of the cancer includes careful examination of locoregional structures and liver function tests every 3 months for the first 2 to 3 years, then every 6 months for an additional 3 to 5 years. Radiographic imaging of the chest and abdominal–pelvic CT scan should be obtained at least at every other evaluation.

THERAPY OF PRIMARY DISEASE

Very early lesions of the anal margin and distal anal canal may be treated with wide local resection and skin graft with cure rates of 60 to 80% These T0 to T1 lesions are found infrequently, however, making up only about 10% of all tumors. An abdominal–perineal resection (APR) is curative in up to one half of all patients but has largely been relegated to the role of salvage therapy after an initial attempt at cure with sphincter-sparing radiation or chemoradiation therapy. Radiation therapy in doses of 60 Gy may achieve cure in more than half of all cases but subsequent APR may be required for recurrent disease or for management of radiation fibrosis and proctitis.

A chemoradiation combination of mitomycin C, 5-FU, and radiation doses to about 50 Gy produce lower long-term toxicity rates, 85 to 95% complete remission rates, and 5-year survival rate in three fourths of patients treated [17,18]. A large clinical trial designed to assess whether the dose of mitomycin C with its associated acute toxicity can be omitted has been completed but reported only in abstract form [19]. The preliminary conclusion suggests that although local control is higher with a regimen that includes mitomycin C, the toxicity from this agent is also substantially increased and, therefore, mitomycin C is not a "mandatory" component of therapy. For patients with residual tumor at biopsy 8 to 12 weeks after initial therapy, additional chemoradiation with cisplatin, 5-FU, and radiation may achieve a complete response. An APR remains a part of the therapeutic plan for patients who, after chemoradiation, do not have biopsy-proven elimination of local disease or who develop recurrent local tumor.

THERAPY FOR ADVANCED DISEASE

Based on high rates of response in other squamous cell tumors, 5-FU and cisplatin or other cisplatin-based regimens have been suggested for metastatic or recurrent disease [20,21]. Other multidrug combinations using bleomycin, nitrosoureas, and anthracyclines are of uncertain benefit. Interstitial radiation therapy alone or with chemotherapy can be effective in controlling initial or relapsed local disease but its success is very dependent on individual techniques and expertise.

REFERENCES

1. Moertel CG, Loprinzi CL, Witzig TE, *et al.*: The dilemma of Stage B-2 colon cancer. Is adjuvant therapy justified? A Mayo Clinic/North Central Cancer Treatment Group Study. *Proc ASCO* 1990, 9:108.

2. American Joint Committee on Cancer: Manual for Staging of Cancer, 4th Ed. 1992, Philadelphia: JB Lippincott.

3. Steele G, Bleday R, Mayer RJ, *et al.*: A prospective evaluation of hepatic resection for colorectal carcinoma metastases to the liver. Gastrointestinal Tumor Study Group Protocol 6584. *J Clin Oncol* 1991, 9:1105–1112.

4. Moertel CG, Fleming TR, Macdonald JS, *et al.*: Levamisole and fluorouracil for adjuvant therapy of resected colon carcinoma. *N Engl J Med* 1990, 322:352–358.

5. Moertel CG, Fleming TR, Macdonald JS, *et al.*: The intergroup study of fluorouracil (5-FU) plus levamisole (Lev) and levamisole alone as adjuvant therapy for stage C colon cancer. *Proc ASCO* 1992, 11:101.

6. Fisher B, Wolmark N, Rockette H, *et al.*: Postoperative adjuvant chemotherapy or radiation therapy for rectal cancer: Results from NSABP R-01. *J Natl Cancer Inst* 1988, 80:21–29.

7. Krook J, Moertel C, *et al*: Effective surgical adjuvant therapy for high risk rectal carcinoma. *N Engl J Med* 1991, 324:709–715.

8. Advanced Colorectal Cancer Meta-analysis Project: Modulation of fluorouracil by leucovorin in patients with advanced colorectal cancer: Evidence in terms of response rate. *J Clin Oncol* 1992, 10:896–903.

9. Gertsner J, O'Connell MJ, Wieand HS, *et al.*: A prospectively randomized clinical trial comparing 5-FU combined with either high or low dose leucovorin for the treatment of advanced colorectal cancer. *Proc ASCO* 1991, 10:134.

10. Peters GJ, van Groeningen CJ: Clinical relevance of biochemical modulation of 5-fluorouracil. *Ann Oncol* 1991, 2:469–480.

11. Lokich JJ, Ahlgren JD, Gullo JJ, *et al.*: A prospective randomized comparison of continuous infusion fluorouracil with conventional bolus schedule in metastatic colorectal carcinoma: A Mid-Atlantic Oncology Program Study. *J Clin Oncol* 1989, 7:425–432.

12. Wagman LD, Kemeny MM, Leong L, *et al.*: A prospective, randomized evaluation of the treatment of colorectal cancer metastatic to the liver. *J Clin Oncol* 1990, 8:1885–1893.

13. Mahood DJ, Dose AM, Loprinzi CL, *et al.*: Inhibition of fluorouracil-induced stomatitis by oral cryotherapy. *J Clin Oncol* 1991, 9:449–452.

14. Casinu S, Fedeli A, Fedeli SA, *et al.*: Control of chemotherapy-induced diarrhea with octreotide in patients receiving 5-fluorouracil. *Eur J Cancer* 1992, 28:482–483.

15. Dazing JR, Weiss NS, Hislop TG, *et al.*: Sexual practices, sexually transmitted diseases and the incidence of anal cancer. *N Engl J Med* 1987, 317:973–977.

16. Penn I: Cancer of the anogenital region in renal transplant recipient: Analysis of 65 cases. *Cancer* 1986, 58:611–616.

17. Sischy B, Duggett RL, Krall JM, *et al.*: Definitive irradiation and chemotherapy for radiosensitization in management of anal carcinoma: Interim report of the Radiation Therapy Oncology Group (study no. 8314). *J Nat Cancer Inst* 1989:850–856.

18. Cummings BJ: Anal cancer. *Int J Rad Oncol Biol Phys* 1990, 19:1309–1315.

19. Flam MS, John MJ, Peters T, *et al.*: Radiation and 5-fluorouracil (5-FU) vs radiation, 5-FU, and mitomycin-C (MMC) in the treatment of anal carcinoma: Preliminary results of a phase III randomized RTOG/ECOG intergroup trial. *Proc ASCO* 1993, 12:192.

20. Majoubi M, Sadek H, Francois E, *et al.*: Epidermoid anal canal carcinoma (EACC): Activity of cisplatin (P) and continuous 5-fluorouracil (5-FU) in metastatic and/or local recurrent (LR) disease. *Proc ASCO* 1990, 9:114.

21. Roca E, DeSimone G, Barugel M, *et al.*: A phase II study of alternating chemoradiotherapy including cisplatin (DDP) in anal canal carcinoma (ACC). *Proc ASCO* 1990, 9:128.

5-FU AND LEUCOVORIN

5-Fluorouracil (5-FU) is a fluorine-substituted uracil that blocks the methylation reaction of deoxyuridylic acid to thymidylic acid, interfering with DNA synthesis. It may be incorporated as a false nucleotide into DNA and RNA. The drug is most active against growing cell populations. Leucovorin (folinic acid, citrovorum factor, or 5-formyl-tetrahydrofolic acid) acts, after further metabolism, as a one-carbon (methyl) donor in the conversion of uridylate to thymidylate. Most preparations (oral or parenteral) are racemic mixtures of the compound but only the L-isomer is biologically active. Oral preparations have lower bioavailability than parenteral forms.

DOSAGE AND SCHEDULING

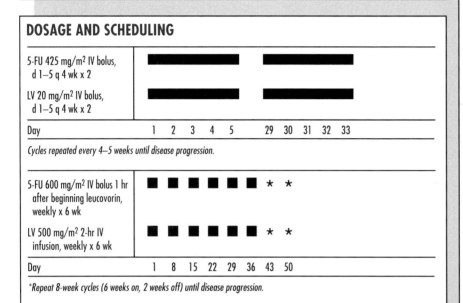

5-FU 425 mg/m² IV bolus, d 1–5 q 4 wk x 2											
LV 20 mg/m² IV bolus, d 1–5 q 4 wk x 2											
Day	1	2	3	4	5	29	30	31	32	33	

Cycles repeated every 4–5 weeks until disease progression.

5-FU 600 mg/m² IV bolus 1 hr after beginning leucovorin, weekly x 6 wk								
LV 500 mg/m² 2-hr IV infusion, weekly x 6 wk								
Day	1	8	15	22	29	36	43	50

*Repeat 8-week cycles (6 weeks on, 2 weeks off) until disease progression.

RECENT EXPERIENCES AND RESPONSE RATES

Study	Evaluable Patients, n	Regimen	Response (%)	Median Survival (mo)
Poon, *et al.*, J Clin Oncol 1991, 9:1967–1972	153	5-FU 425 mg/m² 5-FU-LV 20 mg/m²	42	12.7
	149	5-FU 370 mg/m² 5-FU-LV 200 mg/m²	31	12.7
	155	5-FU-MTX	14	8.4
Petrelli, *et al.*, J Clin Oncol 1989, 7:1419–1426	113	5-FU 600 mg/m² LV 500 mg/m²	30	12.5
	115	5-FU 600 mg/m² LV 25 mg/m²	19	10.4
	115	5-FU 1000 mg/m²	12	10.5

CANDIDATES FOR TREATMENT
Patients with advanced colorectal cancer

SPECIAL PRECAUTIONS
Full recovery from surgery
Pregnant/nursing patients
Elderly patients

ALTERNATIVE THERAPIES
Other 5-FU-based regimens

TOXICITIES
Daily-x-5 regimen: stomatitis and myelosuppression (dose-limiting). **Weekly regimen:** dose-limiting diarrhea (especially in patients over 70 years). **Other:** loss of appetite, abdominal cramps, difficulty with coordination, mouth sores, dry skin or nose, splitting fingernails, metal taste in mouth, watery eyes, nausea, vomiting, temporary alopecia, leukopenia leading to an increased risk of infection, erythrocytopenia leading to anemia, photosensitivity, skin rash, hyperpigmentation, local tissue irritation if drug extravasation occurs

DRUG INTERACTIONS
5-FU: Allopurinol, cimetidine, folinic acid, methotrexate, thymidine; **Leucovorin:** methotrexate, phenobarbitol, phenytoin, primidone

NURSING INTERVENTIONS
Assess patient performance and mental status; monitor weight, encourage adequate fluid, caloric, and protein intake; give antiemetics, antidiarrheals, food supplements as necessary; monitor blood counts and liver function; **Weekly regimen:** question weekly about loose or frequent stools; dose should be held if patients have any early diarrhea

PATIENT INFORMATION
Patient should report diarrhea > 3 × d, soreness in mouth, difficulty swallowing, rash, fever. Patient should minimize sun exposure and avoid alcohol consumption. Weekly regimen: patient should report on stools before the dose is given

5-FU AND LEVAMISOLE

5-Fluorouracil (5-FU) is a fluorine-substituted uracil that blocks the methylation reaction of deoxyuridylic acid to thymidylic acid, interfering with DNA synthesis; it may be incorporated as a false nucleotide into DNA and RNA. The drug is most active against growing cell populations. Levamisole was introduced into clinical practice in 1973 as an antihelmintic. Early *in vivo* research suggested immune modulatory properties; however, its mechanism of action in adjuvant treatment remains undefined. Levamisole as a single agent is not effective for adjuvant therapy, and the combination of 5-FU and levamisole is not effective in advanced (Stage IV) colon cancer.

DOSAGE AND SCHEDULING

5-FU 450 mg/m² IV bolus, daily x 5; starting d 28, weekly for 48 wk	▬▬▬▬▬ ▪ ▪
Levamisole 50 mg PO TID x 3 d, q other wk	▬▬ ▬▬ ▬▬
Day	1 2 3 4 5 15 16 17 29 30 31 36

5-FU 450 mg/m² IV bolus, daily x 5; starting d 28, weekly for 48 wk	▪ ▪ ▪ ▪ ▪
Levamisole 50 mg PO TID x 3 d, q other wk	▬▬ ▬▬ ▬▬
Day	43 44 45 50 57 58 59 64 71 72 73*

*Continue weekly 5-FU and every other week levamisole (x 3 days) for a total of 1 year.

RECENT EXPERIENCE AND RESPONSE RATES

Study	Evaluable Patients, *n*	Regimen	3.5-yr Survival (%)
Moertel, *et al.*, N Engl J Med 1990, 322:352–358	929	Surgery alone	55
		Levamisole	55
		5-FU/levamisole	71

CANDIDATES FOR TREATMENT

Adjuvant therapy for patients who have undergone resection for Stage III (node-positive) colon cancer

SPECIAL PRECAUTIONS

Full recovery from surgery
Pregnant/nursing patients

ALTERNATIVE THERAPY

5-FU and leucovorin

TOXICITIES

5-FU: loss of appetite, diarrhea, abdominal cramps, difficulty with coordination, mouth sores, dry skin or nose, splitting fingernails, metal taste in mouth, watery eyes, nausea, vomiting, temporary alopecia, leukopenia leading to an increased risk of infection, erythrocytopenia leading to anemia, photosensitivity, skin rash, hyperpigmentation, local tissue irritation if drug extravasation occurs
Levamisole: metallic taste (2%), arthralgias/myalgia (1%), mood change/dizziness (3%), exfoliative dermatitis (rare), leukoencephalopy with change in mental status (rare)
Combination: severe nausea, vomiting, diarrhea, myelosuppression (1.5%)

DRUG INTERACTIONS

5-FU: allopurinol, cimetidine, folinic acid, methotrexate, thymidine; **levamisole:** phenytoin, warfarin, ethanol

NURSING INTERVENTIONS

Assess patient performance and mental status; monitor weight, encourage adequate fluid, caloric, and protein intake; give antiemetics, antidiarrheals, food supplements as necessary; monitor blood counts and liver function; inform patients of possible skin reactions; because of levamisole schedule, develop calendar or reminder for patient

PATIENT INFORMATION

Patient should report diarrhea > 3 × d, soreness in mouth, difficulty swallowing, rash, fever. As with all oral medications, reinforce compliance frequently

PROLONGED CONTINUOUS IV 5-FU

5-Fluorouracil (5-FU) is a fluorine-substituted uracil that blocks the methylation reaction of deoxyuridylic acid to thymidylic acid, interfering with DNA synthesis. Direct incorporation of fluoropyrimidine nucleotide into DNA and RNA also occurs. With continuous daily infusion, the activity and toxicity profiles are different than those seen with bolus therapy. The mechanism responsible for these differences is not completely understood.

DOSAGE AND SCHEDULING

5-FU 300 mg/m²/24 hr via ambulatory pump	███	███		
Day	1 – 7 71 – 84	85 – 155	156 – 169*	

*1 to 2 week interruptions may be required for recovery from toxicity before 10 weeks of infusion; continue therapy until disease progression.

RECENT EXPERIENCES AND RESPONSE RATES

Study	Evaluable Patients, *n*	Regimen	Response (%)
Lokich JJ, *et al.*, J Clin Oncol 1989, 7:425–432	87	5-FU bolus	7
	87	5-FU cont. IV	30

CANDIDATES FOR TREATMENT
Patients with colorectal cancer

SPECIAL PRECAUTIONS
Pregnant/nursing patients

ALTERNATIVE THERAPY
Other 5-FU-based regimens

TOXICITIES
Myelosuppression and mucositis are *less* severe, palmar planter erythrodysesthesia with peripheral neuropathy and desquamation (possibly dose-limiting); loss of appetite, diarrhea, abdominal cramps, difficulty with coordination, mouth sores, dry skin or nose, splitting fingernails, metallic taste, watery eyes, nausea, vomiting, temporary alopecia, leukopenia leading to an increased risk of infection, erythrocytopenia leading to anemia, photosensitivity, skin rash, hyperpigmentation, local tissue irritation if drug extravasation occurs

DRUG INTERACTIONS
5-FU: allopurinol, cimetidine, folinic acid, methotrexate, thymidine

NURSING INTERVENTIONS
Instruct patient in care of semipermanent IV access and ambulatory pump; assess patient performance and mental status; monitor weight, encourage adequate fluid, caloric, and protein intake; give antiemetics, antidiarrheals, food supplements as necessary; monitor blood counts and liver function

PATIENT INFORMATION
Patient should report diarrhea > 3 × d, soreness in mouth, difficulty swallowing, rash, fever. Patient should be informed of possible skin reactions

INTERFERON ALPHA-2 AND 5-FU

Interferon alpha-2 (IFN α-2) is a biologic response modifier, curently used in a purified, recombinant form. It has demonstrated both antitumor and immunomodulatory effects.

5-Fluorouracil (5-FU) is a fluorine-substituted uracil that blocks the methylation reaction of deoxyuridylic acid to thymidylic acid, interfering with DNA synthesis. The drug is most active against growing cell populations.

Synergism of this regimen may be attributable to IFN-decreased tumor cell thymidylate synthetase production after 5-FU, protracted metabolism of 5-FU, and serum clearance of 5-FU catabolites, or to additional effects upon the 5-fluorodeoxyuridine monophosphate (FdUMP)–thymidylate synthetase complex formulation. Recombinant IFN α-2 enhances the cytotoxic effects of 5-FU against two human colon cancer cell lines in a dose- and schedule-dependent manner, demonstrating therapeutic synergism when used in a strict regimen. IFNs biochemically modulate the activity of 5-FU *in vitro*, enhancing intracellular levels of FdUMP and the binding of FdUMP to thymidylate synthetase, the target enzyme. Additionally, phase I clinical trials indicated decreased clearance of 5-FU with increased serum levels with IFN α-2 therapy. Finally, IFN α-2 enhances natural killer cell and macrophage activity, although it is unclear if this contributes to enhanced antitumor effects.

CANDIDATES FOR TREATMENT
Patients with advanced colorectal cancers, and carcinoma of the stomach, colon, pancreas, liver, and breast

SPECIAL PRECAUTIONS
Enhanced mucositis, severe diarrhea

ALTERNATIVE THERAPIES
5-FU and leucovorin, 5-FU and levamisole

TOXICITIES
5-FU: loss of appetite, diarrhea, abdominal cramps, difficulty with coordination, mouth sores, dry skin or nose, splitting fingernails, metal taste in mouth, watery eyes, nausea, vomiting, temporary alopecia, leukopenia leading to an increased risk of infection, erythrocytopenia leading to anemia, photosensitivity, skin rash, hyperpigmentation, local tissue irritation if drug extravasation occurs; **IFN α-2:** fever, fatigue, flu-like symptoms, pancytopenia, changes in consciousness, changes in liver function tests, changes in blood pressure, numbness and tingling in fingers and toes; Less frequent: convulsions, confusion, stupor, irregular heart beat, blood clotting abnormalities; anemia more severe than that normally seen with 5-FU alone

DRUG INTERACTIONS
IFN α-2: aspirin, NSAIDs, prostaglandin synthetase inhibitors, antihistamines, immunomodulators; **5-FU:** methotrexate, allopurinol, oxypurinol, thymidine

NURSING INTERVENTIONS
Give acetaminophen prior to IFN for flu-like symptoms and every 4 hr as needed thereafter; assess patient performance and mental status; monitor weight, encourage adequate fluid, caloric, and protein intake; give antiemetics, antidiarrheals, food supplements as necessary; monitor blood counts and liver function; educate on central venous access device and pump and malfunctions

PATIENT INFORMATION
Patient may experience flu-like symptoms; fatigue likely (arrange activities in the morning and allow for frequent rest); nausea/vomiting likely; patient should report diarrhea > 3 × d, soreness in mouth, difficulty swallowing, rash, fever. If diarrhea develops, contact doctor (fluid replacement therapy may be necessary); possible skin reactions

DOSAGE AND SCHEDULING

	Day 1	2	3	4	5	6	7	8	9	10	11	12	13	14
5-FU 750 mg/m²/d by continuous infusion (inpatient), d 1–5	■	■	■	■	■									
5-FU 750 mg/m² bolus (outpatient), d 8								■						
IFN 9 × 10⁶ U sc , d 1, 3, 5, 8, 10, 12	■		■		■			■		■		■		
CBC , d 1, 4, 8, 11	□			□				□			□			
LFT, ECG, d 7, 14							□							□

RECENT EXPERIENCES AND RESPONSE RATES

Study	Evaluable Patients, n	Regimen	CR/PR (%)
Wadler, *et al.*, Cancer Res 1990, 50:2056–2059	18	5-FU: 750 mg/m²/d x 5 d (cont IV infusion); then weekly IFN α-2a: 6, 9, 12, 15, or 18 x 10⁶ U sc	1/4 (28)
Pazdur, *et al.*, J Clin Oncol 1990, 8:2027–2031	45	5-FU: 750 mg/m²/d x 5 d (cont IV infusion); then weekly IFN α-2a: 9 x 10⁶ U sc TIW	1/15 (36)
Kemeny, *et al.*, Cancer 1990, 66:2470–2475	36	5-FU: 750 mg/m²/d x 5 d (cont IV infusion); then weekly IFN α-2a: 9 x 10⁶ U sc TIW	0/9 (26)
Wadler, Wiernik, Semin Oncol 1990, 17(suppl 1):16–21, 38–41	32	5-FU: 750 mg/m²/d x 5 d (cont IV infusion); then weekly IFN α-2a: 9 x 10⁶ U sc TIW	0/20 (63)
Fornasiero, *et al.*, Tumori 1990, 76:385–388	21	5-FU: 1000 mg/wk; IFN α-2a: 6, 9, 12, 18 x 10⁶ U sc TIW (dose escalated each month)	4/5 (43)

RADIATION THERAPY, 5-FU, AND MITOMYCIN C

The combination of 5-FU and mitomycin C with radiation has at the very least an additive cytotoxic effect, and it may have a synergistic "radiosensitizing" effect. 5-Fluorouracil is a fluoride-substituted uracil that blocks the methylation reaction of deoxyuridylic acid to thymidylic acid, interfering with DNA synthesis; it may be incorporated as a false nucleotide into DNA and RNA. The drug is most active against growing cell populations. Mitomycin C is an antibiotic isolated from *Streptomyces caespitosus*. Its antitumor effect results from DNA crosslinking and suppression of RNA and protein synthesis.

DOSAGE AND SCHEDULING

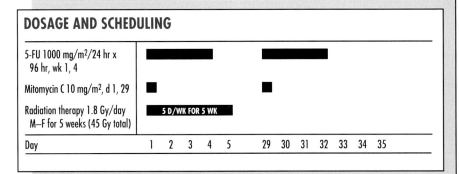

5-FU 1000 mg/m²/24 hr x 96 hr, wk 1, 4													
Mitomycin C 10 mg/m², d 1, 29													
Radiation therapy 1.8 Gy/day M–F for 5 weeks (45 Gy total)	5 D/WK FOR 5 WK												
Day	1	2	3	4	5	29	30	31	32	33	34	35	

RECENT EXPERIENCES AND RESPONSE RATES

Study	Evaluable Patients, *n*	Regimen	Locoregional Control (%)	2-yr Survival (%)
Sishy B, *et al.*, JNCI 1989, 81:850–856	79	RT + 5-FU/MMC	90	87
Flam MS, *et al.*, Proc ASCO 1993, 12:192 (#A557)	151	RT + 5-FU/MMC	92	79
	148	RT + 5-FU	86	81

CANDIDATES FOR TREATMENT
Patients with Stage II or III anal carcinoma in whom sphincter preservation is option

SPECIAL PRECAUTIONS
Pregnant/nursing patients

ALTERNATIVE THERAPY
Mitomycin C may be optional component to regimen

TOXICITIES
5-FU: loss of appetite, diarrhea, abdominal cramps, difficulty with coordination, mouth sores, dry skin or nose, splitting fingernails, metal taste in mouth, watery eyes, nausea, vomiting, temporary alopecia, leukopenia leading to an increased risk of infection, erythrocytopenia leading to anemia, photosensitivity, skin rash, hyperpigmentation, local tissue irritation if drug extravasation occurs
Mitomycin C: fever, nausea, vomiting; myelosuppression, mucositis, alopecia, increased creatinine, pulmonary infiltrates/fibrosis
Chemoradiation: fatal toxicities (1–5%)

DRUG INTERACTIONS
5-FU: Allopurinol, cimetidine, folinic acid, methotrexate, thymidine; **mitomycin C:** vinblastine (worsened lung toxicity)

NURSING INTERVENTIONS
Moderate-to-severe pelvic/perineal skin toxicities from combined therapy; ointments and salves should not be applied to skin (mitomycin C is vesicant); good skin hygiene and Domeboro solution may provide relief

PATIENT INFORMATION
Patient should be informed about skin care. Patient should report diarrhea > 3 × d, soreness in mouth, difficulty swallowing, rash, fever.

ETIOLOGY AND RISK FACTORS

Cancer of the head and neck accounts for approximately 5% of malignancies in the United States. Its incidence is higher in blacks and males and is currently declining in white males [1]. Tobacco and alcohol are the two major risk factors (Table 1). Increasing tobacco consumption is responsible for a rising incidence of head and neck cancer in women. Tobacco chewing is a common risk factor in Asia, resulting in a high incidence of head and neck cancer in parts of the Far East. Although alcohol and tobacco are independent risk factors, they are frequently present together with a synergistic potentiation of the carcinogenic risk [1]. Nasopharyngeal carcinoma is associated with the Epstein–Barr virus and is endemic in regions of North Africa and Asia.

STAGING AND PROGNOSIS

Head and neck cancer represents a heterogeneous group of cancers originating from different primary localizations. Squamous cell carcinoma is the most common histologic type in the adult (Table 2). Treatment depends on localization, resectability, and histology. For squamous cell carcinoma, local and regional extension usually determine the stage and prognosis; in squamous cell carcinoma, distant metastases occur late and are infrequent. Thus, locoregional control is the most important goal in the therapy of squamous cell head and neck cancer.

The tumor (T) staging is dependent on the exact anatomic localization of the tumor. Lesions considered to be T1 and T2 are small primary tumors, whereas T3 and T4 lesions are locally advanced, with T4 invading surrounding structures (eg, bone, cartilage, skin). Regional lymph nodes are staged uniformly for all anatomic sites as N1 to N3, according to increasing size and frequency of nodes (Table 3). Stages I and II represent T1, N_0 and T2, N_0 lesions, respectively. Stages III and IV represent locally advanced disease (T3, T4) and regional involvement (N1–N3). Distant metastases are present in 10% of patients at diagnosis and are included in Stage IV. Lungs, bones, and liver are the most commonly involved sites.

The majority of patients (60%) have at presentation a locoregionally advanced disease (T3, T4 or N1–N3). The majority of these patients die, indicating the inability of currently available therapy to consistently achieve cure. Up to 25% of the patients with advanced squamous cell carcinoma will relapse with distant metastases, and autopsy series suggest 40 to 50% of the patients to have occult metastatic disease. Cure in locally advanced stages is achieved in less than 30% following standard therapy. In early-stage disease, cure rates are 60 to 90%. Nasopharyngeal and laryngeal cancers appear to have a somewhat better prognosis than other tumor sites. Poor tissue vascularization and hoarseness as symptoms leading to early diagnosis may be contributing factors to higher cure rates in laryngeal cancer. Nasopharyngeal cancer with its distinct histology appears to be more radiation-sensitive and may also be more responsive to chemotherapy.

STANDARD THERAPY

Standard therapy for head and neck cancer includes surgery, radiotherapy, and chemotherapy (Fig. 1). The first two modalities are used with a curative intent in newly diagnosed nonmetastatic cases. Chemotherapy and sometimes surgery or radiation have important roles in recurrent disease. Newer investigational approaches include combined modality therapy and focus on better local control and higher cure rates, especially in advanced disease. Organ preservation through less extensive surgery, but without jeopardizing the overall outcome, is a second important goal.

To determine standard or investigational therapy three different settings need to be distinguished: early-stage tumors (Stages I and II), locally advanced tumors (Stages III and IV), and metastatic or recurrent disease (M1+). For the first two groups, treatment is given with curative intent. In metastatic or recurrent disease the usual goal of treatment is palliation and prolongation of survival (Table 4). Only occasionally will those patients to be able to undergo a second successful surgical procedure.

Early-Stage Disease

Early-stage tumors (T1, T2) can be cured with surgery or radiotherapy alone in 60 to 90% of cases. If surgery is done, it frequently includes an elective dissection of the regional lymph nodes. This procedure allows for more accurate pathologic staging, with important prognostic and therapeutic implications. In over 50% of cases, the pathologic stage will be higher than the clinical stage. Newer radiologic procedures (including CT and MRI scans) also have an increasing role in the staging of this disease.

A similar outcome in early-stage disease can be achieved with radiation therapy. Radiation therapy has the advantage of avoiding surgery in a group of patients with underlying morbidities (eg, chronic obstructive pulmonary disease, coronary artery disease, or liver cirrhosis). It also allows for organ preservation. But the therapy is a lengthy process, running over 6 to 7 weeks, with associated mucositis, xerostomia, and loss of taste as the major secondary effects. This modality with curative intent should only be chosen for reliable and compliant patients. For cancer of the larynx, radiation offers significantly better organ preservation and is often the first

Table 1. Risk Factors of Head and Neck Tumors

Tobacco
Alcohol
Poor orodental care
Smokeless tobacco (chewing)
Malnutrition
Epstein-Barr virus

Table 2. Differential Diagnosis of Tumors in the Head and Neck

Benign	Malignant
Cyst	Squamous cell carcinoma
Adenoma	Lymphoepithelioma
Lipoma	Lymphoma
	Sarcoma
	Melanoma
	Adenocarcinoma

Table 3. TMN Staging of Head and Neck Tumors

		N_0	N_1	N_2	N_3
Stage I	T_1				
Stage II	T_2				
Stage III	T_3				
Stage IV	T_4	(any M_1)			

Stages I and II	Early stage
T_3, T_4, and N_1–N_3, M_0	Locally regionally advanced

choice. Nasopharyngeal cancer is considered unresectable and is thus primarily treated with radiation.

Locally Advanced Disease

In locally advanced disease (Stages III and IV), bimodal therapy of surgery followed by radiotherapy is usually administered in patients with resectable disease who are medically operable. This approach results in low cure rates of 20 to 30%. Depending on the extent of the tumor, surgery may lead to impaired or lost organ function, muscle atrophy, and disfigurement.

Recurrent or Metastatic Disease

Chemotherapy has a limited role within standard therapy of head and neck cancer. Traditionally it is used only in recurrent or metastatic disease. In this setting the following drugs have been found active: methotrexate, cisplatin, carboplatin, 5-FU, bleomycin, mitomycin C, cyclophosphamide, doxorubicin, hydroxyurea, and most recently paclitaxel [2]. The response rates as single agents are approximately 30%, with a short response duration of only 2 to 6 months.

In the past, a combination of cisplatin and 5-FU has frequently been used for recurrent disease. Phase II and III trials have shown response rates of 20 to 70% [2–4]. Recently, a randomized trial has shown a significant improvement in response with this combination, compared to the use of single-agent 5-FU or cisplatin. Although the response rate in this trial increased from 13% for single-agent 5-FU and 17% for single-agent cisplatin to 32% for the combination of the two agents, an improved survival rate has not been shown [4]. Another randomized trial compared cisplatin and 5-FU and carboplatin and 5-FU with methotrexate [3]. The response rates were 32, 21, and 10%, respectively. Complete responses were more frequent (6%) in the cisplatin arm. However, median response duration was only 4.2, 5.1, and 4.1 months, respectively, and no difference in over-

all survival was observed. The combination increased toxicity—nausea and vomiting, nephrotoxicity, and ototoxicity. Patients receiving 5-FU experienced significant mucositis. Patients with a poor performance status usually tolerate chemotherapy less well and are more prone to complications. Based on these survival data, methotrexate continues to be the standard chemotherapy, with cisplatin (alone or in combination with 5-FU) as possible alternatives.

EXPERIMENTAL AND MULTIMODALITY THERAPY

Up to 70% of patients initially present with locally advanced disease. Of these, a high percentage will recur locally or regionally. New strategies have been developed in order to improve local control rates and overall survival. Another goal of new and multimodality treatment approaches is to reduce morbidity associated with standard therapy. However, it is important to recognize that these new approaches are still experimental and their benefit not yet proven for the most part.

Induction Chemotherapy

Induction chemotherapy or neoadjuvant chemotherapy is often used in head and neck cancer protocols. The theoretic advantage of early use of chemotherapy is an intact vascular bed (with improved delivery of chemotherapy) and early control of systemic micrometastases [5]. With improvements in locoregional disease control, the latter may be important for long-term survival. Induction chemotherapy also might facilitate less extensive surgery or allow for organ preservation. On the other hand, a delay in performing surgery might result in incomplete resectability due to tumor progression (Table 5).

In phase II trials, induction chemotherapy results in complete response rates of 20 to 50% and a overall response rate of 80 to 100%. The survival rate is improved for complete responders, but whether this is an overall improvement or only represents a selection

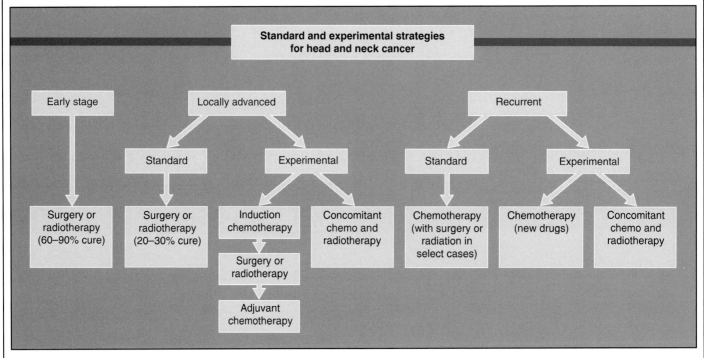

FIGURE 1

of a favorable prognostic group remains unclear. One area of controversy was the number of induction chemotherapy cycles before surgery. Rooney *et al.* have shown that three cycles of chemotherapy result in higher complete response rates than two cycles [6]. In sequential studies by Clark *et al.*, the patients were re-evaluated after two, three, and four cycles of neoadjuvant chemotherapy, with an increase in complete response rates from 2 to 3, but not from 3 to 4 [7]. The University of Chicago data show similar results for an induction regimen with methotrexate, cisplatin, and 5-FU [8,9].

Although induction chemotherapy with cisplatin and 5-FU results in high response rates, this has not translated into a significant survival advantage in randomized trials [10–15]. In four conclusive trials, no improvement in survival was demonstrated. However, a reduction in distant metastasis was demonstrated, thus suggesting systemic activity against early micrometastatic disease [10–12,15] (Table 6).

Organ preservation has been an important end point in one randomized study. The VA Laryngeal Cancer Study Group has shown that, in patients responding to chemotherapy, induction chemotherapy followed by radiation therapy is as effective a treatment for locally advanced laryngeal carcinoma as is standard surgery followed by radiotherapy when measured by survival [15]. In this study, larynx preservation was achieved in 64% of the patients receiving chemotherapy and radiation.

Adjuvant Chemotherapy

In head and neck cancer the most common site of treatment failure is locoregional relapse in up to 60% of the cases, with only 25% developing distant metastatic disease. Adjuvant therapy might have a role in the management of head and neck cancer, especially if locoregional control improves with more aggressive and multimodality therapies. A randomized study with only 46 evaluable patients suggested that adjuvant chemotherapy with cisplatin, bleomycin, and methotrexate

leads to prolonged disease-free, but not overall, survival. Only patients who initially responded to neoadjuvant chemotherapy and had final surgery and/or radiation therapy received adjuvant treatment. The difference was only significant in a subgroup of patients who achieved a partial response, although no additional benefit was seen in patients' complete response rates. The estimated failure-free survival at 3 years was 35% for patients without adjuvant chemotherapy compared to 84% for patients receiving chemotherapy; patients with complete response did well anyhow [16]. However, patients achieving a complete response had a failure-free survival rate of 85%, with or without adjuvant treatment. The numbers in each subgroup were small, and this advantage may only be artifactual.

Subset analysis of the Head and Neck Contracts program found a survival advantage for patients with N2 disease after receiving adjuvant chemotherapy with cisplatin for 6 cycles. In patients with oral cavity cancer, an improved disease-free survival rate of 67% at 3 years compared favorably with 49% for the surgery and radiotherapy standard arm. When site of failure was analyzed, a significantly lower distant failure rate was noted [17]. The recently published Intergroup Study trial also showed a lower incidence of local and distant failures. However, no prolongation in overall survival nor time to progression has been demonstrated [11]. In this trial, the chemotherapy was given after surgery, but before radiotherapy.

Concomitant chemoradiotherapy

In advanced cancer of the head and neck, an aggressive approach with concomitant chemoradiotherapy shows great potential in influencing overall or disease-free survival. It has been postulated that concomitant chemotherapy might eradicate radiation-resistant tumor cells, presumably by making the tumor cells more susceptible to radiation. The rationale for concomitant chemoradiation therapy has been reviewed extensively [18]. Even though concomitant chemoradiotherapy enhances treatment efficacy, unfortunately it also adds significantly to toxicity levels. Mucositis, neutropenia, and infections can be severe and occasionally produce life-threatening complications [19,20]. Not infrequently, these secondary effects lead to an interruption of radiotherapy, thus potentially neutralizing the increased intensity of therapy.

Initially, single-agent chemotherapy in low doses was added to radiation treatment with a pure radiosensitizing objective. More recently, full doses of chemotherapy have been used synchronous with radiation therapy, fully exploiting the possible contribution of the chemotherapy modality at improving local and systemic control rates. A randomized trial with 313 patients using methotrexate and radiotherapy versus radiotherapy alone showed a trend toward prolonged survival for the

Table 4. Standard Therapies for Metastatic or Recurrent Disease

Methotrexate 40–60 mg/m² IV weekly
Cisplatin 100 mg/m² IV every 3–4 wk
Cisplatin 100 mg/m² and 5-FU 800–1000 mg/m² continuous X 4–5 d every 3–4 wk

Table 5. Rationale for Induction Chemotherapy

Potential advantages
  Intact vascular bed; therefore, better drug delivery
  Reduced bulk results in less extensive surgery, or conversion of an unresectable tumor into a resectable status
  Identify chemosensitive tumors, thus better prognosis, organ preservation surgery, and adjuvant chemotherapy
  Identify poor prognostic patients for intensified therapy
  Better performance status, better tolerance of chemotherapy
  Early therapy for micrometastatic disease
Potential disadvantages
  Delay of potentially curative surgery
  Noncompliance after a complete response (refusing surgery) thus missing opportunity for cure
  Overtherapy and morbidity from therapy, increased cost

Table 6. Site of Recurrence After Induction Chemotherapy

| | VA Laryngeal [15] | | SWOG [12] | | |
	Surgery (%)	Preop Chemo (%)	Surgery (%)	Preop Chemo (%)	Degree of Significance
Primary disease	2	12	40	48	ns
Regional disease	5	8	14	24	ns
Distant metastasis	7	11	49	28	ns (p=0.07)

ns—not significant.

concomitant group at a median follow-up of 32 months. The difference in response was significant in a subgroup of patients with oropharyngeal cancer. However, in this trial only submaximal radiation (4500–5000 cGy) was delivered over a 3-week period [21].

5-Fluorouracil has been widely used with concomitant radiation. The response rate correlates with dosage and schedule of administration (continuous infusion being superior to intravenous bolus) [22]. Cisplatin, hydroxyurea, bleomycin, and mitomycin C have also been shown to have radiosensitizing and antitumor activity [23].

More recent trials focus on full-dose chemotherapy combinations with simultaneous radiotherapy once or twice daily. Several phase II trials using 5-FU and hydroxyurea [24–27]; cisplatin and 5-FU [28,29]; and cisplatin and 5-FU enhanced by leucovorin [14,30] suggest a survival benefit. However, these results need to be confirmed in randomized trials.

Ongoing trials attempt to improve response and overall outcome by using hyperfractionated radiation therapy with chemotherapy. By further fractionation of the XRT (eg, smaller doses per fraction at an increased frequency) less normal tissue damage is observed, and more importantly, repair of sublethal damage is less likely. Accelerated radiotherapy gives the same XRT fraction at an increased frequency, thus further diminishing the potential of regeneration of the tumor at the price of more acute reactions [30].

CHEMOPREVENTION

Oral leukoplakia is a recognized premalignant condition that can lead to invasive squamous cell carcinoma. A recent study has shown the efficacy of cis-retinoic acid in reversing this precancerous condi-

tion [31] (Table 7). The response rate was 67%, with a clinical complete response rate of 54% and a histologic one of 38%. In the high dosages used (1–2 mg/kg), the retinoic acid has significant toxicity, particularly dry and peeling skin, facial erythema, cheilitis (79%), hypertriglyceridemia (71%), conjunctivitis (54%), as well as headaches, fatigue, anorexia, and pruritus. After discontinuation of the therapy, a high incidence of relapse after a few months is noted. Recent data suggest benefit from maintenance therapy of 0.5 mg/kg/d, which produces only mild side effects [32]. Over 9 months, only 8% of the patients receiving maintenance therapy with low-dose retinoic acid progressed, compared to a control group treated with beta-carotene, in which 55% of the patients had progression.

In the first 2 to 3 years, local recurrence is the most common site of relapse. In subsequent years, a higher percentage of patients present with secondary malignancies (eg, a second head or neck cancer, or lung cancer). Therefore regular monitoring and follow-up focusing on other disease sites are mandatory in these patients. Instructions and support in order to avoid further risk factor exposure (smoking, alcohol) are needed. Hong et al. showed that the incidence of second primary tumors can be markedly reduced by a daily high-dose of 13-cis-retinoic acid (isotretinoin) (50–100 mg/m²). This therapy, however, does not prevent recurrence of the original tumor [33]. Large long-term chemoprevention trials are currently being conducted by several cooperative groups (Table 8).

ACKNOWLEDGMENT

The authors thank Mrs. Susan Jarman for assistance in preparation of the manuscript.

Table 7. Tables with 13-Cis-retinoic Acid

Oral Leucoplakia	Evaluable patients, n	Regimen	Response Rates
Induction—3 mo [31]	24 20	cis-RA 1–2 mg/kg Placebo	16 (67%) 2 (10%) (p=0.0002)
Maintenance—9 mo [32]	26 33	cis-RA 0.5 mg/kg beta-carotene	Progression 2 (8%) 16 (55%) (p<0.001)
2nd Malignancies Maintenance—12 mo [33]	49 51	cis-RA 50–100 mg/m² Placebo	2nd primary 2 (4%) 12 (24%) (p=0.05)

Table 8. Current Chemoprevention Trials

Agent	Regimen
Isotretinoin	30 mg p.o. QD*
Isotretinoin	10–20 mg p.o. QD†
Beta carotene	30 mg p.o. QD‡
Beta carotene/Vitamin A	50 mg/2500 U p.o. QD§

*Ongoing Intergroup (RTOG, MDA, NCI) trial with low-dose 13-cis retinoic acid (placebo versus isotretinoin for 3 y).
†ECOG/NCCTG randomized placebo controlled trial.
‡SWOG placebo controlled trial (5 y).
§Randomized versus isotretinoin 0.5 mg/kg/d in oral leucoplakia (3 y intervention) (M.D. Anderson).

REFERENCES

1. Sloan D, Goepfert H: Conventional therapy of head and neck cancer. *Hem Oncol Clin North Am* 1991, 5:601–625.

2. Pinto HA, Jacobs C: Chemotherapy for recurrent and metastatic head and neck cancer. *Hem Oncol Clin North Am* 1991, 5:667–686.

3. Forastiere AA, Metch B, Schuller DE, *et al.*: Randomized comparison of cisplatin plus fluorouracil and carboplatin plus fluorouracil versus methotrexate in advanced squamous cell carcinoma of the head and neck: A Southwest Oncology Group Study. *J Clin Oncol* 1992, 10:1245–1251.

4. Jacobs C, Lymen G, Velez-Garcia E, *et al.*: A phase III randomized study comparing cisplatin and 5-fluorouracil in single agents and in combination for enhanced squamous cell carcinoma of the head and neck. *J Clin Oncol* 1992, 10:257–263.

5. Forastiere AA: Randomized trials of induction chemotherapy. A critical review. *Hem Oncol Clin North Am* 1991, 5:725–736.

6. Rooney M, Kish J, Jacobs J, *et al.*: Improved complete response rate and survival in advanced head and neck cancer after three-course induction therapy with 12-hour 5-FU infusion and cisplatin. *Cancer* 1985, 55:1123–1128.

7. Clark JR, Fallon BC, Dreyfuss AI, *et al.*: Chemotherapeutic strategies in multidisciplinary treatment of head and neck cancer. *Semin Oncol* 1988, 15 (Suppl 3):35–44.

8. Vokes EE, Moran WJ, Mick R, *et al.*: Neoadjuvant and adjuvant methotrexate, cisplatin and fluorouracil in multimodal therapy of head and neck cancer. *J Clin Oncol* 1989, 7:838–845.

9. Vokes EE, Panje WR, Mick R, *et al.*: A randomized study comparing two regimens of neoadjuvant and adjuvant chemotherapy in multi-modal therapy for locally advanced head and neck cancer. *Cancer* 1990, 66:206–213.

10. Head and Neck Contracts Program: Adjuvant chemotherapy for advanced head and neck squamous carcinoma. Final Report. *Cancer* 1987, 60:301–311.

11. Laramore GE, Scott CB, Al-Sarraf M, *et al.*: Adjuvant chemotherapy for resectable squamous cell carcinomas of the head and neck: Report on Intergroup Study 0034. *Int J Radiat Oncol Biol Phys* 1992, 23:705–713.

12. Schuller DE, Metch B, Mattox D, *et al.*: Prospective chemotherapy in advanced resectable head and neck cancer: Final report of the Southwest Oncology Group. *Laryngoscope* 1988, 98:1205–1211.

13. Vokes EE, Schilsky RL, Weichselbaum RR, *et al.*: Induction chemotherapy with cisplatin, fluorouracil, and high-dose leucovorin for locally advanced head and neck cancer: A clinical and pharmacologic analysis. *J Clin Oncol* 1990, 8:241–247.

14. Vokes EE, Weichselbaum RR, Mick R, *et al.*: Favorable long-term survival following induction chemotherapy with cisplatin, fluorouracil, and leucovorin and concomitant chemoradiotherapy for locally advanced head and neck cancer. *J Natl Cancer Inst* 1992, 84:877–882.

15. Department of Veterans Affairs Laryngeal Cancer Study Group: Induction chemotherapy plus radiation compared with surgery plus radiation in patients with advanced laryngeal cancer. *N Engl J Med* 1991, 324:1685–1690.

16. Ervin TJ, Clark JR, Weichselbaum RR, *et al.*: An analysis of induction and adjuvant chemotherapy in the multidisciplinary treatment of squamous cell carcinoma of the head and neck. *J Clin Oncol* 1987, 5:10–20.

17. Jacobs C, Makuch R: Efficacy of adjuvant chemotherapy for patients with resectable head and neck cancer: A subset analysis of the Head and Neck Contracts Program. *J Clin Oncol* 1990, 8:838–847.

18. Vokes EE, Weichselbaum RR: Concomitant chemoradiotherapy: Rationale and clinical experience in patients with solid tumors. *J Clin Oncol* 1990, 8:911–934.

19. Denham DW, Abbott RL: Concurrent cisplatin, infusional fluorouracil, and conventionally fractionated radiation therapy in head and neck cancer: Dose limiting mucosal toxicity. *J Clin Oncol* 1991, 9:458–463.

20. Taylor SG, Murthy AK, Caldarelli DD, *et al.*: Combined simultaneous cisplatin/fluorouracil chemotherapy and split course radiation in head and neck cancer. *J Clin Oncol* 1989, 7:846–856.

21. Gupta NK, Pointer RCS, Wilkinson PM: A randomized trial to contrast radiotherapy with radiotherapy and methotrexate given synchronously in head and neck cancer. *Clin Radiol* 1987, 38:575–581.

22. Kish JA, Ensley JF, Jacobs J, *et al.*: A randomized trial of cisplatin and 5-FU infusion and cisplatin and 5-FU bolus for recurrent and advanced squamous cell carcinoma of the head and neck. *Cancer* 1985, 56:2740–2744.

23. Vokes EE, Awan AM, Weichselbaum RR: Radiotherapy with concomitant chemotherapy for head and neck cancer. *Hem Oncol Clin North Am* 1991, 5:753–767.

24. Vokes EE, Panje WR, Schilsky RL, *et al.*: Hydroxyurea, fluorouracil, and concomitant radiotherapy in poor prognosis head and neck cancers: A phase I-II study. *J Clin Oncol* 1989, 7:761–768.

25. Vokes EE, Moormeier JA, Ratain MJ, *et al.*: 5-fluorouracil, leucovorin, hydroxyurea, and escalating doses of continuous-infusion cisplatin with concomitant radiotherapy: A clinical and pharmacologic study. *Cancer Chemother Pharmacol* 1992, 29:178–184.

26. Weppelman B, Wheeler RH, Peters GE, *et al.*: Treatment of recurrent head and neck cancer with 5-fluorouracil, hydroxyurea, and reirradiation. *Int J Radiat Oncol Biol Phys* 1992, 22:1051–1056.

27. Gandia D, Wibault P, Guillot T, *et al.*: Simultaneous chemoradiotherapy as salvage treatment in locoregional recurrences of squamous head and neck cancer patients. *Head Neck* 1993, 15:8–15.

28. Adelstein DJ, Sharan VM, Earle AS, *et al.*: Long-term results after chemoradiotherapy for locally confined squamous-cell head and neck cancer. *Am J Clin Oncol* 1990, 13:440–447.

29. Adelstein DJ, Sharan VM, Earle AS, *et al.*: Simultaneous versus sequential combined technique therapy for squamous cell head and neck cancer. *Cancer* 1990, 65:1685–1691.

30. Wendt TG, Hartenstein RC, Wustrow TPU, *et al.*: Cisplatin, fluorouracil with leucovorin calcium enhancement, and synchronous accelerated radiotherapy in the management of locally advanced head and neck cancer: A phase II study. *J Clin Oncol* 1989, 7:471–476.

31. Hong WK, Endicott J, Itri LM, *et al.*: 13-cis-retinoic acid in the treatment of oral leukoplakia. *N Engl J Med* 1986, 315:1501–1505.

32. Lippman SM, Batsakis JG, Toth BB, *et al.*: Comparison of low dose isotretinoin with beta carotene to prevent oral carcinogenesis. *N Engl J Med* 1993, 328:15–20.

33. Hong WK, Lippman SM, Itri LM, *et al.*: Prevention of second primary tumors with isoretinoin in squamous cell carcinoma of the head and neck. *N Engl J Med* 1990, 323:795–801.

34. Vokes EE, Ratain MJ, Mick R, *et al.*: Cisplatin, fluorouracil, and leucovorin augmented by interferon alfa-2beta in head and neck cancer: A clinical and pharmacologic analysis. *J Clin Oncol* 1993, 11:360–368.

35. Vokes EE, Ratain MJ, Mick R, *et al.*: Cisplatin, fluorouracil and leucovorin augmented by interferon alfa-2B in head and neck cancer: A clinical and pharmacological analysis. *J Clin Oncol* 1992, 11:360–368.

CISPLATIN AND 5-FU

Platinum compounds are complex molecules, which covalently bind to DNA and also interact with proteins. The two available agents in this class, cisplatin (CDDP) and carboplatin, have different toxicity profiles. For both, single-agent activity has been positively shown in head and neck cancer. Most commonly used in this disease group is cisplatin, with an overall response rate of 30% and a complete response rate of less than 10%.

The antimetabolite 5-FU is commonly used in combination regimens and as a single agent. This pyrimidine analogue interferes with DNA and RNA synthesis by binding to thymidylate synthase, or it is incorporated into RNA as a false messenger. In head and neck cancer, 5-FU alone has not commonly been used, but a recent trial reported response rates of 15% [4]. The response rate depends on the dosage and schedule. A randomized trial has shown that continuous infusion therapy over 4 to 5 days is superior to IV bolus administration (when given in combination with cisplatin) in recurrent disease [22].

The combination of the two agents can significantly improve the overall response rate. Several trials using this combination showed an overall response rate of 25 to 40%, with 15% complete responders in recurrent disease. However, randomized trials have failed to demonstrate improved survival using this combination compared to single-agent chemotherapy.

CANDIDATES FOR TREATMENT

Recurrent, metastatic and locally advanced squamous cell carcinomas of the head and neck (in combination with radiation and/or surgery)

SPECIAL PRECAUTIONS

Hydration for 6–12 hr before and after cisplatin administration, antiemetic prophylaxis during initial 48 hr after CDDP administration

ALTERNATIVE THERAPIES

Methotrexate, carboplatin and 5-FU, cisplatin (single agent)

TOXICITIES

Cisplatin: highly emetogenic, nephrotoxicity, cumulative ototoxicity; late chronic neuropathy (up to 40% of the patients); myelosuppression (nadir after approx. 10 d); electrolyte wasting (K, Mg, Ca); **5-FU:** diarrhea, mucositis, loss of appetite, nausea/ vomiting, metallic taste in mouth, myelosuppression, increased liver enzymes

DRUG INTERACTIONS

CDDP: Antimetabolites, nephrotoxic agents (*eg*, aminoglycoside); **5-FU:** leucovorin, interferon alpha [34,35], dipyridamole

NURSING INTERVENTIONS

Agents can be administered by a peripheral venous access, extravasation causes local irritation; monitor fluid status, watch for dehydration and overhydration, do not administer CDDP if urine output <100 ml/hr over the last 4 hr prior to start; monitor electrolytes including magnesium QOD and start supplements early, blood counts need to be checked 1–2 times/wk.

PATIENT INFORMATION

Patient may experience delayed nausea/vomiting with CDDP, antiemetic must be available at all times; contact physician immediately for fevers (neutropenia possible), bleeding (thrombocytopenia rare), and diarrhea (electrolyte wasting, dehydration)

DOSAGE AND SCHEDULING

	Day 1	2	3	4	5	6	7	8
CDDP 100 mg/m² iv over 2–6 hr, d 1	■							
5-FU 1000 mg/m²/d x 5 d by continuous infusion	▬▬▬▬▬▬▬▬▬							
CBC, platelets, d 1,5,8	☐				☐			☐
Na, K, Mg, Ca, BUN, Crea, d 1, 3, 5, 8	☐		☐		☐			☐
SGOT, SGPT, alk. phos., alb., d 1	☐							

Repeat every 3–4 weeks

DOSAGE MODIFICATIONS: For impaired renal function, reduce CDDP to 75% for creatinine clearance of 50–75 ml/min, to 50% for clearance of 25–50 ml/min. Do not administer if clearance <25 ml/min. Dose reduction to 80% of 5-FU necessary for grade III mucositis.

RECENT EXPERIENCE AND RESPONSE RATES

Study	Evaluable Patients, *n*	Regimen	Response Rates
Jacobs *et al.* J Clin Oncol 1992, 10:257–263	79, eval. 63	CDDP 100 mg/m² x 1 + 5-FU 1000 mg/m² x 4 d ci	CR=5, PR=20, RR=32%
	83, eval. 80	CDDP 100 mg/m² x 1	CR=3, PR=11, RR=17%
	83, eval. 75 recurrent or metastatic	5-FU 1000 mg/m² x 4 d	CR=2, PR=9, RR=15%
Vokes *et al.* J Clin Oncol 1991, 9:1376–1384	51, neoadjuvant and adjuvant	CDDP 100 mg/m² x 1 + 5-FU 1000 mg/m² x 5 d ci	CR=22 (43%), pCR=24% PR=24 (47%), RR=90%
Kish *et al.* Cancer 1985, 56:2740–2744	18 randomized	CDDP 100 mg/m² + 5-FU 600 mg/m² bolus d 1 + 8	CR=2, PR=2, RR=20%
	20 locally adv. + recurrent	CDDP 100 mg/m² + 5-FU 1000 mg/m² x 4 d ci	CR=4, PR=9, RR=72%
Liverpool Head and Neck Oncology Group, Br J Cancer 1990, 61:311–315	36	CDDP 100 mg/m²	RR=39%
	34	MTX 40 mg/m²	18%
	39	CDDP + 5-FU 1000 mg/m² x 4 d ci	30%
	45	CDDP + MTX	24%
	total = 200, randomized to 4 groups of 50 patients each	overall survival analysis	28%
Forastiere *et al.* J Clin Oncol 1992, 10:1245–1251	87 randomized	CDDP 100 mg/m² + 5-FU 1000 mg/m² x 4 d ci	RR 32%, surv. 6.6 mo
	86	Carboplatin 300 mg/m² + 5-FU 1000 mg/m² x 4 d ci	RR 21% (ns), surv. 5.0 mo
	88 recurrent or metastatic	MTX 40 mg/m² iv q wk	RR 10%, surv. 5.6 mo

PFL
Cisplatin, 5-FU, and Leucovorin

Interaction and synergy of 5-FU and leucovorin is based on the inhibition of the enzyme thymidylate synthase. The active metabolite 5-FdUMP binds covalently to the thymidylate synthase and in the presence of reduced folates forms a stable ternary complex. Cellular 5-FU resistance is also reduced by the presence of high doses of reduced folates.

Cisplatin is thought to increase intracellular folates and therefore enhance the efficacy of 5-FU. Based on these *in vitro* data, clinical investigations were started combining these three agents, respectively adding leucovorin to the known effective regimen of cisplatin and 5-FU.

Leucovorin is a synthetic tetrahydrofolic acid and can be given IV or PO. Only L-leucovorin is biologically active and absorbed by the gut epithelium. As a vitamin and regular component of our diet there are virtually no side effects.

When leucovorin is added to the combination of cisplatin and 5-FU, the toxicity is increased. Therefore the maximally tolerated dose of 5-FU is only 800 mg/m^2 (compared to 1000 mg/m^2 without leucovorin). Treatment delays and dose adjustments due to toxicity are more often necessary. These limitations reduce the dose intensity of the therapy and may therefore neutralize the potential benefit of this more active combination.

CANDIDATES FOR TREATMENT

Patients with metastatic and recurrent squamous cell carcinoma of the head and neck, induction (neoadjuvant) therapy for locally advanced stages

SPECIAL PRECAUTIONS

Hydration for 6–12 hr before and after cisplatin administration, antiemetic prophylaxis during initial 48 hr after CDDP administration

TOXICITIES

Severe mucositis (dose-limiting) leading to profound dehydration; hand–foot syndrome with skin breakdown; myelosuppression with leucopenia and thrombocytopenia (nadir after 10–14 days); prolonged and delayed nausea/vomiting, diarrhea, electrolyte wasting

DRUG INTERACTIONS

CDDP: Antimetabolites, nephrotoxic agents (*eg*, aminoglycoside); **5-FU:** leucovorin, interferon alpha [34,35], dipyridamole

NURSING INTERVENTIONS

Watch for skin changes, good skin care with lipophilic ointment; prophylaxis for skin breakdown with silvadene and dromboro soaks: good oral hygiene with nonalcoholic antiseptic mouthwashes (4x/d), fungal prophylaxis with nystatin mouthwash or clotrimazole troches; insufficient food and fluid intake may require feeding tube

PATIENT INFORMATION

Patient should be aware of mucositis potential; mouth care needs to be emphasized; dry and peeling skin requires local skin care; call physician if diarrhea, nausea with impaired oral intake, fever (neutropenia), and bleeding (thrombocytopenia) develop

DOSAGE AND SCHEDULING

	Day 1	2	3	4	5	6	7	8
CDDP 100 mg/m^2 IV over 2–6 hr, d 1	■							
5-FU 800 mg/m^2/d x 5 d by continuous infusion	▬▬▬▬▬							
Leucovorin 300 mg/m^2/d mixed with 5-FU, or Leucovorin 100 mg po q 4–6 hr x 5 d	▬▬▬▬▬							
CBC, platelets, d 1,5,8	☐				☐			☐
Na, K, BUN, Crea, Ca, Mg, d 1, 3, 5, 8	☐		☐		☐			☐
SGOT, SGPT, alk. phos., alb., d 1	☐							

Repeat every 3–4 weeks.

RECENT EXPERIENCES AND RESPONSE RATES

Study	Evaluable Patients, *n*	Regimen	Response Rate
Vokes *et al.* J Clin Oncol 1988, 8:618–626	25, eval. 18 Recurrent or metastatic (dose escal.)	CDDP 100 mg/m^2 x 1, 5-FU 800 mg/m^2 x 5 d ci Leucovorin 50 mg/m^2 po q 4–6 hr	CR=1, PR=9, RR 56%
Dreyfuss *et al.* Ann Int Med 1990, 118:167–172	35	CDDP 25 mg/m^2 d x 5 d ci 5-FU 800 mg/m^2 d x 5 d ci Leucovorin 500 mg/m^2 d x 6 d ci	CR=23 (66%), PR=5 (14%), RR 80%
Loeffler *et al.* Adv Exp Med Biol 1988, 244:267–273	58 Untreated 45, prior tx 13	CDDP 20 mg/m^2 d x 5 d IVP 5-FU 400 mg/m^2 d x 5 d IVP Leucovorin 100 mg/m^2 d x 5 d IVP	RR 91%, RR 95%, CR 23, PR 20 RR 77% CR 4, PR 6
Vokes *et al.* J Clin Oncol 1992, 84:877–882	31, eval. 29 locally advanced, neoadjuvant + concomitant	CDDP 100 mg/m^2 x 1 5-FU 1000 mg/m^2 x 4–5 d ci Leucovorin 100 mg po Q4hr	CR=29%, PR=52%, RR=81%. med. surv. not reached, 18 alive at 35 mo, metastatic 3%

CISPLATIN, 5-FU, HYDROXYUREA, AND CONCOMITANT RADIATION

Cisplatin, 5-FU, and hydroxyurea have long been known for their radiosensitizing effects. The mechanism of this interaction is not completely known. Theoretically several mechanisms have been postulated. Ideally both the chemotherapeutic agent and the radiation must have independent antitumor activity. These drugs have been used as single agents with simultaneous radiation therapy in a variety of malignant diseases. Often the use was purely to enhance the radiation effects; therefore the drugs have often been given in a suboptimal fashion at subtherapeutic doses. Only lately has the consequent use of concomitant chemoradiation therapy been pursued.

Cisplatin, like ionizing radiation, causes direct DNA damage by intrastrand crosslinks and breaks. It acts mainly with synergistic cytotoxicity by inhibiting DNA repair from sublethal cell damage.

5-FU is either incorporated into RNA or binds to thymidylate synthase and thus inhibits DNA synthesis. Synergy with radiation has been shown in several *in vitro* studies, where subtherapeutic doses of radiation or 5-FU were not able to induce cell death, but the combination showed increased cytotoxicity. The mechanism of this interaction remains unclear, possibly the cells become more sensitive to the radiation by modification of the cell kinetics. Hydroxyurea (HU) inhibits ribonucleotide reductase specifically in the S phase. It alters the cell kinetics by inhibiting entry into the radioresistant S phase. Hydroxyurea as an antimetabolite inhibits DNA synthesis or repair. Although it has single-agent activity in head and neck cancer, it is rarely used other then as a radiosensitizer. Concomitant radiation therapy with full-dose chemotherapy significantly increases toxicities.

DOSAGE AND SCHEDULING

	1	2	3	4	5	6	7
CDDP 100 mg/m² IV over 2–6 hr, d 1	■						
5-FU 800 mg/m²/d x 5 d continuous infusion		███████████					
HU 1000 mg po bid x 11 doses, first dose 12 hr before RT, d 1–6		███████████					
XRT 200 cGY QD x 5 d		███████					
CBC, platelets, d 1,5	□				□		
Na, K, BUN, Crea, Ca, Mg, d 1,3, 5	□		□		□		
Crea, K, Mg, Ca, d 3, 5			□		□		
Day	1	2	3	4	5	6	7

Repeat cycle every other week. CDDP every other cycle.

CANDIDATES FOR TREATMENT

Patients with locally advanced and recurrent head and neck carcinomas (investigational)

TOXICITIES

Severe mucositis, weight loss (forced feeding commonly necessary)

NURSING INTERVENTIONS

Good oral hygiene with antiseptic mouthwashes (4x/d); insufficient food intake—possible forced feeding required

RECENT EXPERIENCES AND RESPONSE RATES

Study	Evaluable Patients, n	Regimen	Response Rates
Haraf et al. Am J Clin Oncol 1991, 14:419–426	20; recurrent (prior tx) 19; advanced, (no prior tx)	5-FU 800 mg/m² x 5 d ci, HU 1000 mg po BID, XRT 200cGy QD x 5 d	CR 40%, PR 53% CR 71%, PR 29%
Taylor IV et al. J Clin Oncol 1989, 7:846–856	53, locally advanced, recurrent or metastatic	CDDP 60 mg/m² x 1, 5-FU 800 mg/m² x 5 d ci, XRT 200 cGy QD, repeat every 2nd wk	CR 29 (55%), PR 23 (43%), RR 98%
Wendt et al. J Clin Oncol 1989, 7:471–476	62, eval. 59 locally advanced	CDDP 60 mg/m² x 1, 5-FU 350 mg/m² x 4 d ci, LV 50 mg/m² x 4 d ci, XRT 180 cGy QD x 11 d	CR 48 (81%), PR 11 (19%), RR 100%
Adelstein et al. Cancer 1990, 65:1685–1691	48 (Stage II, III, IV) simultaneous therapy (24) randomized versus sequential therapy (24)	CDDP 75 mg/m² x 1, 5-FU 1000 mg/m² x 4 d ci (repeat chemo on d 28) XRT 200 cGy QD x 15 d (3000 cGy total), possibly surgery and repeat above CDDP 100 mg/m² x 1, 5-FU 1000 mg/m² x 5 d ci x 3 cycles, followed by possible surgery and XRT 6000 cGy total	CR 16, PR 8, RR 100%, Grade IV neutropenia 10 (42%), death 1 CR 7, PR 13, RR 83%, Grade IV neutrope-nia 140 (58%), death 2 Trend for improved DFS in simult. group
Adelstein et al. Am J Clin Oncol 1990, 13:440–447	55, eval. 54 (48 locally advanced) no prior chemo- or radiotherapy	CDDP 75 mg/m² x 1, 5-FU 1000 mg/m² 4 d ci (repeat chemo on d 28 and after possible surgery), XRT 200 cGy QD x 15 d (3000 cGy total)	CR 30 (56%), (pCR 19), PR 24 (44%), RR 100%, Surv. 56%, (median >43 months)
Weppelmann et al. Int J Radiat Oncol Biol Phys 1992, 22:1051–1056	21, eval. 20 recurrent or metastatic, after previous surgery and radiation	5-FU 300 mg/m² x 5 d ci, HU>1500 mg/m² QD x 5 d, XRT 200 cGy QD x 5 d every other week	CR 9, PR 6, RR 75% 1 y. surv. 56%
Merlano et al. N Engl J Med 1992, 327:115–121	80 locally advanced, unresectable vs 77 randomized	CDDP 20 mg/m² x 5 d, 5-FU 200 mg/m² x 5 d bolus alternating with XRT 200 cGy x 5 d x wks vs XRT 200 cGy QD (70 Gy total)	CR 43%, PR 29%, 3 y. surv. 41% (p<0.05), CR 22%, PR 43%, 3 y. surv. 23%

With more than 60% of men and 45% of women being current or former smokers in the United States, lung cancer unfortunately is going to remain a major health care problem for the foreseeable future [1]. Treatment with chemotherapy for lung cancer is beset with the same problem encountered with other solid tumors in regard to controlling disseminated disease. Cancer-related mortality for lung cancer has not substantially changed during the last three decades despite intensive clinical investigative effort. The average patient with lung cancer is approaching the sixth decade of life, usually after a significant history of tobacco exposure. Such individuals often have overt or subclinical cardiovascular and respiratory disease, which makes the potential for morbidity associated with chemotherapy administration much more significant. As a result, efforts to increase dose intensity beyond conventional doses for these cancers has not been associated with clinical benefit. Innovations for this disease have focused on attempting to achieve patient benefit while minimizing side effects, identifying new active agents, and refining the approach to the management of subsets of patients who are to receive a particular treatment modality.

STAGES AND RESPONSE RATES

In this chapter, the range of chemotherapeutic options for the clinician treating patients with lung cancer is considered. Specific management issues are focused on, including dose, schedule, and complications, which distinguish this discussion from a superb overview on the subject by Idhe [2]. The recommendations made are tempered by the dichotomy in chemoresponsiveness of the two forms of lung cancer. Non–small cell lung cancer, which comprises 75% of all the cases, is associated with an objective response rate of roughly 20% for good performance in patients with metastatic disease [3]. The administration of chemotherapy for patients with advanced non–small cell lung cancer is not considered standard care, although it is a reasonable option in the appropriate setting. The response rate for small cell lung cancer is at least several times higher than for non–small cell lung cancer, and chemotherapy generally is accepted as standard care in that setting [2].

In considering chemotherapy for a patient with lung cancer, the cost to benefit ratio for the two forms of lung cancer is different. It also appears that the response rate for chemotherapy in patients with regionally advanced lung cancer is higher than for patients with widely metastatic lung cancer (Table 1). In patients with Stage III non–small cell lung cancer, response rates of greater than 50% are frequently reported [4,5]. Although it is not a foregone conclusion that a higher response rate invariably results in enhanced patient survival, a clinician may be more comfortable with an aggressive chemotherapy regimen in this setting compared with aggressive treatment of a patient with metastatic lung cancer. Clearly, clinical judgment in managing care for patients with lung cancer is extremely important in balancing all the relevant treatment factors.

CHEMOTHERAPY

New Active Agents

New drugs either represent analogues of agents with demonstrated activity in lung cancer or drugs that work by novel mechanisms. Analogue development is often driven by the effort to modify toxicity profiles—such as with nephrotoxicity for cisplatin compared with carboplatin [6]. Occasionally, rational design enables a compound to improve on the cytotoxic effect of the parent compound, which may

be the case with the design of 10-methyl-10-ethyl-10-deaza-aminopterin in which the recognition of the importance of polyglutamination and drug uptake has led to the identification of a potentially more active antifol [7].

Three new drugs of potential interest for lung cancer therapy involve novel mechanisms of action. The first is paclitaxel, which has a unique effect on microspindle organization during cell division [8]. It has shown activity in lung cancer cell lines and in phase I trials and is currently undergoing phase II clinical trials. Chang *et al.* studied 119 patients with Stage IV metastatic non–small cell lung cancer who had received no previous chemotherapy (25 of the 119 received paclitaxel) [9]. Murphy *et al.* studied 27 chemotherapy-naive patients with non–small cell lung cancer [10]. All patients received paclitaxel. 200 to 250 mg/m^2 in 24-hour continuous IV infusions, repeated every 3 weeks. The response rates in both trials were similar (20–24%).

An old drug that has sparked new interest is the plant alkaloid camptothecin [11]. Camptothecin inhibits the specific DNA repair actions mediated by topoisomerase I. This compound was originally rejected as being too toxic in the 1970s, but has been reevaluated recently as a result of the elucidation of its mechanism of action. An analogue of camptothecin, CPT-11, which may be a more effective topoisomerase inhibitor, has been the lead compound for this therapeutic strategy.

Vinorelbine (Navelbine) is a new drug recently approved by the FDA for parenteral use in advanced non–small cell lung cancer. This vinca alkaloid analogue inhibits polymerization of microtubules resulting in cell death. While response rates for this drug were only comparable to other available chemotherapies, its low toxicity profile makes it an attractive option. Myelosuppression is the dose-limiting factor, with hair loss and nausea occurring infrequently. Combinations of Navelbine with other drugs used for non–small cell lung cancer are currently under investigation.

The success of these compounds in the treatment of lung cancer will be related to the extent that the mechanisms of drug action effect a central aspect of the biologic make-up of lung cancer cells. Mechanisms of drug resistance for human lung cancer cells are poorly understood to date but it is likely that a multiple drug-resistance phenotype (MDR-I) does not play a significant role in lung

Table 1. Staging Classification for Lung Cancer

	Stage				
	I	II	IIIa	IIIb	IV
TNM Components	T1, N0 T2, N0	T1, N1 T2, N1	T3, N0 T3, N1 T1–3, N2	Any T, N3 T4, any N	M1

TNM Criteria
 T1—Tumor < 3 cm
 T2—Tumor > 3 cm or visceral pleural involvement, > 2 cm from corina
 T3—Circumscribed extrapulmonary (*eg*, chest wall or superior sulcus) but resectable
 T4—SVC syndrome, malignant effusion, unresectable soft tissue invasion
 N1—Ipsilateral peribronchial and hilar nodes (including direct extension)
 N2—Ipsilateral mediastinal or subcorinal nodes
 N3—Supraclavicular or contralateral hilar/mediastinal nodes
 M1—Metastases beyond scope of T4 or N3 classification

cancer [12]. Further research into the nature of chemoresistance for lung cancer cells taken directly from patients instead of from artificially generated resistance models may be a crucial step in the search for more effective anti–lung cancer drugs.

Treatment Strategies

Some general principles are emerging from consideration of the wealth of clinical trial experience with patients with lung cancer. For patients with non–small cell lung cancer, the potential for benefit is small and therefore only patients with good functional status (equivalent to Eastern Cooperative Oncology Group [ECOG] performance status 0–1 [see appendix]) should be considered for combination chemotherapy [5]. The patient with small cell lung cancer has a higher probability of response, and more aggressive management of advanced symptoms seems justified. At the National Cancer Institute, for critically ill patients initially presenting with debilitating small cell lung cancer, we often begin regimens with half the usual initial dose of chemotherapy. If the patient's status improves, the second cycle is delivered at full dose. We would not offer chemotherapy to a patient with non–small cell lung cancer who was not fully ambulatory but would focus on providing that patient appropriate supportive care.

Despite considerable discussion, there is no credible evidence to suggest that a clinically meaningful dose-response relationship exists for the use of chemotherapy in patients with lung cancer [13,14]. The immediate caveats include both that the appropriate concentration of the relevant drugs are administered (usually around the concentration identified in the phase II trials) and that the possibility that a small benefit of dose intensification exists, but only very large trials would demonstrate such a benefit. Again, the ultimate dose intensification has already been applied in non–small cell lung cancer in a trial involving intensive chemotherapy given with bone marrow transplantation support. This effort resulted in a duration of treatment response of approximately 14 weeks, with an induction mortality of 15% [15]. This important report from the University of Chicago group highlights the difficulty in managing this very fragile population of patients.

Clinical data regarding the issue of drug scheduling are minimal. With the exception of one provocative report of cisplatin given daily with concurrent radiation therapy [16], no consistent benefit of drug scheduling has been evident. Again, current trial results do not exclude the possibility of a slight benefit associated with dose scheduling, but it is unlikely that a major benefit of dose scheduling will be found. Because the potential benefit is likely to be small, the enthusiasm for such trials is limited.

The issue of interaction between chemotherapy and radiation therapy is an area of intense research, but because of the lack of mature results from randomized trials, inadequate information exists to justify a change in clinical practice. Referral of patients with Stage III disease to centers participating in randomized phase III trials of neoadjuvant therapy should be considered to assist completion of the current intergroup studies so that patient management decisions can be based on firm data. The one exception is hyperfractionated-dose radiation therapy as used in combined modality therapy for limited small cell lung cancer. The benefit of this approach has been reported by independent groups [17,18].

The duration of chemotherapy treatment has not been rigorously established for the major types of lung cancer but the trend has been for shorter numbers of administered cycles–with about six being the norm for small cell lung cancer [19]. Patients with non–small cell lung cancer usually tolerate only about three cycles of standard chemotherapy, and no data exist to suggest the optimal length of therapy. A practical approach for the treatment of non–small cell lung cancer in a nonstudy setting is to give two courses of chemotherapy and do a limited assessment of response (repeat of initially abnormal pretreatment imaging studies). If a patient has responded (achieving a complete or partial response), a total of six cycles of drug may be given. Chemotherapy in patients with progressive disease is discontinued after two cycles. If, after two cycles, a patient has stable disease, then the decision to proceed to four more cycles of drug is individualized, based on the patient's overall condition and tolerance of the first two cycles of chemotherapy.

TUMOR MARKERS

Performance status, histologic features, and stage of disease remain the most significant determinants of overall outcome with chemotherapy for lung cancer. Other variables have been proposed to select the patients who are most likely to benefit from chemotherapy. An example is the proposal to evaluate a patient's tumor for the expression of neuroendocrine markers [2]. Small cell lung cancer is the most common neuroendocrine tumor in humans, and this cancer is often initially responsive to chemotherapy. Non–small cell lung cancer is not thought to be a neuroendocrine tumor and is not typically as responsive to chemotherapy. We have found that a small percentage of non–small cell lung cancer tumors do express the biochemical markers of neuroendocrine differentiation and we postulate that these "small cell–like" non–small cell tumors may be the more chemoresponsive of the non–small cell tumors [20]. We have evaluated this prospectively but because the neuroendocrine phenotype occurs in only about 12% of the non–small cell cancers, a very large clinical experience is required to evaluate this possibility. As reported, the response rate for the neuroendocrine non–small cell tumors at the National Cancer Institute is higher than that for the remaining patients but data from many more patients will have to be analyzed prior to having the requisite power to determine if this is an important clinical discriminant [21].

We and others have looked at the clinical consequences of deregulation for various oncogenes [22–24] but, despite provocative preliminary reports, knowledge of oncogene status is not an established marker that should influence the selection of chemotherapeutic regimen. Further research is required to identify and validate which molecular markers are most closely linked to chemosensitivity status before molecular probes can be responsibly applied to the management of chemotherapeutic administration. The use of such markers of prognosis might come into practice as discriminants to determine which patients are most appropriate for adjuvant chemotherapy approaches.

In vitro drug sensitivity testing of candidate drugs with actual patient tumor specimens has been proposed to aid in the selection of chemotherapeutic agents [25]. We have evaluated the benefit of such an approach by using a dye exclusion or semiautomated colorimetric assay [21,25]. Although this is an important research question and, generally, such assays provide fairly reliable information in defining true-negative results (patients that will not respond to chemotherapy), this information is of limited value in a clinical situation. The clinical problem, especially for non–small cell lung cancer is that there are no particularly effective drugs; therefore, the issue of the assay selection is not important. Our own experience demonstrates that patients who are going to respond (*ie*, showed good cytotoxicity results *in vitro*) generally would have responded to the standard arm of the trial, which consisted of the administration of etoposide and cisplatin.

The options for the clinician in selecting conventional chemotherapeutic agents for patients with lung cancer are relatively limited. In the protocol pages in this chapter, several common chemotherapy combinations and several new drugs used for lung cancer are discussed. Unfortunately, although these new agents may result in improved anti–lung cancer cytotoxicity, it is unlikely that any of the drugs currently being tested hold the potential for significantly affecting overall mortality from lung cancer. Given the vast numbers of patients with newly diagnosed lung cancer, however, it is incumbent on the oncologic community to attempt to optimize the use of existing therapeutic tools for patients with lung cancer despite the inherent limitations.

REFERENCES

1. Shopland DR, Eyre HJ, Pechacek TF: Smoking-attributable cancer mortality in 1991: Is lung cancer now the leading cause of death among smokers in the United States? *J Nat Cancer Inst* 1991, 83:1142–1148.

2. Idhe DC: Chemotherapy of lung cancer. *N Engl J Med* 1992, 327:1434–1441.

3. Mulshine JL, Glatstein E, Ruckdeschel JC: Treatment of non–small-cell lung cancer. *J Clin Oncol* 1986, 4:1704–1715.

4. Ruckdeschel JC, Holmes EC: Preoperative chemotherapy for locally advanced non–small-cell lung cancer. In Pass HI, (ed): *Chest Surgery Clinics of North America*. 1991, Philadelphia: WB Saunders; 1–12.

5. Mulshine JL, Ruckdeschel JC: The role of chemotherapy in the management of disseminated non–small cell lung cancer. In Roth JA, Ruckdeschel JC, Weisenburger TH (eds): *Thoracic Oncology*. 1989, Philadelphia: WB Saunders; 220–228.

6. Rossof AH, Bearden JD III, Coltman CA Jr: Phase II evaluation of cis-diamminedichloroplatinum (II) in lung cancer. *Cancer Treat Rep* 1976, 60:1679–1680.

7. Sirotnak FM, Degraw JI, Schmid FA, et al.: New folate analogs of the 10-deaza-aminopterin series. Further evidence for markedly increased antitumor efficacy compared with methotrexate in ascitic and solid murine tumor models. *Cancer Chemother Pharmacol* 1984, 12:26–30.

8. McGuire WP, Rowinsky EK, Rosenshein Neil B, et al.: Taxol: A unique antineoplastic agent with significant activity in advanced ovarian epithelial neoplasms. *Ann Intern Med* 1989, 111:273–279.

9. Chang A, Kim K, Glick J, et al.: Phase II study of taxol, merbarone, and piroxantrone in patients with stage IV non–small cell lung cancer (NSCLC): The Eastern Cooperative Oncology Group (ECOG) results. *J Nat Cancer Inst* 1993, 85:388–393.

10. Murphy WY, Fossella FV, Winn RJ, et al.: Phase II study of taxol in patients with untreated advanced non–small cell lung cancer. *J Nat Cancer Inst* 1993, 85:384–388.

11. Muggia FM, Creaven PJ, Hansen HH, et al.: Phase I clinical trials of weekly and daily treatment with camptothecin (NSC 100880): Correlations with clinical studies. *Cancer Chemother Rep* 1972, 56:515–521.

12. Lai SL, Goldstein L, Gottesman M, et al.: MDR1 gene expression in lung cancer. *J Nat Cancer Inst* 1989, 81:1144–1150.

13. Souhami RL, De Elvira MCR: Dose intensity in small cell lung cancer. *Chest*, in press.

14. Seifter EJ, Ihde DC: Therapy of small cell lung cancer: A perspective on two decades of clinical research. *Sem Oncol* 1988, 15:278.

15. Williams S, Bitran J, Hoffman P, et al.: High dose, multiple alkylator chemotherapy with autologous bone marrow reinfusion in patients with advanced non–small cell lung cancer. *Cancer* 1989, 63:238–242.

16. Schaake-Konig C, van den Bogaert W, Dalesio O, et al.: Effect of concomitant cisplatin and radiotherapy on inoperable non–small-cell lung cancer. *N Engl J Med* 1992, 326:524–530.

17. Turrisi AT, Glover DJ, Mason BA: A preliminary report: Concurrent twice-daily radiotherapy plus platinum–etoposide chemotherapy for limited small cell lung cancer. *Int J Radiat Oncol Biol Phys* 1988, 15:183.

18. Ihde DC, Grayson J, Woods E, et al.: Twice daily chest irradiation as an adjuvant to etoposide/cisplatin therapy of limited stage small cell lung cancer. In Salmon SE (ed): *Adjuvant Therapy of Cancer VI*. 1990, Philadelphia: WB Saunders; 162.

19. Feld R, Ginsberg RJ, Payne DG: Treatment of small cell lung cancer. In Roth JA, Ruckdeschel JC, Weisenburger TH (eds): *Thoracic Oncology*. 1989, Philadelphia: WB Saunders; 229–262.

20. Gazdar AF, Kadoyama C, Venzon D, et al.: The effects of histological type and neuroendocrine differentiation on drug sensitivity of lung cancer cell lines. *J Nat Cancer Inst*, in press.

21. Shaw GL, Gazdar AF, Phelps R, et al.: *In vitro* analysis of non–small cell lung cancer (NSCLC) specimens predicts patient response. *Proc ASCO* 1992, 11:293.

22. Rodenhuis S, van de Wetering M, Mooi W, et al.: Mutational activation of the K-ras oncogene: A possible pathogenetic factor in adeno-carcinoma of the lung. *N Engl J Med* 1987, 317:929–935.

23. Mitsudomi T, Steinberg SM, Oie HK, et al.: ras Gene mutations in non–small cell lung cancers are associated with shortened survival irrespective of treatment intent. *Cancer Res* 1991, 51:4999–5002.

24. Mitsudomi T, Steinberg SM, Nau MM, et al.: p53 Gene mutations in non–small cell lung cancer cell lines and their correlation with the presence of ras mutations and clinical features. *Oncogene* 1992, 7:171–180.

25. Mulshine JL, Johnson BE, Gazdar AF, et al.: Biological studies related to circumventing non–small cell lung cancer drug resistance. *Chest* (suppl), in press.

26. Gazdar AF, Steinberg SM, Russell EK, et al.: Correlation of *in vitro* drug-sensitivity testing results with response to chemotherapy and survival in extensive-stage small cell lung cancer: A prospective clinical trial. *J Nat Cancer Inst* 1990, 82:117–124.

27. Tsai C-M, Gazdar AF, Venzon DJ, et al.: Lack of *in vitro* synergy between etoposide and cis-diammine-dichloroplatinum(II). *Cancer Res* 1989, 49:2390–2397.

28. Ihde DC, Minna JD: Non–small lung cancer. *Curr Prob in Cancer* 1991, 15:63–104.

29. Minna JD, Pass H, Gladstein E, et al.: Cancer of the lung. In DeVita VT, Hellman S, Rosenberg SA (eds): *Cancer: Principles and Practices of Oncology*, 3rd ed. 1989, Philadelphia: JB Lippincott, 1989; 668–671.

30. Ruckdeschel JC, Day R, Weissman CH, et al.: Chemotherapy for metastatic non–small cell bronchogenic carcinoma: Cyclophosphamide, doxorubicin, and etoposide vs mitomycin and vinblastine. *Cancer Treat Rep* 1984, 68:1325–1329.

31. Pouillart P, Hoang HT, Brugerie E, et al.: Sequential administration of two oncostatic drugs: Study of modalities for pharmacodynamic potentiation. *Biomedicine* 1974, 21:471–479.

32. Levin ML, Clark PI, Joel S, et al.: A randomized trial to evaluate the effect of schedule on the activity of etoposide in small cell lung cancer. *J Clin Oncol* 1989, 7:1333–1340.

PE
Cisplatin and Etoposide

Cisplatin, a platinum analogue, appears to be one of the most active antineoplastic agents in the armamentarium for lung cancer. It inhibits DNA synthesis by producing intrastrand and interstrand cross-links, which is similar to the process performed by bifunctional alkylating agents. Etoposide exerts its effect on DNA by forming a complex with DNA and the DNA unwinding enzyme, topoisomerase II, causing strand breakage. Studies in animals and clinical trials in humans have indicated that the antineoplastic activity of PE demonstrates synergy against small cell lung cancer and non–small cell lung cancer [26,27], but, as determined by appropriate analytic methods, the drug interaction is actually only additive [28,29].

DOSAGE AND SCHEDULING

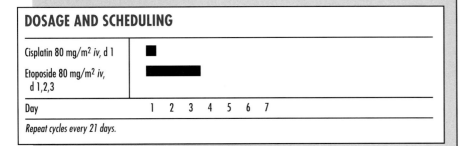

Cisplatin 80 mg/m² *iv*, d 1	■							
Etoposide 80 mg/m² *iv*, d 1,2,3	▬▬▬							
Day	1	2	3	4	5	6	7	

Repeat cycles every 21 days.

RECENT EXPERIENCES AND RESPONSE RATES

Study	Evaluable patients, *n*	Dose/Schedule Cisplatin (mg/m²)	Etoposide (mg/m²)	CR (%)	PR (%)	Comments
Wolf, *et al.*, J Clin Oncol 1987, 5:1880–1889	73	80, Day 1	150, Days 3–5	32	33	Extensive: 22% CR Limited: 50% CR
Idhe, *et al.*, Proc ASCO 1991, 10:240 (Extensive stage SCLC)	42 39	80, Day 1 27, Days 1–5	80, Days 1–3 80, Days 1–5	21 24	60 61	No significant differ. in resp. or surv.

CANDIDATES FOR TREATMENT
Non–small cell lung cancer with excellent performance status: adjuvant (experimental)—Stages I, II, IIIA; neoadjuvant (experimental)—Stages IIIA, IIIB; metastatic (optional)—Stages V; small cell lung cancer: limited stage (with radiation therapy); advanced stage

SPECIAL PRECAUTIONS
Dose modifications in patients with renal dysfunction

ALTERNATIVE THERAPIES
CAV, MVP, edatrexate alone or in combination with mitomycin C or vinblastine, oral etoposide, paclitaxel alone, phase I agents, navelbine-based combinations

TOXICITIES
Myelosuppression, nausea, vomiting, nephrotoxicity with electrolyte wasting, neurotoxicity (peripheral neuropathy), hypotension, hypersensitivity, including anaphylactic reactions, auditory impairment, alopecia, mucositis, diarrhea

DRUG INTERACTIONS
Cisplatin: systemic thiosulfates (IV thiosulfate, WR-2721); other nephrotoxic and ototoxic drugs (*eg* aminoglycosides)

NURSING INTERVENTIONS
Hypersensitivity—anaphylactic reactions have been documented with both agents, benedryl and epinephrine should be readily available as well as crash cart. Myelosuppression—emphasize importance of reporting symptoms of infection, assess for bleeding episodes; nausea, vomiting—give antiemetics before administration and as needed; nephrotoxicity—monitor renal function indices (BUN, serum creatinine, urine output), monitor electrolytes, especially magnesium and calcium, encourage adequate hydration and high urine flow during therapy; neurotoxicity—assess for weakness/numbness of arms hands, legs, and feet, encourage ambulation and range-of-motion exercises, give baseline hearing test for high-risk patients (children, high-dose regimens, baseline hearing impairment); hypotension—usually attributed to fast infusion rate of etoposide (due to vehicle), stop infusion and give supportive care, restart infusion at slower rate; local—phlebitis may occur with IV administration

PATIENT INFORMATION
Patient should drink plenty of fluids and urinate frequently; report prolonged upset stomach and heed advice to relieve these symptoms (although proactive suppression of emesis is part of initial patient management); maintain good nutrition; report symptoms of infection (fever, chills, sore throat); report unusual bleeding or bruising

CAV
Cyclophosphamide, Doxorubicin, Vincristine

The combination of cyclophosphamide, doxorubicin, and vincristine is a well-established chemotherapy regimen in the treatment of small cell lung cancer. This regimen repeatedly produces optimal response rates, median survival, and long-term survival in both limited and extensive-stage small cell lung cancer [27].

DOSAGE AND SCHEDULING

Cyclophosphamide, 1000 mg/m^2 iv, d 1	■	
Doxorubicin, 50 mg/m^2 iv, d 1	■	
Vincristine* 1.4 mg/m^2 iv, 1 d	■	
Day	1 2 3 4 5 6 7	

Repeat cycles every 21 days
*Maximum total dose per injection: 2 mg

RECENT EXPERIENCES AND RESPONSE RATES

Study	CTX (mg/m^2)	ADRIA (mg/m^2)	VCR (mg/m^2)	CR (%)	PR (%)	Comments
Dinwoodie, et al., Proc ASCO 1981, 22:505	750	50	1.4	54	46	Differ. in resp. not statistically significant
	1200	70	1.4	30	55	
Figueredo, et al., J Clin Oncol 1985, 3:54–64	1000	50	1 weekly × 4 doses, then q 3 wks × 2 doses	22	39	Differ. in resp. not statistically significant
	1500 (escalating to 2250)	60	1 weekly × 4 doses, then q 3 wks × 2 doses	21	50	
Comis, Sem Oncol 1986, 13(3):40–44	1000	50	2 mg max			Response rates: extensive— 44%, limited— 66%
Feld, et al., J Clin Oncol 1984, 2:294–304*	900	45	2 mg max			Response rates: extensive— 73%, limited— 84%

*Includes local radiation.
CTX—cyclophosphamide; ADRIA—doxorubicin; VCR—vincristine.

CANDIDATES FOR TREATMENT
Non–small cell lung cancer with excellent performance status: adjuvant (experimental)—Stages I, II, IIIA; neoadjuvant (experimental)—Stages IIIA, IIIB; metastatic (optional)—Stages V; small cell lung cancer: limited stage (with radiation therapy); advanced stage

SPECIAL PRECAUTIONS
Obtain baseline cardiac ejection fraction before beginning doxorubicin therapy; dose modification in patients with hepatic dysfunction

ALTERNATIVE THERAPIES
PE, MVP, edatrexate alone or in combination with mitomycin C or vinblastine, oral etoposide, paclitaxel alone, phase I agents, navelbine-based combinations

TOXICITIES
Myelosuppression, cardiac toxicity (acute arrhythmias, delayed congestive heart failure), hemorrhagic cystitis, nephrotoxicity, neurotoxicity (peripheral neuropathy, cranial nerve paralysis, autonomic effects, central nervous system effects), alopecia, mucositis, diarrhea, local reactions

DRUG INTERACTIONS
Cyclophosphamide: drugs that may interfere with microsomal enzyme activity in liver (*eg*, cimetidine) (monitor such patients closely and dosage changes cautiously); **vincristine**: digoxin

NURSING INTERVENTIONS
Myelosuppression—emphasize importance of reporting symptoms of infection, assess for bleeding episodes; neurotoxicity—assess for weakness/numbness of arms, hands, legs, and feet; assess for jaw pain, foot drop, loss of deep tendon reflexes; encourage ambulation and exercise; constipation—assess bowel habits and nutritional patterns, perform abdominal assessment, institute a bowel regimen *early* in chemotherapy regimen, encourage a high-fiber diet and fluid intake, monitor narcotic usage; cardiac toxicity—know patient's lifetime cumulative dose (max 450 mg/m^2), high-risk patients include those receiving concurrent cyclophosphamide therapy and radiation (obtain baseline cardiac ejection fraction), monitor signs and symptoms of congestive heart failure; local—doxorubicin and vincristine are vesicants: Check for good blood return before and during administration, monitor for clinical manifestations of extravasation (pain, burning, swelling, erythema, absence of blood return), be prepared for emergency procedures for extravasation

PATIENT INFORMATION
Patient should drink plenty of fluids and urinate frequently; report prolonged upset stomach and heed advice to relieve symptoms; maintain good nutrition; report symptoms of infection (fever, chills, sore throat); report unusual bleeding or bruising

MVP
Cisplatin, Mitomycin C, Vinblastine

A frequently used regimen in patients with non–small cell lung cancer is the combination of cisplatin, mitomycin C, and vinblastine. The mechanism of anti-neoplastic activity for cisplatin and mitomycin C is similar to that of the alkylating agents; these agents cause cross-linking of DNA. Vinblastine exerts its cytotoxic effects by interfering with the microtubular proteins of the mitotic spindle, which inhibits mitosis. These drugs have all demonstrated single-agent activity in non–small cell lung cancer, as well as an additive effect when cisplatin was added to the mitomycin C and vinblastine regimen [30,31].

DOSAGE AND SCHEDULING

Mitomycin C 10 mg/m² *iv*, d1	■							
Vinblastine 6 mg/m² *iv*, d1	■							
Cisplatin 40 mg/m² *iv*, d1	■							
Day	1	2	3	4	5	6	7	

Repeat cycles every 21 days

RECENT EXPERIENCES AND RESPONSE RATES

Study	Evaluable patients, *n*	Regimen	RR (%) (CR/PR)	Comments
Ruckdeschel, *et al.*, J Clin Oncol 1985, 3:72–79	112	CBP	20 (4/18)	Differ. in resp. and surv. not statistically significant
	109	AFP	17 (0/18)	
	107	CAP	23 (1/23)	
	104	MVP	26 (5/22)	

CBP—cyclophosphamide, bleomycin, cisplatin; AFP—doxorubicin, 5-FU, cisplatin; CAP—cyclophosphamide, doxorubicin, cisplatin; MVP—mitomycin C, vinblastine, cisplatin.

CANDIDATES FOR TREATMENT
Non–small cell lung cancer with excellent performance status: adjuvant (experimental)—Stages I, II, IIIA; neoadjuvant (experimental)—Stages IIIA, IIIB; metastatic (optional)—Stages V; small cell lung cancer: limited stage (with radiation therapy); advanced stage

SPECIAL PRECAUTIONS
Patients with renal dysfunction

ALTERNATIVE THERAPIES
CAV, PE, edatrexate alone or in combination with mitomycin C or vinblastine, oral etoposide, paclitaxel alone, phase I agents, navelbine-based combinations

TOXICITIES
Myelosuppression (thrombocytopenia, leukopenia); nausea, vomiting; nephrotoxicity and electrolyte wasting. Pulmonary toxicity has been reported with mitomycin C such that coordination with the anesthesiologist is recommended prior to surgery for combined modality approaches. Neurotoxicity (peripheral neuropathy); hematologic, including hemolytic uremic syndrome, especially associated with protracted administration; fever; malaise; alopecia; mucositis; auditory abnormalities; local reactions; hypersensitivity

DRUG INTERACTIONS
Cisplatin: systemic thiosulfates (IV thiosulfate, WR-2721); other nephrotoxic and ototoxic drugs (*eg* aminoglycosides); **vinblastine**: digoxin and phenytoin

NURSING INTERVENTIONS
Myelosuppression—emphasize importance of reporting symptoms of infection, assess for bleeding episodes; nausea, vomiting—use antiemetics before administration and as needed; nephrotoxicity—monitor renal function indices (BUN, serum creatinine, urine output), monitor electrolytes, especially magnesium and calcium, encourage adequate hydration and high urine flow during therapy; local—mitomycin C and vinblastine are vesicants. Use caution during administration, check for good blood return before and during administration, monitor for clinical manifestations of extravasation (pain, burning, swelling, erythema); be prepared with emergency procedures for vesicant extravasation

PATIENT INFORMATION
Patient should drink plenty of fluids and urinate frequently; report prolonged upset stomach and heed advice to relieve symptoms; maintain good nutrition when not debilitated by anorexia; report symptoms of infection (fever, chills, sore throat); report unusual bleeding or bruising

EVM
Edatrexate, Vinblastine, Mitomycin C

Edatrexate (10-ethyl-10-deaza-aminopterin, 10EdAM) is an analogue of methotrexate, an antifolate antimetabolite. This class of agents inhibits dihydrofolate reductase (DHFR), a key enzyme in the production of reduced folates, which play a necessary role in the synthesis of DNA precursors. Other factors that contribute to the cytotoxicity of these agents are the metabolism of parent compounds to toxic polyglutamate derivatives and the accumulation of inactive folates. Compared with methotrexate, 10EdAM has more selective entry into malignant cells versus normal proliferating cells and greater conversion to polyglutamate forms in neoplastic cells. These features lead to increased inhibition of purine synthesis in malignant cells and enhanced cytotoxicity, activities that demonstrate 10EdAM to be therapeutically superior to methotrexate. Edatrexate has been used in clinical trials for the treatment of non–small cell lung cancer as a single agent as well as in combination regimens.

CANDIDATES FOR TREATMENT

Non–small cell lung cancer with excellent performance status: adjuvant (experimental)—Stages I, II, IIIA; neoadjuvant (experimental)—Stages IIIA, IIIB; metastatic (optional)—Stages V; small cell lung cancer: limited stage (with radiation therapy); advanced stage

SPECIAL PRECAUTIONS

Patients exhibiting significant "third-spacing" of fluid; patients may experience more severe adverse effects if heavily pretreated with radiation therapy or chemotherapy

ALTERNATIVE THERAPIES

CAV, MVP, edatrexate alone or in combination with mitomycin C or vinblastine, oral etoposide, paclitaxel alone, phase I agents, navelbine-based combinations

TOXICITIES

Mucositis (dose-limiting), myelosuppression, elevated AST, fatigue, nausea, vomiting, diarrhea, rash, alopecia; pulmonary fibrosis and pleural effusions (rare); stomatitis (self-limiting, dose-related)

DRUG INTERACTIONS

No drug interactions have been noted to date; however, because of the similarities between 10EdAM and methotrexate elimination pathways, drugs known to compete for or interfere with renal elimination of methotrexate should be avoided.

NURSING INTERVENTIONS

Nephrotoxicity—10EdAM is eliminated renally: obtain baseline renal function values (BUN, serum creatinine), monitor urine output and encourage adequate hydration and frequent voiding: stomatitis—use of ice chips will possibly minimize, symptoms, frequently examine patient's mouth and give instructions for mouth care, stress importance of good nutrition, aggressive pain management may be necessary; skin reactions—assess for appearance of rash; myelosuppression—emphasize importance of reporting symptoms of infection, assess for bleeding episodes

PATIENT INFORMATION

Patient should drink plenty of fluids; maintain good nutrition; report symptoms of infection (fever, chills, sore throat); report unusual bleeding or bruising

DOSAGE AND SCHEDULING

Combination

Edatrexate 80 mg/m² *iv*, d1, 15, 22, 29, 71, then q 2 weeks

Edatrexate 40 mg/m² *iv*, d8

Vinblastine 4 mg/m² *iv*, d1

Vinblastine 2 mg/m² *iv*, d8

Vinblastine 4.5 mg/m² *iv*, d15, 22, 29, then q 2 weeks

Mitomycin C 8 mg/m2, *iv*, d1, 29, 71

Single agent

Edatrexate 80 mg/m² *iv*, weekly

Day: 1 8 15 22 29 71 weekly q 2 weeks

RECENT EXPERIENCES AND RESPONSE RATES

Study	Evaluable Patients, n	Dosage	RR (%) (CR/PR)	Median Survival (mo)
Single agent				
Shun, *et al.*, J Clin Oncol 1988, 6:446–450	20	10EdAM 80 mg/m²/wk × 5 wk IV	32 0/6	10.8
Combination				
Grant, *et al.*, In Bernal, *et al.*, Lung Cancer Differentiation 1992, Marcel Dekker, p.337	99	EVM (see above table)	58 3/55	13.6

ORAL ETOPOSIDE

Etoposide is a semisynthetic podophyllotoxin-derivative, antineoplastic agent that has been widely used for the treatment of small cell lung cancer, usually in combination with other chemotherapeutic agents. It has also shown single-agent activity in NSCLC and has been used in combination with cisplatin. The damaging effects of etoposide are cell-cycle specific (G2) and reversible when therapy is discontinued; however, the minimal etoposide concentration for antitumor activity is not known. This evidence suggested that etoposide activity may be influenced by schedule dependency. Although etoposide has been approved by the Food and Drug Administration since 1971, until recently this phenomenon had not been demonstrated clinically. Levin and coworkers [32] demonstrated clinically the schedule dependency of etoposide. They compared etoposide at 500 mg/m^2 in a 24-hour infusion with daily infusions at 100 mg/m^2. The response rates for the continuous infusion and daily infusions were 10% and 84%, respectively, even though the total area under the curve was identical. The addition of an oral formulation has allowed researchers to study the effects of etoposide activity when administered on a chronic, low-dose schedule.

DOSAGE AND SCHEDULING

Etoposide 50 mg/m^2 PO, d 1–21	████████████
Day	1 5 10 15 20 21

Repeat cycles every 28 to 35 days

DOSAGE MODIFICATIONS: *discontinue therapy if WBC < 2.0 or platelets < 75,000; reinitiate when WBC > 3.0. Administer subsequent cycles at 75% dose reduction if WBC nadirs < 2.0 or therapy was discontinued before day 21.*

RECENT EXPERIENCES AND RESPONSE RATES

Study	Evaluable Patients, n	Etoposide (mg/m^2)	RR (%) (CR/PR)	Comments
Johnson, *et al.,* J Clin Oncol 1990, 4:1780–1786	22	50 q d PO × 21 days	46 (2/8)	8 of 18 patients who had previously received IV etoposide responded
Clark, *et al.,* Proc ASCO 1990, 9:226	20	50 BID PO × 14 days q21d	85 (2/15)	

CANDIDATES FOR TREATMENT

Non–small cell lung cancer with excellent performance status: adjuvant (experimental)—Stages I, II, IIIA; neoadjuvant (experimental)—Stages IIIA, IIIB; metastatic (optional)—Stages V; small cell lung cancer: limited stage (with radiation therapy); advanced stage

SPECIAL PRECAUTIONS

Patients with increased serum bilirubin

ALTERNATIVE THERAPIES

CAV, MVP, edatrexate alone or in combination with mitomycin C or vinblastine, paclitaxel alone, phase I agents, navelbine-based combinations

TOXICITIES

Myelosuppression (dose limiting), nausea and vomiting (mild-to-moderate), alopecia; fever, bronchospasm, hypersensitivity, diarrhea, and mucositis (rare)

DRUG INTERACTIONS

None noteworthy

NURSING INTERVENTIONS

GI—nausea and vomiting more frequent with oral than with IV administration (55 vs 5%); sensitivity reactions—not reported with oral formulation

PATIENT INFORMATION

Oral medication may be taken with food; if vomiting occurs (< 15 min) after taking a dose, contact physician for advice; if medication is forgotten, do not take missed days; continue with regular schedule and inform physician; report symptoms of infection (fever, chills, sore throat); if upset stomach persists, heed advice to relieve symptoms; etoposide may cause total loss of hair, which usually reverses when discontinued

Although squamous cell and basal carcinomas are the most frequent tumors of the skin, they are largely curable by local surgical approaches. Melanoma is less frequent, but more lethal, with more than 15% of the patients who develop this tumor ultimately succumbing to metastatic disease [1,2]. The incidence of melanoma has risen more rapidly than other solid tumors, and 1 in 90 Caucasians are expected to be at risk in the year 2000. In 1994, 38,000 patients will develop melanoma. It represents a fascinating tumor with some patterns suggesting genetic predisposition [3,4]. Its association with ultraviolet exposure [5] and its interaction with the host [6] as well as response to immunologic therapies provide insights into tumorigenesis and possible strategies for prevention and therapy. Although surgery remains the mainstay of treatment for localized melanoma, patients with regional and systemic spread have recently responded to biological and cytotoxic therapies that may be capable of prolonging life. Spontaneous regression is observed in less than 1% of patients, and as many as 10% of patients may develop metastases without a known primary.

ETIOLOGY AND RISK FACTORS

Evidence for an inherited predisposition to melanoma includes observations of family history, presence of a characteristic precursor lesion (termed the *dysplastic nevus*), and information suggesting localization on one of several chromosomes, including chromosomes 1, 6, 7, and 10. Dysplastic nevi are suspected precursors in 25 to 40% of sporadic cases [3]. Congenital melanocytic nevi are precursors less frequently related to melanoma in the population at large. Ten percent of all melanomas are associated with a family history and the dysplastic nevus syndrome. Of note, the total number of all moles is an independent risk factor beyond the presence of dysplastic nevi. With the presence of dysplastic nevi and two cases of melanoma in the family history the risk for an individual to develop melanoma approaches 100% at age 70. With dysplastic nevi and a personal history of melanoma, the risk of a second primary melanoma increases eightfold.

Ultraviolet exposure clearly plays a role in the development of melanoma. Evidence for this is found in the topographic distribution of melanoma, which is directly related to sun exposure. The incidence of melanoma is associated with latitude and the intensity of solar exposure among susceptible populations. Fair-skinned individuals who have migrated to Australia and New Zealand are at particularly high risk because of the extensive solar radiation and the constitutional susceptibility of this population.

The evidence for host immune reactivity to melanoma includes the frequent observation of disappearance of acquired nevi, and, on rare occasion, melanoma. A variety of conditions associated with immunodeficiency are also associated with increased risk of melanoma, including ataxia telangiectasia, chronic lymphocytic leukemia and Hodgkin's disease, immunosuppression for organ transplantation, and the acquired immunodeficiency syndrome. Histologic evidence of an immunologic role in the course of melanoma includes the frequent finding of lymphocytic infiltrates in primary lesions, as well as dysplastic nevi. Lymphocytic infiltrates are also clearly observed with metastatic lesions, although less frequently. Melanoma is responsive to many immunologic therapies, including interferon alpha and interleukin 2 (see protocol page). Both serologic and cellular reactivity to melanoma is detectable in as many as 20 to 40% of patients. A number of melanoma antigens recognized by T cells have been identified (MAGE-1, tyrosinase, Aa). Loss of class I MHC antigens (HLA-ABC), as well as B_2 microglobulin, has been found in many melanomas.

CLINICAL AND PATHOLOGIC APPEARANCE

The characteristics of melanoma include *a*symmetry and changes in *b*order, variation in *c*olor, and enlarging *d*iameter or height (ABCD). Bleeding and ulceration are findings suggesting a particularly poor prognosis. Evolution in the characteristics of a lesion should always prompt investigation and possible biopsy. The pathologic components of the progression in human melanoma appear to involve a series of morphologic stages: 1) an acquired or congenital melanocytic nevus, 2) melanocytic nevus with architectural atypia, 3) histologically dysplastic nevus with cytologic atypia and architectural atypia, 4) primary melanoma in radial growth phase, 5) primary melanoma in vertical growth phase with or without transit metastases, 6) regional lymph node metastatic melanoma (lymphatic), and 7) distant metastatic melanoma (hematogenous). A patient can often give a clear history of progression from a nevus to a tumor or the appearance of nodularity associated with a vertical growth phase. A variety of different morphologic types of melanoma have been recognized (Table 1).

PROGNOSIS AND STAGING

The treatment of melanoma may be decided according to its stage (Table 2). Melanoma may be simply divided in three general subgroups: 1) local disease, for which surgical ablation is the predominant therapy, 2) regional disease, for which evolving concepts of adjuvant interferon-alpha therapy in addition to surgery are currently being definitively tested, and 3) systemic disease, for which a variety of experimental chemotherapeutic and immunologic approaches exist.

A workup for primary melanoma includes a physical examination with attention to skin pigmentation, including the presence of hypopigmentation. The latter may reflect scarring, which in some circumstances obliterates the primary site or paraneoplastic vitiligo-like destruction of the normal pigment cells in the skin. If the patient presents with lymph nodal or distant metastatic disease in the absence of an obvious primary lesion, it is particularly important to examine the mucosal surfaces and the uveal tract of the eye. A chest radiograph and liver function test, including lactic dehydrogenase should be performed. Evaluation for more intensive protocols may specify CT or MR imaging of the head, chest, and abdomen and a gallium tomoscan (SPECT) to more completely identify potential sites of metastasis.

Table 1. Morphologic Types of Melanoma

Superficial spreading melanoma	Acral lentiginous melanoma
Nodular melanoma	Ocular melanoma
Lentigo maligna melanoma	

Table 2. Staging of Cutaneous Melanoma

Stage	TNM	Criteria
IA	T1	Breslow ≤ 0.75 mm (Clark II)
IB	T2	Breslow 0.76–1.50 mm (Clark III)
IIA	T3	Breslow 1.51–4.0 mm (Clark IV)
IIB	T4	Breslow ≥ 4.1 (Clark V) or satellite(s) (within 2 cm)
III	Any T,N_1	One regional node station, node(s) mobile, diameter ≤ 5 cm *in transit* metastases # < 5
IV	Any T,N_2	More than one LN station involved; or LN > 5 cm or fixed; or *in transit* metastases ≥ 5
IV	Any T,N,M_1	Involvement of skin or subcutaneous tissue beyond site of primary tumor and its drainage
IV	Any T,N,M_2	Visceral metastasis

The recognition of primary melanoma and its precursor lesions (including dysplastic nevi) depends upon awareness of a change in pigmented lesions. An incisional (punch) or excisional (surgical) biopsy is required to fully evaluate lesions that are suspected of harboring melanoma. Patients with regional lymphadenopathy in the absence of evidence of systemic spread are best treated with regional lymphadenectomy. Dye and scintigraphic methods to ascertain the drainage of melanoma to specific nodal sites are currently undergoing evaluation. Documentation of tumor at suspected metastatic sites can often be obtained with needle biopsy. There is little evidence to support excision of visceral metastases from most patients with melanoma. Limited cutaneous or nodal tumor resection does appear to have a role in palliation of symptomatic mass lesions, and it may, in subsets of patients, even have an impact upon survival, although this is unproven.

Prognostic factors important for determining survival include sections with stage of disease as dictated by tumor thickness (Breslow depth) and skin layer penetration (Clark level) (Tables 2 and 3). Mitotic rate, ulceration, and the presence of satellites are histologic determinants. Patients who are young, female, and have lesions on the extremities (as opposed to the head, neck, and trunk) do better than do those who are older, male, and have truncal tumors. Although the presence of T-cell infiltrate is a favorable prognostic factor, expression of the class II MHC molecule, (DR, DP, DQ) and certain adhesion molecules (ICAM-1, or intercellular adhesion molecule 1) are unfavorable prognostic findings.

TREATMENT

The optimal surgical treatment [7–9] for primary melanoma has been under study for many years. It was demonstrated by the World Health Organization that 1 cm margins are adequate for melanomas of less than 1 mm. It is reasonable to conclude that a wide local excision should be performed for lesions deeper than 4.0 mm. Margins of 2cm have recently been evaluated and shown to be equivalent to 4-cm margins in a prospective intergroup randomized trial for primary tumors of 1 to 4 mm depth. Therapeutic lymphadenectomy is indicated for isolated regional lymph node metastases. Prophylactic regional lymph node dissection has not been demonstrated to be of value in prolonging survival or time to relapse. It may be indicated in certain experimental protocols, especially in the context of new lymphographic procedures to better define lymph node drainage and the "sentinel" node for a given primary. Patients with isolated brain metastases or with tumors of the gastrointestinal tract may obtain significant benefit from resection. In general resection of metastases, particularly in the lung, liver, and other abdominal viscera, provide little benefit [10,11].

Radiation therapy has been evaluated as an alternative modality for palliation of inoperable visceral sites of metastasis. In high-dose fractions given for metastatic brain disease, steroid premedication should be used to prevent edema. Bleeding into brain tumors is a problem in patients with melanoma. Intensive local irradiation using a stereotactic delivery in special multibeam units (gamma knife therapy) appears to offer an advantage for treatment of patients with unresectable isolated or limited numbers of small (< 2.5-cm) lesions [11,12].

Dacarbazine is the single FDA-approved chemotherapeutic agent for treatment of metastatic melanoma in the United States [13]. Complete and partial responses occur in upwards of 20% of patients, with a mean duration of response of 5 to 7 months. Patients with soft tissue disease and women generally exhibit the highest rate of response to therapy with dacarbazine. No benefit has been demonstrated for adjuvant chemotherapy with dacarbazine alone or in combination with other agents. No other single chemotherapeutic agent has shown results suggesting a true response rate significantly greater (ie, 15%) than dacarbazine. Patients presenting with asymptomatic or minimally symptomatic metastatic melanoma can be treated by a variety of investigational treatment programs. Combination chemotherapy has historically been associated with increased toxicity, outweighing modest gains in response rates obtained with a variety of different protocols. The combination of dacarbazine with tamoxifen appears to have benefited subjects in one randomized trial [10]. This impact was greatest in women and individuals of higher body mass. High-dose chemotherapy with bone marrow rescue using melphalan, thiotepa, or bischloroethyl nitrosurea have achieved an improved short-term response rates but not durable complete remissions.

Evidence to support use of immunologic reagents has come initially from the use of non-specific immunostimulants, such as the microbial agents (Coley's toxin, *C. parvum*, BCG, OK-432). More recently the use of these agents have been employed to enhance the immune response to experimental vaccines.

Interferon alpha is a biologic antineoplastic agent associated with a response rate in 16 to 22% of collected series of patients with metastatic melanoma [14]. Treatment can be associated with durable complete remissions, and there is other evidence that interferon has an immunologic impact. Response is associated with smaller size disease and soft tissue or pulmonary disease–dominant sites. A variety of combinations with chemotherapy have been investigated, with contradictory results, which may be due to the dose and sequence of agents utilized. Although adjuvant protocols are being evaluated, they are not yet approved by the FDA for use following diagnosis and surgical excision of regional disease.

Interleukin 2 is a T-cell growth factor that has been employed since 1984 in the treatment of patients with melanoma. It has achieved response rates of approximately 20 to 25%, with a subset of patients who experience durable complete response [12]. Treatment with IL-2 (which has recently been approved by the FDA for metastatic renal cell cancer) requires very high dosages for induction of response. This is associated with vascular leak syndrome, hypotension, and rarely with myocardial infarction, and reversible renal failure; toxicity has tempered the application of this agent. Other cytokines, including IL-4, tumor necrosis factor, and IL-1 [15], have attractive rationals for therapeutic application—but no clinical evidence of benefit yet exists for melanoma.

Significant interest in vaccines has existed in the field of melanoma for many years. A variety of different vaccine preparations have been tested, but none has yet shown evidence of an increase in survival in properly controlled trials. Adoptive immunotherapy with transfer of cellular reagents, including tumor infiltrating lymphocytes or lymphokine-activated killer cells, have been shown to induce response rates of up to 50% in limited series, but substantiation of their role in larger multicenter trials has not been obtained. Gene therapy, employing cytokine genes transferred into lymphocytes, or directly into tumors, are currently undergoing evaluation at a number

Table 3. Adverse Prognostic Factors of Cutaneous Melanoma

1. Increased tumor thickness (Breslow depth) or skin layer penetration (Clark level), increased imitotic rate, presence of ulceration or satellites
2. Advanced age, male gender, trunk or head and neck as site of origin, mucosal melanoma, or morphology of the primary tumor (nodular as opposed to superficial spreading)
3. Lack of lymphoid inflammatory infiltrate beneath the primary lesion, HLA antigen expression, or serum antibody response to melanoma antigens

of larger centers. Perfusion of melanoma localized to the extremity is being evaluated for evidence of benefit, with control response rates of 80 to 100% with combination of melphalan and TNF [16,17].

NONMELANOMA SKIN CANCERS

The most frequent tumors in caucasians are nonmelanomatous skin tumors [18]. There are about 500,000 new cases of basal cell carcinoma per year and approximately 100,000 squamous cell carcinomas. The incidence appears to be increasing by as much as 65% since 1980, probably due to increased sun exposure. [19]. Most of the tumors occur on skin that is exposed to the sun, and there is clearly a relationship between latitude and cumulative solar exposure and incidence of these tumors. Deaths due to these tumors are extremely infrequent, allowing most cancer protocols treating tumors at other sites to permit these as a preceding malignancy. There are approximately 1500 deaths per year, due largely to squamous cell carcinoma (about 1 in 500 patients will die of their tumor). This incidence of death is about one fourth of that due to melanoma.

The multiple associated causes of nonmelanoma skin cancers are listed in Table 4. Clearly, efforts to decrease exposure to sun and carcinogenic factors associated with a concomitant decrease in skin tumors. The most common sites of metastases (which occur rarely) are regional lymph nodes. Rarely, liver, lung, bone, and brain metastases can be found. The primary treatment for skin tumors is local ablative therapy, currently consisting of simple excisional surgery,

electrodesiccation and curettage, cryosurgery, Mohs' surgery, or radiation therapy. Each procedure is designed to ablate the tumor totally. Since local recurrence is the major complication, especially in cosmetically sensitive areas, Moh's surgery attempts to remove a minimal amount of tissue yet completely excise the tumor, allowing albeit normally, for a better cosmetic result. It is, however, a very time-consuming procedure to perform. Radiation therapy is perhaps best used in older patients. Topical fluorouracil can be used to treat multiple basal cell carcinomas or actinic keratosis [20,21]. Beta carotene and isoretinan have been surgically applied in dermal trials [22,23].

Table 4. Factors Associated with Increased Risk of Nonmelanoma Skin Cancer	

1. Host factors
a. Older age
b. Male sex
c. Skin that tans poorly or burns easily
d. Freckling
e. Light complexion
f. Inherited disorders
  i. Xeroderma pigmentosum (autosomal recessive)
  ii. Basal-cell nevus syndrome (autosomal dominant)
  ii. Albinism (autosomal recessive)
	iv. Epidermodysplasia verruciformis (autosomal recessive)
	2. Environmental factors
	a. Sun exposure (high ultraviolet B)
	b. Radiation therapy or other sources of ionizing radiation
	c. Cigarette smoking or exposure to other hydrocarbons (squamous cell carcinoma)
	d. Chronic scars or cutaneous ulcers
	e. Immunosuppression especially in the context of AIDS or immunosuppression in the context of transplantation

REFERENCES

1. Balch CM, Houghton AN, Milton GW, *et al.* (eds): *Cutaneous Melanoma.* 1992, Philadelphia: JB Lippincott.

2. Rumke P (ed): *Therapy of Advanced Melanoma.* 1990, Basel: Karger.

3. Bale SJ, Dracopoli NC, Tucker MA, *et al.*: Mapping the gene for hereditary cutaneous malignant melanoma-dysplastic nevus to chromosome 1p. *N Engl J Med* 1989, 320(21):1367–1372.

4. Lotze MT: National institutes of health consensus development conference, diagnosis and treatment of early melanoma. Keystone symposium. Melanoma and biology of neural crest. *Melanoma Res* 1992, 2:131–138.

5. Stretch JR, Gatter KC, Ralfkiaer E, *et al.*: Expression of mutant p53 in melanoma. *Cancer Res* 1991, 51:5976–5979.

6. Topalian SL, Hom SS, Kawakami Y, *et al.*: Recognition of shared melanoma antigens by human tumor-infiltrating lymphocytes. *J Immunother* 1992, 12:203–206.

7. Sim FH, Taylor WF, Ivins JC, *et al.*: A prospective randomized study of the efficacy of routine elective lymphadenectomy in management of malignant melanoma: Preliminary results. *Cancer* 1978, 41:948–956.

8. Veronesi U, Adamus J, Bandiera DC, *et al.*: Inefficacy of immediate node dissection in stage I melanoma of the limbs. *N Engl J Med* 1977, 297:627–630.

9. Balch CM, Urist MM, Karakousis CP, *et al.*: Efficacy of 2-cm surgical margins for intermediate-thickness melanomas (1-4 mm): Results of a multi-institutional randomized surgical trial. *Ann Surg* 1993, 218:262–269.

10. Harpole DH, Johnson CM, Wolfe WG, *et al.*: Analysis of 945 cases of pulmonary metastatic melanoma. *J Thorac Cardiovasc Surg* 1992, 103:743–750.

11. Somoza S, Kondziolka D, Lansford D, *et al.*: Stereostatic radiosurgery for cerebral metastatic melanoma. *J Neurosurg* 1993, 79:661–666.

12. Lotze MT, Rosenberg SA: Interleukin-2: Clinical applications. In DeVita VT Jr, Hellman S, Rosenberg SA (eds): *Biologic Therapy of Cancer.* Philadelphia: JB Lippincott, 1991, p 159–179.

13. Cocconi G, Bella M, Calabresi F, *et al.*: Treatment of metastatic malignant melanoma with dacarbazine plus tamoxifen. *N Engl J Med* 1992, 327(8):516–523.

14. Kirkwood JM, Ernstoff MS, Hunt M: A randomized controlled trial of high-dose IFN alpha-2b for high-risk melanoma. *Proc ASCO* 1993, 12:390.

15. Smith JW, Urba WJ, Curti BD, *et al.*: The toxic and hematologic effects of interleukin-1 alpha administered in a phase I trial of patients with advanced malignancies. *J Clin Oncol* 1992, 10:1141–1152.

16. Ghussen F, Nagel K, Groth W, *et al.*: A prospective randomized study of regional extremity perfusion in patients with malignant melanoma. *Ann Surg* 1984, 200:764–770.

17. Lienard D, Lejeune FJ, Ewalenko P: In transit metastases of malignant melanoma treated by high dose rTNFa in combination with interferon-gamma and melphalan in isolation perfusion. *World J Surg* 1992, 16:234–240.

18. Preston DS, Sterns RS: Nonmelanoma cancers of the skin. *N Engl J Med* 1992, 327:1649–1662.

19. Glass AG, Hoover RN: The emerging epidemic of melanoma and squamous cell skin cancer. *JAMA* 1989, 262:2097–2100.

20. Cullen SI: Topical fluorouracil therapy for precancer and cancers of the skin. *J Am Geriatr Soc* 1979, 27:529–535.

21. Ashton H, Beveridge GW, Stevenson CJ: Topical treatment of skin tumors with 5-flourouracil. *Br J Dermatol* 1970, 82:207–209.

22. Greenberg ER, Baron JA, Stukel TA: A clinical trial of beta carotene to prevent basal-cell and squamous-cell cancers of the skin. *N Engl J Med* 1990, 323:189–795.

23. Tangrea JA, Edwards BK, Taylor PR: Long-term therapy with low-dose isotretinoin for prevention of basal cell carcinoma: A multicenter clinical trial. *J Nat Cancer Inst* 1992, 84:328–332.

24. Creech O, Krementz ET, Ryan RF, Wibled JN: Chemotherapy of cancer: Regional perfusion utilizing an extracorporeal circuit. *Ann Surg* 1958, 148:616–632.

25. Coit DG: Hyperthermic isolation limb perfusion for malignant melanoma: a review. *Cancer Invest* 1992, 10:277–284.

26. Ghussen F, Kruger I, Smalley R, Groth W: Hyperthermic perfusion with chemotherapy for melanoma of the extremities. *World J Surg* 1989, 13:598–602.

27. Kirkwood JM, Ernstoff MS, Ginliano A, *et al.*: Interferon alpha-2b and dacarbazine in melanoma. *J Nat Cancer* 1991, 82:1062–1063.

INTERFERON ALPHA-2

Interferon α-2 has shown modest levels of antitumor activity as a single agent in patients with metastatic melanoma, ranging from 15% to 20% in multiple trials. The highest response rates with IFN α-2 were noted in patients with the smallest bulk of disease. Immune mechanisms of antitumor response have their greatest impact in the setting of microscopic (or adjuvant) therapy, rather than in the advanced disease setting.

DOSAGE AND SCHEDULING

Arm A: high-dose IFN α-2b for 1 yr
Induction therapy: 20 MU/m^2 QID IV for 5 d × 4 wk
Maintenance: 10 MU/m^2/d 3 × weekly SC × 48 wk
Arm B: chronic low-dose IFN α-2b for 2 yr
      3 MU/m^2/d 3 × weekly SC
Arm C: Observation: studies at serial intervals (control)

DOSAGE MODIFICATION: *Reduce dose if bilirubin is elevated (2.6–5 x ULN) or SGOT, alkaline phosphatase is elevated (2.6–5 x ULN).*

CANDIDATES FOR TREATMENT

High-risk patients with deep primary melanoma (> 4 mm Breslow depth) with or without lymph node involvement (T4, NO, MO)

TOXICITIES

Fever, chill, myalgia/arthralgia, fatigue, headache; neutropenia, anemia, thrombocytopenia (not dose-limiting unless severe); hepatotoxicity (at high doses), hyperbilirubinemia, apparent hepatic necrosis (rare); proteinuria, elevated creatinine or BUN (at high doses)

ALTERNATIVE THERAPIES

Vaccination with cultured irradiated lines of tumor cells or partially purified proteins, whole tumor cells, partially purified proteins shed from cultured tumor cells, virus-modified tumor cell vaccine, defined gangliosides for immunization against melanoma, defined peptides and proteins for immunization against melanoma, anti-idiotype antibodies as vaccine

ENTRY TO THE INTERGROUP STUDY

Patients may be formally entered into study by investigators in the Eastern Cooperative Oncology Group, Cancer and Leukemia Group B, and Southwest On-cology Group or at the MD Anderson and Memorial Sloan-Kettering Cancer Centers (see appendix)

DRUG INTERACTIONS

Aspirin, prostaglandin synthetase inhibitors, antihistamines, other immunomodulators, NSAIDs

DACARBAZINE ALONE OR IN COMBINATION

The ECOG study group is conducting a phase III trial of dacarbazine alone versus pairwise combinations with interferon treatment-2, tamoxifen, or a combination of these agents for surgically incurable metastatic melanoma. This trial is designed to confirm or refute initial reports using dacarbazine combined with IFN α-2 in South Africa and with tamoxifen in Italy to a reasonably high level of confidence.

Dacarbazine is the only single agent that is FDA-approved for the indication of palliative therapy of metastatic melanoma. Combined chemotherapy for melanoma has not previously induced remissions significantly more frequently (> 15%) than dacarbazine nor prolonged survival of tested patients. However, two approaches have suggested prolonged survival of patients with metastatic melanoma through combined-modality treatment: tamoxifen plus dacarbazine [12] and IFN α-2 plus dacarbazine.

TRIAL DESIGN

Phase III comparison of dacarbazine or dacarbazine combined with either IFN α-2, tamoxifen, or both: dacarbazine alone, dacarbazine plus tamoxifen, dacarbazine plus IFN α-2, or dacarbazine plus IFN α-2 plus tamoxifen

This efficient trial design will allow analysis of groups separately and collapsed into larger groups with or without tamoxifen and with or without IFN.

CANDIDATES FOR TREATMENT

Histologically confirmed surgically incurable metastatic melanoma; measurable disease; performance status of 0–2 (see appendix); normal hematologic and biochemical values; SGOT < 3 times the upper limit of normal (unless deviation due to metastases); no prior chemotherapy; no prior radiotherapy to measurable disease; and no brain metastases
Exclusion Criteria: ocular melanoma; angina pectoris, ventricular arrhythmias or myocardial infarction within 6 mo; prior malignancy; history of clinical depression

TOXICITIES

Flu-like syndrome (anorexia, fatigue/malaise, chills or rigors, myalgias and arthralgias); hematologic, renal, hepatic, CNS, and GI toxicities; weight gain (fluid retention) or loss (anorexia)

ALTERNATIVE THERAPIES

Three-drug regimen of cisplatin, vinblastine, decarbazine, with response rates of 50%, four-drug regimen of cisplatin, BCNU, tamoxifen, and dacarbazine with response rates of 50%; six-drug regimen with IFN alpha-2 and IL-2 added to the four day combination: response rates of up to 57%

HYPERTHERMIC PERFUSION WITH MELPHALAN

Locoregional spread of melanoma of the extremity is a problem for a subset of approximately 10% of patients. In spite of the lack of systemic spread, many patients develop local complications related to in-transit spread that are difficult to manage. Creech developed a method to apply locoregional perfusion using cytotoxic agents [18]. The application of chemotherapy, heat, and/or immunotherapy using this method has been used by a variety of surgeons [19]. One prospective randomized study showing benefit was carried out by Ghussen *et al.*from 1980 to 1983. In a control group (n = 54) the tumors were widely excised and the regional lymph nodes removed. The perfusion group received this treatment, as well as hyperthermic (42°) perfusion with melphalan. After a median observation time of 5 years, 11 months, 26 recurrences were diagnosed in the control group and 6 noted in the perfusion group (p < 0.001). A survival advantage was also noted for the perfusion group (p < 0.01). Other studies have not shown a significant advantage, however. Recent variations that have used this approach have included coadministration of TNF and interferon gamma.

Hyperthermic perfusion alone has been used with apparent antitumor effects. Subsequently, Stehlin reported that the antitumor effect could be increased by adding chemotherapy. Melphalan (L-phenylalanine mustard) is used most frequently in perfusates. Recently cisplatin has also been tested in some protocols. The maximally tolerated dose used in the randomized study was 1 mg/kg for the upper extremity and 1.5 mg/kg for the lower extremity. Morbidity and mortality for the isolation limb perfusion have been reported. A 6 to 39% morbidity, including requirement for major skin grafting and limb loss due to a compartment syndrome, has been reported in various series. Mortality is unusual but has been reported up to 3% in some series.

DOSAGE AND SCHEDULING

Upper extremity (UE): The axillary vein and artery are exposed through an incision from the clavicle to the anterior axillary line. The patient is heparinized systemically (100 u/kg), and the vessels are occluded and catheters inserted. The initial perfusate is whole blood using an extracorporeal heater/bubble oxygenator/low flow pump. Flow rates range from 250 to 400 ml/min.

Lower extremity (LE): The femoral vessels are exposed through an incision from a point medial to the anterosuperior iliac spine to the femoral triangle. The inferior epigastric and circumflex iliac vessels are temporarily occluded and catheters inserted into the external iliac vessels so that the catheters are lying in the proximal femoral vessels. An Esmarch is applied around the root of the limb to prevent circulation through cutaneous or subcutaneous blood vessels. Leakage is measured using dye dilution techniques.

The perfusate temperature is maintained at 42.5°C, monitored by thermistor probes between the muscles and in the subcutaneous tissues of the thigh and calf. Melphalan is given in the UE (1.0 mg/kg) and in the LE (1.5 mg/kg). The first half of the dose is administered when the limb has reached 40°C, and the balance is injected in 3 equal aliquots at 15, 30, and 45 minutes, the entire procedure taking place over 1 hour.

CANDIDATES FOR TREATMENT

Patients with deep primary melanoma of the extremity, or *in transit*, advanced locoregional melanoma; other advanced locoregional diseases confined to the extremity (squamous carcinomas, sarcomas)—currently under investigation.

DRUG INTERACTIONS

TNFα and IFNγ (septic shock-like syndrome and death in some instances [5]) appear to enhance melphalan activity

TOXICITIES

Wound healing (5.7%), lymphatic fistulas (7.5%), low-grade fever, mild pain and erythema of the extremity, compartment syndrome (approximately 10%, amputation possibly required)

Give acetaminophen and/or indomethacin in the first 24–48 hr to control fever and chills; observe perfusion of the extremities to assess circulation, swelling, and presence of pulse (using handheld Doppler device); monitor vital signs every 4 hr during immediate postoperative period; refrain from movement of the extremity until drains are removed.

PATIENT INFORMATION

Patient should be informed of benefits and side effects. Possible injury to the skin or other structures in the extremity may require additional operations and even amputation. The procedure is done under anesthesia and a hospital stay of approximately 1–2 weeks is required.

TOPICAL APPLICATIONS OF 5-FU

Patients with multiple actinic solar keratoses are at risk for development of nonmelanoma skin cancers. In addition, patients with established basal cell carcinomas or multiple basal cell carcinomas may be treated with a 5% fluorouracil cream.

Fluorouracil blocks the methylation reaction of deoxyuridylic acid to thymidylic acid. It inhibits the synthesis of DNA and, to a lesser extent, RNA. The primary effect of 5-FU is on rapidly growing cells, and topical application has been shown to lead to insignificant absorption and primarily local antitumor effects.

DOSAGE AND SCHEDULING

When Efudex is applied to a tumor, local inflammation occurs associated with erythema, blister formation, ulceration, local necrosis and ultimately re-epitheliazation [3]. 5-FU cream or solution is applied twice daily in an amount sufficient to cover lesions [4]. The treatment is continued until inflammation resolves, usually for a period of 2 to 4 weeks. For treatment of basal cell carcinomas, applications for as long as 12 weeks may be required. A patient should be followed to determine the antitumor effects.

CANDIDATES FOR TREATMENT

Patients with Bowen's disease, patients with actinic keratosis, patients with multiple basal cell carcinomas

SPECIAL PRECAUTIONS

Patients must not have a known hypersensitivity to any components of the drug

DRUG INTERACTIONS

None known

TOXICITIES

Local reactions: pain, pyrites, hyperpigmentation, burning at the site of application; other reactions: contact dermatitis, scarring, tenderness, local infection, swelling

NURSING INTERVENTIONS

Instruct the patient in the expected side effects and to keep the area clean, dry, and potentially bandaged to prevent exposure to exogenous pathogens

PATIENT INFORMATION

This treatment is useful for patients thought to be at high risk for development of tumors of the skin or those who have had multiple previous tumors of the skin. In addition, some people with very early tumors, such as Bowen's disease or some basal cell carcinomas, will benefit from application of the cream. The cream should be applied in amounts sufficient to cover the lesions and the area lightly bandaged. Treatment may continue as long as 10 to 12 weeks and will cause redness, swelling, some pain, and itching. The patient should be followed closely by the physician during the course of treatment and thereafter to insure that tumor eradication has occurred.

Sarcomas are a group of diverse tumors arising primarily from mesenchymal structures. These cancers are rare, representing 1% of adult malignancies and 15% of malignancies in children and adolescents. Most sarcomas develop in tissues of mesodermal embryologic origin and are collectively called soft tissue sarcomas. Neurosarcomas, peripheral neuroectodermal tumors (PNET), and probably Ewing's sarcomas arise from tissues of ectodermal origin. Sarcomas derived in soft tissue, bone, and ectoderm are considered separately in this chapter because each of their treatment strategies differ.

ETIOLOGY AND RISK FACTORS

Sarcomas have been associated with a number of conditions, including genetic syndromes and toxic exposures (Table 1). In addition, many sarcomas have characteristic cytogenetic abnormalities [1].

STAGING AND PROGNOSIS

Staging for sarcomas is largely dependent on grade [2], which relies on the number of mitoses per 10 high-power microscopic fields (Table 2). Regional lymph node involvement is less than 10%. The most important prognostic parameters for localized disease are (in order of importance): tumor grade, the extent of the surgical margins, the size of the gross lesion in the unfixed pathology specimen, tumor size greater or less than 5 cm, and the histologic subtype. The lungs are the most frequent site of metastasis, with evidence of bone, liver, and central nervous system spread much less common. Preoperative staging evaluation should include a chest CT scan. Marrow is frequently involved in Ewing's sarcoma and rhabdomyosarcoma.

Sarcomas are typically pseudoencapsulated tumors that grow along histologic planes with microscopic neoplastic projections beyond the apparent margin or "capsule." Because local recurrences follow "shelling out" procedures in about 80% of cases, wide excisions are indicated (although tumor location strongly influences resectability). There are many histologic subtypes of sarcoma (Tables 3 and 4), and

the treatment is generally similar grade-for-grade, as histologic grade has proven to be more important than histopathologic type in predicting biologic behavior. The major exceptions are rhabdomyosarcoma, bone sarcomas (which are treated routinely with combined modality therapy including chemotherapy), and Kaposi's sarcoma.

SOFT TISSUE SARCOMAS

PRIMARY DISEASE THERAPY

An incisional biopsy is indicated prior to staging and resection. Surgery is the primary therapy for all localized soft tissue sarcomas (with the notable exceptions of rhabdomyosarcoma and Kaposi's sarcoma) (Fig. 1). Wide excision (> 3 cm histologically normal tissue) is optimal for curative intentions. In the event that one margin is

Table 2. Staging Schema for Sarcomas

Stage	Grade	Criteria
1	Low	<1 mitoses/10 HPF
2	Intermediate	1–4 mitoses/10 HPF
3	High	>5 mitoses/10 HPF
Limited disease (1–3)	Lesion size	A<5 cm
		B>5 cm
4A	Lymph node involvement	
4B	Metastases	

HPF—high-power microscopic field.

Table 3. Histologic Subtypes of Soft Tissue Sarcoma

Histology*	Comment
Malignant fibrous histiocytoma	Derived from cells of fibroblastic origin
Liposarcomas	Commonly single lesions in thigh or retroperitoneum; variable behavior
Fibrosarcomas	Now called spindle cell sarcomas, or MFH
Synovial sarcomas	Developed in extremities adjacent to joints
Neurosarcomas	
Malignant schwannomas	Patients with von Recklinghausen's neurofibromatosis
PNETs	Same chromosome translocation as Ewing's sarcoma and treated as Ewing's
Vascular sarcomas	
Angiosarcomas	Found in scalp in elderly males (may behave in indolent fashion), breast, liver, heart, and lungs (aggressive)
Kaposi's sarcoma	Indolent cutaneous lower extremity lesions in elderly men; aggressive variant is seen in patients with HIV infection
Leiomyosarcomas	Smooth muscle of gut, uterus, retroperitoneum, blood vessels
Rhabdomyosarcomas	Found in skeletal muscle elements of young patients; presumed to be systemic at diagnosis

*Histologic types are listed in order of frequency.

Table 1. Risk Factors for the Development of Sarcoma

Risk Factor	Predominant Histology
Genetic condition	
Li-Fraumeni syndrome	Osteosarcoma, soft tissue sarcoma
Familial retinoblastoma	Osteosarcoma
Familial osteochondroma	Osteo/chondrosarcoma
Toxic exposure	
Prior radiation therapy	Osteosarcoma, rare soft tissue sarcoma
Alkylating agents	Osteosarcoma, soft tissue sarcoma
Polyvinyl chloride	Hepatic angiosarcoma
Arsenic	Hepatic angiosarcoma
Iron overload	Hepatic angiosarcoma
Thorium	Hepatic angiosarcoma
Immunosuppression	
Renal transplantation	Kaposi's sarcoma, soft tissue sarcoma
AIDS	Kaposi's sarcoma
CLL	Soft tissue sarcoma
Paget's disease	Osteosarcoma

pathologically uninvolved but less than 3 cm (a deep margin or one adjacent to a major nerve or bone), radiotherapy is required to increase the chance for local control.

Because of the likelihood of occult metastasis, rhabdomyosarcoma is presumed to be systemic at diagnosis. The multimodality approach to therapy includes resection (when possible), followed by regional radiotherapy and chemoradiotherapy in a sequential/combination schedule [3].

Table 4. Histologic Subtypes of Bone Sarcoma

Histology*	Comment
Osteosarcoma	Biphasic incidence: elderly (associated with Paget's), adolescence (epiphyses of growing long bones)
Ewing's sarcoma	Often disseminated at presentation; long bones of the extremities, flat bones of the pelvis/ribs
Chondrosarcomas	Relatively resistant to both radiotherapy and chemotherapy, should be adequately resected at the time of diagnosis
Giant cell tumors of bone (osteoclastomas)	"Benign," but malignant behavior after multiple recurrences

*Histologic types are listed in order of frequency.

THERAPY FOR REGIONAL DISEASE

In patients with high-grade extremity lesions, a combined modality approach, including limb-sparing surgery (< 3-cm margin) followed by adjuvant postoperative radiation therapy, provides good local control rates. More recently, preoperative radiation therapy has been combined with conservative surgery and may be of value in patients with otherwise borderline resectable lesions. Retroperitoneal sarcomas frequently cannot be completely resected, and radiation therapy is difficult to deliver due to gastrointestinal toxicity. Consequently, this disease site is associated with the lowest 5-year survival rates.

THERAPY FOR ADVANCED DISEASE

In a review of individual chemotherapeutic agents (Table 5), doxorubicin and ifosfamide are the most active in soft tissue sarcomas. Dacarbazine has a single-agent response rate of 16% and is particularly active in leiomyosarcomas. The response rate of single-agent doxorubicin at 70 mg/m^2 is higher than that of cyclophosphamide with doxorubicin at 50/m^2 (dose reduced to accommodate the myelosuppression of cyclophosphamide).

Combination Chemotherapy

In a randomized European trial, doxorubicin alone was tested against doxorubicin and ifosfamide versus cyclophosphamide, vincristine, doxorubicin, and dacarbazine [4]. Although there was a trend toward an increased response duration for the combination, there was no significant difference in survival. A more recent EORTC trial showed a 45% response rate for a doxorubicin and ifosfamide regimen [5]. An Intergroup trial (ISSG) and an ECOG study randomizing a doxoru-

FIGURE 1

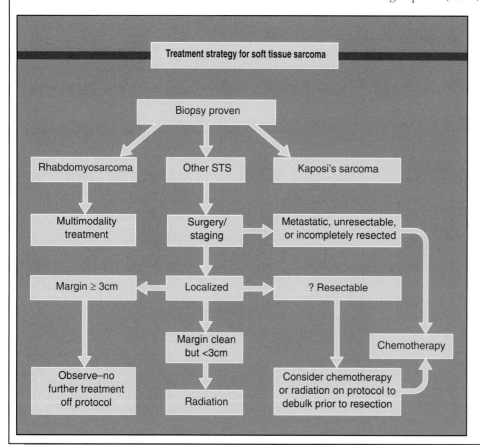

Treatment strategy for soft tissue sarcoma

The information here is provided as guidance only. Prescribers should always consult the manufacturer's current prescribing information.

138

bicin-containing regimen with or without ifosfamide showed a significantly increased response rate for the ifosfamide regimen; however survival was not affected [6,7]. This combination regimen of doxorubicin, ifosfamide (at higher dose, 7.5 g/m²), and dacarbazine was given at the Dana-Farber Cancer Institute with a response rate of 50% [8]. Currently, this regimen yields the highest response rates in soft tissue sarcomas. An improved response rate may be particularly important in the management of high-grade, borderline-resectable lesions or pulmonary metastases, particularly in younger patients who are more likely to tolerate significant myelosuppression.

Relapsed Metastatic Disease

Surgical resection of pulmonary metastases can be curative in 15 to 30% of selected patients, particularly those with a few, isolated, slowly-growing nodules (disease free interval > 12 months). This approach, however, has not been particularly useful in rhabdomyosarcoma.

Kaposi's sarcomas generally respond to radiotherapy or low doses of vinblastine or doxorubicin. An aggressive variant of Kaposi's sarcoma is seen in patients with acquired immune deficiency syndrome (AIDS). These patients may be treated locally with radiation therapy, given chemotherapy (weekly vinblastine or vincristine; monthly doxorubicin, bleomycin, and vinblastine, or liposomal doxorubicin), or started on immunotherapy (interferon) for widespread disease.

BONE SARCOMAS

PRIMARY TUMOR THERAPY

Patients with possible osteosarcoma should be referred to an institution with sarcoma experience, as an improperly placed biopsy may

limit subsequent limb-sparing surgery. Primary lesions must be excised with several centimeters of microscopically clear margins, and patients with a significant soft tissue component or neurovascular involvement generally require amputation. Unlike soft tissue tumors, there is convincing evidence for adjuvant therapy in this disease based on significantly improved 2-year disease-free survivals after five- and six-drug adjuvant regimens, respectively [10] (Fig. 2).

Ewing's sarcoma is a primitive, small blue cell tumor of bone, and extraosseous presentations are staged and treated like primary bony disease. Although clinically detectable metastases are present in about one-third of patients at diagnosis, the 90% mortality after surgical resection alone suggest dissemination at presentation. Initial treatment consists of combination chemotherapy concurrent with radiotherapy to the involved bone or resection if possible (Fig. 3). Survival rates of patients with localized disease correlate inversely with age.

THERAPY FOR REGIONAL DISEASE

Selected patients with osteosarcoma who receive limb-sparing surgery have local control rates (90-97%) and survival rates similar to those

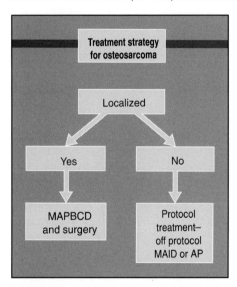

FIGURE 2

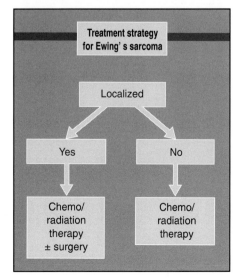

FIGURE 3

Table 5. Efficacy of Commercially Available Single Agents in Soft Tissue Sarcomas

Agents by Class	Studies, *n*	Cases	Response Rates (%)*
Anthracyclines			
Doxorubicin	7	356	26
Antimetabolites			
High-dose methotrexate	6	76	13
Standard-dose methotrexate	3	81	21
Bleomycin	1	32	6
Actinomycin D	1	30	17
5-Fluorouracil	1	8	12
Vincas			
Vincristine	2	103	12
Etoposide	2	40	8
Alkylating agents			
Ifosfamide	10	218	30
Dacarbazine	1	109	16
Cisplatin	6	103	12
Cyclophosphamide	2	82	8

*When the denominator includes at least 10 cases.
Modified from Chang et al. [9]; with permission.

found with patients receiving amputation. Radiotherapy alone does not improve the rate of successful limb-sparing surgery nor decrease the risk of local recurrence for close or involved surgical margins.

Preoperative (neoadjuvant) combination chemotherapy with local resection and postoperative chemotherapy is under evaluation. Patients require close observation during preoperative chemotherapy and prompt resection if response is suboptimal, because of the potential for increased local or distant failure. Preoperative chemotherapy theoretically may more effectively eradicate early occult metastatic deposits, and the response to preoperative chemotherapy can be evaluated histologically. Patients with less than 90% tumor necrosis at resection may benefit from receiving other effective agents postoperatively. In selected centers, intra-arterial use of chemotherapy has been effective.

THERAPY FOR ADVANCED DISEASE

Palliative Treatment

Adult patients presenting with metastatic osteosarcoma may be treated palliatively with doxorubicin and cisplatin alone or with the MAID regimen, instead of the intensive sequential six-drug protocol. Pediatric patients are given the protocol therapy that may contain phase II agents in addition to the core regimen.

As Ewing's sarcoma is generally a chemosensitive disease, patients treated for strictly palliative intent may receive lower doses of the active drugs. The MAID regimen has been effective in the treatment of these sarcoma subtypes, but the numbers of treated patients are small. Radiation therapy also affords palliation for Ewing's sarcoma.

Fibrosarcomas, chordomas, angiosarcomas, and malignant fibrous histiocytomas of bone are generally treated the same way as the corresponding histologic soft tissue sarcomas. In contrast, extraosseous presentations of primary bony tumors (including Ewing's sarcoma) are treated like the tumor of bone.

Relapsed Metastatic Disease

Surgical resection of pulmonary metastases can be curative in 15 to 30% of selected patients, particularly those with a few isolated, slowly growing nodules (disease free interval > 12 months), but has not been particularly useful in Ewing's sarcoma.

REFERENCES

1. Fletcher JA, Weidner N, Corson JM: Laboratory investigation and genetics in sarcomas. *Curr Sci* 1990, 2:467–473.

2. Russell W, Cohen J, Enzinger F, *et al.*: A clinical and pathologic staging system for soft tissue sarcomas. *Cancer* 1977, 40:1562–1570.

3. Mauer HM, Gehan EA, Beltangady M, *et al.*: The Intergroup Rhabdomyosarcoma Study—II. Cancer 1993, 71:1904–1922.

4. Santoro A, Rouesse J, Steward W, *et al.*: A randomized EORTC study in advanced soft tissue sarcomas (STS): ADM vs. ADM + IFX vs. cyvadic. *Proc ASCO* 1990, 9:309.

5. Steward W, Verweij, Somers R, *et al.*: Granulocyte-macrophage colony-stimulating factor allows safe escalation of dose intensity of chemotherapy in metastatic adult soft tissue sarcomas: A study of the EORTC soft tissue and bone sarcoma group. *J Clin Oncol* 1993, 11:15–21.

6. Antman K, Crowley J, Bolcerzak, *et al.*: An intergroup phase III randomized study of doxorubicin and dacarbazine with or without ifosfamide and mesna in advanced soft tissue and bone sarcomas. *J Clin Oncol* 1993, 7:1276–1285.

7. Edmonson JH, Ryan LM, Blum RH, *et al.*: Randomized comparison of doxorubicin alone versus ifosfamide plus doxorubicin or mitomycin, doxorubicin, and cisplatin against advanced soft tissue sarcomas. *J Clin Oncol* 1993, 7:1269–1275.

8. Elias A, Eder JP, Shea T, *et al.*: High dose ifosfamide with mesna uroprotection: A phase I study. *J Clin Oncol* 1990, 8:170–178.

9. Chang A, Rosenberg SA, Glatstein E, Antman K: Sarcomas of soft tissue. In DeVita VT, Hellman S, Rosenberg SA (eds): *Cancer Principles and Practice of Oncology*, 3rd ed. 1990, Philadelphia: JB Lippincott, pp 1345–1398.

10. Mazanet R, Antman K: Adjuvant therapy of soft tissue sarcomas. *Sem Oncol* 1991, 18:603–612.

11. Miser JS, Kinsella TJ, Triche TJ, *et al.*: Ifosfamide with mesna uroprotection and etoposide; an effective regimen in the treatment of recurrent sarcomas and other tumors of children and young adults. *J Clin Oncol* 1987, 5:1191–1198.

12. Kung FH, Pratt CB, Vega RA, *et al.*: Ifosfamide/etoposide combination in the treatment of recurrent malignant solid tumors of childhood. *Cancer* 1993; 71:1898–1902.

MAID

Mesna, Doxorubicin, Ifosfamide, Dacarbazine

Doxorubicin and ifosfamide have the highest single-agent response rates for soft tissue sarcoma. Ifosfamide has activity in patients who fail doxorubicin. This combination regimen of doxorubicin, ifosfamide, and dacarbazine (MAID) has shown a response rate of 50%. Hematopoietic growth factors have been given with this regimen as part of clinical trials and may ameliorate the neutropenia.

CANDIDATES FOR TREATMENT
Patients with soft tissue sarcoma

SPECIAL PRECAUTIONS
Give doxorubicin by central venous access; patients with abnormal hepatic function (reduce doxorubicin); patients with renal or urinary tract disease or obstruction

ALTERNATIVE THERAPIES
Initial use of doxorubicin and dacarbazine followed by ifosfamide upon progression is preferred approach for older patients or those with low-grade lesions; single-agent doxorubicin for palliation in patients who may not tolerate combination therapy

DOSAGE AND SCHEDULING

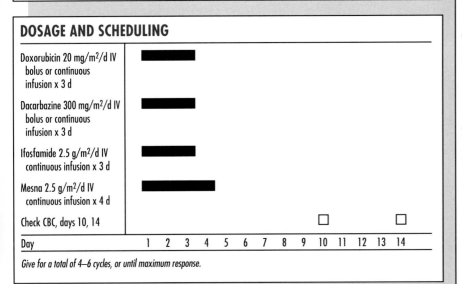

Doxorubicin 20 mg/m²/d IV bolus or continuous infusion x 3 d

Dacarbazine 300 mg/m²/d IV bolus or continuous infusion x 3 d

Ifosfamide 2.5 g/m²/d IV continuous infusion x 3 d

Mesna 2.5 g/m²/d IV continuous infusion x 4 d

Check CBC, days 10, 14

Day 1 2 3 4 5 6 7 8 9 10 11 12 13 14

Give for a total of 4–6 cycles, or until maximum response.

TOXICITIES
Drug combination: very myelosuppressive, which can lead to life-threatening infections and bleeding; nausea and vomiting; infertility; alopecia; **Doxorubicin:** red/orange urine; tissue damage/phlebitis with extravasation; late side effects (mucositis, hyperpigmentation of skin and nails, photosensitivity); possibly radiosensitizing, causing reactivation of toxicity in previously irradiated sites; cumulative toxicity—cardiac damage; **Ifosfamide:** hemorrhagic cystitis (given with mesna); possible neurotoxicity (reversible confusion, somnolence, visual hallucinations); proximal RTA with HCO_3, potassium, and magnesium wasting (reversible); **Dacarbazine:** delayed emesis; flu-like symptoms and fever

RECENT EXPERIENCES AND RESPONSE RATES

Study	Regimen	Evaluable Patients, *n*	CR (%)	RR (%)
Elias *et al.*, J Clin Oncol 1990, 8:170–178	IAD (I, 7.5 g/m²)	108	10	47
Schutte *et al.*, Proc ASCO 1986, p. 145	IA (I, 6 g/m²)	125	NA	36
Mansi *et al.*, Eur J Cancer Clin Oncol 1988, 24:1439–1443	IA	54	6	22

CR—complete response; RR—response rate.

DRUG INTERACTIONS
Doxorubicin: digitalis glycosides, barbiturates; **Ifosfamide:** barbiturates; **Drug combination:** NSAIDs, live vaccines

NURSING INTERVENTIONS
Give prophylactic antiemetics for chemotherapy; avoid sedation (do not mask neurotoxicity); monitor urinalysis daily for hematuria during ifosfamide administration; avoid extravasation of doxorubicin; instruct patients in the care of central venous access device, to use prophylactic mouth care to minimize mucositis, to call physician if they experience symptoms of infection, bleeding, or congestive heart failure

PATIENT INFORMATION
Nausea and vomiting are likely. Fall in blood counts 10–14 days after chemotherapy, which will gradually increase on their own, but transfusion may be required; call physician if fever of 101°F or above, chills, abnormal bleeding, redness or soreness around central venous access device, shortness of breath, or swelling in the ankles develops

MABCDP
Methotrexate, Doxorubicin, Bleomycin, Cyclophosphamide, Actinomycin D, Cisplatin

This regimen consists of high doses of active drugs administered in a sequential/combination fashion over 42 weeks. Based on the results from randomized trials, chemotherapy with a doxorubicin- and cisplatin-based regimen has become standard treatment for osteosarcoma. The question currently under study is the impact of neoadjuvant (preoperative chemotherapy in resectable patients) chemotherapy followed by surgery versus the traditional approach of surgical treatment of the primary tumor followed by adjuvant chemotherapy.

CANDIDATES FOR TREATMENT
Patients with resectable osteosarcoma; patients with advanced osteosarcoma who warrant aggressive therapy

SPECIAL PRECAUTIONS
Provide appropriate support and leucovorin rescue for high-dose methotrexate; patients with abnormal renal or hepatic function (reduce dosage)

ALTERNATIVE THERAPIES
Investigational approaches such as intra-arterial chemotherapy for limb salvage; adult patients with metastatic disease may be treated palliatively with doxorubicin/cisplatin alone or MAID; pediatric patients are treated on protocol therapy that may contain phase II agents in addition to core regimen

TOXICITIES
Drug combination: cumulative myelosuppression, which can lead to life-threatening infections and bleeding; infertility; alopecia; **Methotrexate:** renal failure (in high doses and without allopurinol and leucovorin); severe myelosuppression, mucositis, hepatic toxicity, cumulative toxicities—hepatic fibrosis, pulmonary dysfunction, osteoporosis; **Doxorubicin:** red/orange urine; local tissue damage/phlebitis with extravasation; late side effects (mucositis, hyperpigmentation, photosensitivity); possibly radiosensitizing; cumulative toxicity—cardiac damage; **Cisplatin:** nephrotoxicity, ototoxicity, peripheral neuropathy; nausea and vomiting; myelo-suppression; **Bleomycin:** anaphylactic or hypersensitivity reaction (give test dose); pneumonitis can progress to pulmonary fibrosis, particularly with cumulative dosing > 400 U; discontinue drug for significant decrease in DLCO; avoid high-inhaled oxygen concentrations; **Cyclophosphamide:** hemorrhagic cystitis (give with adequate hydration); myelo-suppression; **Actinomycin D:** nausea and vomiting; local tissue damage and phlebitis if extravasated; rash

DRUG INTERACTIONS
Drug combination: NSAIDs, live vaccines; **Doxorubicin:** digitalis glycosides, barbiturates; **Methotrexate:** cholestyramine, ethanol, PABA, probenecid, salicylates, 5-FU, live vaccines

NURSING INTERVENTIONS
Prophylactic antiemetics; hydrate vigorously; become familiar with leucovorin rescue schedule; avoid doxorubicin and actinomycin D extravasations; instruct patients to follow complicated inpatient/outpatient 42 week schedule, to care for access device, to use prophylactic mouth care to minimize mucositis, to call physician if infection, bleeding, volume depletion, or congestive heart failure develops

PATIENT INFORMATION
Nausea and vomiting are likely; mouth sores 5–10 days after therapy; fall in blood counts 10–14 days after chemotherapy, which gradually increase, but transfusion may be required; call physician if fever of 101°F, chills, abnormal bleeding, redness or soreness around access device, inability to take adequate fluids, shortness of breath, or ankle swelling develops

DOSAGE AND SCHEDULING

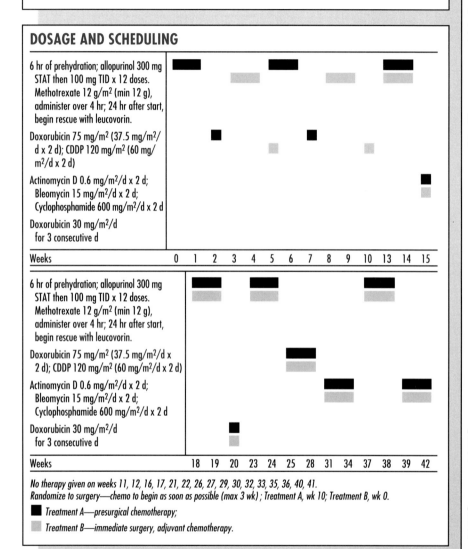

6 hr of prehydration; allopurinol 300 mg STAT then 100 mg TID x 12 doses. Methotrexate 12 g/m² (min 12 g), administer over 4 hr; 24 hr after start, begin rescue with leucovorin.

Doxorubicin 75 mg/m² (37.5 mg/m²/d x 2 d); CDDP 120 mg/m² (60 mg/m²/d x 2 d)

Actinomycin D 0.6 mg/m²/d x 2 d; Bleomycin 15 mg/m²/d x 2 d; Cyclophosphamide 600 mg/m²/d x 2 d

Doxorubicin 30 mg/m²/d for 3 consecutive d

Weeks: 0 1 2 3 4 5 6 7 8 9 10 13 14 15

6 hr of prehydration; allopurinol 300 mg STAT then 100 mg TID x 12 doses. Methotrexate 12 g/m² (min 12 g), administer over 4 hr; 24 hr after start, begin rescue with leucovorin.

Doxorubicin 75 mg/m² (37.5 mg/m²/d x 2 d); CDDP 120 mg/m² (60 mg/m²/d x 2 d)

Actinomycin D 0.6 mg/m²/d x 2 d; Bleomycin 15 mg/m²/d x 2 d; Cyclophosphamide 600 mg/m²/d x 2 d

Doxorubicin 30 mg/m²/d for 3 consecutive d

Weeks: 18 19 20 23 24 25 28 31 34 37 38 39 42

No therapy given on weeks 11, 12, 16, 17, 21, 22, 26, 27, 29, 30, 32, 33, 35, 36, 40, 41. Randomize to surgery—chemo to begin as soon as possible (max 3 wk) ; Treatment A, wk 10; Treatment B, wk 0.

■ *Treatment A—presurgical chemotherapy;*
▨ *Treatment B—immediate surgery, adjuvant chemotherapy.*

RECENT EXPERIENCES AND RESPONSE RATES

Study	Regimen	Observation			Chemotherapy			
		N	DFS (%)	S (%)	N	DFS (%)	S (%)	p
Taylor et al., Mayo Clin Proc 1978, 53:695–700	MV	18	44	62	20	40	80	NS
Link et al., N Engl J Med 1986, 314:1600–1606	MABCDP	18	17	NA	18	66	NA	<.001
Eilber et al., J Clin Oncol 1987, 5:21–26	MABCAd	28	39	65	27	59	86	.005

DFS—disease-free survival; S—survival.

VACD
Vincristine, Doxorubicin, Cyclophosphamide, Actinomycin D

Because 80 to 90% of patients with locally controlled disease in the absence of chemotherapy develop disseminated disease, Ewing's sarcoma and rhabdomyosarcoma are presumed to be systemic at diagnosis. Patients are generally treated with combination chemotherapy developed on pediatric protocols, including vincristine, doxorubicin, cyclophosphamide, and actinomycin D (VACD). The multimodality approach also includes resection (when possible), followed by regional radiotherapy in a sequential/combination schedule over the course of a year. Although children with metastatic disease can be cured, the prognosis in adults, even with localized disease, is poor despite excellent initial responses to aggressive chemotherapy.

DOSAGE AND SCHEDULING

Drug	0	3	6	9	10*	11*	12*	13*	14*	15	18	21	24	27	30
Vincristine 2 mg/m² (max 2 mg) IV push, wk 0,3,6,9,12–15,18, 21,24,27,30,33,36,39,42,45, 48,51	■	■	■	■			■	■	■	■	■	■	■	■	■
Doxorubicin 75 mg/m² IV over 15 min (total cumulative dose 375 mg/m²)†, wk 0,3,6,9,18	■	■	■	■							■				
Actinomycin D 1.25 mg/m² IV push, wk 21,24,27,30,33, 36,39,42,45,48,51												■	■	■	■
Cyclophosphamide 1200 mg/m² IV over 30 min with mesna, wk 0,3,6,9,18,21,24,27,30, 33,36,39,42,45,48,51	■	■	■	■							■	■	■	■	■
Weeks	0	3	6	9	10*	11*	12*	13*	14*	15	18	21	24	27	30

Drug	33	36	39	42	45	48	51
Vincristine 2 mg/m² (max 2 mg) IV push	■	■	■	■	■	■	■
Doxorubicin 75 mg/m² IV over 15 min (total cumulative dose 375 mg/m²)†							
Actinomycin D 1.25 mg/m² IV push	■	■	■	■	■	■	■
Cyclophosphamide 1200 mg/m² IV over 30 min with mesna	■	■	■	■	■	■	■
Weeks	33	36	39	42	45	48	51

No therapy given on weeks 1, 2, 4, 5, 7, 8, 10, 11, 16, 17, 19, 20, 22, 23, 25, 26, 28, 29, 31, 32, 34, 35, 37, 38, 40, 41, 43, 44, 46, 47, 49, 50, 52, 53, 54.

*Local control measures
†If the patient receives ≥ 2000 cGy to any portion of the heart, the doxorubicin dose should not exceed 300 mg/m²

CANDIDATES FOR TREATMENT
Patients with rhabdomyosarcoma or Ewing's sarcoma

SPECIAL PRECAUTIONS
Give doxorubicin by central venous access; patients with abnormal hepatic function (reduce doxorubicin)

ALTERNATE THERAPIES
Lower doses of active drugs in patients treated for strictly palliative intent; MAID; radiation therapy for palliation of Ewing's sarcoma; investigational approaches—alternating ifosfamide and etoposide with vincristine, doxorubicin, and cyclophosphamide in Ewing's sarcoma; high-dose (noncross–resistant) chemotherapy with autologous hematopoietic stem cell support

TOXICITIES
Drug combination: myelosuppression can lead to life-threatening infections and bleeding; nausea and vomiting; infertility; alopecia; **Doxorubicin:** red/orange urine; local tissue damage/phlebitis with extravasation; late side effects (mucositis, hyperpigmentation of skin and nails, and photosensitivity); possibly radiosensitizing, causing reactivation of toxicity in previously irradiated sites; cumulative toxicity—cardiac damage; **Vincristine:** ileus, peripheral neuropathy; local tissue damage/phlebitis with extravasation; **Cyclophosphamide:** mild hemorrhagic cystitis; **Actinomycin D:** delayed nausea and vomiting, mucositis

DRUG INTERACTIONS
Doxorubicin: digitalis glycosides, barbiturates; **Drug combinations:** NSAIDs, salicylates, live vaccines

NURSING INTERVENTIONS
Give prophylactic antiemetics for chemotherapy; avoid extravasation of doxorubicin and vincristine; Instruct patients to use prophylactic mouth care to minimize mucositis, to call physician if they experience symptoms of infection, bleeding, or congestive heart failure

PATIENT INFORMATION
Nausea and vomiting are likely; fall in blood counts 10–14 days after chemotherapy, which will gradually increase on their own, but transfusion may be required; constipation may occur; call physician if fever of 101°F or above, chills, abnormal bleeding, redness or soreness around central venous access device, shortness of breath, or swelling in the ankles develops

IE
Ifosfamide and Etoposide

Ifosfamide has activity in patients who fail doxorubicin. It is not clear if patients treated with an ifosfamide/doxorubicin combination regimen as first-line therapy benefit from further ifosfamide therapy. Trials utilizing carboplatin or cisplatin in addition to ifosfamide and etoposide, with hematopoietic growth factors to potentially ameliorate neutropenia, for refractory/relapsed sarcomas are ongoing.

DOSAGE AND SCHEDULING

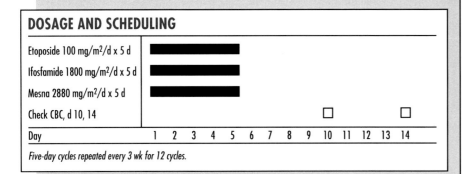

	1	2	3	4	5	6	7	8	9	10	11	12	13	14
Etoposide 100 mg/m²/d x 5 d														
Ifosfamide 1800 mg/m²/d x 5 d														
Mesna 2880 mg/m²/d x 5 d														
Check CBC, d 10, 14										☐				☐
Day	1	2	3	4	5	6	7	8	9	10	11	12	13	14

Five-day cycles repeated every 3 wk for 12 cycles.

RECENT EXPERIENCES AND RESPONSE RATES

Responses ranging from 54–94% in untreated pediatric sarcomas. Good responses in recurrent sarcomas [11,12].

CANDIDATES FOR TREATMENT

Patients with relapsed sarcomas

SPECIAL PRECAUTIONS

Patients with history of renal or urinary tract disease or obstruction (continue mesna for at least 12 hours after ending therapy)

ALTERNATIVE THERAPIES

Investigation therapy may be explored (because patients have already failed with doxorubicin); resection may benefit patients with isolated pulmonary metastasis

TOXICITIES

Drug combination: myelosuppression, which can lead to life-threatening infections and bleeding; nausea; infertility; alopecia; **Etoposide:** anaphylactic reactions; **Ifosfamide:** hemorrhagic cystitis (must give with mesna); possible neurotoxicity (reversible confusion, somnolence, visual hallucination); proximal RTA with HCO_3, potassium, magnesium wasting (reversible)

DRUG INTERACTIONS

Ifosfamide: digitalis glycosides, barbiturates; **Drug combination:** NSAIDs, live vaccines

NURSING INTERVENTIONS

Give antiemetics as needed; avoid sedation (do not mask neurotoxicity); monitor urinalysis daily for hematuria during ifosfamide administration; instruct patients to call physician if they experience symptoms of infection or bleeding

PATIENT INFORMATION

Nausea and vomiting are likely; fall in blood counts 10–14 days after chemotherapy, which will gradually increase on their own, but transfusion may be required; call physician if fever of 101°F or above, chills, or abnormal bleeding develops

VACD AND IE
Vincristine, Doxorubicin, Cyclophosphamide, Actinomycin D and Ifosfamide, Etoposide

The combination of surgery and radiotherapy in the absence of chemotherapy for Ewing's sarcoma gives a failure-free survival rate of 10%; this poor result indicates the need for treatment upfront with combination chemotherapy. Attempts to improve survival in Ewing's sarcoma have centered around the addition of ifosfamide and etoposide to standard therapy (VACD). Actinomycin D is substituted for doxorubicin when the total cumulative dose is 375 mg/m². The multimodality approach also includes resection (when possible), followed by regional radiotherapy in a sequential/combination schedule over the course Of a year. Although children with metastatic disease can be cured, the prognosis in adults, even with localized disease, is poor, despite excellent initial responses to aggressive chemotherapy.

CANDIDATES FOR TREATMENT
Patients with Ewing's sarcoma

SPECIAL PRECAUTIONS
Patients with renal or urinary tract disease or obstruction; give doxorubicin by central venous access; patients with abnormal hepatic function (reduce doxorubicin dose)

ALTERNATIVE THERAPIES
Standard VACD; investigational approaches—high-dose (noncross–resistant) chemotherapy with autologous hematopoietic stem cell support

TOXICITIES
Drug combination: myelosuppression leading to life-threatening infections and bleeding, nausea and vomiting; infertility; alopecia; **Doxorubicin:** red/orange urine; local tissue damage/phlebitis with extravasation; late side effects (mucositis, hyperpigmentation of skin and nails, and photosensitivity); possibly radiosensitizing, causing reactivation of toxicity in previously irradiated sites; cumulative toxicity—cardiac damage; **Vincristine:** ileus, peripheral neuropathy; local tissue damage/phlebitis with extravasation; **Cyclophosphamide:** mild hemorrhagic cystitis; **Actinomycin D:** delayed nausea and vomiting, mucositis, **Etoposide:** anaphylactic reactions; **Ifosfamide:** hemorrhagic cystitis (give with mesna); possible neurotoxicity (reversible confusion, somnolence, visual hallucinations); proximal RTA with HCO_3, potassium, magnesium wasting (reversible)

DRUG INTERACTIONS
Doxorubicin: digitalis glycosides, barbiturates; **Drug combination:** NSAIDs, salicylates, live vaccines

NURSING INTERVENTIONS
Give prophylactic antiemetics for chemotherapy; avoid sedation (do not mask neurotoxicity); monitor urinalysis daily during ifosfamide administration; avoid extravasation of doxorubicin and vincristine; instruct patients to use prophylactic mouth care to minimize mucositis, to call physician if they experience symptoms of infection, bleeding, or congestive heart failure

PATIENT INFORMATION
Nausea and vomiting are likely; fall in blood counts 10–14 days after chemotherapy, which will gradually increase on their own, but transfusion may be required; constipation may occur; call physician if fever of 101° F or above, chills, abnormal bleeding, redness or soreness around central venous access device, shortness of breath, or swelling in the ankles develops

DOSAGE AND SCHEDULING

	0	3	6	9	10*	11*	12*	13*	14*	15	18	21	24	27	30
Ifosfamide 1.8 g/m² IV over 1 hr/d x 5 d with mesna, wk 0, 6,12,15,21,27,33,39,45,51	■	■	■				■			■		■		■	■
Etoposide 100 mg/m² IV over 1 hr/d x 5 d, wk 0,6,12,15, 21,27,33,39,45,51	■	■	■				■			■		■		■	■
Vincristine 2 mg/m² (max 2 mg) IV push, wk 3,9,18,24,30, 36,42,48		■	■								■		■		■
Doxorubicin 75 mg/m² IV over 15 min (total cumulative dose 375 mg/m²)†, wk 3,9,18,24,30		■	■								■		■		■
Actinomycin D 1.25 mg/m² IV push, wk 36,42,48															
Cyclophosphamide 1200 mg/m² IV over 30 min with mesna, wk 3,9,18,24,30,36,42,48		■	■								■		■		■
Weeks	0	3	6	9	10*	11*	12*	13*	14*	15	18	21	24	27	30

	33	36	39	42	45	48	51
Ifosfamide 1.8 g/m² IV over 1 hr/d x 5 d with mesna	■	■	■	■			
Etoposide 100 mg/m² IV over 1 hr/d x 5 d	■	■	■	■			
Vincristine 2 mg/m² (max 2 mg) IV push		■	■	■			
Doxorubicin 75 mg/m² IV over 15 min (total cumulative dose 375 mg/m²)†							
Actinomycin D 1.25 mg/m² IV push		■	■	■			
Cyclophosphamide 1200 mg/m² IV over 30 min with mesna		■	■	■			
Weeks	33	36	39	42	45	48	51

No therapy given on weeks 1, 2, 4, 5, 7, 8, 10, 11, 13, 14, 16, 17, 19, 20, 22, 23, 25, 26, 28, 29, 31, 32, 34, 35, 37, 38, 40, 41, 43, 46, 47, 49, 50, 52–54

*Local control measures

†If the patient receives ≥ 2000 cGy to any portion of the heart, the doxorubicin dose is not to exceed 300 mg/m²

While tremendous strides have been made in the treatment of genitourinary malignancies in the past 10 to 15 years, the recent explosion of new findings in cell biology, physiology, biochemistry, pharmacology, immunology, and radiobiology have broadened and deepened our understanding of the treatment of these malignancies. This chapter summarizes present medical and surgical therapies employed for prostate, urinary bladder, testicular, and renal cancers. Highlighted are salient basic and clinical observations that have formed the foundation of our current therapeutic strategies in genitourinary cancers.

TESTICULAR CANCER

ETIOLOGY AND RISK FACTORS

Germ cell cancers of gonadal and extragonadal origin, arise from pleuripotent cells capable of differentiating along five embryonic lines. These tumors are commonly grouped into seminoma and nonseminoma. Seminoma arise from the spermatocyte, the earliest cell with the greatest ability to differentiate into embryonic or placental tissue. Nonseminoma tumors are commonly mixed and contain elements of embryonal cells, teratoma, yolk sac, and choriocarcinoma. The risk factors associated with testicular tumors are listed in Table 1.

STAGING AND PROGNOSIS

The diagnosis and therapeutic approaches to germ cell tumor of the testis must consider the anatomy of lymphatic drainage, course of the neurovascular bundles, stage of disease, histologic type, and the presence of vessel invasion. In addition, the relative sensitivity to chemotherapy or radiation therapy may dictate choice of treatment for these tumors. Following the clinical suspicion of a testicular malignancy, a routine battery of laboratory and radiologic evaluations should be performed including a complete blood count, lactate dehydrogenase (LDH), beta human chorionic gonadotropin (βHCG), alpha-fetoprotein (AFP), urine analysis, and computed tomography (CT) of the chest and abdomen. Other tests that may prove useful in the diagnosis and management of testicular tumors include testicular ultrasound and intravenous pylography.

Accurate tumor markers for assessment of germ cell cancers have become essential for the correct management of these malignancies [5]. Elevation of AFP, βHCG, or both are found in 85% of nonseminomatous germ cell cancer, whereas 10% of seminomas may show mild elevation in βHCG. False elevations in serum markers are rare but should be recognized because treatment decisions are based,

in part, on these measurements. Although LDH is a nonspecific marker, it is helpful in suggesting bulky lymph node involvement.

Traditional staging of patients with testicular disease is provided in Table 2. For patients with metastatic disease a number of prognostic factors have been identified and used in devising staging systems. The commonly used systems, M.D. Anderson Classification, Memorial Sloan—Kettering Cancer Institute Classification, and Indiana Classification, attempt to estimate the bulk of disease and do so relatively well. We use the Indiana system, which classifies patients with testicular cancer into three categories (Table 3).

PRIMARY DISEASE THERAPY

There is no controversy over the appropriate initial therapeutic approach to suspected testicular malignancies (Table 4). An inguinal orchiectomy allows for control of blood and lymphatic vessels and *en bloc* removal of the affected testicle. Trans-scrotal biopsies or orchiectomy may lead to locoregional recurrences in as many as one quarter of patients and are discouraged. Lymphatic pathways from the testicle pass first to the peri- and preaortic lymph nodes on the left and interaortocaval, preaortic, and precaval lymph nodes on the right. Identification of the sympathetic nerves, which supply the ejaculatory muscles, and understanding of which nodal groups are likely to be involved with tumor have allowed for an effective and more-limited retroperitoneal lymph node dissection (RPLND), preserving fertility. More recently, laproscopic techniques for lymph node dissections have become available. As these techniques become more popular, their role in evaluation of nodal status will need to be assessed.

Table 1. Risk Factors for Testicular Cancers

Genetic Factors
Association of Lewis antigen Le(a-b-) with germ cell tumors [1]
Association of HLABw41 with seminoma [1]

Acquired Factors
Cryptorchidism (relative risk of 7.4) [2]
Exposure to diethylstilbesterol *in utero* (relative risk 9.8) [3]
Decreased risk with birth order (for fourth or later child compared to firstborn a relative risk of 0.3) [4]

Table 2. Staging of Testicular Cancers

Stage*	TNM Staging	Criteria
0	Tis	Intratubular, preinvasive tumor
	N0	
	M0	
I	T1	Tumor limited to testes and/or rete testis
(A)	T2	Invasion beyond tunica albuginea or into epididymis
	N0	
	M0	
II	T3	Invasion of spermatic cord
(A)	T4	Invasion of scrotum
	N0	Invasion of scrotum
	M0	
III	Any T	
(B1)	N1	Metastasis to one lymph node ≤ 2 cm in dimension
	M0	
IV	Any T	
(B2)	N2	Metastasis to one lymph node 2–5 cm in size or multiple lymph nodes < 5 cm
(B3)	N3	Metastasis to lymph node ≥ 5 cm in diameter
	M0	
(C) or	Any T	
	Any N	
	M1	Distant metastases

*AUA staging in parentheses.

ADJUVANT THERAPY FOR REGIONAL DISEASE

The success of platinum-based multichemotherapy for the treatment of nonseminomatous testicular cancers has been the foundation for the treatment of early stage disease as well. The question in Stage I nonseminomatous disease following an inguinal orchiectomy and demonstration of no other metastases by serologic, radiologic, and physical examinations is whether to do an elective RPLND or to recommend surveillance. Studies of surveillance suggest that disease progression will occur in approximately 30% of patients who will frequently present with bulkier disease. Embryonal, yolk sac, and choriocarcinoma histologic elements are highly prone to metastatic spread. Venous or lymphatic invasion and tumor outside the tunica albuginea or involving the epididymis (T2) suggest a tumor with the ability to metastasize. Vessel invasion was the single, most important histologic risk factor in a report by the Testicular Cancer Intergroup Study. Individuals with this finding are poor candidates for surveillance [8].

Table 3. Indiana Staging System for Metastatic Testicular Malignancies

Minimal disease
  Elevated βHCG and or AFP
  Palpable cervical nodes with or without nonpalpable retroperitoneal nodes
  Unresectable, but nonpalpable, retroperitoneal nodes
  Less than five metastatic lesions per lung field with none > 2 cm in largest diameter, with or without nonpalpable retroperitoneal nodes

Moderate disease
  Palpable abdominal mass as only anatomical disease
  Five to ten pulmonary metastases per lung field < 3 cm in largest diameter, or a mediastinal mass < 50% of the intrathoracic diameter, or a solitary pulmonary metastasis > 2 cm in largest diameter with or without nonpalpable retroperitoneal nodes

Advanced disease
  Mediastinal mass > 50% of the intrathoracic diameter, or > 10 pulmonary nodules per lung field, or multiple pulmonary metastases > 3 cm with or without nonpalpable retroperitoneal nodes
  A palpable abdominal mass with any pulmonary or intrathoracic metastases
  Liver, bone, or CNS metastases

Other factors identified with poor outcome [6]
  AFP > 500 IU/L
  βHCG > 1000 IU/L
  Age > 35 yr

Factors associated with poor outcome in patients with low-volume disease (ie, minimal disease)
  AFP > 1000 IU/L
  βHCG > 10,000 IU/L

Adapted from Birch et al. [7]; with permission.

Table 4. Management of Early-stage Primary Testicular Disease

Inguinal orchiectomy
Surveillance for good candidates
RPLND for nonseminomatous tumors to determine adjuvant chemotherapy
For seminoma, radiotherapy to nodal groups at risk

Approximately 25% of patients who undergo RPLND for clinical Stage I disease will have evidence of microscopic metastases. Approximately 10 to 15% of patients undergoing a RPLND will relapse with cancer that is usually outside the operative field. Randomized studies have shown that two cycles of cisplatin, vinblastine, and bleomycin chemotherapy following RPLND for Stage II disease will yield a cure in approximately 98% of patients. We currently recommend adjuvant therapy for those patients with positive nodes at the time of RPLND. Newer markers and histopathologic factors may identify high-risk patients in this category that will allow for a more selective approach to adjuvant therapy.

THERAPY FOR ADVANCED DISEASE

Modern multiagent chemotherapy has had a significant impact on the treatment of testicular tumors. In the early 1970s, investigators at Memorial Sloan-Kettering Cancer Center began to evaluate the combination of vinblastine, actinomycin D, and bleomycin (VAB-I) in patients with metastatic nonseminomatous cancers demonstrating a 36% objective response rate (14% complete response rate). The addition of cyclophosphamide and cisplatin to this regimen (VAB-VI) improved the complete response rate to 78%. Concomitantly, the group at Indiana University began using the combination of cisplatin, vinblastine, and bleomycin (PVB) demonstrating a 70% complete response rate and a 60% 10-year survival rate. Toxicity of PVB chemotherapy was principally due to the high dose of vinblastine (0.4 mg/kg). Subsequent trials evaluated the vinblastine dosage and led to a comparative randomized study of PVB chemotherapy versus cisplatin, etoposide, and bleomycin (PEB). The study demonstrated a significant reduction of toxicity in the PEB arm, with equal or better response and survival rates (83% complete response rate for PEB versus 71% complete response rate for PVB). More recent studies have continued to focus on diminishing toxicity.

Removing bleomycin from PEB chemotherapy was tested in a randomized study. The initial study evaluating PEB versus cisplatin and etoposide (PE) performed through the Eastern Cooperative Oncology Group in good-prognosis metastatic nonseminomatous cancers (Indiana Stage "Minimal Disease") was discontinued after it was felt that response rates were lower in the PE arm. The Australasian Germ Cell Trial Group compared PVB to cisplatin and vinblastine (PV) in 222 patients with inoperable gonadal tumors. Patients were matched on prognostic risk factors. The minimum duration of follow-up was 4 years. Although relapse rates (7% for PV and 5% for PVB) and overall survival rates were not different for the two groups, tumor-related deaths occurred in 16 patients (15%) in the PV group and in 6 patients (5%) in the PVB arm ($p = 0.02$). Toxicity was greater in the PVB arm with two deaths related to lung toxicity due to bleomycin. Although both hematologic and nonhematologic toxicity was worse in the PVB group, bleomycin does significantly enhance the therapeutic benefit of PV [9].

Response rates in patients with metastatic seminoma to platinum-based combination chemotherapy regimens have proven to be as good as those found in patients with nonseminomatous cancers, with better than 80% cure rates. This has lead to a rethinking of recommendations for radiotherapy, which is the traditionally employed modality for the treatment of early-stage seminoma. Initial treatment of Stage I and II disease entails the use of involved-field and extended-field radiation therapy. Trials of radiation therapy for Stage II disease reveal a 70 to 90% 5-year survival rate. In Stage II disease, approximately 30% of patients will fail outside the radiation ports. Salvage of patient failures with combination chemotherapy may be compromised by radiation damage to the bone marrow. We suggest treating Stage II seminoma patients with upfront chemotherapy, followed by radiation therapy for patients with evidence of residual cancer. Treatment strategies for Stage I seminoma is more controversial. It appears that prophylactic radiation of the mediastinum does not provide survival advantage and adds to morbidity and late toxicity, and also causes difficulty in administering chemotherapy at a later time if needed. Inguinal orchiectomy and postsurgery radiation therapy to abdominal lymph nodes have a 5-year survival rate of better than 98%. Chemotherapy is reserved for the few patients who relapse.

With the use of platinum-based multiagent chemotherapy, extragonadal testicular tumors are treated with equal success, stage for stage, to primary gonadal tumors that have metastasized [10].

Long-term follow-up for patients with testicular cancers should include evaluation for secondary leukemia in patients treated with chemotherapy, and solid organ malignancies, such as gastric carcinoma, in patients who received abdominal radiation therapy.

PROSTATE CANCER

ETIOLOGY AND RISK FACTORS

Therapy for prostate cancer continues to generate much controversy. One thing is sure, a significant number of men will be diagnosed with this cancer and will die from their illness each year. In the United States, 132,000 men with prostate cancer were diagnosed in 1992 and 32,000 deaths were attributed to this disease. In autopsy studies, 30% of men between the ages of 50 and 70 with no overt evidence of prostate cancer before death had pathologic evidence of prostate carcinoma. The risk factors associated with this disease are listed in Table 5.

For the most part, prostate cancers are slow growing and metastasize late in their natural history. This presents to the treating clinician a therapeutic dilemma in patients with early-stage disease: which patients will have aggressive cancers needing treatment and which patients will have indolent disease requiring no further therapy? Furthermore, if treatment is chosen, which treatment will provide the best outcome with the least morbidity? While radical prostatectomy or radiotherapy have remained the keystones for initial therapy for early-stage prostate cancer (Stages A and B), recent outcome analyses have questioned these time-honored approaches, raising more questions than answers [15,16]. The controversies over treatment for early-stage prostate cancer will continue for some time.

Table 5. Etiology and Risk Factors for Prostate Cancer

Age
Race
Family history
Testosterone level [11]
Suspected risk factors
Vasectomy (methodologic issues remain in the major studies evaluating vasectomy and prostate cancer) [12]
Dietary fat [13]
5-Alpha reductase activity [14]

Treatment for metastatic disease remains palliative but the question of when to begin therapy is unresolved at this time.

SCREENING

Early diagnosis of prostate cancer is the focus of numerous screening modalities, including digital rectal examination, transrectal ultrasound, and serum prostate-specific antigen. No study to date has documented that screening will have an impact on overall survival from prostate cancer [17]. Furthermore, the controversy over treatment requirements for early-stage disease will cause increasing difficulty in assessing the role of screening. The American Cancer Society recommends screening for prostate cancer with digital rectal examinations beginning at age 50. Assessment of PSA levels using 4 ng/ml as the upper limits of normal has been shown to improve prostate cancer detection [18,19]. A survey of 4.7% practicing urologists who are members of the American Urological Association found that screening for prostate cancer was recommended to men between the ages of 50 and 80 [20].

STAGING AND PROGNOSIS

With early diagnosis comes the dilemma of identifying clinically aggressive cancer that will cause significant morbidity by metastasizing or that will result in premature death. Except for invasion outside the capsule of the gland (T3, Stage C) and histologic grade, which portend a bad prognosis, other factors have failed to further delineate aggressive from indolent disease, causing considerable difficulty in interpreting screening results and confounding treatment decision (Table 6). A number of recent studies have suggested that HER2/neu expression is associated with more aggressive disease.

Evaluation of prostate cancer should consist of technitium pyrophosphate bone scan for patients with PSA above 10, chest radiograph, CT or magnetic resonance imaging of the prostate, and evaluation of blood work, including complete blood cell counts, and coagulation profile measurement of tumor markers (prostatic acid phosphatase, PSA, and LDH). Usually PSA alone, if elevated, is used in following patients with prostate cancer. More recently, evaluation of lymph node involvement is being assessed by peritoneoscopy with lymph node sampling. Approximately 90% of nodal tissue can be examined using this technique. The best clinical setting for the use of laproscopic node dissection still needs to be determined. Another modality being tested for staging purposes is radiolabeled murine monoclonal antibodies. Small published series employing CYT-356 antibody have not yet adequately defined the role of this imaging technique.

PRIMARY DISEASE THERAPY

Initial treatment recommendations are dependent on clinical staging, radiographic findings, level of serum tumor markers and histology. Assessment of clinical stage, PSA level, and histologic grade can be used to determine the likelihood of invasion outside the confines of the prostate gland or for metastatic spread. Survival rates for men with Stage A1 (T1a) disease appear about the same as age-matched controls; these patients are followed with close observation and repeat biopsies of the prostate when clinically indicated. A mathematical model of patients with localized prostate cancer (Stages A2, B1, B2 or T1b, T2a, T2b) suggests a benefit with therapeutic intervention (surgery or radiotherapy) for men younger than 65 only. The model is provocative and suggests that a clinical trial needs to be performed to confirm these predictions. The best initial treatment of Stage A2 or B disease continues to be hotly debated between surgeons and radiotherapists. The only randomized study between radiation therapy and radical prostatectomy in patients with Stage A2 and B disease was reported by Paulson in 1982 but remains controversial due to the methodologic approach. Although the study suggests a survival advantage to surgery, the patients treated with radiotherapy appear to have a worse outcome than reports of other radiotherapy programs. The Veterans Administration Cooperative Urologic Research Group (VACURG) reported a small study of Stage A and B patients randomized to radical prostatectomy plus placebo versus placebo alone. Although there appears to be a survival advantage for the patients treated on the placebo-alone arm the study is flawed by its small patient sample and high percentage of poorly differentiated tumors in the surgery arm with none in the placebo arm. With the controversy continuing, it is unlikely that an answer to this timeworn question will be forthcoming in the foreseeable future.

Both surgical and radiation techniques continue to be improved for the treatment of early-stage disease. One technique that will most likely yield a lower morbidity and higher dose of radiation is three-dimensional conformal radiotherapy, which allows specifically for more accurate delivery of the radiation dose. More recent attention has focused on the timing of adjuvant hormonal intervention.

ADJUVANT THERAPY FOR REGIONAL DISEASE

Regional disease defined as penetration through the capsule of the prostate gland (T3) with or without spread to neighboring organs (T4) or first-tier pelvic lymph nodes (N1) is incurable with surgical or radiotherapy techniques. Treatment choices must again reflect the natural history of the disease and development of symptoms. It remains speculative whether early hormonal intervention improves survival.

THERAPY FOR ADVANCED DISEASE
Hormonal Therapy

The concept of complete androgen blockade was introduced by Labrie; with the advent of both leutinizing hormone-releasing hormone (LHRH) agonists (or orchiectomy) and dihydrotestosterone (DHT) receptor blockers the question could be studied. A randomized, double-blind study comparing the combination of flutamide and leuprolide with leuprolide and placebo demonstrated a small but statistically significant superior progression-free and overall survival with total androgen blockade. Because leuprolide and goserelin are LHRH agonists, initial stimulation of the pituitary–testis axis may cause a disease flare, resulting in worsening symptoms or, in extremely rare isolated cases, sudden death. We suggest the addition of flutamide to beginning concomitantly with LHRH agonists to prevent disease flare.

There has been a suggestion of survival advantage in advanced disease with hormonal therapy in the VACURG study that evaluated placebo to three different doses of DES. A retrospective analysis of patients treated on the Eastern Cooperative Oncology Group prostate protocols suggested that continued androgen blockade despite progression of disease is associated with better survival rates.

The discovery of receptors for other growth factors such as epidermal growth factor receptor (EGFr) provide foundation for alternative treatment strategies. Suramin sodium is a polysulfonated naphthylurea used to treat African tyrpanosomiasis and onchocerciasis and has been found to bind to EGFr and block growth. In addition, suramin has been shown to decrease circulating androstenedione, dehydroepiandrosterone, and dehydroepiandrosterone sulfate by 40% in patients with metastatic prostate cancer who failed previous hormonal therapy. *In vitro*, suramin can block the proliferation of prostate cancer cells as well as inhibit testosterone and fibroblast growth factor–induced proliferation. Pilot studies of this agent in hormonal refractory patients have reported a response rate as high as 54% and suggest that suramin may be useful in the treatment of metastatic prostate cancer. Current trials used the observation of nonandrogen autocrine/paracrine growth factors as a rationale to test the combination of LHRH analogue, DHT receptor blockade, and EGFr receptor blockade.

Table 6. Staging of Prostate Cancer

Stage*	TNM Staging	Criteria
0 (A1)	T1a	Tumor is incidental histologic finding in < 3 microscopic foci
(B1)	T2a	Tumor ≤ 1.5 cm with normal tissue on at least three sides in one lobe of the prostate gland
	N0	
	M0	
	G1	Well-differentiated cancer
I (A1)	T1a	
(B1)	or T2a	
	N0	
	M0	
	G2,G3–4	Moderately differentiated or poorly differentiated, respectively
II (A2)	T1b	Tumor is incidental histologic finding in > 3 microscopic foci
(B2)	or T2b	Tumor > 1.5 cm or in > 1 lobe
	N0	
	M0	
	Any G	
III	T3	Invasion of prostatic apex, or into or beyond prostatic capsule, bladder neck, or seminal vesicle, but not fixed
(C1 or C2)	N0	
	M0	
	Any G	
IV	T4	Tumor is fixed or invades adjacent structure other than those for T3
(C2)	N0	
	M0	
	Any G	
or		
(D)	Any T	
	N1	Single lymph node, ≤ 2 cm involved with cancer
	N2	Metastasis in a single lymph node 2–5 cm in diameter or multiple lymph nodes < 5 cm
	N3	Metastasis to lymph node > 5 cm
	M0	
	Any G	
or		
(D)	Any T	
	Any N	
	M1	Distant metastases
	Any G	

*AUA staging in parentheses.

Chemotherapy

Single-agent chemotherapy has had little effect on the outcome of prostate cancer. Studies of doxorubicin, mitoxantrone, cisplatin, cyclophosphamide, methotrexate, estramustine, and 5-fluorouracil have demonstrated minimal single-agent activity, and combination chemotherapies have had no impact on this disease. Studies evaluating newer manipulations of these agents, alone or in combinations, are underway and may provide better insight into the role of chemotherapy.

Radiation Therapy

One of the most devastating complications from prostate cancer is the pain and dysfunction from bone metastases. External beam irradiation is useful in palliating isolated bone metastases. Unfortunately, patients with metastatic prostate cancer usually have multiple bone metastases. Two newer approaches to the treatment of bone disease using radiation include hemibody irradiation and bone-seeking compounds such as strontium 89 or rhenium 186-hydroxyethlidene diphosphonate.

TRANSITIONAL CELL CARCINOMA OF THE UROTHELIUM

ETIOLOGY AND RISK FACTORS

There are three major histologies of cancers arising from the urothelium. Squamous cell carcinoma and adenocarcinoma of the bladder require different therapeutic strategies and are not discussed in this chapter.

The major risk factor for transitional cell carcinomas remains tobacco use, particularly in association with a slow acetylator phenotype and exposure to beta-naphthylamine (Table 7). Although dietary factors have been implicated in bladder cancer formation, there is no definitive evidence to date. Chlorine has been implicated in the carcinogenesis of bladder cancer. Meta-analysis has confirmed that the consumption of highly chlorinated water (chlorination by-products) is associated with a 1.21 relative risk for bladder cancer.

Screening tests for bladder cancer have not yet been developed fully. Preliminary results from the Drake Health Registry suggest that in high-risk individuals exposed to beta-naphthylamine screening with Papanicolaou cytology, fluorescence image analysis, and urinalysis may be capable of identifying early changes, but the specificity of these changes is uncertain.

STAGING AND PROGNOSIS

Transitional cell carcinoma of the bladder may be divided by superficial or invasive tumors. Superficial tumors of the bladder represent local disease with little or no capability for metastases and thus can be treated with local therapies. Histologic grading, tumor type (papillary or carcinoma *in situ*), muscle invasion, and differentiation are important clinicopathologic features that need to be evaluated in determining prognosis in clinical practice (Table 8).

Recurrence of superficial tumors (Stage 0 or I) and the need for intravesical therapy is determined by tumor grade, size, and number [28,29]. True squamous differentiation in the tumor usually predicts for poor response to systemic chemotherapy.

PRIMARY DISEASE THERAPY

Most uroepithelial tumors will present with either gross or microscopic hematuria. Urinary cytology is therefore an important part of the evaluation. Full assessment of the uroepithelium is indicated and is accomplished with cystoscopy and intravenous or retrograde pyelography. Transurethral resection of the bladder tumor (TURBT) is the initial treatment. Intravesical therapy is usually considered for high-grade tumors, carcinoma *in situ*, or recurrent low-grade tumors. Recent genetic evaluation of multiple simultaneous tumors arising in women suggest a clonal origin, that is, the probability that tumors arise from a single cell that seeds other areas of uroepithelium. This process is well established in experimental animal models.

Table 7. Risk Factors for Transitional Cell Carcinoma

ß-napthylamine
Tobacco [23]
Slow acetylator phenotype [22]
Chlorination by-products [25,27]
Diet (questionable) [21,24,26]
　High caloric intake from fat in those under 65
　Decrease risk with consumption of carotenoid in those under 65
　High sodium intake

Table 8. Staging of Transitional Cell Carcinoma of Urinary Badder

Stage*	TNM Staging	Criteria
0	Tis	Carcinoma *in situ*
	Ta	Noninvasive papillary cancer
	N0	
	M0	
I	T1	Invasion of subepithelial connective tissue
(A)	N0	
	M0	
II	T2	Invasion of muscle not extending beyond the inner half
(B1)	N0	
	M0	
III	T3a	Invasion of deep muscle—outer half of the bladder wall
(B2)	T3b	Invasion of perivesical fat
	N0	
	M0	
IV	T4	Invasion of neighboring anatomical structures: prostate, uterus, vagina, pelvic wall, abdominal wall
(C)		
	N0	
	M0	
or		
(D)	Any T	
	N1	Metastasis to a single lymph node ≤ 2 cm
	N2	Metastasis to a single lymph node 2–5 cm in size or multiple lymph nodes < 5 cm in diameter
	N3	Metastasis in any lymph node > 5 cm in diameter
	M0	
or		
	Any T	
	Any N	
	M1	Distant metastasis

*AUA staging in parentheses.

Treatment for superficial bladder cancers is not only directed at tumor regression but reduction of the subsequent recurrence rate and prevention of tumor invasion. TURBT alone, for low-grade papillary disease, or in combination with intravesical chemotherapy and immunotherapy can control local superficial tumor and prevent recurrences and invasion. Many therapeutic agents have been used in the treatment of superficial disease with bacillus Calmette–Guérin (bCG) considered the best of these agents, although not without morbidity.

Thiotepa, mitomycin C, and doxorubicin are the most common intravesical chemotherapies employed today and have been shown to be effective and safe agents. Burnand et al. reported a randomized trial demonstrating a single dose of thiotepa (90 mg over 0.5 hr) can reduce recurrences by 40% at 1 year follow-up compared to TURBT alone. Weekly thiotepa given for established superficial tumor can cause complete regression in approximately 30% of cases. The low molecular weight of thiotepa allows absorption across the bladder epithelium and may cause toxicity, specifically, mild leukoneutropenia.

Mitomycin C appears to give the same clinical results as thiotepa with less risk of leukoneutropenia but with increased risk of bladder irritation. Of intravesical chemotherapy, doxorubicin appears to give the best response rates in patients with established tumors, with a complete response rate as high as 66%.

A randomized study of 262 patients with Stage Ta and T1 papillary tumors or carcinoma in situ treated with either doxorubicin or bCG was reported by Lamm et al. Estimated 5-year disease-free survival was 17% for the doxorubicin-treated patients and 37% for bCG-treated patients with Ta or T1 lesions without carcinoma in situ ($p = 0.015$). The median time to treatment failure in patients with carcinoma in situ disease was 5.1 months for doxorubicin and 39 months for bCG. Estimated 5-year disease-free survival in patients with carcinoma in situ was 18% for doxorubicin and 45% for bCG.

Other randomized studies comparing bCG to mitomycin C are currently underway and results have not been reported to date. Other forms of intravesical immunotherapy, specifically interferon alpha, have been used and appear to have benefits in superficial bladder cancer as well. We have conducted pilot studies of intravesical tumor necrosis factor. Although this agent can be given with a high degree of safety, clinical benefit has not yet been proven.

Phototherapy of superficial bladder tumors is an alternative treatment but has not been tested against standard agents. Phototherapy employs laser treatments with photosensitizing agents such as photofrin poly porphyrin. This approach is under investigation in refractory superficial tumors.

ADJUVANT THERAPY FOR REGIONAL DISEASE

The current standard therapy for locally invasive transitional cell carcinoma of the bladder remains cystectomy. Patient's risk to relapse is dependent on the depth of invasion into the wall of the bladder. There is approximately a 40 to 60% chance of failure overall from cystectomy alone, raising the question of the need and effectiveness of adjuvant therapies. Newer pathologic techniques are becoming available to help distinguish metastatic potential of invasive bladder cancers, including NM23 RNA levels, DNA ploidy, and expression of the antigen T138 on the cell surface. Another issue relates to the desire to provide bladder-sparing treatments.

The role of radiotherapy combined with multiagent chemotherapy (cisplatin, vinblastine, and methotrexate) has been explored by Shipley et al. A pilot study of 53 patients demonstrated a 77% survival rate at 54 months [30]. A confirmatory study evaluating the role of radiotherapy with and without preradiation chemotherapy is currently underway in the Radiation Therapy Oncology Group (RTOG).

The role of adjuvant or neoadjuvant chemotherapy has not been definitively proven at this time, but preliminary reports of randomized trials suggest that cisplatin-based multiagent chemotherapy may have a significant impact on the treatment of high-risk invasive bladder cancer. Stockle et al. reported a study of 49 patients with pathologically staged T3b and T4a bladder cancer with or without lymph node involvement randomized to receive methotrexate, vinblastine (or epirubicin), doxorubicin, and cisplatin following cystectomy or cystectomy alone. Although time of follow-up is limited, only 3 of 18 patients treated with adjuvant chemotherapy have relapsed compared to 18 of 23 patients in the control arm. Trials involving neoadjuvant multiagent cisplatin-based chemotherapy have not been completed as of this time. Preliminary data suggest that major pathologic responses of the primary tumor to chemotherapy is seen in approximately 40% of patients [31–33]. These patients have a much improved survival rate compared to those patients who did not achieve a response to treatment prior to cystectomy. Our current recommendations to patients with invasive bladder cancer are to participate in one of the multigroup (South Western Oncology Group [SWOG] or RTOG) studies evaluating adjuvant chemotherapy.

The RTOG study (89-03) employs MCV (methotrexate, cisplatin, vinblastine) and radiation therapy. Complete responders undergo close follow-up without cystectomy. The SWOG study (8710) compares three cycles of preoperative M-VAC (methotrexate, vinblastine, doxorubicin, cisplatin) plus cystectomy with cystectomy alone. Both trials will provide answers to the question of whether cisplatin-based multichemotherapy regimens succeed as adjuvant therapy for high-risk invasive bladder cancer.

THERAPY FOR ADVANCED DISEASE

Advances in chemotherapy have been sought in the setting of metastatic transitional cell carcinoma of the urinary bladder. Phase II studies of single agents demonstrated significant activity (> 15%) for methotrexate, vinblastine, doxorubicin, cisplatin, and 5-fluorouracil. Cisplatin has emerged as the single best agent and is used in combination chemotherapy regimens. The most commonly used combinations today are M-VAC and MCV. Although response rates to M-VAC were significantly lower than those reported in single institution studies (33 vs. 60%), M-VAC was found to be superior to cisplatin alone (objective response rates of 33 versus 15% respectively, $p = 0.001$) in a randomized trial evaluating the treatment of metastatic bladder cancer conducted by the Eastern Cooperative Oncology Group [34].

In an attempt to improve the toxicity profile of M-VAC, colony-stimulating factors have been employed. Although G-CSF and GM-CSF can reduce the length of leukoneutropenia and improve mucositis, response and survival rates have not differed significantly from those with M-VAC.

RENAL CELL CARCINOMA

ETIOLOGY AND RISK FACTORS

In 1992, approximately 26,000 individuals in the United States were diagnosed with renal cell carcinoma (RCC) and nearly 50% of them had metastatic disease at presentation. Although there are reports of long-term survivors with metastatic disease, the 5-year survival curves predict that virtually all patients will die from their disease by that time. Radical nephrectomy for local disease remains the only curative approach. Investigation of systemic therapies has provided insight into newer treatment methods that may have an impact on survival of a subset of patients.

Molecular genetic evaluation has yielded more information on the nature of renal cell carcinoma. The most common chromosomal abnormality is the loss of heterozygosity of 3p14–26, which is found in 66 to 98% of clear cell RCC tumors. Papillary tumors do not appear to have this abnormality. Patients with von Hippel–Lindau syndrome have a similar loss of heterozygosity of 3p. Further molecular genetic studies may uncover markers for metastatic behavior (Table 9).

STAGING AND PROGNOSIS

Many prognostic schema have been used to attempt to predict survival and outcome (Tables 10 and 11). The sarcomatoid variant of renal cell carcinoma tends to have a worse prognosis with median survival of less than 1 year. Performance status, disease-free survival greater than 1 year (or in some schema greater than 2 years), number of sites of metastases (one vs. more than one), and the presence of central nervous system metastases are common prognostic factors in most schema.

PRIMARY DISEASE THERAPY

A radical nephrectomy may be performed via a number of different approaches and includes complete resection of Gerota's fascia, kidney, and adrenal gland. The role of regional lymph node dissection remains unknown. Although no definitive proof exists that lymph node dissection will prolong life, it is usually performed because, in the context of adjuvant therapy trials, accurate staging is imperative. In the usual dissection, the ipsilateral nodes from the diaphragm to the origin of the common iliac arteries and the renal hilar lymph nodes are removed. Kidney-sparing operations are being performed that include partial nephrectomy and excisional resection of the tumor. Although reports of these less radical procedures appear good, a number of pathologic series suggest that renal cell tumors may be multicentric.

Table 9. Risk Factors for Renal Cell Carcinoma

Genetic [35,36]
    von Hippel—Lindau disease
    Familial RCC
Acquired traits
    Cystic kidney disease
    End-stage renal failure requiring dialysis
Environmental factors [37,38]
    Tobacco use
    Asbestos exposure
    Analgesic abuse (phenactin)
    Obesity
    Thorotrast

Table 10. Staging of Renal Cell Carcinoma

Stage*	TNM Staging	Criteria
I (A)	T1	Limited to the kidney, ≤ 2.5 cm, surrounded by normal renal parenchyma
	N0	
	M0	
II (A)	T2	Tumor > 2.5 cm, limited to the kidney
	N0	
	M0	
III (C)	T1	Metastasis to a single lymph node ≤ 2 cm
	N1	
	M0	
or		
(C)	T2	Metastasis to a single lymph node 2–5 cm or multiple lymph nodes < 5 cm
	N2	
	M0	
or		
(B)	T3a	Tumor involving perinephric fat
	T3b	Tumor involving renal vein
	T3c	Involvement of infradiaphragmatic vena cava
	N0	
	M0	
or		
(C)	T3a	Tumor involving perinephric fat
	T3b	Tumor involving renal vein
	T3c	Involvement of infradiaphragmatic vena cava
	N1	
	M0	
or		
IV (D)	T4a	Tumor invasion beyond Gerota's fascia into surrounding organs
	T4b	Tumor involving supradiaphragmatic vena cava
	Any N	
	M0	
or		
	Any T N2 or N3	Metastasis to a lymph node > 5 cm
	M0	
or		
	Any T Any N	
	M1	Distant metastases

* Robson staging in parentheses.

Table 11. Prognostic Factors in Renal Cell Carcinoma

Histology (sarcomatoid variant)
Performance status
Disease-free survival
Central nervous system disease
Number of metastatic sites [39]

Partial nephrectomies should be considered in patients where preservation of renal function is an important goal of therapy, such as in patients with von Hippel–Lindau syndrome or unilateral kidney.

Radiation therapy for RCC has been directed at the palliation of metastatic sites, specifically, bone, spine, and brain. Sterotatic radiation or gamma knife therapy may be useful in conjunction with whole brain radiation for palliation of single brain metastases of 2–3 cm or less. Initial reports of this modality suggest high sterilization rates. There is no clear evidence to date that adjuvant radiotherapy to the bed of the kidney improves survival rates, and we do not routinely give adjuvant radiation therapy to patients following nephrectomy.

THERAPY FOR ADVANCED DISEASE

Treatment of metastatic disease remains difficult. Biologic response modifiers have had the most impact on treatment of metastatic disease with high-dose interleukin-2 (IL-2) recently approved by the FDA for the treatment of this condition.

Common toxicities to IL-2 (> 50%) in patients treated with high doses include chills, pruritus, nausea, vomiting, diarrhea, hyperbilirubinemia, oligouria with an increase in blood urea nitrogen and creatinine, weight gain, edema, hypotension, and lymphopenia with eosinophilia. Respiratory distress with pulmonary edema secondary to leaky capillary syndrome, bronchospasm, pleural effusion, somnolence, disorientation anemia, thrombocytopenia, hypothyroidism, and arrhythmias are seen in 10 to 50% of patients. Rare toxicity includes myocardial infarction, central line sepsis, severe hypotension, renal failure, and death. In centers with experience with high-dose IL-2, much of the toxicity can be managed with noninvasive monitoring and fluid replacement, antibiotics, H-2 blockers, antiemetics, and antihistamines. Awareness of early warning signals, such as a slight change in mental status, and skipping one or two doses have improved the overall toxicity profile of high-dose IL-2. Blood pressure support is maintained with fluid replacement and adrenergic agonists such as dopamine and norepinephrine. Rarely, intubation and mechanical ventilatory support are required. IL-2 dose is held until the patient has cardiopulmonary stabilization. Usually this requires skipping a dose or two over the course of 1 week.

Although response rates to high-dose IL-2 alone or with adoptively transferred lymphokine-activated killer cells (LAK) vary from 4 to 35%, the duration of the response in those achieving a complete remission is significantly long. The summary of 255 cases treated with high-dose IL-2 demonstrated an overall response rate of 14%. Approximately one-third of responses are complete and patients usually maintain their response for about 2 years.

Trials employing interferon alpha suggest a response rate from 10 to 20%. Initial studies employing human leukocyte interferon reported by Quesada et al. and Kirkwood et al. suggested a clinical role for interferon alpha. These studies were limited by availability and specific activity of the material. Subsequent trials of recombinant DNA–produced interferon alpha and lymphoblastoid interferon alpha have confirmed activity of this cytokine in metastatic RCC with response rates of 18%.

At present, interferon alpha is a reasonable alternative for treatment in patients with metastatic renal cell carcinoma. We recommend subcutaneous treatment with 3 μ/m^2 three times weekly, with dose escalation to 10 μ/m^2 tiw as tolerated. We continue treatment for a minimum of 2 to 3 months when possible. Patients with non–life-threatening minimal progression of disease, stable disease, or evidence of response during the first 2 to 3 months continue on this treatment for up to 1 year.

Flu-like symptoms are the most common acute toxicity to the interferons and are seen in virtually 100% of patients. Flu-like symptoms begin about 1 to 2 hours following a dose and include fever, chill or rigor, myalgias, low backache, arthralgias, headache, and malaise. Acetaminophen pretreatment usually blunts the flu-like symptom. Tachyphylaxis of the flu-like symptoms occurs with repetitive doses. Patients may have chronic low-grade fever, and with the associated decrease in appetite, may develop subclinical dehydration, contributing to the malaise. We recommend vigorous oral fluid intake to improve the tolerance of the agent. Occasionally, outpatient intravenous hydration may be warranted.

Gastrointestinal symptoms to interferon alpha are rare. Central nervous system toxicities include slight confusion, minimal paranoia, stupor, and coma and are associated with diffuse slowing on the EEG. These effects are reversible, but stupor and coma may take as long as 3 to 4 weeks to reverse. Peripheral neuropathy is also uncommon and is associated with the typical hand-glove paresthesias with slowing of nerve conduction.

Cardiovascular toxicity is usually characterized by supraventricular tachyarrhythmias, which may be controlled with beta-blockers or calcium channel blockers. Cardiac toxicity is usually seen at dosages of over 10 μ/d, in older patients (> 70 years), and in patients with underlying heart disease.

REFERENCES

1. Dieckmann KP, Klan R, Bunte S: HLA antigens, Lewis antigens, and blood groups in patients with testicular germ-cell tumors. *Oncology; J Clin Exp Cancer Res* 1993, 50:252–258.

2. Pinczowski D, McLaughlin JK, Lackgren G, *et al.*: Occurrence of testicular cancer in patients operated on for cryptorchidism and inguinal hernia. *J Urol* 1991, 146:1291–1294.

3. Marselos M, Tomatis L: Diethylstilbestrol: I, Pharmacology, toxicology and carcinogenicity in humans. *Eur J Cancer* 1992, 28A:1182–1189.

4. Prener A, Hsieh CC, Engholm G, *et al.*: Birth order and risk of testicular cancer. *Cancer Causes Cont* 1992, 3:265–272.

5. Klepp O, Olsson AM, Henrikson H, *et al.*: Prognostic factors in clinical Stage I nonseminomatous germ cell tumors of the testis: Multivariate analysis of a prospective multicenter study. Swedish-Norwegian Testicular Cancer Group. *J Clin Oncol* 1990, 8:509–518.

6. Aass N, Klepp O, Cavallin-Stahl E, *et al.*: Prognostic factors in unselected patients with nonseminomatous metastatic testicular cancer: A multicenter experience. *J Clin Oncol* 1991, 9:818–826.

7. Birch R, Williams S, Cone A, *et al.*: Prognostic factors for favorable outcome in disseminated germ cell tumors. Southeastern Cancer Group. *J Clin Oncol* 1986, 4:400–407.

8. Sesterhenn IA, Weiss RB, Mostofi FK, *et al.*: Prognosis and other

clinical correlates of pathologic review in Stage I and II testicular carcinoma: A report from the Testicular Cancer Intergroup Study. *J Clin Oncol* 1992, 10:69–78.

9. Levi JA, Raghavan D, Harvey V, *et al.*: The importance of bleomycin in combination chemotherapy for good-prognosis germ cell carcinoma. *J Clin Oncol* 1993, 11:1300–1305.

10. McAleer JJ, Nicholls J, Horwich A: Does extragonadal presentation impart a worse prognosis to abdominal germ-cell tumours? *Eur J Cancer* 1992, 28A:825–828.

11. Pienta KJ, Esper PS: Risk factors for prostate cancer. *Ann Intern Med* 1993, 118:793–803.

12. DerSimonian R, Clemens J, Spirtas R, Perlman J: Vasectomy and prostate cancer risk: Methodological review of the evidence. *J Clin Epidemiol* 1993, 46:163–172.

13. Hankin JH, Zhao LP, Wilkens LR, Kolonel LN: Attributable risk of breast, prostate, and lung cancer in Hawaii due to standard fat. *Cancer Causes Cont* 1992, 3:17–23.

14. Ross RK, Bernstein L, Lobo RA, *et al.*: 5-Alpha-reductase activity and risk of prostate cancer among Japanese and US white and black males. *Lancet* 1992, 339:887–889.

15. Fleming C, Wasson JH, Albertsen PC, *et al.*: A decision analysis of alternative treatment strategies for clinically localized prostate cancer. The Prostate Patient Outcome Research Team. *JAMA* 1993, 269:2650–2658.

16. Lu-Yao GL, McLerran D, Wasson J, Wennberg JE: An assessment of radical prostatectomy. Time trends, geographic variation, and outcomes. The Prostate Patient Outcome Research Team. *JAMA* 1993, 269:2633–2636.

17. Littrup PJ, Lee F, Mettlin C: Prostate cancer screening: Current trends and future implications. *CA* 1992, 42:198–211.

18. Roetzheim RG, Herold AH: Prostate cancer screening. Primary care: *Clin Off Prac* 1992, 19:637–649.

19. Gerber GS, Thompson IM, Thisted R, Chodak GW: Disease-specific survival following routine prostate cancer screening by digital rectal examination. *JAMA* 1993, 269:61–64.

20. Thompson IM, Zeidman EJ: Current urological practice: Routine urological examination and early detection of carcinoma of the prostate. *J Urol* 1992, 148:326–329.

21. Vena JE, Graham S, Freudenheim J, *et al.*: Diet in the epidemiology of bladder cancer in western New York. *Nut Cancer* 1992, 18:255–264.

22. Vineis P, Ronco G: Interindividual variation in carcinogen metabolism and bladder cancer risk. *Ehp Environ Health Persp* 1992, 98:95–99.

23. Kadlubar FF, Butler MA, Kaderlik KR, *et al.*: Polymorphisms for aromatic amine metabolism in humans: Relevance for human carcinogenesis. *Ehp Environ Health Persp* 1992, 98:69–74.

24. Elcock M, Morgan RW: Update on artificial sweeteners and bladder cancer. *Reg Toxicol Pharmacol* 1993, 17:35–43.

25. Morris RD, Audet AM, Angelillo IF, *et al.*: Chlorination, chlorination by-products, and cancer: A meta-analysis. *Am J Pub Health* 1992, 82:955–963.

26. Mills PK, Beeson WL, Phillips RL, Fraser GE: Bladder cancer in a low risk population: Results from the Adventist Health Study. *Am J Epidemiol* 1991, 133:230–239.

27. Marsh GM, Callahan C, Pavlock D, *et al.*: A protocol for bladder cancer screening and medical surveillance among high-risk groups: the Drake Health Registry experience. *J Occup Med* 1990, 32:881–886.

28. Kiemeney LA, Witjes JA, Verbeek AL, *et al.*: The clinical epidemiology of superficial bladder cancer. Dutch South-East Cooperative Urological Group. *Br J Cancer* 1993, 67:806–812.

29. Tachibana M, Deguchi N, Baba S, *et al.*: Prognostic significance of bromodeoxyuridine high labeled bladder cancer measured by flow cytometry: Does flow cytometric determination predict the prognosis of patients with transitional cell carcinoma of the bladder. *J Urol* 1993, 149:739–743.

30. Prout GR Jr, Shipley WU, Kaufman DS, *et al.*: Interval report of a phase I-II study utilizing multiple modalities in the treatment of invasive bladder cancer. A bladder-sparing trial. *Urol Clin North Am* 1991, 18:547–554.

31. Splinter TA, Scher HI, Denis L, *et al.*: The prognostic value of the pathological response to combination chemotherapy before cystectomy in patients with invasive bladder cancer. European Organization for Research on Treatment of Cancer—Genitourinary Group. *J Urol* 1992, 147:606–608.

32. Wallace DM, Raghavan D, Kelly KA, *et al.*: Neo-adjuvant (pre-emptive) cisplatin therapy in invasive transitional cell carcinoma of the bladder. *Br J Urol* 1991, 67:608–615.

33. Skinner DG, Daniels JR, Russell CA, *et al.*: The role of adjuvant chemotherapy following cystectomy for invasive bladder cancer: A prospective comparative trial. *J Urol* 1991, 145:459–467.

34. Loehrer PJ Sr, Einhorn LH, Elson PJ, *et al.*: A randomized comparison of cisplatin alone or in combination with methotrexate, vinblastine, and doxorubicin in patients with metastatic urothelial carcinoma: A cooperative group study. *J Clin Oncol* 1992, 10:1066–1073.

35. McCredie M, Stewart JH: Risk factors for kidney cancer in New South Wales. IV. Occupation. *Br J Indus Med* 1993, 50:349–354.

36. McCredie M, Stewart JH, Day NE: Different roles for phenacetin and paracetamol in cancer of the kidney and renal pelvis. *Int J Cancer* 1993, 53:245–249.

37. McCredie M, Stewart JH: Risk factors for kidney cancer in New South Wales–I. Cigarette smoking. *Eur J Cancer* 1992, 28A:2050–2054.

38. La Vecchia C, Negri E, D'Avanzo B, Franceschi S: Smoking and renal cell carcinoma. *Cancer Res* 1990, 50:5231–5233.

39. Palmer PA, Vinke J, Philip T, *et al.*: Prognostic factors for survival in patients with advanced renal cell carcinoma treated with recombinant interleukin-2. *Ann Oncol* 1992, 3:475–480.

PEB
Cisplatin, Etoposide, and Bleomycin

Although not exactly known, cisplatin's anticancer action is thought to be similar to that of a bifunctional alkylating agent. Cisplatin binds to plasma protein, and although serum half-life is calculated in hours, tissue levels have been detected as far out as 4 months.

Etoposide (VP-16) is a podophyllotoxin from the mandrake plant. Although podophyllotoxins bind to tubulin, there is little discernible effect of VP-16 on microtubular assembly. VP-16 blocks cell division at G2. Stable terniary complexes are formed with DNA and topoisomerase II causing single-strand DNA breaks. Recent studies suggest that etoposide may be carcinogenic and lead to second malignancies.

Bleomycin is an antibiotic derived from the fungus *Streptomyces verticullus*. The major isoform in the mixture is A_2. Bleomycin binds to DNA and ferrous ion. Ferrous ion is oxidized ultimately leading to oxygen radicals that cause DNA single- and double-strand breaks.

CANDIDATES FOR TREATMENT
Patients with testicular neoplasms—Stage II nonseminomatous cancers, metastatic seminomas, nonseminoma testicular malignancies

SPECIAL PRECAUTIONS
Patients with renal failure
Patients with allergy to bleomycin

ALTERNATIVE THERAPIES
PVB, VAB-6

TOXICITIES
Cisplatin: leukopenia, thrombocytopenia, anemia, hemolytic anemia, nephrotoxicity, hyperuricemia, uric acid nephropathy, ototoxicity, anaphylaxis, neurotoxicity, optic neuritis, papilledema, stomatitis, SIADH, nausea, vomiting, diabetes insipidus, Franconi's syndrome, magnesium wasting;
Bleomycin: urticaria, Raynaud's phenomenon, pulmonary fibrosis, pneumonitis, burning at injection site, nail loss, fever, chills, anaphylaxis, stomatitis, confusion, wheezing, hepatotoxicity, pleuropericarditis, renal toxicity, cerebral arteritis, cerebral vascular accidents, myocardial infarction, thrombotic microangiopathy, rash, alopecia;
Etoposide: anemia, leukopenia, thrombocytopenia, stomatitis, anaphylaxis, chemical phlebitis, neurotoxicity, anorexia, nausea, vomiting, lethargy, diarrhea, alopecia

DRUG INTERACTIONS
Cisplatin: allopurinol, colchicine, probenicid, sulfinpyrazone, antihistamines, buclizine, cyclizine, loxapine, meclizine, phenothiazines, thioxanthinese, trimethobenzamid, bleomycin, radiation therapy, aminoglycosides, furosemide, vaccines, erythromycin, ethacrynic acid, salicylates, vancomycin; **Etoposide:** radiation therapy, vaccines; **Bleomycin:** general anesthetics, concurrent radiation, cisplatin, vincristine

DOSAGE AND SCHEDULING

	Day 1 2 3 4 5 6 7 8 9 10 11 12 13 14
Cisplatin 20 mg/m²/d x 5, every 3 wk	▬▬▬▬▬
VP-16, 100 mg/m²/d x 5, every 3 wk	▬▬▬▬▬
Bleomycin 30 U/wk	■ (d1) ■ (d8)
Chemistries, tumor markers with each cycle, d 1	□
CBC weekly and daily on subsequent doses if CBC counts are low, d 1,8	□ □
CXR prior to therapy every 2 months	

DOSAGE MODIFICATIONS: *Maintain PEB schedule regardless of CBC counts; for granulopenic fever, reduce VP-16 dosage by 25%; for granulocytopenia on day 1 of 2nd, 3rd, or 4th cycle of therapy, do daily CBC counts and if WBC counts do not recover adequately, hold VP-16 on day 5; discontinue bleomycin if signs of pulmonary fibrosis develop*

NURSING INTERVENTIONS
Give antiemetics, maintain adequate intravenous fluid intake, monitor ins and outs closely, monitor weight; assess patient performance, mental and pulmonary status; use antidiarrheals as needed; monitor blood counts, liver function tests, renal function; advise patients on delayed nausea, development of fever and urinary symptoms, cessation of smoking (if appropriate)

PATIENT INFORMATION
Patient should inform physician of history of allergic reaction; watch for and report to physician fever, chills, change in urinary habits, tarry stool, blood in the stool, change in hearing, pins and needles, rash, diarrhea, and sores in mouth

RECENT EXPERIENCES AND RESPONSE RATES

Study	Evaluable Patients, *n*	Dose and Schedule	Complete Response Rates (%)
Williams *et al.*, N Engl J Med 1987, 316:1435–1440	121 nonseminoma	Cisplatin 20 mg/m²/d x 5 q3 wk Vinblastine 0.15 mg/kg d1 & 2q3 wk Bleomycin 30 U/wk	(61)
	123 nonseminoma	Cisplatin 20 mg/m²/d x 5 q3 wk VP-16 100 mg/m²/d x 5 q3 wk Bleomycin 30 U/wk	(60)
Einhorn *et al.*, J Clin Oncol 1989, 7:387–391	88 nonseminoma	Cisplatin 20 mg/m²/d x 5 q3 wk VP-16 100 mg/m²/d x 5 q3 wk Bleomycin 30 U/wk 3 cycles	66(75)
	vs 96 nonseminoma	Cisplatin 20 mg/m²/d x 5 q3 wk VP-16 100 mg/m²/d x 5 q3 wk Bleomycin 30 U/wk 4 cycles	70(73)

VAB-6
Vinblastine, Cyclophosphamide, Dactinomycin, Bleomycin, and Cisplatin

Vinblastine is an alkaloid from the plant *Vinca rosea*. Vinblastine binds to tubulin, inhibits microtubule formation, and disrupts cells during the M phase of mitosis. Dose modifications are required for hyperbilirubinemia. One mechanism of resistance to vinblastine is through the ATP-dependent efflux pump P-170.

Cyclophosphamide is an alkylating agent activated in the hepatic microsomal system. 4-hydroxycyclophosphamide enters the cell where it is converted to aldophosphamide and ultimately phosphoramide mustard and acrolein. Acrolein, excreted unchanged in the urine, is principally responsible for hemorrhagic cystitis. Phosphoramide mustard cross-links to strands of DNA and RNA, inhibiting cell division and protein synthesis.

Dactinomycin is an antibiotic from the *Streptomyces* species and is not cell cycle–specific in its antitumor mechanisms. It intercalates into DNA and prevent RNA template formation, and causes single-stranded DNA breaks.

Bleomycin is an antibiotic derived from the fungus *Streptomyces verticullus*. The major isoform in the mixture is A_2. Bleomycin binds to DNA and ferrous ion. Ferrous ion is oxidized ultimately leading to oxygen radicals that cause DNA single- and double-strand breaks.

Although cisplatin's anticancer action is not exactly known, it is thought to be similar to that of a bifunctional alkylating agent. Cisplatin binds to plasma protein and although serum half-life is calculated in hours, tissue levels have been detected as far out as 4 months.

DOSAGE AND SCHEDULING

Vinblastine 4 mg/m² d 1
Cyclophosphamide 600 mg/m² d 1
Dactinomycin 1 mg/m² d 1
Bleomycin 30 U IV push d 1
Bleomycin 20 U/m² continuous infusion d 1,2,3
Cisplatin 120 mg/m² d 4
Chemistries, tumor markers with each cycle, d 1
CBC, daily and on subsequent doses if CBC counts are low, d 1
CXR prior to therapy q 2 mo

Day 1 2 3 4 5 6 7

Cycle repeated every 4 weeks.

DOSAGE MODIFICATIONS: *Maintain VAB-6 schedule regardless of CBC counts; for granulocytic fever, reduce dactinomycin and vinblastine by 25%; discontinue bleomycin should signs of pulmonary fibrosis develop.*

RECENT EXPERIENCES AND RESPONSE RATES

Study	Evaluable Patients, *n*	Dose and Schedule	Complete Response Rates (%)
Bosl *et al.*, J Clin Oncol 1988, 6:1231–1238	82	VAB-6 vs	83
	82 (good-risk pts) nonseminoma	Etoposide 100 mg/m²/d x 5 Cisplatin 20 mg/m²/d x 5 q 3–4 weeks	88
Bosl *et al.*, J Clin Oncol 1986, 4:1493–1499	125 met. nonsem. & 22 met. sem.	VAB-6	69
	19 extragonadal	VAB-6	53
Stanton *et al.*, J Clin Oncol 1985, 3:336–339	28 sem.	VAB-6	86

CANDIDATES FOR TREATMENT
Patients with testicular neoplasms

SPECIAL PRECAUTIONS
Patients with renal failure or allergy to bleomycin

ALTERNATIVE THERAPIES
PEB, PVB

TOXICITIES
Cisplatin: leukopenia, thrombocytopenia, anemia, hemolytic anemia, nephrotoxicity, hyperuricemia, uric acid nephropathy, ototoxicity, anaphylaxis, neurotoxicity, optic neuritis, papilledema, stomatitis, SIADH, nausea, vomiting, diabetes insipidus, Franconi's, magnesium wasting; **Bleomycin:** urticaria, Raynaud's, pulmonary fibrosis, pneumonitis, burning at injection site, nail loss, fever, chills, anaphylaxis, stomatitis, confusion, wheezing, hepatotoxicity, pleuropericarditis, renal toxicity, cerebral arteritis, cerebral vascular accidents, myocardial infarction, thrombotic microangiopathy, rash, alopecia; **Dactinomycin:** aplastic anemia, leukopenia, esophagitis, pharyngitis, diarrhea, proctatitis, GI ulceration, anaphylaxis, phlebitis, hepatitis, hyperpigmentation, nausea, vomiting, skin rash, alopecia; **Cyclophosphamide:** gonadal depression, leukopenia, thrombocytopenia, myocarditis, hemorrhagic cystitis, pneumonitis, pulmonary fibrosis, SIADH, anaphylaxis, stomatis, hyperglycemia, hyperpigmentation, nausea, vomiting, headache, alopecia; **Vinblastine:** leukoneutropenia, thrombocytopenia, cellulitis, stomatitis, jaw pain, loss of ankle jerk, peripheral neuropathy, nausea, vomiting, ileus, alopecia

DRUG INTERACTIONS
Cisplatin: allopurinol, colchicine, probenicid, sulfinpyrazone, antihistamines, buclizine, cyclizine, loxapine, meclizine, phenothiazines, thioxanthinese, trimethobenzamid, bleomycin, radiation, aminoglycosides, furosemide, vaccines, erythromycin, ethacrynic acid, salicylates, vancomycin; **Vinblastine:** radiation, vaccines, allopurinol, colchicine, probenecid, sulfinpyrazone; **Bleomycin:** general anesthetics, concurrent radiation, cisplatin, vincristine; **Dactinomycin:** allopurinol, colchicine, probenecid, sulfinpyrazone, radiation therapy, vaccines, vitamin K; **Cyclophosphamide:** allopurinol, colchicine, probenecid, sulfinpyrazone, anticoagulants, radiation, cocaine, hepatic enzyme inducers, lovastatin, succinylcholine, vaccines

NURSING INTERVENTIONS
Give antiemetics, maintain adequate IV fluid intake, monitor ins and outs closely, monitor weight; assess patient performance, mental and pulmonary status; use antidiarrheals as needed; monitor blood counts, liver function, pulmonary function, and renal function; advise patients on delayed nausea, fever and urinary symptoms, cessation of smoking place patient on bowel regimen

PATIENT INFORMATION
Patient should inform physician of history of allergic reactions; report fever, chills, change in urinary habits, tarry stool, blood in the stool, change in hearing, pins and needles, rash, diarrhea, sores in mouth, pain in jaw, constipation

M-VAC
Methotrexate, Vinblastine, Doxorubicin, and Cisplatin

In a randomized trial evaluating the treatment of metastatic bladder cancer conducted by ECOG, M-VAC was found to be superior to cisplatin alone (objective response rates of 33 vs. 15% respectively, p = 0.001). The role of M-VAC in the treatment of metastatic transitional cell carcinoma is well documented, but its use, or the use of other combination chemotherapy, as adjuvant therapy for high-risk local disease has not yet been proven.

Methotrexate, an antimetabolite, inhibits dihydrofolic acid reductase, thus interfering with DNA synthesis. It is polyglutamated within cells, allowing it to remain in cells for prolonged periods of time. Vinblastine is an alkaloid from the plant *Vinca rosea*. Vinblastine binds to tubulin, inhibits microtubule formation, and disrupts cells during the M phase of mitosis. Dose modifications are required for hyperbilirubinemia. Doxorubicin is an anthracycline antibiotic from *Streptomyces peucetius* var. *caesius*. Although all of doxorubicin's mechanisms of action have not been elucidated, it is known to enter the cell quickly and intercalate with DNA, thus inhibiting cellular division. Although cisplatin's anticancer action is not exactly known, it is thought to be similar to that of a bifunctional alkylating agent. Cisplatin binds to plasma protein and although serum half-life is calculated in hours, tissue levels have been detected as far out as 4 months.

DOSAGE AND SCHEDULING

Methotrexate 30 mg/m² d 1, 15, 22
Vinblastine 3 mg/m² d 2, 3, 4
Doxorubicin 30 mg/m² d 2
Cisplatin 70 mg/m² d 2
Chemistries d 1
BUN/creatinine d 1, 15, 22
24 hr CrCl d 1
CBC d 1

Day: 1 2 3 4 5 6 7 10 15 20 22

Cycle repeated every 3 weeks.

DOSAGE MODIFICATIONS: Give full-dose methotrexate and vinblastine on day 15 and 22 if WBC count is 1999/mm³ and platelet count is > 74,999/mm³. If counts fall below, dose is held and restarted at 67% when counts return to normal. Omit days 15 and 22 if blood counts take more than 2 weeks to recover. On days 15 and 22 methotrexate should be given on schedule regardless of CBC counts. For granulocytic fever, reduce dactinomycin and vinblastine dosage by 25%; discontinue bleomycin should signs of pulmonary fibrosis develop

RECENT EXPERIENCES AND RESPONSE RATES

Study	Evaluable Patients, n	Dose and Schedule	Response Rates (%) Complete/Partial
Sternberg *et al.*, J Urol 1988, 139:461–69	92	Methotrexate 30 mg/m² d 1, 15, 22 Vinblastine 3 mg/m² d 2, 15, 22 Doxorubicin 30 mg/m² d 2 Cisplatin 70 mg/m² d 2	34/28
Sternberg *et al.*, J Urol 1990, 144:396–397	121	Methotrexate 30 mg/m² d 1, 15, 22 Vinblastine 3 mg/m² d 2, 15, 22 Doxorubicin 30 mg/m² d 2 Cisplatin 70 mg/m²	36/36
Connor *et al.*, J Urol 1990, 144:397	14	Methotrexate 30 mg/m² d 1, 15, 22 Vinblastine 3 mg/m² d 2, 15, 22 Doxorubicin 30 mg/m² d 2 Cisplatin 70 mg/m²	31/37
Scher *et al.*, J Urol 1988, 139:470–477	41 neoadjuvant	Methotrexate 30 mg/m² d 1, 15, 22 Vinblastine 3 mg/m² d 2, 15, 22 Doxorubicin 30 mg/m² d 2 Cisplatin 70 mg/m²	24/39
Scher *et al.*, J Urol 1988, 139:478–487	5 extragonadal	Methotrexate 30 mg/m² d 1, 15, 22 Vinblastine 3 mg/m² d 2, 15, 22 Doxorubicin 30 mg/m² d 2 Cisplatin 70 mg/m²	60/—

CANDIDATES FOR TREATMENT
Patients with metastatic transitional cell carcinoma of the uroepithelium

SPECIAL PRECAUTIONS
Patients with liver dysfunction or renal failure

ALTERNATIVE THERAPIES
MVC

TOXICITIES
Methotrexate: nausea, vomiting, gigivitis, pharyngitis, stomatitis, diarrhea, enteritis, lukopenia, thrombocytopenia, hypogammaglobulinemia, erythematous rash, pruritus, urticaria, photosensitivity, depigmentation, alopecia, acne, hepatic atrophy and necrosis, cirrhosis, renal failure, cystitis, defective oogenesis or spermatogenesis, menstrual dysfunction, infertility, fetal defects, abortion, nephropathy, blurred vision, seizures, arachnoiditis, leukoencephalopathy, conjunctivitis; **Vinblastine:** leukoneutropenia, thrombocytopenia, cellulitis, stomatitis, jaw pain, loss of ankle jerk, peripheral neuropathy, nausea, vomiting, paralytic ileus, alopecia; **Doxorubicin:** leukoneutropenia, cardiotoxicity, arrhythmias, phlebosclerosis, facial flushing, alopecia, hyperpigmentation of the nail beds and dermal creases, recall reaction to radiation, erythematous streaking at IV site, tissue necrosis from extravasation, mucositis, conjunctivitis, nausea, vomiting, allergy (including anaphylaxis); **Cisplatin:** leukopenia, thrombocytopenia, anemia, hemolytic anemia, nephrotoxicity, hyperuricemia, uric acid nephropathy, ototoxicity, anaphylaxis, neurotoxicity, optic neuritis, papilledema, stomatitis, SIADH, nausea, vomiting, diabetes insipidus, Franconi's syndrome, magnesium wasting.

DRUG INTERACTIONS
Methotrexate: alcohol, acetaminophen, amiodirone, estrogens, erythromycin, isoniazid, methyldopa, phenothiazines, phenytoin, piperacillin, rifampin, allopurinol, colchicine, sulfinpyrazones, NSAIDs, folic acid, oral neomycin, salicylates, sulfonamides, vaccines; **Vinblastine:** radiation therapy, vaccines, allopurinol, colchicine, probenecid, sulfinpyrazone; **Doxorubicin:** allopurinol, colchicine, alcohol, amiodirone, estrogens, isoniazid, methyldopa, phenothiazines, phenytoin, piperacillin, rifampin, vaccines; **Cisplatin:** allopurinol, colchicine, probenicid, sulfinpyrazone, antihistamines, buclizine, cyclizine, loxapine, meclizine, phenothiazines, thioxanthinese, trimethobenzamid, bleomycin, radiation therapy, aminoglycosides, furosemide, vaccines, erythromycin, ethacrynic acid, salicylates, vancomycin

NURSING INTERVENTIONS
Give antiemetics, maintain adequate IV fluid intact, monitor ins and outs closely, monitor weight; assess patient performance, mental and pulmonary status; use antidiarrheals as needed; monitor blood counts, liver function tests, renal function; advise patients on delayed nausea, development of fever and urinary symptoms, and adequate bowel regimen

PATIENT INFORMATION
Patient should inform physician of history of allergic reaction; watch for and report to physician fever, chills, change in urinary habits, tarry stool, blood in the stool, change in hearing, paresthesia, rash, diarrhea, sores in the mouth, jaw pain; patient should be informed that if constipation develops it must be treated aggressively.

The information here is provided as guidance only. Prescribers should always consult the manufacturer's current prescribing information.

Tumors of the female reproductive organs are heterogeneous with regard to histology, natural history, clinical behavior, and methods of treatment. Appropriate treatment requires careful diagnostic evaluation to distinguish them from other malignancies of the pelvis, including sigmoid and rectal cancers and bladder cancer, as well as from metastatic lesions, such as Krukenburg tumors. Accurate staging is critical because therapy is virtually always guided by extent of spread. Treatment of these malignancies requires a thorough understanding of their natural history and should not be attempted by those with little experience in this field. Optimal diagnosis, staging, and therapy require excellent communication between the medical and radiation oncologists, the radiologist, and the surgeon—this is particularly true in instances where multimodality therapy is contemplated.

Tumors discussed in this section include the common tumors of the ovary, uterine cervix, uterus, and vulva, and gestational trophoblastic neoplasms (Table 1).

EPITHELIAL TUMORS OF THE OVARY

ETIOLOGY AND RISK FACTORS

Epithelial tumors of the ovary comprise approximately 95% of all ovarian malignancies. They occur most commonly in women in their 50s and 60s. Etiology and risk factors for ovarian cancer are listed in Table 2.

STAGING AND PROGNOSIS

The course of the disease is dominated by locoregional spread, with peritoneal involvement being most common. Precise histologic diagnosis and accurate staging are required prior to treatment (Tables 3–5).

TREATMENT STRATEGIES

Goals of therapy for early-stage disease (International Federation of Gynecology and Obstetrics [FIGO] Stages I to III) include cure and for later-stage disease (suboptimal Stages III to IV), include palliation, particularly reduction of ascites, preservation of bowel function, adequate nutrition, and prevention of pain, although rarely do these more advanced-stage patients enjoy prolonged survival.

The cornerstone of treatment for epithelial ovarian tumors is surgery performed by an experienced gynecologic oncologist. Patients require a staging laparotomy with thorough inspection of the entire peritoneal cavity including the gutters, the pelvis, and the domes of the diaphragm, total abdominal hysterectomy and bilateral salpingo-oophorectomy, liver palpation and biopsy, lymph node sampling, omentectomy, and peritoneal washings. All gross disease should be removed if possible. If surgical debulking is incomplete, the surgeon must estimate the size and extent of residual tumor. Patients who have had a biopsy only or incomplete debulking may be referred to an experienced gynecologic oncologist for consideration for repeat

Table 1. Common Tumors of the Female Reproductive Tract

Ovary	Cervix
Epithelial	Vulva
Stromal	Gestational trophoblastic
Germ cell	neoplasm
Metastatic	Hydatidiform mole
Uterus	Invasive mole
Adenocarcinoma	Choriocarcinoma
Sarcoma	
Leiomyosarcoma	
Carcinosarcoma (mixed mesodermal tumors)	
Endometrial stromal sarcoma	

Table 2. Etiology and Risk Factors For Epithelial Tumors of the Ovary

Heredity
  Site-specific familial ovarian cancer syndrome
  Breast-ovarian cancer family syndrome
  Cancer family syndrome (Lynch syndrome II)

Hormonal
  Decreased risk with birth control pill use
  Increased risk nulligravidas

Environmental
  Higher risk in industrialized countries
  Higher risk in Western countries than in Japan
  Higher risk in Japanese who emigrate to the United States

Table 3. Staging of Epithelial Tumors of the Ovary

Stage	Criteria
I	Disease confined to the ovary
II	Disease confined to the pelvis
III	Disease confined to the abdominal cavity, including surface of the liver, pelvic, inguinal or paraaortic lymph node, omentum, or bowel
IV	Spread to liver parenchyma, lung (if effusion only, with positive cytologic test results), or other extra-abdominal site

Table 4. Prognosic Outcome of Epithelial Tumors of the Ovary

Stage	3-Yr Survival (%)
Ia, Ib	90.4
Ic, II	66.5
III	28.1
IV	10.4

Table 5. Unfavorable Prognostic Factors for Epithelial Tumors of the Ovary

Inability to surgically debulk to < 2 cm
Visceral involvement
Gross residual tumor after first-line chemotherapy
Stage III, IV
Grade 3
Aneuploidy, ?increased S phase
Elevated Her 2/*neu*

surgery because clinical outcome may be affected. Staging is performed per FIGO criteria.

PRIMARY DISEASE THERAPY

Primary therapy for patients with early-stage ovarian cancer, either confined to the ovary (FIGO Stage I) or confined to the pelvis (FIGO Stage II), is surgery. Nevertheless, among selected subgroups, the failure rate is high enough to warrant adjuvant therapy with either radioisotopes, external-beam irradiation, or chemotherapy. The Gynecologic Oncology Group (GOG) has attempted to define precisely the subgroups that would benefit from adjuvant therapy and determine the optimal form of therapy for these patients. Two clinical trials were initiated in 1976 to accomplish these goals.

Stage Ia and Ib

GOG 7601 included patients with Stage Ia or Ib disease (growth limited to one or both ovaries with no ascites and negative peritoneal washings) with well- or moderately differentiated histologic patterns. Patients were randomly assigned to observation or to receive melphalan, 0.2 mg/kg of body weight orally for 5 days every 4 to 6 weeks for 12 cycles. At a follow-up of 6 years, there was no difference between the two groups. Furthermore, the 5-year disease-free survival rate in the observation arm was 91% and the overall survival rate was 94%, suggesting that this subset of patients does well and should not receive adjuvant therapy [1].

Stages Iaii, Ibii, Ic-IIc, and Ia or Ib with Poorly Differentiated Histologic Features

GOG 7602 included patients with either a ruptured capsule or excrescences on the ovarian surface, high-grade histologic patterns, positive ascites or peritoneal washings, or spread to the uterus, fallopian tubes, or other pelvic tissues. Patients were randomly assigned to receive melphalan as noted previously or 15 mCi of intraperitoneal ^{32}P as chromic phosphate. The failure rate with 6 years of follow-up was 20%, with failures distributed evenly between both groups. Toxicities were modest in both groups; however, the authors concluded that treatment with ^{32}P was preferred because of the limited toxicity and no risk of developing leukemia, which has been observed with alkylating agents. In the replacement trial for the GOG, treatment with ^{32}P is compared with three cycles of cyclophosphamide and cisplatin administration. Optimal therapy for these patients remains unknown; when feasible, they should be entered into clinical trials.

THERAPY FOR ADVANCED OR SUBOPTIMAL DISEASE

Single agents with activity against ovarian cancer are shown in Table 6. The first combination regimen to demonstrate an impact on survival superior to that achieved with melphalan was HexaCAF (hexamethylmelamine, cyclophosphamide, methotrexate, 5-fluorouracil) [2], although reanalysis of this data by Ozols et al. [3] suggested that the benefit was confined to patients with high-grade tumors only. Subsequent studies have failed to confirm a benefit for HexaCAF.

The introduction of cisplatin in ovarian clinical trials in the 1970s had an important impact on the treatment of this disease. Cisplatin combinations appear to result in higher response rates, especially among patients with poor prognoses who have bulky tumors or poorly differentiated tumors.

Two-Drug Cisplatin Combinations

Cisplatin and doxorubicin (AP)

This combination resulted in a response rate of 80% when tested at Mt. Sinai Hospital [4], a rate better than that seen with treatment with nonplatinum combinations and similar to that seen with some four-drug combinations.

Cisplatin and cyclophosphamide (CP)

This regimen became a standard treatment combination for ovarian carcinoma since its introduction in the early 1980s [5]. It has activity similar to that of the AP combination and avoids some toxicities associated with doxorubicin, including cardiac toxicities—especially congestive heart failure, which may develop at dosages of more than 400 mg/m², and extravasation injuries. Doses of cyclophosphamide of 750 to 1000 mg/m² are required for full activity.

Carboplatin and cyclophosphamide

A preliminary report from the Southwest Oncology Group demonstrated equal efficacy for this combination versus CP but a lower incidence of irreversible toxicities associated with cisplatin treatment, including nephrotoxicity and neurotoxicity. The carboplatin and cyclophosphamide combination became a standard regimen for the treatment of ovarian cancer. Doses of carboplatin are 350 to 400 mg/m² and of cyclophosphamide are 600 to 750 mg/m². This treatment regimen has now been supplanted by the combination of paclitaxel and cisplatin.

Three-Drug Regimens: The Role of Doxorubicin

Cisplatin, doxorubicin, and cyclophosphamide (CAP or PAC)

PAC I uses a single dose of cisplatin, 50 mg/m², on day 1 and PAC V uses cisplatin, 20 mg/m² daily for 5 days. PAC I was compared with HexaCAF and single-agent melphalan and was shown to be superior to both [6].

Table 6. Single-agent Activity in Ovarian Cancer

Drug	Patients, n*	Response Rate (%)
Cisplatin (mg/m²)		
Low dose (30–50)	71	45
Intermediate (60–90)	31	55
High dose (100–120)	21	52
Carboplatin	18	50
Cyclophosphamide		
Low dose	355	43
High dose	36	61
Melphalan	541	47
Thiotepa	337	48
Chlorambucil	40	23
Doxorubicin	58	34
5-Fluorouracil	92	20
Methotrexate	25	20
Hexamethylmelamine	59	34
Vinblastine	20	10
Paclitaxel	124	24†
Ifosfamide	40	20†

*Previously untreated patients, except as noted.
†Most patients heavily pretreated.

CAP was not shown to be superior to CP, however, in a large trial by the Gynecologic Oncology Group [7]. When cyclophosphamide is used at full doses, therefore, doxorubicin does not add to the efficacy of the regimen.

Four-Drug Regimens: The Role of Hexamethylmelamine

Hexamethylmelamine (HMM) has been added to multiple CAP-type regimens because it is relatively marrow sparing, can be given orally, and has activity against ovarian carcinoma. These regimens are similar in efficacy and appear to be superior to single-agent therapies or to non-platinum–containing regimens. Their superiority to two-drug platinum-containing regimens remains to be demonstrated.

Cyclophosphamide, HMM, doxorubicin, and cisplatin (CHAD)
This regimen was more effective than single-agent melphalan in producing objective responses and prolonging progression-free survival, but the effect on overall survival was blunted because of the efficacy of cisplatin-containing regimens as salvage therapy [8].

CHAP-2 (same drugs)
CHAP-2 involves the use of doxorubicin and cyclophosphamide on day 3 and escalates the dose of doxorubicin, then HMM, to patient tolerance. This program has resulted in higher response and salvage rates, longer progression-free survival, and negative second-look surgery as compared with historical controls treated at Mt. Sinai. Comparison with two-drug therapy is necessary to confirm the benefits of this regimen.

CHAP-5 (same drugs)
CHAP-5 alternates cisplatin and doxorubicin and cyclophosphamide and HMM every 15 days. The regimen has been shown to be superior to HexaCAF [9], but not superior to the two-drug combination, CP [10].

Paclitaxel-based Regimens

Paclitaxel is a complex molecule derived from the bark of the Western yew. It has been currently approved for use as a salvage agent in patients with advanced ovarian carcinoma. Recent clinical trials suggest that paclitaxel in combination with cisplatin may be as active or more active than combinations of alkylating agents and cisplatin. Thus, the precise role for paclitaxel is currently under investigation. Paclitaxel is one of the most active agents against ovarian cancer, demonstrating response rates of 20 to 40% as a salvage agent in patients who had not responded to one or more prior treatments.

A recent phase III trial by the GOG compared treatment of advanced ovarian cancer with cyclophosphamide and cisplatin or paclitaxel and cisplatin. The dose of paclitaxel was 135 mg/m^2 as a 24-hour infusion every 3 weeks and the dose of cisplatin was 75 mg/m^2 administered after the paclitaxel. This combination was superior to cyclophosphamide-based regimen in terms of overall clinical response rates (77 vs 62% [*p*= 0.02]) and in progression-free interval, but not in complete response rate or overall survival. Thus, there appears to be a benefit to the paclitaxel/cisplatin combination, although the results of this trial require confirmation and questions remain unanswered regarding cost and quality of life. Nevertheless, the combination of paclitaxel and cisplatin appears to be the preferred first-line therapy.

A study by the National Cancer Institute of Canada compared high-dose (175 mg/m^2) and low-dose paclitaxel (135 mg/m^2) and a 24-hour versus a 3-hour infusion in women with advanced ovarian cancer. All patients had failed at least one prior cisplatin-containing regimen. The major findings in this study were no increase in toxicity with the shorter, outpatient infusion of paclitaxel and unaffected response rates. The higher dose of paclitaxel resulted in higher response rate. These data are preliminary and also remain to be confirmed in previously untreated patients.

Major clinical research issues in the treatment of ovarian cancer include the role of intensification of therapy by using autologous bone marrow transplantation, hematopoietic growth factors or other protective agents, such as WR2721 (ethiofos), to support patients' bone marrow or by combining cisplatin and carboplatin. These approaches remain experimental.

Following surgery for advanced ovarian cancer (Stage III or IV) patients are commonly treated with a platinum-based regimen, such as paclitaxel and cisplatin or cyclophosphamide and carboplatin. The Eastern Cooperative Oncology Group is currently testing the combination of carboplatin and paclitaxel administered in the outpatient setting. The preliminary toxicities of these regimens are myelosuppression and emesis. Emesis may be controlled with newer antiemetic agents, such as ondansetron. A hematopoietic growth factor, such as granulocyte–colony-stimulating factor (G-CSF) or granulocyte-macrophage–colony-stimulating factor (GM-CSF), may decrease the duration of neutropenia and number of days of necessary antibiotic administration, but has not been shown to improve survival or response duration and should not be considered standard therapy. The use of a single alkylating agent, such as melphalan, is suboptimal therapy, and should only be considered in patients who cannot receive standard therapy.

Before treatment, levels of the ovarian tumor marker, CA-125, should be measured and used as adjunctive evidence of response to therapy. Levels should be measured routinely during the course of treatment.

Treatment usually consists of four to eight cycles of therapy administered monthly. Residual disease should be measured before the initiation of therapy by visual inspection at the time of surgery, by computed tomographic scan if bulk disease remains, or by physical examination or chest roentgenography when appropriate. Levels of CA-125 are followed as described previously. If these levels rise or fail to decrease, resistance to treatment should be suspected.

SECOND-LOOK SURGERY

Patients who are clinical complete responders may be candidates for second-look surgery to re-stage their disease, although the utility of this approach has never been proven and practice of such should be confined to a clinical trial. Patients who have clinically evident disease after initial treatment may be candidates for second-debulking surgery. Like second-look surgery, this approach remains experimental and should not be routinely practiced.

SALVAGE CHEMOTHERAPY

Patients who do not respond to first-line therapy may be candidates for salvage therapy with single agents or combinations of etoposide, conventional dose or high-dose doxorubicin, cisplatin, ifosfamide, etoposide, hexamethylmelamine, or 5-fluorouracil and leucovorin, although optimal second-line therapy remains to be defined. Paclitaxel has demonstrated excellent salvage activity against ovarian carcinomas [11].

INTRAPERITONEAL THERAPY

For patients who are free of disease or have minimal disease at the time of second-look surgery, intraperitoneal therapy may be considered. This therapy remains an experimental approach whose efficacy has not yet been proved and so should be used within the confines of a formal clinical trial.

CARCINOMA OF THE UTERINE CERVIX

ETIOLOGY AND RISK FACTORS

Cancer of the cervix has a biphasic age distribution, with peaks in the fourth and fifth decades and eighth and ninth decades of life. It is more common in lower socioeconomic groups and in women who have been sexually active (Table 7).

Goals of treatment in early-stage disease are cure, and in late stage disease are prevention of pain, preservation of renal function, and prevention of disease progression, which can result in fistula formation, malodorous discharge, and thromboembolic events. As opposed to carcinoma of the ovary, diagnosis is usually straightforward because the cervix can be visually inspected and easily biopsied. Thus, 75% of cervical cancers are diagnosed at early stages, whereas only 25% of ovarian carcinomas are diagnosed before abdominal spread.

STAGING AND PROGNOSIS

As with ovarian cancers, precise staging is required because the stage correlates well with prognosis (Table 8). Long-term survival rates are 76% for Stage I (confined to the cervix), 55% for Stage II (local spread to adnexa or upper vagina), 31% for Stage III (spread to pelvic sidewalls or lower vagina), and 7% for Stage IV (spread beyond the pelvis). Furthermore, accurate staging is the foundation for further approaches to therapy. In addition to clinical staging, a chest roentgenogram is required to rule out pulmonary spread and a computed tomographic scan of the abdomen and pelvis is required to rule out lymph node and liver involvement. The role of nuclear magnetic resonance imaging remains unresolved.

PRIMARY DISEASE THERAPY

For patients with disease confined to the pelvis, radiation therapy is recommended. Radiation consists of external-beam therapy at doses of 5000 to 6000 cGy, followed by brachytherapy with a cesium source to deliver 6500 to 7200 cGy to point A (the bulkiest portion of the tumor). Recent studies suggest a benefit for the addition of cisplatin or either cisplatin or mitomycin C plus 5-fluorouracil to radiation therapy, although this benefit remains to be proved in a randomized trial. Early-stage cervical cancer (Stage I or IIA) can also be treated with radical hysterectomy with equivalent results to those of radiation therapy. Radical hysterectomy includes, in addition to total hysterectomy, *en bloc* resection of the parametrial connective tissues and the upper vagina, ureteral dissection, and total pelvic lymphadenectomy. The risks for surgical complications are markedly increased compared with total hysterectomy.

For patients with abnormal paraaortic lymph nodes, therapy is controversial. Treatment of microscopic disease in paraaortic nodes prolonged survival in one study; however, this finding does not necessarily imply a clinical benefit for patients with macroscopic involvement. These patients may be considered candidates for treatment of advanced disease; control of the primary lesion is indicated to prevent local complications.

Patients who do not response to local radiation therapy and have no evidence of distant disease may be candidates for pelvic exenteration, a morbid procedure that should only be attempted by those with expertise in this area. Partial exenterative procedures (anterior or posterior) may be associated with less morbidity. Reconstructive procedures include construction of continent conduits, creation of a neovagina, and low rectal anastomosis.

ADJUVANT THERAPY FOR REGIONAL DISEASE

Patients who have not responded to local therapy or present *de novo* with disease at distant sites, such as liver, bone, or lung, are candidates for systemic therapy. The utility of single agents is limited, and the activity for selected single agents is shown in Table 9.

The GOG conducted a randomized trial of three different doses and schedules of cisplatin [12]. The higher dose, 100 mg/m^2, produced higher response rates but no improvement in duration of response or survival.

Table 7. Etiology and Risk Factors for Carcinoma of the Uterine Cervix

Lower socioeconomic status, underdeveloped countries

First coitus at early age

Multiple sexual partners

Human papillomavirus types 16, 18, 31, 33, 35, and others

AIDS-related malignancy

Table 8. Staging and Prognosis of Carcinoma of the Uterine Cervix

Stage	Criteria
I	Microscopic or macroscopic disease confined to the cervix
II	Disease confined to the pelvis but not to the pelvic sidewall, or to the upper two thirds of the vagina
III	Disease that has spread to the pelvic sidewall or the lower third of the vagina, or that presents with hydronephrosis
IV	Disease that has invaded the bladder or rectum or has spread outside the pelvis

Table 9. Single-agent Activity in Carcinoma of the Uterine Cervix

Drug	Patients, *n*	Response Rate (%)
Cisplatin	52	40
Vincristine	44	23
Doxorubicin	78	10
Bleomycin	172	10
Cyclophosphamide	228	14
5-Fluorouracil	348	20
Methotrexate	77	16

The role of combination chemotherapy in cervical cancer is controversial. Although many prefer a cisplatin-based regimen, there is no standard therapy. Most combinations use cisplatin plus bleomycin with one or more additional agents. Combination chemotherapy has not been shown to be more effective than single-agent therapy and may accrue substantial toxicities. The introduction of ifosfamide and the use of infusional schedules has resulted in an increase in complete responses and high overall response rates [13], but this approach remains to be rigorously compared with single-agent cisplatin therapy.

Recent results with the combination of the vitamin A derivative, cis-retinoic acid, and the biologic response modifier, interferon, have been reported, and this combination has demonstrated activity. Although it remains to be confirmed, the activity of this combination may be equivalent to more toxic cisplatin-based treatments. Patients may be considered for experimental therapy once the risks and benefits have been fully explained. Inhibitors of the enzyme topoisomerase I, which helps regulate DNA unwinding, include the camptothecin derivatives topotecan, CPT-II, and 9-aminocamptothecin. CPT-II has demonstrated activity against cervical cancer in a Japanese study and is currently being tested in the United States.

Palliation of symptoms may be achieved with local radiation therapy. Renal function may be preserved with a percutaneous renal stent; however, prolonged survival or palliation have not been demonstrated with this approach. Adequate pain control may be achieved with opiates, such as morphine sulfate or fentanyl patches. Patients with fistula formation often present with intractable problems including malodorous discharge, which may be partially controlled with charcoal-impregnated pads, or they present with infection, requiring antibiotic therapy. Cachexia requires dietary counseling and nutritional supplementation.

ENDOMETRIAL CARCINOMA

ETIOLOGY AND STAGING

Carcinoma of the endometrium is the most common tumor of the female genital tract, yet it accounts for fewer deaths than does carcinoma of the ovary. This lower mortality rate results from the vastly higher incidence of early-stage disease at the time of diagnosis compared with ovarian carcinoma. In fact, at the time of diagnosis, 80% of cases are classified as Stage I disease, confined to the uterine corpus.

The peak age group is 60 to 70 years, and the disease is associated with obesity and diabetes, making these patients somewhat older and less healthy than other patients with gynecologic malignancies. This accounts for the lesser role played by chemotherapy in the treatment of this disease. Tables 10–12 list etiology and risk factors and staging and prognostic factors.

PRIMARY DISEASE THERAPY
Stage I

For patients with disease confined to the uterine corpus, the treatment is total abdominal hysterectomy (TAH) and bilateral salpingo-oophorectomy (BSO) (Table 13). The ovaries are removed because of occasional implants on ovaries or fallopian tubes. Suspicious pelvic nodes are also excised; if the frozen section shows disease, paraaortic lymph node dissection is indicated. For patients at high risk for recurrence, adjuvant radiation therapy may be given. For patients who are not candidates for surgery, radiation therapy may provide equivalent results.

ADJUVANT THERAPY FOR REGIONAL DISEASE
Stages II and III

For patients with gross involvement of the uterine cervix, either a radical hysterectomy or preoperative radiation therapy is indicated, followed by total abdominal hysterectomy and bilateral salpingo-oophorectomy. For patients with microscopic cervical spread, treatment includes TAH-BSO followed by postoperative radiation therapy. For patients with spread to other pelvic tissues, treatment includes TAH-BSO followed by pelvic radiation treatment.

THERAPY FOR ADVANCED DISEASE
Stage IV

For patients with disease that has spread beyond the pelvis, TAH-BSO plus pelvic radiation therapy may be required to prevent complications from hemorrhage. Systemic therapy would include either hormonal therapy or chemotherapy.

Hormonal Therapy

Hormonal therapy is most successful in patients with a long disease-free interval (≥ 2 years), well-differentiated tumors, and progesterone-receptor– "rich" tumors. There is a high degree of progesterone-receptor positivity in endometrial carcinomas, ranging

Table 10. Etiology and Risk Factors for Endometrial Carcinoma
Increased risk: obesity, nulliparity, late menopause, estrogen use, hypertension, diabetes Decreased risk: combination oral contraceptives?

Table 11. Staging and Prognosis of Endometrial Carcinoma	
Stage	**Criteria**
I	Disease confined to the corpus
II	Disease involves the corpus and cervix
III	Disease confined within the pelvis
IV	Spread of disease to bladder, rectum, small bowel, sigmoid colon, or distant organs

Table 12. Unfavorable Prognostic Factors for Endometrial Carcinoma
Histology: clear cell, papillary, adenosquamous Increased grade Increased uterine size Myometrial invasion Positive peritoneal cytologic test results Pelvic or paraaortic lymph nodes Adnexal spread

from 33 to 64% in undifferentiated tumors to 81 to 95% in well-differentiated tumors, and 70 to 72% overall [14]. The definition of "receptor-rich" is unclear. Overall, response to hormonal therapy with progestational agents is observed in 71% of patients with positive cytosolic progesterone receptors and 8% in patients without progesterone receptor protein [14]. One caveat is that the assay for progesterone receptors must be performed properly—*ie*, on fresh tissue that has been rapidly frozen at -70°C with appropriate controls.

The most commonly used single agent is the progestational agent megestrol acetate, which is administered at higher doses than are used for breast cancer (320 mg daily). Progestational agents, such as 17-hydroxyprogesterone caproate or 6-α-methyl-hydroxy progesterone acetate, are administered by injection. Toxicities with progestational agents are modest, with the most common side effects being fluid retention and weight gain. Response rates initially reported at 35% [15] were not confirmed in later studies [16], with response rates in the range from 11 to 16% being more common. The antiestrogenic agent, tamoxifen, also has activity against endometrial carcinoma, similar to that of progestational agents.

Chemotherapy

For patients who have not responded well to treatment with progestational agents or who have life-threatening visceral involvement and are candidates for systemic chemotherapy, treatment with cytotoxic drugs is indicated. Single-agent activity is shown in Table 14.

It is unclear that treatment with combination chemotherapy increases response rates over single-agent therapy with doxorubicin, and toxicities are increased. Two-drug therapy with doxorubicin and cisplatin has resulted in response rates of 33% [17]. Several studies have used CAP (cyclophosphamide, doxorubicin, cisplatin) or cyclophosphamide, doxorubicin, and vinblastine with response rates of 31 to 47%. In a randomized phase II study of cisplatin versus CAP conducted by the North Central Cancer Treatment Group, 3 of 14 patients responded to cisplatin and 5 of 16 to CAP. Only 7 and 12% of patients survived 2 years, and the authors concluded that treatment with experimental phase II agents was warranted [18]. Combinations of cytotoxic agents plus progestational agents have been tested and do not appear more active than does single-agent chemotherapy.

GESTATIONAL TROPHOBLASTIC NEOPLASM

Although uncommon in North America, gestational trophoblastic neoplasm (GTN) is an important neoplasm to the medical oncologist because it is highly curable with chemotherapy. The incidence of GTN varies widely in different parts of the world, being five times more common in Africa and Asia than in Europe or North America.

ETIOLOGY AND RISK FACTORS

The etiology of GTN is not well established (Table 15). Patients with a prior molar pregnancy have a higher risk for developing trophoblastic disease. Risk factors for the development of a molar pregnancy include a uterus large for dates, although a molar pregnancy can occur in a normal-sized uterus. Time of evacuation may also increase the incidence of malignant sequelae, with evacuations occurring earlier than 10 weeks being less likely to result in a malignancy.

PRIMARY AND REGIONAL DISEASE THERAPY

The clinical features of GTN have been reviewed previously [19]. The prognosis for this disease and approaches to treatment are directly related to the clinical and histopathologic features of GTN.

Table 13. Treatment Strategies by Stage for Endometrial Carcinoma

Stage	Treatment
I, II	TAH-BSO (*en bloc*)
	Paraaortic lymph node sampling (myometrial invasion only)
	± pelvic node sampling
	Peritoneal washings
	Postoperative radiation therapy for:
	High risk: + lymph nodes or adnexal spread ?Intermediate risk: myometrial invasion > 1/2, spread to cervix or vascular space, + peritoneal washings, grade 3, incomplete surgical staging
	Adjuvant chemotherapy for papillary serous histology
III	Radiation alone or surgery + radiation therapy
IV	Radiation therapy ± hormonal therapy ± chemotherapy

Table 14. Single-agent Activity in Carcinoma of the Endometrium

Agent	Response Rate (%)
Cisplatin	42
Doxorubicin	37
Cyclophosphamide	21
5-Fluorouracil	23
Idarubicin	10
Mitoxantrone	5

Table 15. Risk Factors Involved in Gestational Trophoblastic Neoplasm (GTN)

Mole	Nonmetastatic GTN
Asia > North America or Europe	Low risk
Age > 50 yr or < 16 yr	Serum βHCG < 40,000 mU/ml
Prior hydatidiform mole	Duration < 4 mo
Postmolar GTN	No antecedent term pregnancy, prior chemotherapy, or brain or liver metastases
Increased human chorionic gonadotropin	
Increased maternal age	High risk
Uterine enlargement	Serum βHCG > 40,000 mU/ml
Theca lutein cysts	Duration > 4 mo
	Antecedent term pregnancy, failed prior chemotherapy, or brain or liver metastases

Clinical features include degree of invasiveness (localized to uterine cavity, invasion into uterine myometrium, or metastatic to lungs or vagina [low risk] or metastatic to brain or liver [high risk]), disease-free interval, and bulk of tumor (best assessed by levels of the tumor marker, βHCG). The important histopathologic features include the presence of complete or partial mole and the presence of choriocarcinoma.

Methotrexate was first reported to be curative in patients with metastatic choriocarcinoma in 1956 and has remained the mainstay of therapy for low-risk disease. The most commonly used regimen is the New England Trophoblastic Disease Center regimen: methotrexate (MTX), 1 mg/kg given intramuscularly every other day for 8 days, alternating with leucovorin rescue, 0.1 mg/kg given intramuscularly every other day for 8 days. MTX has also been administered as a 12-hour intravenous infusion, orally, and as weekly intramuscular therapy. Cure rates are high with all regimens; however, the accepted regimen is the alternating 8-day treatment. Actinomycin is also an active drug in the treatment of GTN but is more toxic than is the combination of MTX and leucovorin.

THERAPY FOR ADVANCED DISEASE

Patients with high-risk disease include patients with brain or liver metastases, large tumor burdens or high βHCG levels, prior resistance to chemotherapy, or long disease intervals. These patients require treatment with combination chemotherapy. Early regimens combined methotrexate and actinomycin with other agents (MAC, CHAMOCA). More recently, etoposide (VP-16) has been incorporated into GTN regimens with equivalent results to those seen with CHAMOCA, but with less toxicity [20]. The two most important regimens are EMA/CO and EMA/EP. EMA/CO incorporates etoposide with methotrexate, leucovorin, and actinomycin (EMA) and cyclophosphamide with vincrisitine (CO), and each is administered on alterate weeks. High-risk patients had a survival rate of 84%; those who had not responded to previous therapy had a response rate of 74%. In a subsequent series, responses were observed in 76% of chemotherapy-naive, high-risk patients and in 57% of patients who had not responded previously to treatment [21]. Currently, EMA/CO would be considered acceptable for patients with high-risk GTN.

REFERENCES

1. Young RC, Walton LA, Ellenberg SS, *et al.*: Adjuvant therapy in Stage I and Stage II epithelial ovarian cancer: Results of two prospective randomized trials. *N Engl J Med* 1990, 322:1021–1027.

2. Young RC, Chabner BA, Hubbard SP, *et al.*: Advanced ovarian adenocarcinoma: A prospective clinical trial of melphalan (L-PAM) versus combination chemotherapy. *N Engl J Med* 1978, 299:1261–1266.

3. Ozols RF, Garrin AJ, Costa J, *et al.*: Advanced ovarian cancer: Correlations of histologic grade with response to therapy and survival. *Cancer* 1980, 45:572–581.

4. Bruckner HW, Cohen CJ, Goldberg JD, *et al.*: Improved chemotherapy for ovarian cancer with cis-diamminedichloroplatinum and adriamycin. *Lancet* 1981, 47:2288–2294.

5. Decker DG, Fleming TR, Malkasian GD, *et al.*: Cyclophosphamide plus cisplatinum in combination: Treatment program for Stage III and IV ovarian carcinoma. *Obstet Gynecol* 1982, 60:481–487.

6. Sturgeon JFG, Fine S, Gospodarowicz MK, *et al.*: A randomized trial of malphalan alone versus combination chemotherapy in advanced ovarian cancer. *Proc ASCO* 1982, 1:108.

7. Omura GA, Bundy DA, Berek JS, *et al.*: Randomized trial of cyclophosphamide plus cisplatin: A Gynecologic Oncology Group study. *J Clin Oncol* 1989, 7:457–465.

8. Vogl SE, Kaplan B, Pagano M: Diamminedichloroplatinum (D)-based combination chemotherapy (CT) is superior to melphalan for advanced ovarian carcinoma (OVCA) when age is over 50 and tumor diameter over 2 cm. *Proc ASCO* 1982, 1:119.

9. Neijt JB, ten Bokkel Huinink WW, van den Burg MEL, *et al.*: Randomized trial comparing two combination chemotherapy regimens (HexaCAF v CHAP-5) in advanced ovarian carcinoma. *Lancet* 1984, 2:594–600.

10. Neijt JP, ten Bokkel Huinink WW, van den Burg MEL, *et al.*: Randomized trial comparing two combination chemotherapy regimens (CHAP-5 v CP) in advanced ovarian carcinoma. *J Clin Oncol* 1987, 5:1157–1168.

11. McGuire WP, Rowinsky EK, Rosenshein NB, *et al.*: Taxol: A unique antineoplastic agent with significant activity in advanced ovarian epithelial neoplasms. *Ann Intern Med* 1989, 111:273–279.

12. Bonomi P, Blessing JA, Stehman FB, *et al.*: Randomized trial of three cisplatin dose schedules in squamous cell carcinoma of the cervix: A Gynecologic Oncology Group study. *J Clin Oncol* 1985, 3:1079–1085.

13. Buxton EJ, Meanwell CA, Hilton C, *et al.*: Combination bleomycin, ifosfamide and cisplatin chemotherapy in cervical cancer. *J Natl Cancer Inst* 1989, 81:359–361.

14. Richardson GS, MacLaughlin DT: The status of receptors in the management of endometrial cancer. *Clin Obstet Gynecol* 1986, 29:628–637.

15. Reifenstein EC: The treatment of advanced endometrial cancer with hydroxyprogesteron caproate. *Gynecol Oncol* 1974, 2:377–414.

16. Podratz KC, O'Brien PC, Malkasian GD: Effects of progestational agents in the treatment of endometrial carcinoma. *Obstet Gynecol* 1985, 66:106–115.

17. Seltzer V, Vogl SE, Kaplan BH: Adriamycin and cis-diamminedichloroplatinum in the treatment of metastatic endometrial adenocarcinoma. *Gynecol Oncol* 1984, 19:308–313.

18. Edmonson JH, Krook JE, Hilton JF, *et al.*: Randomized phase II studies of cisplatin and a combination of cyclophosphamide-doxorubicin-cisplatin (CAP) in patients with progestin-refractory advanced endometrial carcinoma. *Gynecol Oncol* 1987, 28:20–24.

19. Berkowitz RS, Goldstein DP: Gestational trophoblastic diseases. *Sem Oncol* 1989, 16:410–416.

20. Newlands ES, Bagshawe KD, Begent RJH, *et al.*: Developments in chemotherapy for medium-and high-risk patients with gestational trophoblastic tumors (1979–1984). *Br J Obstet Gynecol* 1986, 93:63–69.

21. Bolis G, Bonazzi C, Landoni F, *et al.*: EMA/CO regimen in high-risk gestatational trophoblastic tumor. *Gynecol Oncol* 1988, 31:439–444.

EMA/CO

Etoposide, Methotrexate, Leucovorin, Actinomycin D, Vincristine, and Cyclophosphamide

EMA/CO is an intensive 6-drug combination regimen in which activity is centered on etoposide. The design of this regimen incorporates the principle of alternating non–cross-resistant chemotherapy by using multiple agents in alternating weekly cycles with the intent of preventing the emergence of drug resistance. The design also incorporates features such as leucovorin "rescue"—to prevent methotrexate-induced mucositis and myelosuppression—and cycling in the marrow-sparing agent, vincristine, to prevent myelosuppression with the goal of intensifying the doses that can be safely administered.

Actinomycin D is an antibiotic that intercalates DNA and causes DNA strand breaks. At low concentrations actinomycin D inhibits RNA synthesis. Etoposide (VP-16) is a topoisomerase II inhibitor that causes DNA strand breaks. Methotrexate is an antimetabolite that blocks the enzyme, dihydrofolate reductase. The inability to synthesize reduced folates results in inhibition of one-carbon metabolism, thus blocking purine synthesis. Folinic acid (leucovorin) is a reduced folate that enters the folate cycle past the block at dihydrofolate reductase, thus "rescuing" cells from methotrexate-induced depletion of reduced folates. Vincristine is a vinca alkaloid that blocks mitosis by inhibiting polymerization of tubulin. Cyclophosphamide is an alkylating agent that forms a covalent bond with DNA, thus inhibiting DNA synthesis.

DOSAGE AND SCHEDULING

COURSE 1

Actinomycin D 0.5 mg IV push d 1,2	■■							
Etoposide 100 mg/m^2 IV over 30 min d 1,2	■■							
Methotrexate 100 mg/m^2 IV push d 1	■							
Methotrexate 200 mg/m^2 IV 12-hr infusion d 1	■							
Leucovorin 15 mg orally/IM twice daily x 4 starting 24 hr after start of MTX therapy d 2	■							
Day	1	2	3	4	5	6	7	

COURSE 2

Vincristine 1 mg/m^2 IV push d 1	■							
Cyclophosphamide 600 mg/m^2 IV over 30 min d 1	■							
Day	1	2	3	4	5	6	7	

Alternate courses 1 and 2 every 6 days (if no mucositis develops) until complete remission or drug resistance; patients receiving cranial prophylaxis should receive methotrexate, 12.5 mg intrathecally only on day 1 of course 2; take CBC counts, differential, platelet count, BUN, creatinine, and liver function tests prior to each cycle; modify vincristine dose if liver function tests are elevated

RECENT EXPERIENCES AND RESPONSE RATES

Study	Evaluable Patients, n	Survival Rates (%)	
		No Prior Treatment	Prior Treatment
Newlands et al. Br J Obstet Gynecol 1986, 93:63–69	56 (high risk)	93	74
Bolis et al. Gynecol Oncol 1988, 31:439–444	17 (high risk)	76	57

CANDIDATES FOR TREATMENT

High-risk gestational trophoblastic neoplasm, including patients with brain or liver metastases, patients who have not responded to previous chemotherapy, and patients with bulky disease (βHCG > 100,000 IU/ml)

SPECIAL PRECAUTIONS

Avoid extravasation of actinomycin D and vincristine; give etoposide over 1 to 2 hr to avoid hypotension; patients with pleural effusion should not be given MTX; do not treat patients with prior anaphylactic reaction to any of the agents

ALTERNATIVE THERAPIES

Many alternative therapies tested but none improve survival and all appear more complex and toxic than EMA/CO

TOXICITIES

Actinomycin D: myelosuppression, nausea, vomiting, mucositis, alopecia, rash or hyperpigmentation, extravasation reactions, radiation recall reactions; **Methotrexate:** myelosuppression, nausea, vomiting, anorexia, stomatitis, hepatotoxicity including fibrosis and elevated LFTs, rash, alopecia, dizziness, malaise, renal failure; **Etoposide:** myelosuppression, alopecia, fever, hypotension; uncommon: nausea, vomiting; bronchospasm, phlebitis (rare); **Vincristine:** neurotoxicity, constipation, paralytic ileus, foot drop, cranial nerve palsy, SIADH, alopecia, extravasation reaction; **Cyclophosphamide:** myelosuppression, hemorrhagic cystitis, SIADH, nausea, vomiting, anorexia, pulmonary infiltrates, alopecia, amenorrhea

DRUG INTERACTIONS

Actinomycin D: radiation; **Methotrexate:** salicylates, sulfonamides, phenytoin, other protein-bound drugs, alcohol, coumadin, amphotericin, steroids, cephalothin; **Cyclophosphamide:** allopurinol, barbiturates, phenytoin, chloral hydrate, corticosteroids, general anesthetics

NURSING INTERVENTIONS

Several agents used are highly emetogenic; give adequate antiemetic therapy prior to treatment, prolonged vomiting after EMA can leave patients dehydrated prior to receiving CP, thus making them more susceptible to cyclophosphamide-induced hemorrhagic cystitis, therefore, make sure patients who have been vomiting are hydrated prior to receiving cyclophosphamide; administer actinomycin D and vincristine by slow push through a newly started, well-functioning IV line; if extravasation occurs, stop the infusion immediately, attempt to withdraw extravasated drug, and put ice on the area; advise patients to call physician immediately if fever develops, 8–14 days after each treatment; monitor βHCG on every-other-week schedule.

PATIENT INFORMATION

Possibility of fevers 8–14 days after treatment—call physician immediately; severe mucositis possible; if unable to eat, IV hydration may be required; contraceptives must be used for 1 year after initiation of therapy

PACLITAXEL AND CISPLATIN

Chemotherapy for advanced ovarian carcinoma is based on the combination of a platinum compound with paclitaxel or an alkylating agent. Currently, the combination cisplatin and paclitaxel is preferred. The two-drug combination appears as efficacious as more complex regimens and is less toxic.

Paclitaxel is a derivative of the Western yew tree that inhibits depolymerization of tubulin.

Cisplatin forms DNA adducts composed of intrastrand cross-links, which act much in the same way as do classic alkylating agents, preventing DNA transcription and synthesis and causing DNA strand breaks.

DOSAGE AND SCHEDULING

Paclitaxel 135 mg/m^2 24-hr infusion every 3 wk, followed by cisplatin 75 mg/m^2 2-hr infusion

LAB MONITORING: *Treatment generally continues for 4–8 cycles; take CBC count, differential, platelet count, CA-125, BUN, creatinine prior to each cycle; failure of the CA-125 level to decrease suggests emerging resistance to drug treatment*

RECENT EXPERIENCES AND RESPONSE RATES

Study	Evaluable Patients, *n*	Dose and Schedule	CR/PR (%)
McGuire *et al.*, Proc ASCO 1993, 12:255	209 .	Cyclophosphamide/cisplatin	62
		Paclitaxel/cisplatin	77 (*p*=0.02)

CANDIDATES FOR TREATMENT

Patients with advanced (Stage III or IV) ovarian carcinoma

SPECIAL PRECAUTIONS

Patients with inadequate leukocyte and platelet counts and dehydration prior to initiation of treatment; those with bone marrow suppression (leukocytes or platelets) should not be treated

ALTERNATIVE THERAPIES

Cyclophosphamide and carboplatin combination is second choice

TOXICITIES

Cisplatin: nephropathy, neurotoxicity, ototoxicity, emesis, hemolytic anemia, anaphylaxis; **Paclitaxel:** anaphylaxis (2%), neutropenia, profound granulocytopenia, sensory neuropathy, alopecia, cardiac conduction abnormalities; arthralgias/myalgias, nausea and vomiting, diarrhea, mucositis

DRUG INTERACTIONS

Paclitaxel: ketoconazole

NURSING INTERVENTIONS

Check combined blood count, including platelets, prior to administering drugs; pretreat patients with adequate antiemetic therapy; question patients regarding pregnancy (paclitaxel may be mutagenic)

PATIENT INFORMATION

Caution patients about fevers that may develop 8 to 14 days after therapy; possible hypersensitivity reactions and neutropenia

CRA/IFN
Cis-Retinoic Acid and Interferon α-2b

The role of chemotherapy in the treatment of advanced cancer of the cervix is tenuous. Although responses are achieved, response durations are generally short and cisplatin-based regimens may be toxic. This experimental regimen has resulted in response rates similar to those achieved with cisplatin-based regimens, with less toxicity.

The mechanism of action is unknown. Retinoids are bound by specific cellular receptors and probably act as differentiating agents for epithelial cells. Interferons have antiviral, antiproliferative, and cytotoxic effects. In this regimen, interferon α-2b, which has minimal activity as a single agent in advanced cervical cancer, may modulate the activity of cis-retinoic acid or may be acting independently as a negative growth factor.

The high response rates in Mexican women with cis-retinoic acid and interferon α-2b were achieved in patients who had not received prior treatment. In women in the United States who had failed prior therapy with radiation and/or cisplatin there were no responses. The current status of retinoids combined with interferon in cervical cancer remains to be more thoroughly studied.

DOSAGE AND SCHEDULING

cis-Retinoic acid 1 mg/kg/d orally for at least 2 mo

Interferon α-2b 6 MU/d SC for at least 2 mo

RECENT EXPERIENCES AND RESPONSE RATES

Study	Evaluable Patients, n	Dose and Schedule	CR/PR(%)
Lippman et al., J Natl Cancer Inst 1992, 84:241	26	13-cis-retinoic acid 1 mg/kg/d orally IFN α-2b 6MU SC daily	4/46
Alberts et al., Proc ASCO 1993, 12:266	13	13 cRA (same as above) IFNα-2b 3MU/m²/d	0

CANDIDATES FOR TREATMENT

Patients with advanced cervical cancer (Stage IV) and squamous cell carcinoma of the skin—investigational regimen; exclude pregnant patients

SPECIAL PRECAUTIONS

Patients with pre-existing dementia or with previous thromboembolic events

ALTERNATIVE THERAPIES

Single-agent cisplatin (50–75 mg/m²)

TOXICITIES

cis-Retinoic acid: mucocutaneous toxicities including skin dryness, cheilitis, xerosis, epistaxis, rashes; ocular toxicities including dry eyes, blepharoconjunctivitis, corneal erosions; myalgias and arthralgias; hepatic toxicity with elevations of liver enzymes; hyperlipidemias; teratogenicity; **Interferon α-2b:** fevers, myalgias, flu-like syndrome, fatigue, depression, anemia, thrombocytopenia, leukopenia, diarrhea, LFT abnormalities, elevated creatinine, encephalopathy, seizure, coma

DRUG INTERACTIONS

None noteworthy

NURSING INTERVENTIONS

Teach patients to self-inject interferon

PATIENT INFORMATION

Patients must be cautioned to not become pregnant, because retinoids are potent teratogens

The diagnosis and management of disease in patients with primary neoplasms of the central nervous system (CNS) pose special problems and offer unique treatment opportunities to clinicians involved in the care of patients with cancer. Primary brain tumors represent approximately 2% of all cancers in adults in the United States; 17,500 new primary brain tumors were diagnosed in 1992. Brain tumors are a heterogeneous group of neoplasms that can arise from any of the constituent elements of the central nervous system—neurons, glia, endothelia, meninges—and the biologic behavior of a given brain tumor is very much predicated on its cell of origin. The most common primary brain tumors in adults are glial neoplasms, which account for approximately 65% of all primary CNS tumors.

Remarkable advances during the past 15 years in the fields of neuroimaging, neurosurgery, and neuropathology have greatly increased the accuracy of detection of brain tumors. Similar advances in the neurosciences have increased our understanding of brain tumor neurobiology. During that same interval, the development of chemotherapeutic agents with improved CNS penetration and the development of improved drug delivery systems have focused interest on the role of chemotherapy in the treatment of brain tumors. Despite these advances, the prognosis for patients with primary brain tumors has not improved significantly. New and promising protocols continue to be developed, however, and a review of the latest treatment strategies for patients with brain tumors is therefore especially pertinent now.

HISTOLOGY

Glial cells—astrocytes, oligodendrocytes, and ependymocytes—are the support cells of the central nervous system. They perform important nutritive, metabolic, and electrophysiologic functions that are prerequisite for normal neuronal activity. Normal glial cells have a very low rate of division except in response to brain injury. When these cells become malignant, their rate of proliferation increases markedly, and they can spread rapidly throughout the brain.

In a broad sense, gliomas can originate from any cell of glial origin and therefore include astrocytic neoplasms—astrocytomas and anaplastic astrocytomas—which arise from astrocytes, oligodendrogliomas, which arise from oligodendrocytes, and ependymomas and choroid plexus papillomas, which arise from ependymocytes. The cell of origin of the glioblastoma, the most primitive and malignant of the gliomas, is not always clear. Evidence points to an astrocytic origin in most cases. In the usual sense, however, gliomas include only astrocytomas, anaplastic astrocytomas, and glioblastomas because these tumors constitute approximately 90 to 96% of all glial neoplasms. Gliomas exhibit characteristic age-specific incidence patterns. Both astrocytomas and glioblastomas have small peaks in incidence during childhood followed by a steady rise in incidence until larger adult peaks are reached in the fifth and sixth decades, respectively [1]. There is a slight male predominance but no racial predilection in patients with gliomas.

ETIOLOGY AND RISK FACTORS

The environmental and genetic factors that may lead to the development of gliomas are poorly understood. There is substantial evidence that previous cranial radiation treatment increases the incidence of malignant gliomas after a latent period of 3 to 30 years [2]. Children are most vulnerable to the effects of ionizing radiation on the central nervous system. Head trauma has been cited, but most studies have failed to demonstrate an increased incidence of gliomas after head injury. The concurrence of gliomas with progressive multifocal leukoencephalopathy and multiple sclerosis has led to unconfirmed speculation regarding the role of demyelination in the genesis of gliomas. Smoking, alcohol consumption, and dietary patterns have not been shown to be risk factors for gliomas. Thirty-three percent of patients with glioblastoma have a family history of cancer, but instances of familial gliomas are rare. Certain genetic disorders are clearly associated with the occurrence of glial neoplasms. Patients with tuberous sclerosis, Turcot's syndrome, and the central form of neurofibromatosis (NF, type II) are predisposed to subependymal astrocytomas, glioblastomas, and optic nerve gliomas, respectively. The genetic basis of this association, however, has not been identified.

Although the cause of gliomas is not known, the molecular biologic characteristics of gliomas suggest clues regarding their pathogenesis. Specific oncogenes, genes that promote neoplastic cell transformation by encoding growth factors, growth factor receptors, intracellular transducers, or nuclear transcription factors, have been identified in astrocytomas. These oncogenes include c-sis, which encodes the B-subunit of platelet-derived growth factor and a homologue of c-erbB, which encodes the epidermal growth factor receptor. Alternatively, a role for tumor suppressor genes, genes that suppress cell growth, in glioma ontogeny has also been proposed. The two best characterized tumor suppressor genes in human cancers, Rb^3 and p53, are located on chromosomes 13 and 17, respectively. Deletion loci on chromosomes 13 and 17, as well as chromosomes 9, 10, and 22, have been identified in astrocytomas, and inactivation of p53 and Rb^3, either by deletion or by "unmasking" of a mutant allele, has been demonstrated in high-grade gliomas [3]. These findings implicate the loss of a tumor suppressor gene in the pathogenesis of glial neoplasms, although the specific mechanism by which their inactivation promotes oncogenesis remains unknown.

Patients with gliomas may develop a variety of clinical symptoms ranging from insidiously evolving cognitive impairment to the apoplectic onset of status epilepticus. In general, patients present with either a change in mental function, headaches, seizures, focal neurologic signs such as hemiparesis or aphasia, or evidence of increased intracranial pressure. In such patients, and increasingly in asymptomatic patients, computed tomography (CT) scan or magnetic resonance (MR) imaging of the brain provide sensitive, accurate detection of the tumor mass. The diagnosis of a glioma, as with other tumors, is established by surgical resection or biopsy, and histopathologic examination.

GRADING AND PROGNOSIS

The identification of those factors that affect survival is critical in determining the appropriate treatment and counsel for a given patient. During the past 15 years, multi-institutional randomized clinical trials, including those conducted by the Brain Tumor Study Group (BTSG), the Radiation Therapy Oncology Group–Eastern Cooperative Oncology Group (RTOG-ECOG), and other large retrospective surveys have established several factors as predictive of survival in patients with gliomas [1,4,5]. These factors can be classified into clinical, pathologic, and treatment categories.

The clinical factors of prognostic significance in patients with gliomas include age at the time of diagnosis, performance status, and seizures. Survival is longer for patients who are less than 40 years at the time of diagnosis, patients who initially have a high performance status, and, possibly, patients who present with seizures [4,5].

Performance status is rated using the Karnofsky Scoring System, a clinical grading scale based on the patient's ability to perform activities of daily living. Scores range from 10 to 100 and patients with normal or near normal scores (80–100) have an improved prognosis.

The single most important prognostic factor in predicting outcome for patients with glial neoplasms is the histopathologic appearance of the tumor. Several different grading systems have been used by neuropathologists in evaluating gliomas, which has led to some confusion in determining which histologic features are most predictive of survival in patients with gliomas. The two most frequently used grading systems are three-tier systems (such as those proposed by Burger, WHO, and Rubenstein [6–8]), which classify astrocytic neoplasms as astrocytomas, anaplastic astrocytomas, and glioblastoma multiforme, and the Kernohan system, which grades astrocytomas from grade I through IV—grade IV astrocytomas being the most malignant [6,9]. Kernohan grades I and II astrocytoma roughly correspond with the WHO designation of astrocytoma, whereas grades III and IV correspond with the classifications for anaplastic astrocytoma and glioblastoma, respectively (Table 1). Low-grade (I and II) astrocytomas are better differentiated and show less evidence of cytologic atypia than do high-grade astrocytomas (III and IV), which are more poorly differentiated and which show increasing evidence of such anaplastic features as nuclear atypism, mitoses, endothelial proliferation, or coagulative necrosis. Regardless of which grading system is used, the presence of coagulative necrosis is the single histologic feature most predictive of survival [6]. Patients with astrocytomas containing necrosis found at biopsy or resection have a median survival of 8 to 10 months, whereas patients with anaplastic astrocytomas survive an average of 18 to 24 months [6]. Patients with astrocytomas lacking anaplastic features have a median survival of 5 to 7 years. High-grade astrocytomas are often called *malignant gliomas* and low-grade astrocytomas, *benign* based on the degree of cellular differentiation these tumors display histologically. As can be seen from the survival data, however, even low-grade astrocytomas behave in a clinically malignant fashion regardless of their histopathologic appearance.

An inherent limitation in the histopathologic examination of gliomas, beyond the lack of consensus regarding grading systems, is that the tissue sampled may not be representative of the tumor. The histologic appearance of the gliomas can vary significantly within the boundaries of the tumor, and because brain resections or biopsies are often limited so as to preserve neurologic function, the subsequent pathologic diagnosis may underestimate the actual degree of malignancy. Mention should also be made of two histologic variants—pilocytic astrocytomas and subependymal giant cell astrocytomas—whose biologic behavior is distinct from that of other astrocytomas. Pilocytic astrocytomas occur primarily in children or young adults, most frequently are located in the cerebellum, and have associated 25-year survival rates in excess of 90%. Subependymal giant cell astrocytomas occur typically in patients with tuberous sclerosis, are periventricular in location, and are also associated with long-term survival after surgery. These two histologic variants are distinguished clinically and pathologically from other astrocytomas and they should be regarded as separate entities when determining the treatment strategies for patients with gliomas.

The location of the glioma within the neuraxis is also important in predicting survival. The topographic nature of a tumor is often closely related to its clinical behavior. For example, as many as 70% of cerebellar gliomas are pilocytic astrocytomas and are associated, as noted previously, with excellent 25-year survival rates. Even for patients with cerebellar astrocytomas with anaplastic features, long-term survival rates are better than for patients with gliomas at other sites. In contrast, patients with localized low-grade gliomas of the brain stem have only a 50% chance of survival at 3 years. The distinction between low-grade and high-grade gliomas remains critical, however, because tumor histology is predictive of survival independent of tumor location. In the series of localized brain stem gliomas just described, the 3-year survival rate for patients with high-grade tumors was less than 10%.

Postoperative ionizing radiation is the treatment factor most important in predicting survival for patients with high-grade gliomas. A BTSG trial that randomly assigned patients with grade III and IV astrocytomas to treatment with surgery alone and treatment with surgery plus radiation showed that median survival was doubled from 14 to 36 weeks by the addition of radiation to surgery [4]. Similar results were recorded by the Scandinavian Glioblastoma Study Group (SGSG), with median survival increased from 5.2 months to 10.8 months by the addition of postoperative radiation therapy. The extent of surgical resection may affect survival. Some investigators have reported that survival is increased in patients who undergo extensive tumor resection at the time of diagnosis [10]. The prognostic significance of adjuvant chemotherapy for high-grade gliomas and radiation therapy for low-grade gliomas has not yet been determined. The impact of these and other treatment strategies on survival is discussed in the following section on primary disease therapy. Table 2 summarizes the factors associated with improved prognoses.

PRIMARY DISEASE THERAPY

Gliomas, like other central nervous system malignancies, occupy a unique position within the spectrum of human cancers. Gliomas have important anatomic and biologic characteristics that distinguish them from cancers of other organ systems. These characteristics greatly influence the clinical behavior and treatment response of gliomas, and their significance should be well understood by clinicians involved in the treatment of patients with glial neoplasms.

Table 1. Histologic Classification of Gliomas

Kernohan Classification	Three-tier Classification	Median Survival
Grades I and II	Astrocytoma	5–7 yr
Grade III	Anaplastic astrocytoma	18–24 mo
Grade IV	Glioblastoma multiforme	8–10 mo

Table 2. Prognostic Factors Associated with Increased Survival in Patients with Gliomas

Prognostic Factor	Increased Survival
Age	Age less than 40 yr at diagnosis
Performance status	High performance status
Histology	Low-grade glioma
Location	Cerebellar glioma
Treatment	Postoperative radiation

These characteristics include the presence of the blood–brain barrier, the absence of draining lymphatics, confinement in a fixed volume by a nondistensible skull, an immunologically privileged state, and a propensity to remain localized and not metastasize outside the central nervous system.

The blood–brain barrier is a selectively permeable barrier between the plasma and the brain interstitium formed by specialized cerebral endothelial cells. Whereas the endothelia of extracerebral vessels permit essentially free passage of macromolecules into parenchymal tissues, the tight junctions of cerebral endothelia markedly limit the entry into the brain of molecules that are water soluble, ionized, or greater than 200 daltons. Although the new cerebral vessels that proliferate within the tumor bed often have an incomplete or inefficient blood–brain barrier, the blood–brain barrier continues to limit significantly the penetration of chemotherapeutic drugs into glial tumors. Conversely, because endothelia supplying the glioma are in many cases abnormally permeable, some passage of plasma proteins into the brain interstitium occurs, which leads to the development of vasogenic edema. The absence of draining lymphatics accelerates edema formation. Because the cranial cavity has a restricted volume, increases in peritumoral edema and the tumor mass itself can result in deleterious increases in intracranial pressure. Fortunately, vasogenic edema responds well to treatment with corticosteroids. Corticosteroid agents are a major adjunct in the management of patients with gliomas and their dose should be carefully titrated to maximize the reduction in morbidity from increased intracranial pressure and minimize the complications of prolonged corticosteroid use.

The incidence of seizures in patients with gliomas reaches 60% in some series and therefore the prophylactic use of anticonvulsants is recommended. Treatment usually is initiated with phenytoin at a dose of 5 to 7 mg/kg/d and drug levels should be maintained in the therapeutic range, which is 10 to 20 µg/ml in most laboratories. Carbamazepine, phenobarbital, or valproic acid can also be used for prophylaxis against secondary generalized seizures. The incidence of deep vein thrombosis ranges from 40% to 45% in patients with high-grade gliomas and, therefore, treatment with anticoagulants is often required [11]. The prevention of pulmonary emboli has traditionally been accomplished by the use of infrarenal inferior vena cava (IVC) filters because of the fear of iatrogenic intracerebral hemorrhage in patients with brain tumors. However, a recent retrospective report found that the complications from IVC filters in patients who do not receive anticoagulant treatment are unacceptably high, reaching 62%, whereas the incidence of anticoagulant-associated intracerebral hemorrhage in patients with high-grade gliomas is no higher—approximately 2%—than in patients not receiving the anticoagulants [11]. Anticoagulants can be safely used in conjunction with IVC filters for the treatment of deep vein thrombosis and the prevention of pulmonary embolism in patients with gliomas, provided that anticoagulant effects are assiduously monitored.

Although the anatomic and biologic characteristics of glial neoplasms pose special problems for clinicians treating patients with gliomas, they also afford potential advantages. Because gliomas remain localized and rarely metastasize, involvement of other vital organ systems almost never occurs. Patients seldom suffer the systemic complications seen frequently with other cancers. The blood–brain barrier, as stated earlier, is abnormally permeable at the site of the tumor. As a result, it limits the penetration of chemotherapeutic drugs into normal brain tissue far more efficiently than into the tumor itself, and significantly higher doses of chemotherapy can be achieved in the tumor than in the adjacent brain parenchyma. Finally, although gliomas are immunologically privileged tumors, this privileged status makes them potentially susceptible to innovative immunologic therapies.

The primary therapies used in the treatment of gliomas are surgery, radiation, and chemotherapy. Brachytherapy may be a potentially useful adjunct therapy. Immunotherapy and gene therapy offer promise for the future but thus far have not proved to be clinically beneficial. Because high-grade gliomas and low-grade gliomas have such distinct natural histories, it is most appropriate to consider their management separately.

Surgery

Surgery is the primary therapy for patients with high-grade gliomas. High-grade gliomas are infiltrative tumors with indistinct margins and they inevitably involve adjacent normal parenchyma. Although complete resection is not possible, most neurosurgeons favor doing an extensive resection of the tumor at the time of diagnosis. Extensive resection improves diagnostic accuracy by providing sufficient tissue for histologic examination, relieves mass effect, and often improves performance status. More importantly, several large clinical trials have shown that survival is increased in patients who undergo extensive surgical resection at the time of presentation.

Radiation Therapy

Radiation treatment after surgery is standard primary therapy for patients with high-grade gliomas. The value of postoperative radiation therapy has been proved in several large clinical trials [4,5,10]. Radiation therapy improves or stabilizes neurologic function in approximately 90% of patients. Median survival, as stated previously, is more than doubled for patients receiving postoperative radiation therapy when compared with patients treated with supportive therapy after surgery.

Whole-brain radiation therapy is no longer considered mandatory for high-grade gliomas [12]. Studies have demonstrated that tumor extent as determined by CT scan correlates well with the pathologic extent of glioblastomas at autopsy, with a margin of 2 cm. Conventional radiation therapy now, therefore, includes the tumor and a 2- to 3-cm margin around the limits of peritumoral edema, as demonstrated by CT scan or MR image, in the radiation field. This approach minimizes damage to the adjacent normal parenchyma.

Studies have determined that the optimal dosing schedule for patients with high-grade gliomas is a total dose of approximately 6000 rad delivered in 172- to 200-rad fractions [4,10]. Larger total doses or the same total dose delivered in fewer, larger fractions results in an unacceptably high incidence of radionecrosis, a progressive late effect of radiation that begins from months to several years after radiation therapy and that results from damage to slowly dividing oligodendroglia and endothelia. Fewer fractions with larger fractionated doses also potentiate the acute effects of radiation—cerebral edema, scalp and cranial soft tissue irritation, and hair losses. Hyperfractionation, the use of two to three daily fractions that are smaller than conventional fractions, has not been shown to improve survival when compared with the use of conventional daily fractionation.

Adjuvant Chemotherapy

In contrast to radiation therapy, no standard chemotherapeutic regimen has been established for the treatment of high-grade gliomas.

The nitrosoureas—bischloroethylnitrosourea (BCNU), lomustine, and semustine—are highly lipophilic chemotherapeutic agents specifically synthesized with characteristics to maximize blood–brain barrier penetration and are the drugs most frequently used. However, virtually every chemotherapeutic drug used to treat systemic malignancies has also been used to treat high-grade gliomas, either as a single agent or in combination [13]. Drugs have been delivered by bolus or continuous intravenous infusion, by intra-arterial bolus, and by direct topical application to tumor.

Chemotherapy is typically administered as adjuvant treatment after surgery either during radiation therapy or after the completion of radiation therapy. A survival benefit from adjuvant chemotherapy for patients with high-grade gliomas has not been unequivocally demonstrated. Studies comparing single-agent or combination chemotherapy in addition to radiation therapy with the use of radiation therapy alone have shown either a limited beneficial effect or no beneficial effect of chemotherapy [4,5,10]. A recent meta-analysis of 16 large prospective randomized chemotherapeutic trials for high-grade gliomas involving more than 3000 patients compared the survival rates of patients who received radiation therapy alone with those who received radiation therapy and adjuvant chemotherapy [14]. Median survival in patients treated with radiation therapy alone was 9.4 months and 12.6 months in patients treated with radiation therapy and adjuvant chemotherapy. The authors concluded that "chemotherapy is advantageous for patients with malignant gliomas." However, questions concerning which subgroup of patients will benefit the most from chemotherapy, which chemotherapeutic agent or agents are most effective, and what route of drug delivery is best remain unanswered and the value of adjuvant chemotherapy remains unclear.

Important arguments against the use of adjuvant chemotherapy can be made. Adjuvant chemotherapy, as noted previously, is administered either concurrent with radiation therapy or after the completion of radiation therapy. Radiation therapy, in the process of reducing tumor volume, actively destroys the vascular supply to much of the tumor bed. Drug delivery to the tumor, which is already impaired by the presence of the blood–brain barrier, is further limited. Because most chemotherapeutic agents are given as a bolus infusion and many have short half-lives, the possibility of delivering therapeutic concentrations of chemotherapy to the tumor is markedly decreased in the setting of the atretic vascular supply produced by radiation therapy. Laboratory studies have demonstrated that sublethal doses of chemotherapeutic agents accelerate the development of resistant cell lines in culture, and therefore the use of adjuvant chemotherapy during or after radiation therapy potentially promotes tumor resistance to chemotherapy. In addition, radiation therapy reduces the growth fraction—the percentage of cells either synthesizing DNA or actively cycling—of high-grade gliomas. Because almost all chemotherapeutic agents are effective at killing only dividing, or soon to be dividing, cells and because the growth fraction of high-grade gliomas is low before treatment begins, radiation therapy decreases the already limited effectiveness of chemotherapeutic agents when it is delivered before or during chemotherapy.

A promising and innovative chemotherapeutic strategy designed to minimize the inherent limitations of drug delivery to glial tumors and to circumvent the potential problems of chemotherapy when used as adjuvant treatment has been developed by investigators at the Pittsburgh Cancer Institute and the Johns Hopkins Oncology Center. This protocol administers chemotherapy—BCNU and cisplatin—as primary therapy for high-grade gliomas after surgery and before radia-

tion therapy. Patients receive three monthly cycles of chemotherapy and then are treated with a standard course of radiation therapy consisting of 6020 rad divided in 35 fractions. Each cycle of chemotherapy is delivered by continuous infusion over a 72-hour period (Fig. 1). Continuous infusion of chemotherapeutic agents provides sustained plasma drug levels, permits the drug to equilibrate more completely between plasma and interstitium, and results in a more homogeneous distribution and higher concentration of drug within the tumor. Because chemotherapy is administered "up front"— after surgery and before radiation therapy—the growth fraction of the tumor is relatively high and the vascular supply of the tumor that persists postoperatively is intact. This strategy maximizes the potential tumor response to chemotherapy and minimizes the possibility of delivering sublethal concentrations of drug to the tumor. Results of two recent studies that used this protocol demonstrated substantial short-term and long-term survival benefits in patients with high-grade gliomas when compared with historical controls treated with standard radiation therapy and adjuvant chemotherapy [15,16].

Other strategies designed to maximize drug delivery to glial neoplasms include intra-arterial chemotherapy, blood–brain barrier disruption, and topical chemotherapy. Intra-arterial administration of

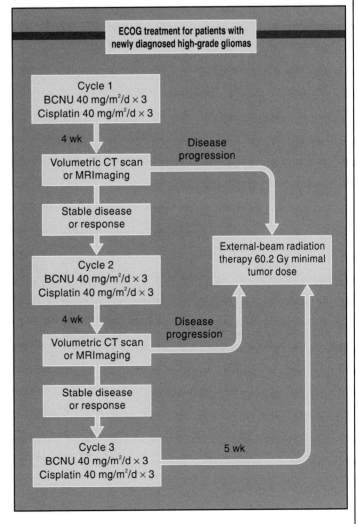

FIGURE 1

chemotherapy potentially permits increased delivery of drug to the tumor without increasing systemic toxicity. Unfortunately, local toxicities have limited the clinical usefulness of intra-arterially administered BCNU. Retinal damage and blindness have followed the administration of BCNU in the carotid artery below the ophthalmic artery, and the supraopthalmic delivery of BCNU, while reducing eye toxicity, has produced coagulative necrosis of white matter and irreversible encephalopathy. A BTSG phase III trial comparing intra-arterial BCNU with intravenous bolus BCNU also showed a lack of efficacy in patients treated with intra-arterial BCNU [17]. The major limitations of intra-arterial chemotherapy may be related to a fluid-dynamic phenomenon called streaming—essentially, unequal arterial mixing of drug with plasma—that results in a markedly heterogeneous distribution and delivery of drug. The development of new superselective arterial catheters may overcome this limitation by generating a more homogeneous arterial distribution of drug. The clinical effectiveness of intra-arterial chemotherapy is yet to be demonstrated, however. Similarly, blood–brain barrier disruption and topical chemotherapy delivery by means of negatively charged liposomes or bioerodible polymers, while theoretically promising, have not proved to be of clinical benefit.

Brachytherapy

Brachytherapy is the stereotactic implantation of radiation sources, usually iodine 125 or iridium 192, in a tumor for 4 to 6 days. This technique provides a local "boost" in the dose of radiation that can be delivered to the tumor beyond conventional radiation therapy while sparing surrounding parenchyma. Brachytherapy can be delivered "up front"—after the completion of conventional radiation therapy—or at the time of tumor recurrence. While some recent studies have shown a clinical benefit in patients with high-grade gliomas treated with brachytherapy, demonstration that brachytherapy is a clinically useful adjunct therapy awaits confirmation in larger randomized trials [18].

Biologic Therapy

Immunotherapy and gene therapy are potential biologic therapies for patients with high-grade gliomas. Lymphokine-activated killer (LAK) cells will lyse autologous high-grade glioma cells in culture, but a recent clinical study of intratumoral LAK cell therapy in human gliomas was terminated early because of neurotoxicity and minimal efficacy [19]. *In vivo* retroviral-mediated gene transfer of the herpes simplex thymidine kinase gene into rat gliomas and subsequent treatment with gancyclovir has produced a 77% cure rate in an animal model [20]. A clinical trial of gene therapy in patients with high-grade gliomas that involves the use of retroviral-mediated gene transfer is presently being conducted at the National Institutes of Health. Although not yet of demonstrated clinical benefit, immunotherapy and gene therapy offer great promise for the treatment of gliomas.

THERAPY FOR LOW-GRADE GLIOMAS

Considerable controversy exists concerning the management of low-grade gliomas [21]. Most patients with low-grade gliomas present with a transient neurologic event, usually a seizure, and have a normal neurologic examination. The tumor is detected on a brain CT scan or on MR imaging as a nonenhancing mass lesion with little or no mass effect. The issue of when to perform a biopsy or resect the mass has not been settled. Some studies have shown that deferring diagnosis and delaying therapy until the tumor progresses does not shorten survival length, but other investigators recommend immediate diagnosis [21,22]. A diagnosis may be pursued by biopsy or resection. Several studies have shown that survival is increased in patients undergoing "complete" resection when compared with patients undergoing subtotal resection. No studies to date have randomly assigned patients to receive biopsy or resection, however, and therefore the impact of the timing and extent of surgery on the natural history of low-grade gliomas remains unanswered.

There is no agreement either on the timing of radiation therapy. Some investigators favor immediate radiation therapy, especially for patients undergoing partial resection, whereas others recommend deferring radiation therapy in patients with low-grade gliomas, especially in view of the risk for delayed radionecrosis. The timing of radiation therapy in the treatment of low-grade gliomas is currently the subject of a national protocol being conducted by the BTSG and the Southwest Oncology Group (SWOG).

Given the lack of consensus regarding the management of patients with low-grade gliomas, the timing of diagnosis and therapy must be made by the patient's physician on the basis of the clinical impression. If a diagnosis is deferred, regular neurologic examinations and neuroimaging studies are required. If a diagnosis is pursued, the patient may be a candidate for entry into the national protocol, which is designed to determine the appropriate timing of radiation therapy for patients with low-grade gliomas.

THERAPY FOR REGIONAL AND ADVANCED DISEASE

High-grade gliomas, as noted earlier, rarely metastasize and the concepts of regional and advanced disease cannot be applied to gliomas as they can to other systemic malignancies. Essentially, all high-grade gliomas recur, however, and most low-grade gliomas progress. Unfortunately, the management of recurrent or progressive disease is hampered by the lack of uniformity in the initial treatment of gliomas. Patients with recurrent disease may or may not have undergone tumor debulking, may or may not have received chemotherapy, and may or may not have been treated with brachytherapy. Developing well-controlled, randomized treatment trials of patients with recurrent glial neoplasms is made difficult by such variability and the management of these patients often, of necessity, becomes individualized.

REFERENCES

1. Mahaley MS, Mettlin C, Natarajan N, *et al.*: National survey of patterns of care for brain-tumor patients. *J Neurosurg* 1989, 71:826–836.

2. Ron E, Modan B, Boice JD, *et al.*: Tumors of the brain and nervous system after radiotherapy in childhood. *N Engl J Med* 1988, 319:1033–1040.

3. Frankel RH, Bayona W, Koslow M, *et al.*: p53 Mutations in human malignant gliomas: Comparison of loss of heterozygosity with mutation frequency. *Cancer Res* 1992, 52:1427–1433.

4. Walker MD, Alexander E, Munt WE, *et al.*: Evaluation of BCNU and/or radiotherapy in treatment of anaplastic gliomas. *J Neurosurg* 1978, 49:333–343.

5. Chang CH, Horton J, Schoenfield D, *et al.*: Comparison of postoperative radiotherapy and combined postoperative radiotherapy and chemotherapy in the multidisciplinary management of malignant gliomas. *Cancer* 1983, 52:997–1007.

6. Burger PC, Vogel FS, Green SB, *et al.*: Glioblastoma multiforme and anaplastic astrocytoma: Pathologic criteria and prognostic implications. *Cancer* 1985, 56:1106–1111.

7. Zülch KJ: *Histologic Type of Tumours of the Central Nervous System.* Geneva: World Health Organization, 1979, pp. 17–57.

8. Rubenstein LJ: Tumors of the central nervous system. In *Atlas of Tumor Pathology*, Series 2, Fasicle G. Washington, DC: Armed Forces Institute of Pathology, 1972.

9. Kernohan JW, Moborn RF, Svien HJ, *et al.*: A simplified classification of gliomas. *Proc Staff Meet Mayo Clin* 1949, 24:71–75.

10. Walker MD, Green SB, Byar DP, *et al.*: Randomized comparisons of radiotherapy and nitrosoureas for the treatment of malignant glioma after surgery. *N Engl J Med* 1980, 303:1323–1329.

11. Levin JM, Schiff D, Loeffler JS, *et al.*: Complications of therapy for venous thromboembolic disease in patients with brain tumors. *Neurology* 1993, 43:1111–1114.

12. Marks JE: Ionizing radiation. *Neurobiol Brain Tumor* 1991, pp. 299–319.

13. Kornblith PL, Walker M: Chemotherapy for malignant gliomas. *J Neurosurg* 1988, 68:1–17.

14. Fine HA, Dear KB, Loeffler JS, *et al.*: Meta-analysis of radiation therapy with and without adjuvant chemotherapy for malignant gliomas in adults. *Cancer* 1993, 71:2585–2597.

15. Gilbert MR, Lunsford LD, Kondziolka D, *et al.*: A phase II trial of continuous infusion chemotherapy, external beam radiotherapy and local boost radiotherapy. *Proc ASCO* 1993, 12:176.

16. Grossman SA, Sheidler VR, Ahn H, *et al.*: Complete and partial response of newly diagnosed malignant astrocytomas following continuous infusion of BCNU and cisplatin. *Proc ASCO* 1989, 8:344.

17. Shapiro WR, Green SB, Burger PC, *et al.*: A randomized comparison of intra-arterial (IA) versus intravenous BCNU for patients with malignant gliomas: Interim analysis demonstrating lack of efficacy for IA BCNU. *Proc ASCO* 1987, 6:69.

18. Larsen DA, Gutin PH, Leibel SA, *et al.*: Stereotaxic irradiation of brain tumors. *Cancer* 1990, 65:792–799.

19. Barba D, Saris SC, Holder C, *et al.*: Intratumoral LAK cell and interleukin-2 therapy of human gliomas. *J Neurosurg* 1989, 70:175–182.

20. Ram Z, Culver KW, Walbridge S, *et al.*: *In situ* retroviral-mediated gene transfer for the treatment of brain tumors in rats. *Cancer Res* 1993, 53:83–88.

21. Recht LD, Lew R, Smith TW: Suspected low-grade glioma: Is deferring treatment safe? *Ann Neurol* 1992, 31:431–436.

22. Shapiro WR: Low-grade gliomas: When to treat? *Ann Neurol* 1992, 31:437–438.

BCNU AND CISPLATIN

An ECOG phase II study of continuous-infusion BCNU and cisplatin with external-beam radiation therapy for the treatment of patients with newly diagnosed glioblastoma multiforme is being conducted to establish the feasibility of a continuous-infusion chemotherapy regimen in a multicenter trial. This trial serves as a prelude to a planned phase III study comparing this continuous-infusion regimen with standard treatment. The response rates and toxicities of three cycles of BCNU and cisplatin therapy in patients with glioblastomas are being evaluated to estimate the proportion of patients who survive for 1 year after the institution of therapy.

The role of "adjuvant" chemotherapy—chemotherapy delivered during or after the completion of radiation therapy—is of uncertain benefit in prolonging survival in patients with glioblastoma multiforme. The use of "upfront" continuous-infusion chemotherapy maximizes the potential tumor response to chemotherapy by improving drug delivery to the tumor.

DOSAGE, SCHEDULING, AND RESPONSE RATES

Study	Evaluable Patients, n	Dosage and Scheduling	Complete Response	Partial Response	Stable Disease	Progressive Disease
Phase II, Pittsburgh Cancer Institute	52	BCNU 40 mg/m²/d × 3 Cisplatin 40 mg/m²/d × 3 for 3 monthly cycles	8 (15%)	33 (64%)	9 (17%)	2 (4%)

CANDIDATES FOR TREATMENT
Patients ≥ 18 years with histologically confirmed supratentorial glioblastoma multiforme, no other malignancy, and no prior therapy

SPECIAL PRECAUTIONS
Patients with WBC count < 4000, platelets < 150,000, creatinine > 1.6, bilirubin > 2.0

ALTERNATIVE THERAPIES
NCI phase III study of radiation therapy alone versus radiation therapy/bromodeoxyuridine followed by PCV in patients with anaplastic astrocytomas; NCI phase III trial of eflornithine plus PCV versus PCV alone in patients with malignant gliomas who have received radiation therapy; NCI phase II study of COP and radiation therapy in patients with subtotal resection of high-grade gliomas; standard radiation therapy and adjuvant BCNU

TOXICITIES
Leukopenia and thrombocytopenia (25–60 d, possibly cumulative); anemia; nausea and vomiting; reversible elevations of aspartate aminotransferase, alanine aminotransferase, bilirubin, elevated serum creatinine and BUN; **BCNU:** pulmonary infiltrates and/or fibrosis, especially with prolonged therapy and higher doses (do not exceed cumulative dose of 1400 mg/m²); hypotension from rapid or concentrated infusion; burning at injection site; facial flushing; **cisplatin:** nephrotoxicity (dose related, relatively uncommon with adequate hydration and diuresis); peripheral neuropathy (common and dose limiting when cumulative dose exceeds 400 mg/m²); seizures (rare); ototoxicity, manifested initially by high-frequency hearing loss (common); coronary vasospasm (rare); hypomagnesemia; hypocalcemia; hyponatremia; vein irritation; fatigue; anaphylaxis (rare)

DRUG INTERACTIONS
BCNU: polyvinyl chloride infusion bags and sodium bicarbonate; **cisplatin:** aluminum

NURSING INTERVENTIONS
Assess lab results prior to therapy—patients may require potassium and magnesium supplements; assess urine output prior to each dose, maintain hydration, monitor intake and output (100–150 ml/hr), order diuretics; premedicate with antiemetics; avoid skin contact with BCNU; assess for burning at IV site, stomatitis, signs of anaphylaxis and neurotoxicity; monitor CBC, liver and renal function tests

PATIENT INFORMATION
Patient will experience 100% asymptomatic high-frequency hearing loss (20% have symptomatic hearing loss); blood/platelet transfusion may be required during treatment; nausea/vomiting and peripheral neuropathy usually improve after completion of treatment

The endocrine cancers comprise a rare and diverse group of neoplasms. Endocrine tumors cannot reliably be diagnosed as benign or malignant neoplasms from histologic criteria. Patients with presumed benign endocrine tumors, therefore, must be followed clinically for evidence of recurrence. Therapeutic regimens differ widely and in most cases are not yet standard. The most commonly used regimens for some of the most frequently or urgently occurring neoplasms are presented in this chapter.

ADRENAL CORTICAL CARCINOMA

ETIOLOGY AND RISK FACTORS

The incidence of adrenal cortical carcinoma (ACC) in the United States is about 2 persons in every million. Except for a very rare association with certain inherited tumor syndromes (such as multiple endocrine neoplasia, type I) the risk factors and etiology of ACC are unknown. There is a bimodal age distribution, with peak incidence in young children and in people between 40 and 60. Patients with ACC present with symptoms related to steroid hormone excess or an enlarging abdominal mass (Table 1).

The endocrinologic evaluation of functional ACC begins with documentation of steroid hormone synthesis and exclusion of pituitary and ectopic sources. Aldosterone-secreting ACC does occur but is exceedingly rare.

In this age of radiologic imaging, clinically silent adrenal "incidentalomas" are identified with increasing frequency. The vast majority of these are benign adenomas. The strategy of Ross and Aron for hormonal evaluation of the patient with an incidentally discovered adrenal mass is efficient and careful [1]. Because subclinical cortisol production can lead to postoperative adrenocortical insufficiency in half such patients, testing is recommended in patients with adrenal incidentalomas [2]. Initial reports from the National Cancer Institute have suggested that magnetic resonance (MR) imaging may be helpful in distinguishing benign adenomas from ACC, pheochromocytoma, or metastases to the adrenal gland based on relative brightness of the T_2-weighted scan [3]. This technique is still experimental. Pheochromocytomas can secrete ACTH, mimicking adrenal cortical cancer. Biochemical screening to exclude pheochromocytoma is obligatory before any needle biopsy or surgery for an adrenal mass that otherwise might precipitate a fatal hypertensive crisis.

STAGING AND PROGNOSIS

The most important factor in staging is tumor size at presentation (Table 2). Although fewer than one in 10,000 adrenal lesions less than 6 cm in size represents ACC, the risk that a 6-cm lesion is malignant is 35 to 98% higher [1]. We currently recommend excision of all nonfunctional adrenal masses greater than 5.0 cm, with close follow-up of lesions 3.5 to 5 cm in size. Clinically functional tumors are resected regardless of size. The hypercortisolism of Cushing's syndrome is itself a seriously morbid condition with a 5-year survival of only 50%, primarily due to infection and stroke.

Prognosis in ACC is related to disease stage and treatment. In recent studies, there has been an overall median survival of 2 years, with 5-year survival rates of 22 to 30% and 10-year survival rates of 10%. As many as 70% of patients present with Stage II to IV disease. Patients with Stage IV disease have a median survival of 11 to 14 months. Patients with anaplastic ACC have a median survival of 5 months. Recent studies document no significant sex- or age-related differences in prognosis.

In addition to tumor size (> 100 g) other factors associated with poor prognosis are vascular invasion, mitotic rate, and necrosis. Factors of limited significance include ploidy, capsular invasion, known immunohistochemical stains, and functional status of the tumor.

PRIMARY DISEASE THERAPY

Because ACC spreads early by local and often silent extension, surgical resection offers the only realistic chance of cure. Somewhat less than one half of patients are resectable at presentation. The goal of initial surgery is *en bloc* resection, which may involve adjacent viscera, vena cava, or diaphragm. Wide resection can be properly accomplished only through an abdominal incision. If the tumor is entered at surgery, seeding of the operative cavity can progress rapidly, with fatal results. Steroid hormone replacement, prophylaxis for deep venous thrombosis, and prevention of infection are required perioperatively. Complete recovery of the hypothalamic–pituitary axis may take up to 2 years after surgery [4]. Slow to resolve depression can be a significant feature of convalescence. Patients with resected Stage I to II disease have a mean survival of 5 years, and patients with invasion of contiguous structures, a mean survival of 2.3 years.

Table 1. Presenting Clinical Features of Adrenal Cortical Carcinoma

Symptom	Rate (%)
Cushing's syndrome	40–60
Virilization or feminization	10–20
Hypertension and hypokalemia	1
Abdominal symptoms only	30

Table 2. Staging Criteria for Adrenal Cortical Carcinoma

	Stage			
	I	II	III	IV
TNM Components	T1, N0, M0	T2, N0, M0	T1 or T2, N1, M0 or T3, N0, M0	Any T, any N, M1 or T3–T4, N1

Criteria
T1—Tumor ≤ 5 cm, no invasion
T2—Tumor > 5 cm, no invasion
T2—Tumor outside adrenal fat
T4—Tumor invading adjacent viscera
N0—No involved lymph nodes
N1—Positive lymph nodes
M0—No distant disease
M1—Distant disease

Adapted from Norton et al. [3]; with permission.

ADJUVANT THERAPY FOR REGIONAL DISEASE

Although surgical resection can be curative, the great majority of patients recur, with a median disease-free interval of 3 to 12 months. The disease-free interval was a significant prognostic factor in a recent report from the National Cancer Institute on efficacy of aggressive re-resection for select patients with recurrent or metastatic disease [5]. In this nonrandomized study, 15 patients treated with chemotherapy alone had a median survival from first recurrence of 11 months, whereas 18 patients whose recurrent disease was resected with intent to cure, plus chemotherapy, had a median survival of 27 months. One third of the operated patients survived more than 5 years from initial re-resection. Pulmonary metastasectomy, wide resection of involved viscera, and in some cases multiple reoperations were employed. Because of the design, this study may suggest only that patients who live long enough for aggressive re-resection may do better. In patients being followed for recurrence or progression of ACC it is useful to follow urine steroid profiles, as well as serial chest and abdominal computed tomographic (CT) scan and bone scan. Because of their toxicities, adjuvant therapies for ACC are generally reserved for patients with inoperable and/or metastatic disease.

THERAPY FOR ADVANCED DISEASE

ACC metastasizes to lung (71%), liver (42%), and bone (26%). Palliative debulking of ACC has not been shown to have a survival benefit but significantly improves quality of life for many patients. Chemotherapy for ACC has been largely ineffective, with most responses anecdotal and with no clear efficacy or documented benefit. Duration of response in all series has been short. The single agent with the most activity appears to be cisplatin (Table 3). The pesticide analogue mitotane has been used for years because of its ability to cause infarction of adrenal tissues, albeit on an inconsistent basis. Mitotane is poorly tolerated and has not been studied in a controlled setting. Although there are isolated reports of long-term survivors, most of the 20 to 30% of patients who respond to mitotane have a partial response of short duration. External beam radiotherapy is ineffective except in the management of painful bony metastases.

The combination of cisplatin and etoposide, with or without bleomycin, appears to have promise. A Southwest Oncology Group study using cisplatin, etoposide, and mitotane in patients with

metastatic ACC is ongoing. Other agents under investigation include suramin (an inhibitor of reverse transcriptase) and gossypol (a mitochondrial uncoupler found in cottonseed oil), but responses have been limited. There is currently no information about immunotherapeutic strategies for metastatic ACC.

THYROID CANCER

ETIOLOGY AND RISK FACTORS

Thyroid cancer usually presents as a thyroid nodule. Thyroid nodules are quite common (4–7% of the population), but only 10% of solid nodules are malignant. Currently there are 12,400 new cases of thyroid cancer diagnosed yearly in the United States (73% are in women). There is a vast amount of subclinical disease; the challenge is early identification of those patients at highest risk.

Important clinical factors that increase the likelihood of malignancy include growth on TSH suppressive therapy, patient age (< 20 or > 50), residence in an iodine-deficient geographic area, and history of thyroiditis, goiter, or head and neck irradiation. Worrisome, but nonspecific clinical features include neck pain, dyspnea, dysphagia, hoarseness, and cervical adenopathy. Although, prior exposure to head and neck radiation is an etiologic factor in the development of papillary thyroid cancer, it is not a prognostic factor in its outcome. The thyroid gland is quite sensitive to ionizing radiation and there is a linear dose-response relation up to 2000 cGy; at higher doses, the incidence of thyroid cancer drops off as thyroid cells are killed. Papillary thyroid cancer occasionally occurs as a feature of inherited tumor syndromes (eg, Gardner's syndrome, familial polyposis coli).

The chances of accurately diagnosing cancer in a thyroid nodule have been at least doubled by the advent of fine needle aspiration biopsy (FNA). With FNA, thyroid scans are now largely unnecessary and the annual number of thyroidectomies is half of what it was formerly. Patients with cytologic indications of malignancy undergo thyroidectomy. Patients with benign-appearing FNA cytology are observed, generally on exogenous L-thyroxine at a dose sufficient to suppress TSH to less than 0.4 mIU/ml. When this strategy is used, the incidence of thyroid cancer in operated nonresponders to suppression is 20 to 40%. FNA currently cannot reliably distinguish between follicular adenoma and follicular thyroid cancer; patients with indeterminate follicular lesions, therefore, undergo thyroid lobectomy for diagnosis, which is based on the pathologic presence of vascular or capsular invasion. The rate of follicular thyroid cancer at surgery is 24% using this strategy. CT scan and MR imaging can be helpful in evaluating the degree of tracheal deviation and compression, extension into the mediastinum, and carotid artery involvement by tumor.

STAGING AND PROGNOSIS

Mortality from thyroid cancer accounts for more than 1100 deaths a year in the United States. The most important factors in staging of thyroid cancer are age and cell type. The staging system is given in Table 4.

There are four primary cell types of thyroid cancer. Papillary (75% of patients) and follicular (10–15% of patients) thyroid cancers arise from thyroid follicular cells and, together with their poorer prognostic variants, Hürthle cell, tall-cell, insular, and diffuse sclerosing papillary cancer, are termed *well-differentiated thyroid cancer*. Mixed

Table 3. Chemotherapy for Advanced Adrenal Cortical Cancer

Study	Agents	Response Rate
Decker et al. [12]	Mitotane, doxorubicin	19% = 3/16 PR
van Slooten et al. [7]	Cisplatin, doxorubicin, cyclophosphamide	18% = 2/11 PR
Schlumberger et al. [11]	Cisplatin, doxorubicin, 5-FU	23% =1/13 CR, 2/13 PR
Bukowski et al. [6]	Mitotane, cisplatin	30% = 1/37 CR, 10/37 PR
Johnson et al. [8]	Cisplatin, etoposide	2/2 PR
Hesketh et al. [9]	Cisplatin, etoposide, bleomycin	1/4 CR, 2/4 PR
Berruti et al. [10]	Cisplatin, etoposide, doxorubicin	2/2 PR

CR—complete remission; PR—partial remission.

papillary–follicular cancer is classified as papillary thyroid cancer because its behavior and prognosis are similar to that histology. Prognosis for well-differentiated thyroid cancer is related primarily to risk group, although papillary histologies have a slightly better prognosis than do the follicular cell types. Several widely used systems for determining risk have been developed based on multivariate analysis (AMES, AGES, MACIS). All systems agree that the most important single factor in predicting survival is age at presentation. Tumor invasion, size of primary tumor, and presence of distant metastases are also significant factors. Nuclear DNA content has also been cited as an important prognostic variable [13]. Table 5 presents the most recent scoring system for papillary thyroid cancer [14]. The prognostic significance of cervical lymph node involvement is controversial; some studies have even reported a univariate survival advantage with local nodal metastases. In general, the presence of cervical metastases is a predictor of local recurrence, but has been shown in many studies not to influence survival. The validity of female sex as a favorable prognostic factor is still controversial.

Isolated papillary lesions less than 1 cm in size represent papillary microcarcinomas and occur in 10% of persons in autopsy series. After thyroid lobectomy is performed, these require no treatment other than expectant follow-up. Follicular cancers today are increasingly uncommon except in iodine-deficient geographic areas. The absence of vascular or capsular invasion marks a benign follicular adenoma. Follicular cancer with capsular invasion alone may have a better prognosis. The relatively uncommon Hürthle cell variant is staged with the other well-differentiated cancers, but may in some cases metastasize earlier to lymph nodes, lung, and bone.

Medullary thyroid cancer (5–10% of patients) arises from the neuroendocrine parafollicular C cells, which secrete calcitonin as part of the amine precursor uptake and decarboxylation system. The decarboxylation serum level of calcitonin can thus serve as a biochemical marker for this disease. Medullary thyroid cancer appears in four unique clinical settings: sporadic (80% of cases, unifocal) or inherited in association with multiple endocrine neoplasia, type IIa, multiple endocrine neoplasia, type IIb, or familial medullary thyroid cancer. The three inherited forms arise from precursor C-cell hyperplasia and can thus be multifocal. Medullary thyroid cancer can present either as a clinical thyroid nodule or as occult disease detected by provocative pentagastrin-stimulated screening in a patient at risk for an inherited form. In the first case, confirmation of the diagnosis by FNA requires immunoreactive staining for calcitonin. Sixty percent of patients with palpable medullary thyroid cancer already have metastases (lymph nodes, liver, lung, bone, abdominal viscera), but the only symptom of high levels of calcitonin may be clinically significant diarrhea. Elevated levels of serum CEA are thought to define a subpopulation of patients who have aggressive metastatic disease and a poorer prognosis.

Anaplastic thyroid cancer (2% of patients) is a highly malignant tumor arising from thyroid epithelium and in some cases from pre-existing well-differentiated thyroid cancer or longstanding goiter. With earlier and more effective treatment of differentiated thyroid cancer, the incidence of anaplastic cancer has dropped dramatically over the past 50 years. A great many "anaplastic" thyroid cancers of years gone by were actually primary thyroid lymphomas. The distinction is made today by immunohistochemistry and flow cytometry and is crucial to prognosis (Table 6) and management. One third to one half of cases of non-Hodgkin's lymphoma of the thyroid gland occur in the setting of pre-existing Hashimoto's thyroiditis.

PRIMARY DISEASE THERAPY

Primary treatment of thyroid cancer is based on histologic type and for papillary and follicular neoplasms is surgical. The extent of surgery has been controversial [15,16], but at present there is a

Table 4. Staging of Thyroid Cancers

Primary Tumor (T)	Nodal Involvement	Metastases
T1—Diameter ≤ 3 cm	NN—Cannot be assessed	MN—Not assessed
T2—Diameter > 3 cm	N0—No involved nodes	M0—No known metastases
T3—Multiple intraglandular tumor foci	N1—Clinically or pathologically positive nodes	M1—Distant metastases
T4—Fixation or direct invasion		

Cancer Type/Stage	< 45 yr	> 45 yr
Papillary/Follicular		
I	Any T, any N, M0	Any T, N0, M0, T1, N1, M0
II	Any T, any N, M1	Papillary T2-4, N1, M0/follicular T2-4, N1, M0
III	None	Papillary none/follicular any T,N1, M0
IV	None	Any T, any N, M1
Medullary		
I	None	None
II	Any T, any N, M0	None
III	None	Any T, any N, M0
IV	Any T, any N, M1	Any T, Any N, M1
Anaplastic		
I–III	None	None
IV	Any T, any N, any M	Any T, any N, any M

Adapted from Norton et al. [3]; with permission.

Table 5. MACIS Prognostic Index for Papillary Thyroid Cancer

Variable	Points Assigned
Age < 39	+ 3.1
Age > 40	+ 0.08 × age
Diameter of primary tumor	+0.3 × cm
Incomplete resection	+ 1
Extrathyroidal invasion	+ 1
Distant metastases	+ 3

MACIS Score	Metastasis at 10 yr (%)	Mortality at 20 yr (%)
< 6	3	1
6–6.9	18	13
7–7.9	40	45
8 +	60	76

Adapted from Hay et al. [14]; with permission.

clear consensus that for low-risk, well-differentiated thyroid cancer the minimum operation is a thyroid lobectomy and isthmusectomy. Total or near-total thyroidectomy should be performed for lesions greater than 1.5 cm in size and for angioinvasive follicular cancer, Hürthle cell cancer, patients over 50, or papillary cancer in association with prior neck irradiation or local invasion. A survival advantage for total thyroidectomy versus subtotal thyroidectomy or lobectomy has never been shown in a prospective randomized study, but was clearly observed in a recent large retrospective series ($P < 0.001$) for low-risk patients not treated with I^{131} [15]. Extirpative surgery also offers the significant advantage of simplifying postoperative surveillance and treatment of thyroid cancer. Occult bony and lung metastases may not be adequately seen on radioiodine scan if the patient has intact thyroid tissue. Modern risks of bilateral thyroidectomy include a 1% chance of permanent recurrent laryngeal nerve injury and a 1 to 3% chance of permanent hypoparathyroidism. These risks are demonstrably lower in the hands of expert surgeons. Neck dissection has no proven or theoretical role in primary treatment of well-differentiated thyroid cancer. Survival rates are given in Table 7.

Primary therapy for medullary cancer is surgical. Because at least 16% of inherited medullary thyroid cancer is not recognized at presentation, every patient with medullary thyroid cancer requires screening preoperatively to exclude pheochromocytoma, which if unrecognized can precipitate disastrous adrenergic crisis during operation. The operation of choice is total thyroidectomy and central node dissection. Modified or radical node dissection should be performed for palpable cervical disease. Patients with multiple endocrine neoplasia, type IIb should undergo total thyroidectomy upon diagnosis of the syndrome, as most will otherwise develop lethal medullary thyroid cancer by their second decade.

Primary therapy for anaplastic cancer is not surgical resection. Initial management entails securing the airway against further rapid growth of the tumor, accomplished by tracheostomy. Core or incisional biopsy may be required to definitively exclude lymphoma. Further surgery only delays the urgent administration of radiation and chemotherapy needed to forestall death from asphyxiation. Primary therapy for thyroid lymphoma is external radiation or combination chemotherapy, depending on stage (*see* the chapter on non-Hodgkin's lymphoma).

ADJUVANT THERAPY FOR REGIONAL DISEASE

Subsequent to surgery, well-differentiated thyroid cancer is treated with hormonal therapy and radioactive iodine, monitoring thyroglobulin levels during the course of therapy (Table 8). All patients with thyroid cancer, regardless of risk status, should receive exogenous L-thyroxine suppressive therapy; considerable indirect evidence demonstrates that long-term TSH suppressive therapy favorably influences tumor recurrence, disease progression, and survival in well-differentiated thyroid cancer. Thyroglobulin is secreted by normal and cancerous thyroid cells and serves as a useful tumor marker for thyroid cancer persistence, recurrence, and progression. The sensitivity of this method is greatest when the patient is hypothyroid with high TSH levels [16]. A poorly differentiated cancer may still secrete thyroglobulin after its iodine-concentrating ability has been lost. A long-awaited new commercial assay (Nichols Institute) excludes the confounding nature of serum antithyroglobulin antibodies.

Normal thyroid tissue concentrates radioiodine much more efficiently than thyroid cancer. For this reason, thyroid remnants remaining after thyroidectomy are usually ablated by administration of a low dose of I^{131} to the intentionally hypothyroid patient. I^{131} (30–200 mCI) is the treatment of choice for recurrent or metastatic differentiated thyroid cancer. In a very important study of 1599 patients with well-differentiated thyroid cancer treated at the M.D. Anderson Cancer Center, radioactive iodine therapy significantly increased both disease-free interval and survival rates ($P < 0.001$) [15].

Differentiated thyroid cancer that has lost affinity for radioiodine can still be successfully treated with large doses; 30 to 90% of patients with detectable thyroglobulin levels and a negative low-dose radioio-

Table 6. Prognosis for Medullary Thyroid Cancer, Anaplastic Thyroid Cancer, and Thyroid Cancer

Thyroid Cancer Subtype	Associated Endocrinopathies	15-yr Survival (%)
Medullary		
Sporadic	None	70–80
MEN-IIa	Pheochromocytoma, parathyroid hyperplasia	85–90
MEN-IIb	Pheochromocytoma, mucosal neuromas	< 40–50
FMCT	None	100%
Anaplastic	None	4–6 mo median survival
Thyroid lymphoma	None	51 at 10-yr survival

FMCT—familial medullary thyroid cancer; MEN-IIa and MEN-IIb—multiple endocrine neoplasia, types IIa and IIb.

Table 7. Survival Rates for Papillary and Follicular Thyroid Cancer

	5 yr (%)	10 yr (%)	Distant Metastases at Presentation (%)
Papillary	95	92	20
Follicular	82	70	18

Table 8. Adjuvant Management of Well-differentiated Thyroid Cancer

1. Postoperative withdrawal of L-thyroxine for 6 wk; administration of tri-iodothyronine (25–50 µg BID-TID) for first 4 wk. (Pregnancy should be prevented during this period.)

2. When TSH is < 35 mIU/ml, obtain I^{131} scan and serum thyroglobulin level.

3. If, after total thyroidectomy, thyroid remnants or metastases are detected, or thyroglobulin level is > 10 mg/dl, administer calculated ablative/therapeutic dose of I^{131}, with post-therapy whole-body scan.

4. Begin/resume long-term L-thyroxine replacement to completely suppress TSH to < 0.1 mIU/ml.

5. Repeat hypothyroid I^{131} scan, thyroglobulin monitoring and radiotherapy every 6–12 mo until normal, then every 3–5 yr (or until total I^{131} dose of 500–800 mCi).

dine scan who are treated with I[131] have uptake on their posttherapy scan. A treatment dose of 150 cGy delivers about 1000 cGy to the lesion. The risks of I[131] include temporary local pain, swelling, and nausea in up to a third of patients, rare myelotoxicity, and very rare leukemia and bladder cancer. Radioiodine is not taken up by Hürthle cell, papillary tall-cell, medullary, or most anaplastic thyroid cancers. I[131] is the most effective therapy for pulmonary metastases and offers effective palliation, although a low cure rate (7%), for bony metastases of thyroid cancer. Thyroid cancers that do not respond to radioiodine therapy are treated as advanced disease. Resection of recurrent regional disease offers no proven or theoretical advantage over I[131], except perhaps in the management of direct tracheal invasion [17]. External radiation therapy is reserved for palliation of bony metastases or for cases in which radioiodine is not taken up by the tumor. For locally advanced thyroid cancer Kim and Leeper observed successful local control in 84% of patients treated with low-dose doxorubicin and hyperfractionated radiotherapy, but no improvement in distant disease or in survival [18].

Treatment selection for regional medullary thyroid cancer is based upon the indolent growth of most tumors. Basal and stimulated calcitonin levels and serum CEA are followed postoperatively as an indicators of recurrence and/or progression. With close surveillance and early reoperation, survival rates as high as 86% have been reported [19]. Most experts recommend resection of clinically or radiologically evident disease, but a minority advocates aggressive search for residual medullary thyroid cancer using invasive imaging techniques, followed by comprehensive resection in an attempt to obtain a biochemical cure [20]. Medullary thyroid cancer is insensitive to I[131] and external radiotherapy.

THERAPY FOR ADVANCED DISEASE

The fact that mortality rates for thyroid cancer have not changed over the years probably reflects improved management of primary disease rather than progress in treatment of relapsed and metastatic thyroid cancer. In 33 to 42% of patients, metastatic disease does not take up radioiodine, and these patients have significantly decreased survival rates (83% versus < 1% at 10 years). The single most active chemotherapeutic agent to date is doxorubicin, which when given alone at doses up to 75 mg/m² produces a 17 to 33% response rate in metastatic nonmedullary thyroid cancer. Responses are partial and of moderate duration (2 yr); most patients die of lung (80%) and/or brain (20%) metastases. The combination of doxorubicin with other agents such as cisplatin or bleomycin has not improved efficacy. Shimoaka did report an increased response rate with combination doxorubicin and cisplatin [21], but other groups were unable to detect an advantage. Although there is much indirect evidence that autoimmune mechanisms may favorably influence the outcome of patients with metastatic thyroid cancer, no trials employing biologic response modifiers have been reported.

If feasible, surgical resection of recurrent medullary thyroid cancer is indicated even for advanced disease. Chemotherapy in advanced medullary thyroid cancer is generally reserved until the development of debilitating diarrhea, which is the main symptom of advanced disease, occurring with calcitonin levels greater than 10,000 pg/ml. Doxorubicin alone or in combination has the highest response rate (30–46%), with mean duration of response 21 months, and no documented survival benefit. Octreotide therapy has produced palliation of symptoms and objective biochemical responses in several recent small studies; however, dose escalation was usually required to main-

tain the effect. Interferon alpha may provide similar palliative benefit to octreotide for advanced medullary thyroid cancer.

Anaplastic thyroid cancer is Stage IV disease by definition (Table 5). Systemic chemotherapy has made no impact on the dismal prognosis. After the diagnosis is made and the airway secured, treatment is focused on local tumor control in the neck. A protocol employing low-dose doxorubicin as a radiosensitizer for hyperfractionated external radiotherapy was introduced in 1983 and has since gained momentum [22]. A subsequent study of multimodality hyperfractionated radiotherapy, surgery, and combination chemotherapy (bleomycin, cyclophosphamide, and 5-FU) provided improved local control but no survival advantage [23].

CARCINOID TUMORS

ETIOLOGY AND RISK FACTORS

Carcinoid tumors arise from neuroendocrine enterochromaffin cells and secrete the biogenic amine serotonin (5-hydroxytryptamine, 5-HT). Enterochromaffin cells secreting amines are part of the amine precursor uptake and decarboxylation system, which is characterized in part by the potential for secretion of multiple amine (and peptide) hormones. Carcinoid tumors therefore can secrete ACTH, somatostatin, alpha- and beta-HcG, gastrin, pancreatic polypeptide, and other substances, which can disguise or complicate the clinical presentation of a carcinoid tumor. Precursor enterochromaffin cells are found submucosally throughout the gastrointestinal tract, bronchial tree, and genitourinary tract, and carcinoid tumors can and do arise from any of these sites.

Carcinoid tumors occur at a reported rate of 3.2 persons per million, a number that, according to one autopsy study, far underestimates their actual incidence (6500 per million) [24]. Known etiologies include 1) an association of thymic carcinoids with multiple endocrine neoplasia, type I; 2) an association of ampullary carcinoids with von Recklinghausen's disease; and 3) an association of gastric carcinoids with hypergastrinemic states such as pernicious anemia, atrophic gastritis, gastrinoma, and chronic omeprazole administration.

Carcinoid tumors are slow-growing. Because the most common clinical presentation is intermittent abdominal pain, many carcinoids are diagnosed late or fortuitously at endoscopy or surgery performed for another reason. Median duration of symptoms prior to diagnosis is 21 months. Although half of symptomatic patients have unresectable disease at diagnosis, half of these patients go on to live 5 years or more after diagnosis. Median survival after onset of symptoms is 3.5 to 8.5 years.

Carcinoid syndrome is caused by the release of serotonin, often with histamine and tachykinins, into the systemic venous system. Symptoms include flushing, diarrhea, bronchospasm, and valvular heart disease (tricuspid regurgitation, pulmonic stenosis). The severity of carcinoid syndrome is directly related to the bulk of tumor draining into the systemic circulation and thus outside the first-pass effect of the portal circulation. The syndrome almost always occurs from foregut tumors or from liver metastases of gastrointestinal carcinoids. Rarely, carcinoid syndrome arises in patients with nonmetastatic gastrointestinal primary tumors, ovarian or testicular carcinoids, medullary thyroid cancer, or pancreatic islet tumors.

Severe symptoms present as carcinoid crisis, which can be precipitated by stress, FNA, anesthesia, or chemotherapy and which can cause intense abdominal pain, hypotension, coma, and death. Carcinoid crisis is well treated with octreotide (100 mg IV), which can also be used prophylactically prior to FNA or surgery (100 µg SQ q 8 hr).

In patients suspected to have a carcinoid tumor, the diagnosis is confirmed by measuring elevated levels of 24-hour urine serotonin and 5-HIAA (serotonin metabolite.) Measurement of platelet serotonin [25], serum chromogranin A, serotonin and substance P, and urinary 5-hydroxytryptophan (5-HTP, a serotonin precursor) can be helpful in ambiguous cases. Bronchial lavage for ACTH and thymic vein sampling are of little value in the diagnosis of bronchial carcinoid. Tumor localization is difficult, relying on endoscopy, colonoscopy, CT, and other studies as appropriate. New reports suggest that I[131] MIBG and I[123] octreotide scans may be reasonably sensitive and specific in the localization of carcinoid tumors [26].

STAGING AND PROGNOSIS

To understand their biological behavior and prognosis, carcinoid tumors can be grouped by primary location (Table 9). Foregut carcinoids usually arise in the bronchial tree as classic "coin lesions" on chest radiographs, but also include tumors of the thymus, stomach, duodenum, and pancreas. Foregut carcinoids have a low 5-HT content and often secrete other agents such as 5-HTP, histamine, or ACTH. Gastric carcinoids are commonly multifocal. Midgut carcinoids secrete 5-HT and arise from the appendix or ileum, and rarely from the jejunum or right colon. Half of appendiceal carcinoids are diagnosed at surgery for acute appendicitis (in about one in 250 acute appendectomies) and 90% are less than 1 cm in size (usually occurring at the tip). Ileal carcinoids are multiple in 25 to 35% of patients; 15% are less than 1 cm in size. Hindgut carcinoid tumors rarely secrete 5-HT. They arise from the rectum and rarely from the bladder, ovary, testis, or left colon; 80% are less than 1 cm in size. With modern clinical screening, rectal carcinoids are recognized much more frequently, typically as a small yellow submucosal nodule protruding from the anterior or lateral rectal wall.

Important prognostic factors for carcinoid tumors are site of primary tumor (Table 9), histologic subtype, size of primary tumor, and extent of tumor at presentation. Of the four histologic subtypes, insular is considered to have the best prognosis, trabecular is intermediate, and glandular and undifferentiated have the worst.

Other histologic criteria cannot be relied upon to differentiate benign from malignant neoplasms. Size of the primary tumor is indicative of malignant potential, but race, sex, age, nuclear DNA content, and function have not proven to be significant prognostic factors. The most important predictor of survival is the presence of metastases (Table 10).

PRIMARY DISEASE THERAPY

The only curative therapy for carcinoid neoplasms is surgery. The extent of surgery is determined by the size and extent of the primary tumor. Lesions of 1 cm or smaller, and without invasion, are generally amenable to simple full-thickness excision. The extent of surgery is still somewhat controversial for lesions 1 to 2 cm in size; other prognostic factors such as site and histology are commonly taken into account. Results of this treatment strategy have been reportedly curative for appendiceal and rectal carcinoids [24]. Perioperative octreotide blockade is recommended for patients with carcinoid syndrome.

THERAPY FOR REGIONAL DISEASE

In these very indolent tumors, patients whose disease recurs have a median disease-free interval of 16 years. Primary resection of involved regional lymph nodes is reportedly associated with improved survival (80% at 5 years). Resection of isolated hepatic metastases may also improve prognosis, with mean survival of 5 years after resection in one series. Only 2 to 5% of patients with carcinoid syndrome are suited for such liver resections, however.

As ileal carcinoids spread to the mesentery and lymph nodes a marked fibrotic reaction can distort or infarct the bowel. Palliative resection is appropriate for bowel obstruction or bowel ischemia, but has never been shown to prolong survival.

THERAPY FOR ADVANCED DISEASE

Carcinoid tumors metastasize to regional lymph nodes, liver, bone, and rarely to breast and myocardium. Patients with carcinoid tumors should be monitored radiologically for the development of liver metastases, which, if isolated, may be resectable. Patients with functional tumors should be monitored biochemically for rise in tumor markers.

When distant or bilobar metastases develop, treatment is concerned both with therapy of advanced tumor and with chemical palliation of the carcinoid syndrome. The carcinoid syndrome develops in about half of patients with distant metastases. Many patients remain well and active for years, except for these debilitating episodes. Treatment is based on the avoidance of precipitating stress, foods, and actions and the administration of palliative pharmaceuticals (Table 11).

Table 9. Prognosis of Carcinoid Tumors

Site	Relative Frequency (%)	Rate of Metastasis (%)	5-yr Survival (%)	Incidence of Carcinoid Syndrome (%)
Foregut				
Bronchi	12	20	87	13
Stomach	2	22	52	9.5
Midgut				
Appendix	40	2	99	< 1
Ileum	25	35	54	9
Hindgut				
Rectum	15	15	83	1

Adapted from Norton et al. [3]; with permission.

Table 10. Prognosis for Carcinoid Tumors by Extent of Disease

	5-yr Survival (%)	10-yr Survival (%)
Localized disease	94	88
Regional lymph node metastasis	64	
Distant metastases	18–30	0

Of these agents octreotide, a long-acting analogue of somatostatin, has the best response rate and also has a modest antitumor effect (partial remission of 14%). Duration of response can be short in some patients (6–30 mos), with a median of about 20 months [27]. Side effects include gallstone formation and acute cholecystitis in up to a third of patients; thus, prophylactic cholecystectomy should be considered if gallstones are present. In patients debilitated by carcinoid syndrome and unresponsive to other therapies, hepatic artery occlusion may result in significant palliation of symptoms (*vide infra*).

Administration of systemic agents to treat advanced disease has conventionally been reserved until significant disability, symptoms, or poor prognosis develop (*eg*, worsening liver function, carcinoid heart disease, or carcinoid syndrome unresponsive to drug therapy). Several agents have modest activity alone or in combination, generally with duration of response under 1 year (Table 12). In contrast to several other endocrine tumor types, the combination of cisplatin and etoposide has not had significant activity against metastatic carcinoid cancer.

Introduced by Oberg in 1983, immunotherapy of carcinoid metastases using leukocyte or recombinant interferon α has produced a good but variable biochemical response rate (29–60%), with occasional complete remissions reported [28]. Median duration of response varies from 6 to 34 months [28]. In addition interferon α can offer excellent palliation of the symptoms of carcinoid syndrome (30–80% response rate) (Table 11). In a randomized study, therapy with interferon α had a significantly higher response rate and fewer side effects than did systemic 5-FU chemotherapy. Prior cytotoxic chemotherapy did not preclude effective treatment with interferon α [28]. In a phase II study, low-dose interferon α-2b (3×10^6 U $3 \times$ wk) produced the same response as higher doses and had less toxicity [29]. The combination of interferon alpha and octreotide recently produced biochemical objective responses in 77% of patients with median duration of remission of 12 months [30]. Therapy with interferon alpha has been less successful in decreasing tumor size (15%) [30]. There is some data that suggest interferon α-2a is less effective than interferon α-2b, perhaps because of more frequent development of interferon antibodies with the former. No trials have combined interferon alpha-2b with cytotoxic drugs.

With or without the use of chemotherapy, hepatic artery embolization or ligation as treatment of advanced carcinoid cancer is controversial. In selected patients, moderately good response rates have been observed, but with short or even transient duration of response [24,31]. HAO is always associated with a postembolization syndrome, including fever, abdominal pain, hepatic dysfunction, and leukocytosis, and may also cause septicemia, liver abscess, gallbladder necrosis, pleural effusion, encephalopathy, and death (5% mortality rate in one series). There is no information to suggest that this type of treatment is superior to systemic chemotherapy. Radiotherapy has been useful only in palliation of bony metastases.

Table 11. Chemotherapy for Carcinoid Syndrome

Agent	Flush	Diarrhea	Dose
Phenoxybenzamine	Better	No change	10–30 mg/d
Chlorpromazine	Better	No change	10–25 mg q 8 hr
Methyldopa	Somewhat better	No change	4–6 g/d
Cyproheptadine	No change	Better	4–8 mg q 8 hr
Ketanserin	Somewhat better	Better	40–160 mg/d
Methysergide	No change	Better	3–8 mg/d
Octreotide	Better (89%)	Better (74%)	50–150 mu g SQ q 8 hr
rIFN α-2b	Better	Better	9–30 X 10_6 U/m^2/wk

Adapted from Norton et al. [3]; with permission.

Table 12. Adjuvant Therapy for Carcinoid Tumors

Agent	Response Rate (%)
Doxorubicin	21
Streptopzocin	30
5-Flourouracil	26
Streptozocin and 5-FU	33
Streptozocin + doxorubicin	40
Interferon alpha	42–47 (median duration 36 months)

REFERENCES

1. Ross NS, Aron DC: Hormonal evaluation of the patient with an incidentally discovered adrenal mass. *N Engl J Med* 1990, 323:1401–1405.

2. Reincke M, Nieke J, Krestin GP, *et al.*: Preclinical Cushing's syndrome in adrenal "incidentalomas": Comparison with adrenal Cushing's syndrome. *J Clin Endocrinol Metab* 1992, 75:826–832.

3. Norton JA, Doppman JL, Jensen RT: Cancer of the endocrine system. In DeVita VT, Hellman S, Rosenberg SA (eds). *Cancer: Principles and Practice of Oncology.* 1989, Philadelphia: JB Lippincott.

4. Doherty GM, Nieman LK, Cutler GB, *et al.*: Time to recovery of the hypothalamic-pituitary-adrenal axis after curative resection of adrenal tumors in patients with Cushing's syndrome. *Surgery* 1990, 108:1085–1090.

5. Jensen JC, Pass HI, Sindelar WF, Norton JA: Recurrent or metastatic disease in select patients with adrenocortical carcinoma. *Arch Surg* 1991, 126:457–461.

6. Bukowski RM, Wolfe M, Levine HS, *et al.*: Phase II trial of mitotane and cisplatin in patients with adrenal carcinoma: A Southwest Oncology Group study. *J Clin Oncol* 1993, 11:161–165.

7. van Slooten H, Moolenaar AJ, van Seters AP, *et al.*: The treatment of adrenocortical carcinoma with o,p-DDD: Prognostic implications of serum levels monitoring. *Eur J Clin Oncol* 1984, 20:47.

8. Johnson DH, Creco A: Treatment of metastatic adrenal cortical carcinoma with cisplatin and etoposide (VP-16). *Cancer* 1986, 58:2198.

9. Hesketh PJ, McCaffrey RP, Finkel HE, *et al.*: Cisplatin-based treatment of adrenocortical carcinoma. *Cancer Treat Rep* 1987, 71:222.

10. Berruti A, Terzolo M, Paccotti P, *et al.*: Favorable response of metastatic adrenocortical carcinoma to etoposide, adriamycin and cisplatin (EAP) chemotherapy: Report of two cases. *Tumori* 1992, 78:345–348.

11. Schlumberger M, Brugierer L, Gicquel C, *et al.*: 5-Fluorouracil, doxorubicin, and cisplatin as treatment for adrenal cortical carcinoma. *Cancer* 1991, 67:2997–3000.

12. Dedier RA, Elson P, Hogan TF, *et al.*: Mitoxane and adriamycin in patients with advanced adrenocortical carcinoma. *Surgery* 1991, 110:1006–1013.

13. Pasieka JL, Zedenius J, Auer G, *et al.*: Addition of nuclear DNA content to the AMES risk-group classification for papillary thyroid cancer. *Surgery* 1992, 112:1154–1160.

14. Hay ID, Goellner JR, Bergstralh EJ, *et al.*: Predicting outcome in papillary thyroid carcinoma: Development of a reliable prognostic scoring system using a cohort of 1,851 patients surgically treated at one institution during 1940–1990. *Surgery*, in press.

15. Samaan NA, Schulta PN, Hickey RC, *et al.*: The results of various modalities of treatment of well differentiated thyroid carcinoma: A retrospective review of 1599 patients. *J Clin Endocrinol Metab* 1992:714–720.

16. Black EG, Sheppard MC, Hoffenberg R: Serial serum thyroglobulin measurements in the management of differentiated thyroid carcinoma. *Clin Endocrinol* 1987, 27:115–120.

17. Grilo HC, Suen HC, Mathisen DJ, Wain JC: Resectional management of thyroid carcinoma invading the airway. *Ann Thorac Surg* 1992, 54:3–10.

18. Kim JH, Leeper RD: Treatment of locally advanced thyroid carcinoma with combination doxorubicin and radiation therapy. *Cancer* 1987, 60:2372–2375.

19. van Heerden JA, Grant CS, Gharib H, *et al.*: Long-term course of patients with persistent hypercalcitonemia after apparent curative primary surgery for medullary thyroid carcinoma. *Ann Surg* 1990, 212:395–401.

20. Tisell L-E, Hansson G, Jansson S, Salander H: Reoperation in the treatment of asymptomatic metastasizing medullary thyroid carcinoma. *Surgery* 1986, 99:60–66.

21. Shimaoka K, Schoenfeld DA, DeWys WK, *et al.*: A randomized trial of doxorubicin versus doxorubicin plus cisplatin in patients with advanced thyroid carcinoma. *Cancer* 1985, 56:2155–2160.

22. Kim JH, Leeper RD: Treatment of anaplastic giant and spindle cell carcinoma of the thyroid gland with combination adriamycin and radiation therapy. *Cancer* 1983, 52:954–957.

23. Werner B, Abele J, Alveryd A, *et al.*: Multimodal therapy in anaplastic giant cell thyroid carcinoma. *World J Surg* 1984, 8:64–70.

24. Moertel CG: An odyssey in the land of small tumors. *J Clin Oncol* 1987, 5:1503–1522.

25. Kema IP, de Vries EGE, Schellings AMJ, *et al.*: Improved diagnosis of carcinoid tumors by measurement of platelet serotonin. *Clin Chem* 1992, 38:534–540.

26. Lamberts SWJ, Bakker WH, Reubi J-C, Krenning EP: Somatostatin-receptor imaging in the localization of endocrine tumors. *N Engl J Med* 1990, 323:1246–1249.

27. Oberg K, Norheim I, Theodorsson E: Treatment of malignant midgut carcinoid tumours with a long-acting somatostatin analogue octreotide. *Acta Oncol* 1991, 30:503–507.

28. Oberg K, Norheim I, Lind E, *et al.*: Treatment of malignant carcinoid tumors with human leukocyte interferon: Long-term results. *Cancer Treat Rep* 1986, 70:1297–1304.

29. Veenhof CHN, de Wit R, Taa BG, *et al.*: A dose-escalation study of recombinant interferon-alpha in patients with a metastatic carcinoid tumor. *Eur J Cancer* 1992, 28:75–78.

30. Tienssu Janson E, Ahlstrom H, Andersson T, Oberg KE: Octreotide and interferon alfa: A new combination for the treatment of malignant carcinoid tumors. *Eur J Cancer* 1992, 28A:1647–1650.

31. Ruszniewski P, Rougier P, Roche A, *et al.*: Hepatic arterial chemoembolization in patients with liver metastases of endocrine tumor. *Cancer* 1993, 71:2624–2630.

MITOTANE AND CISPLATIN

Mitotane (o,p-DDD) is an isomer of the pesticide DDT that inhibits corticosteroid biosynthesis and, at high doses, causes selective adrenocortical atrophy and infarction. It is not effective in bulky retroperitoneal adrenal cortical cancer. Cisplatin is an alkylating agent that acts to cross-link DNA. *In vitro*, mitotane reverses the multidrug resistance mediated by MDR-1 expression that occurs in adrenal cortical cancer cells.

DOSAGE AND SCHEDULING

1. Prehydrate with saline 2 L IV and mannitol 12.5 g IV
2. Cisplatin 100 mg/m^2 IV, mannitol 25 g IV, and saline 1 L IV over 2 hr, d 1
3. o,p-DDD 1 g PO QID, d 1 and daily while on regimen
4. Cortisone acetate and fludrocortisone acetate daily as needed

RECENT EXPERIENCE AND RESPONSE RATES

In a recent phase II clinical trial these two agents in combination produced responses in 11 of 37 (30%) patients, with a median duration of response of 8 months and median time to response of 76 days [6]. Median survival from treatment was 11.8 months. Although patients with complete surgical resection of tumor were not eligible for the study, a significant survival advantage was found for patients who had previously undergone surgical removal of primary tumor or bulky disease and for patients with a performance status of 0 or 1 [6]. Patients over 65, those with extensive prior radiation, and those with poor tolerance to previous chemotherapy were considered "high-risk" and were given a lower dose of cisplatin.

CANDIDATES FOR TREATMENT

Patients with inoperable adrenal cortical cancer, regardless of tumor functionality

ALTERNATIVE THERAPIES

Dose escalation of mitotane to 8–16 g/d; possibly cisplatin and etoposide combination therapy, but currently insufficient data for recommendation [8–10]

SPECIAL PRECAUTIONS

Patients with significantly impaired renal function, myelosuppression, or hearing loss are ineligible

TOXITIES

Drug combination: severe nausea and vomiting (22% of patients), mild mucositis, mild myalgias, weakness
Mitotane: dose-dependent anorexia, nausea, vomiting, diarrhea, confusion, somnolence, depression, dizziness, skin rash, cholestasis, male gynecomastia, visual disturbances;
Cisplatin: nausea and vomiting, nephrotoxicity, irreversible paresthesias and neuropathies, cumulative ototoxicity, myelosuppression, anaphylaxis

DRUG INTERACTIONS

Anticonvulsants, aminoglycoside antibiotics, warfarin, exogenously administered steroids

NURSING INTERVENTIONS

Monitor renal function and obtain CBC, BUN, and creatine frequently throughout treatment; be prepared for anaphylactic reactions; provide proper antiemetics; hydrate well to prevent renal toxicity

PATIENT INFORMATION

Patient should be informed that mitotane may cause adrenal insufficiency

LOW-DOSE DOXORUBICIN AND RADIATION THERAPY

Most anaplastic thyroid cancers are metastatic at presentation and, uncontrolled, produce death from suffocation in 4 to 6 months. Conventional radiotherapy often fails to induce significant regression of tumor around the airway. Doxorubicin is the single most active agent against thyroid carcinoma and, in addition, acts as a radiosensitizer of radioresistant hypoxic tumor cells, particularly at low doses. A hyperfractionated radiation therapy schedule may deliver more efficacious therapy to rapidly dividing tissues, while minimizing tissue morbidity.

DOSAGE AND SCHEDULING

Doxorubicin 10 mg/m^2 IV administered 1 x wk 1.5 hr prior to radiation therapy and hyperfractionated radiation dose of 160 cGy per treatment, 2 x d for 3 d/wk; total tumor dose 5760 cGy delivered over 40 d

DOSAGE MODIFICATIONS: *70% of patients require a 1 wk respite during therapy due to toxicity*

LAB MONITORING: *clinical examination and subjective dyspnea, WBC*

RECENT EXPERIENCE AND RESPONSE RATES

In 1983 Kim and Leeper reported that this regimen, now under further investigation at the National Cancer Institute, resulted in complete tumor regression in 8 of 9 patients with anaplastic giant and spindle cell carcinoma of the thyroid gland [22]. Patients went on to die of distant metastatic disease (median survival from treatment 10 mo) without increased survival by comparison to historical controls. Findings were confirmed in a follow-up study published in 1987 (84% response rate) [18]. Median survival was 1 year from therapy.

CANDIDATES FOR TREATMENT

Patients with confirmed anaplastic thyroid cancer, patients with locally advanced well-differentiated thyroid cancer unresponsive to I^{131} therapy.

ALTERNATIVE THERAPIES

Systemic chemotherapy (with adriamycin-based regimens). A phase II trial of doxorubicin and interferon alpha for metastatic nonmedullary thyroid cancer is currently ongoing at the Pittsburgh Cancer Institute

SPECIAL PRECAUTIONS

Airway must be secured first

TOXICITIES

Therapy combination: increased toxicity to the myocardium, mucosae, skin, and liver with this combination;
Doxorubicin: minimal at this dose;
Radiation: mild-to-moderate pharyngoesophagitis and tracheitis; skin erythema, hyperpigmentation and late desquamation, laryngeal edema, cervical myelopathy

PATIENT INFORMATION

Patient should be informed that therapy may cause local pain and swelling

OCTREOTIDE AND INTERFERON ALPHA-2B

Octreotide, a long-acting analogue of the natural hormone somatostatin, suppresses the secretion of serotonin and gut peptides. It has been used effectively by many clinicians for the symptoms of carcinoid syndrome, but produces tumor regression at a low rate. Interferon alpha-2b (IFN α-2b) is believed to exert direct antiproliferative action against tumor cells as well as to modulate the host immune response to tumor. This protocol was designed to augment the response to octreotide by the addition of IFN α-2b, which itself has a 30 to 60% response rate in malignant carcinoid tumors.

DOSAGE AND SCHEDULING

IFN α-2b 3×10^6 U SQ $3 \times$ wk and octreotide 100 µg SQ BID

DOSAGE MODIFICATIONS: Weeks 8–16—dose escalation of IFN α-2b to 5×10^6 U SQ $\times$ wk, as allowed by side effects and leukocyte count ($> 4 \times 10^9$/l); After week 16—further escalation of IFN α-2b to 10×10^6 U SQ $3 \times$ wk, as allowed by side effects and leukocyte count

LAB MONITORING: Urine 5-HIAA, plasma serotonin, and other tumor markers q 4 wk; CBC, platelet count, glucose, renal function, response q 4 wk; thyroid function, gallbladder ultrasound q 8 wk

RECENT EXPERIENCE AND RESPONSE RATES

In a recent phase II clinical trial, these two agents were administered together to 24 patients who, during initial treatment with octreotide (50–150 µg twice daily), had demonstrated progressive disease [30]. Administration of IFN α-2b together with octreotide produced an objective biochemical 77% response rate with median duration of response of 12 months. Median survival from treatment was 58 months. Symptoms of carcinoid syndrome were ameliorated in 10 of 18 patients (56%). No patient in this trial had significant objective tumor regression. No information is available concerning the efficacy of this regimen in patients not previously nonresponding to octreotide alone.

CANDIDATES FOR TREATMENT

Patients with inoperable metastatic carcinoid neoplasms, regardless of tumor functionality

SPECIAL PRECAUTIONS

Patients with significant pre-existing cardiac disease or renal failure

ALTERNATIVE THERAPIES

Regimens with higher doses of octreotide (50–150 µg SQ TID) and IFN α-2b (10 mIUµ SQ daily); hepatic artery occlusion combined with chemotherapy or IFN α-2b (recently reported with comparable success rate)

TOXICITIES

Octreotide: changes in blood glucose mild and reversible, hypothyroidism, fat malabsorption, migratory thrombophlebitis; gallstones or sludge (15–20% of patients) and acute cholecystitis (up to one third of patients with gallstones), prophylactic cholecystectomy may be appropriate;
IFN alpha-2b: flulike syndrome and nausea and vomiting with first administration; may exacerbate pre-existing cardiac disease; anorexia, mild weight loss, bone marrow suppression, disturbed thyroid function including hypothyroidism and autoimmune thyroiditis, depression

DRUG INTERACTIONS

Octreotide: H_2-antagonists, antidiarrheal agents, insulin, sulfonureas, beta-blockers, antihypertensives, thyroid replacement hormone; **Interferon alpha:** unknown

NURSING INTERVENTIONS

Monitor for development of gallstones and biliary colic; instruct patient in self-injection

PATIENT INFORMATION

Patients may self-administer injection after learning technique

The therapy of acute leukemia involves the use of combinations of cytotoxic drugs in very intense regimens that are intended to be extremely myelotoxic. The regimens used for the acute leukemias employ an induction component followed by variable periods of postremission consolidation therapy designed to eliminate residual occult disease that ultimately would lead to relapse.

ACUTE MYELOID LEUKEMIA

ETIOLOGY AND RISK FACTORS

While certain predisposing factors for the development of acute myeloid leukemia (AML) exist, the majority of patients who develop this disease have no known antecedent risk factor. Rare in childhood, the incidence of AML steadily increases with age, thus accounting for 80% of the cases of acute leukemia in adults. The median age of onset of AML is about 55 years. Overall, there are about 3 cases per year per 100,000 population and a slight male predominance. Occupational exposure to chemicals (eg, benzene in the rubber industry and ionizing radiation) is associated with increased risk of AML.

Inherited genetic disorders are associated with a higher incidence of AML, including Bloom's syndrome, Fanconi's anemia, Down's syndrome, and Li-Fraumeni syndrome. Bloom's syndrome and Fanconi's anemia have DNA instability in common. Kindreds with the Li-Fraumeni syndrome have a mutated recessive oncogene, the p53 gene on chromosome 17.

CLASSIFICATION AND PROGNOSIS

Because the outcome to treatment of AML is variable, it is of value to determine, based on inherent features of the leukemia and the patient, which patients might do better with therapy (Table 1). Determining the prognosis can also contribute to progress in the evolution of therapy, because the therapy could be tailored more appropriately to the patient. Thus, patients with a very poor prognosis could be treated with more aggressive or conceptually different therapeutic modalities in an effort to improve their outlook, whereas patients who would do well with current therapeutic programs would not be subjected to unnecessarily aggressive experimental therapies.

Older patients with AML do not do as well as younger patients. Patients over 60 have a lower complete remission rate than those who are younger. This is due in part to the higher rates of death in these older patients from infection and other complications during remission induction. In addition, the older population contains more patients with secondary leukemias arising from a previous myelodysplastic syndrome or from complications of treatment for a previous disease. These secondary leukemias have a worse outcome, apparently due to inherent features of the leukemic clone that render it more resistant to chemotherapy.

Patients presenting with high blast cell counts (> 100,000/μl) also have a worse prognosis, presumably related to the high proliferative potential of the leukemic clone and the early mortality from leukostasis, a process in which the malignant cells occlude capillaries in the lung and brain leading to respiratory failure and obtundation.

Certain recurring cytogenetic findings have been shown to affect prognosis in AML. Patients whose cells demonstrate translocations of chromosomes 8 and 21 and inversions of chromosome 16 have a better prognosis than other patients. Conversely, those with deletions of chromosomes 5 or 7 do less well. It is not possible to know whether the cytogenetic lesion is a marker of biologic activity or is directly associated with the behavior of the malignant clone.

AML cells express a variety of cell surface markers indicative of cell lineage and state of differentiation. In the lymphoid malignancies, the expression of surface markers associated with lymphoid cells has been helpful in determining subsets (eg, T vs B lineage), and this information has been useful clinically. At this time, it is less clear how surface marker determinations are helpful in AML. In general, AML blasts express antigens associated with the myeloid lineage. In one study, patients whose cells reacted to the My4 (CD14) or My7 (CD13) monoclonal antibodies had a worse prognosis than those whose cells did not. It has also been found that patients whose cells expressed CD2 (OKT11 monoclonal antibody) had a better prognosis than those whose cells were CD2 negative. This example of apparently mixed-lineage leukemia is an exception; most mixed-lineage leukemias behave more poorly than those displaying only myeloid antigens. It is important to note that prognostic markers are related to the therapy used for the disease. Thus, the value of a marker may be dependent on the particular therapy used in the study that revealed the marker. The marker may thus change in value as therapies evolve over time.

THERAPY
Chemotherapy

Acute myeloid leukemia has been treated for many years with cytosine arabinoside (cytarabine or ara-C) (Table 2). Most patients are treated with a regimen consisting of cytarabine as a continuous infusion over 7 days of 100 to 200 mg/m^2 in conjunction with an anthracycline compound, such as daunorubicin [1], idarubicin [2,3], or mitoxantrone [4], for three consecutive days. For many years the

Table 1. Prognostic Factors in AML

Factor	Good Prognosis	Poor Prognosis
WBC	< 100,000/μl	> 100,000/μl
Age	< 60	> 60
Cytogenetic finding	Translocation of chromosomes 8 and 21	Deletions of chromosomes 5 and 7, +8
	Abnormal chromosome 16	Other chromosomal abnormalities

Table 2. Initial Therapy of AML

1. Cytarabine (100–200 mg/m^2 x 7 d)
   plus
   Daunorubicin (45 mg/m^2)
   or
   Idarubicin (12 mg/m^2)
   or
   Mitoxantrone (12 mg/m^2)
   or
2. Cyclophosphamide and etoposide
   or
3. High-dose cytarabine (3 g/m^2) with an anthracycline

standard anthracycline has been daunorubicin. Recently, trials using the synthetic anthracyclines, idarubicin [2,3], and mitoxantrone [4], appear to show equal or possibly greater efficacy, at least in subgroups of patients. Two randomized prospective trials comparing daunorubicin to idarubicin in conjunction with cytarabine demonstrated superior remission induction and survival rates in the idarubicin arm for patients under 60 years of age. However, the daunorubicin arm showed worse survival rates than expected from historical data, thus leaving some skepticism regarding the superior result with idarubicin. Daunorubicin and idarubicin are both cardiotoxic at doses exceeding 450 mg/m^2, whereas mitoxantrone is less cardiotoxic when used in the dose ranges required for efficacy.

An alternative to the standard-dose cytarabine-based induction protocols has been high-dose cyclophosphamide and etoposide [5] or high-dose cytarabine (HIDAC) [6]. Interestingly, a recent study that used high-dose cytarabine with daunorubicin as induction followed by the same regimen as consolidation showed somewhat worse outcome than a previous study by the same group that used standard-dose cytarabine followed by high-dose cytarabine [6]. In the initial report of this group, patients treated with standard induction who then received consolidation with HIDAC had a 3-year disease-free survival rate of 49%. Patients under age 45 years fared especially well. However, when the same HIDAC regimen was employed for initial therapy followed by consolidation with the same regimen, long-term disease-free survival was only 32%. This could be explained by the prospective nature of the high-dose induction protocol compared to the previously reported use of HIDAC after standard-dose induction chemotherapy, which may have been biased toward patients whose disease was stable enough to await entry into the high-dose consolidation study.

Postremission therapy usually involves reiterations of standard-dose cytarabine and anthracycline regimen at least two times, ideally 1 month apart but often requiring more time to allow recovery of marrow function. As mentioned, high-dose cytarabine regimens have also been used as consolidation therapy with promising results when used following standard-dose cytarabine therapy. Administration of the cytarabine regimen, 3 g/m^2 every 12 hours for 12 doses with an anthracycline for one cycle, resulted in 50% of patients remaining in continuous complete remission at 5 years. While two cycles of this therapy were planned, only 25% of patients received the second course due to patient or physician reluctance to continue therapy, alloimmunization, and toxicity. Two cycles of the HIDAC regimen did not significantly increase the proportion of patients remaining in complete remission [7].

The Cancer and Leukemia Group B recently studied three different doses of cytarabine used as consolidation following cytarabine at 100 mg/m^2 [8]. Patients under 60 years old were treated with one of three different doses of cytarabine; 100 mg/m^2 for 5 days, 400 mg/m^2 for 5 days, and 3 g/m^2 every 12 hours for a total of six doses, each given four times over a period of 4 to 6 months, followed by four more cycles of subcutaneous cytarabine (100 mg/m^2 twice a day for 10 doses) and daunorubicin (45 mg/m^2). The high-dose arm (3 g/m^2) resulted in superior disease-free survival in patients from ages 40 to 60, but not for those less than 40. Both the 3 g/m^2 and the 400 mg/m^2 doses were superior to the 100 mg/m^2 dose in patients aged 20 to 40 years.

Thus, optimal therapy of AML is not yet completely defined. Chemotherapy administered in nonmyeloablative doses in protocols using a variety of doses, schedules, and agents cures approximately 25% of all newly diagnosed patients with *de novo* AML. However, relapse still occurs in more than 50% of patients.

Therapy of AML at relapse is generally not satisfactory as long-term disease-free survival is rarely achieved, even if a second remission is obtained. The success of remission-inducing therapy is dependent in part on the length of the first remission. Patients who relapse after a first remission that lasted more than a year can be treated with a cytarabine and anthracycline regimen. Other regimens include single agents, such as mitoxantrone [9] and carboplatinum [10], or high-dose cytarabine and combinations, such as etoposide and mitoxantrone [11], amsa and cytarabine [12] and 1-asparaginase and cytarabine [13] (Table 3). Remissions are induced in about 40 to 50% of patients independent of the agent used. The remainder either relapse or die from therapy-related toxicities. Unfortunately, second remissions are rarely durable. Median disease-free survival is usually for 4 to 5 months. When patients relapse again, similar agents or combinations of agents may be used to reinduce third and even fourth remissions. Therapy becomes palliative at this stage without consideration of marrow transplantation.

New approaches to the treatment of leukemia involve the use of hematopoietic growth factors (HGFs) to induce cells to proliferate and the use of differentiating agents to induce the malignant cells to overcome their block in differentiation.

There are two basic rationales for using HGFs in the treatment of AML. HGFs recruit leukemia cells into active cell division in order to make them more susceptible to S-phase–specific drugs such as ara-C. A note of caution is suggested by a report from the M.D. Anderson Hospital; when GM-CSF was administered prior to chemotherapy for AML, survival was actually worse than that in historical controls [14].

HGFs also ameliorate the toxicity of chemotherapy against normal bone marrow cells when they are used after chemotherapy to stimulate hematopoiesis. Use of GM-CSF following induction chemotherapy for AML accelerated recovery of granulocytes and did not promote leukemia regrowth [15].

The use of differentiation therapy is based on the observation that AML cells have the phenotype of normal myeloid cells that are arrested in an early stage of differentiation and that this block can be overcome by chemical agents, including certain vitamins such as 1,25 dihydroxyvitamin D$_3$ and retinoic acid (RA). It has been shown that some mature myeloid cells in patients with AML in remission are clonal by G6PD isoenzyme or RFLP analysis and that they are, therefore, probably derived from the malignant clone. This observation suggests that the differentiation block can be overcome spontaneously. More support for the concept of differentiation therapy comes from studies of leukemia cell lines. For example, the HL-60 line, derived from a patient with promyelocytic leukemia, displays many of the features of AML cells from this subtype. Cells from this line can be induced to differentiate into either monocytoid or

Table 3. Salvage Regimens in Acute Leukemia

Acute Myeloid Leukemia	Acute Lymphocytic Leukemia
Etoposide and mitoxantrone	High-dose cytarabine and anthracycline
High-dose cytarabine and anthracycline	Teniposide and cytarabine
High-dose cytarabine and L-asparaginase	High-dose methotrexate
Carboplatin	
High-dose cyclophosphamide and busulfan with stem cell support	

neutrophilic cells, depending on the differentiation agent used. One of the compounds that was found to have granulocytic differentiation–inducing activity was RA. This led investigators in France and China to use RA to treat patients with acute promyelocytic leukemia (APL) [16]. All trans-retinoic acid (trans-RA) was found to be superior to cis-retinoic acid *in vitro* and *in vivo* in inducing differentiation of blast cells from patients. In fact, all trans-RA was capable of inducing remissions in patients with APL without the use of cytotoxic therapy [16,17]. It is believed that the mechanism of action of this therapy is pharmacologically induced differentiation of leukemic blasts. It is unclear whether this therapy will work in producing long-term remissions because it has been observed that chronic therapy is necessary to maintain remission. It is of interest that the breakpoint in t(15;17) found in APL involves the gene of the alpha isoform of the RA receptor generating a chimeric fusion messenger transcript comprised of the alpha-RAR and a sequence called PML analogous to the phenomenon in chronic myeloid leukemia involving bcr and the abl oncogene that also generates a fusion mRNA and protein.

Bone Marrow Transplantation

Bone marrow transplantation (BMT), either allogeneic or autologous, is the best therapeutic option for patients who have achieved second or third remissions with AML and may be the optimal treatment for patients in first complete remission. The most common preparative regimens used are those containing cyclophosphamide (CY) (60 mg/kg body weight/d x 2) and total body irradiation (TBI) (200 cGy twice a day for 3 d, 1200 cGY) [18], or busulfan (BU) (16 mg/kg/d x 4 orally) and CY (either 60 mg/kg/d x 2 [BU/CY2] [19] or 50 mg/kg/d x 4 [BU/CY4]). In the initial report of the BU/CY2 regimen there was efficacy equal to results of the BU/CY4 regimen but with less toxicity [19]. It is not clear that any one preparative regimen is superior for disease control because multiple nonrandomized studies have provided conflicting results. Disease-free survival between 30 and 60% can be expected using these regimens in patients in remission. Results are generally better for allogeneic BMT in first remission than in later remissions. Autologous BMT results are not as clearly remission-dependent, with about 50% of patients in first remission and later remissions achieving long-term disease-free survival.

An alternative to awaiting second remission for patients who have failed first-line therapy is to perform high-dose chemotherapy and bone marrow transplantation at first relapse. The same regimens used to prepare patients for BMT in remission (CY/TBI or BU/CY) can be used to induce remission. The advantage of this approach is that more patients achieve complete remissions and enjoy long-term disease-free survival at least as often as patients who are transplanted in second or later remissions. Thus, more patients benefit from this therapy because standard remission–inducing therapy is only effective in 40 to 50% of patients. This concept is under study by the Cancer and Leukemia Group B using the BU/CY2 regimen and monoclonal antibody–purged bone marrow.

Allogeneic Bone Marrow Transplantation

Allogeneic BMT is performed using an HLA-matched donor, usually a sibling. Data from large pooled registries, such as the International Bone Marrow Transplant Registry, have shown that approximately 50% of patients transplanted in this manner will be cured. Performance of the BMT at relapse or in second remission results in lower cure rates [18]. Earlier intervention probably is more effective because the leukemia cells are less drug-resistant at that

time. Other factors may contribute to the worse outcome in second remission, including greater host susceptibility to infection and alloimmunization to platelet antigens, thus leading to more frequent bleeding episodes.

The biggest obstacle to allogeneic BMT is availability of suitable donors and the morbidity/mortality of graft-versus-host disease (GVHD). GVHD is more common and severe in older patients, particularly those over the age of 55 years. Thus most centers will only perform HLA-matched sibling donor allogeneic transplants on patients under the age of 55. Organizations such as the National Marrow Donor Program are attempting to increase the pool of potential donors by maintaining files of HLA-typing on large numbers of potential donors. It is too early to comment on the role that "matched unrelated donor" transplants may play in the approach to the patient with AML. However, there is a greater incidence of GVHD in this type of transplant with its attendant mortality [20].

One theoretical advantage that allogeneic transplantation has over autologous transplantation is the potential of a graft versus leukemia effect mediated by donor cells against the recipient's leukemia cells. This effect is seen most clearly in allogeneic BMT for chronic myeloid leukemia when T-cell depletion is performed to abrogate graft-versus-host disease, resulting in a very high relapse rate.

Autologous Bone Marrow Transplantation

An approach for patients who do not have an HLA-matched donor or who are over 45 years old, an age where allogeneic BMT has greater toxicity, is autologous bone marrow transplantation (ABMT). With ABMT, bone marrow transplantation can be more widely used in AML, avoiding the complication of GVHD and associated problems, such as interstitial pneumonitis. Many centers employ a purging technique, usually with a cytotoxic drug such as 4-hydroperoxycyclophosphamide (4HC) or monoclonal antibodies (mAb) directed to antigens expressed on leukemia cells in order to eradicate residual occult disease from the autologous marrow [21,22]. In a recent analysis of data, the European Bone Marrow Transplant Group has shown a benefit of purging with the chemical mafosfamide (a cyclophosphamide congener) for patients transplanted within 6 months of attaining their first and second complete remission. Despite investigators' optimism for the use of purged marrows, no randomized studies comparing ABMT with and without marrow purging have been reported. However, because AML patients almost invariably relapse after achieving second or later standard chemotherapy-induced remissions, it seems clear that high-dose chemo- and radiation therapy and ABMT have been responsible for the long-term survivors in the BMT studies. Long-term disease-free remissions can be achieved in up to 50% of patients in second and third remission at the time of ABMT, an outcome superior to that from allogeneic BMT from HLA-matched siblings. Lower relapse rates are seen following allogeneic BMT but a greater mortality from GVHD decreases the proportion of long-term survivors [18].

ACUTE LYMPHOBLASTIC LEUKEMIA

ETIOLOGY AND RISK FACTORS

Acute lymphoblastic leukemia (ALL) is more common in children than in adults, the converse of AML. Risk factors include fragile chromosome states, Down's syndrome, and radiation exposure (as in AML) (Table 4).

CLASSIFICATION AND PROGNOSIS

ALL is subclassified into three morphologic groups: L1, L2, and L3 (Burkitt's lymphoma). In addition, the lineage of the cells can be determined by immunophenotyping with monoclonal antibodies to surface antigens characteristic of B- and T-lymphoid cells. The majority of cases are in the B lineage although most have a "pre-B-cell" phenotype (no surface immunoglobulin but positive for B-cell surface antigens).

Cytogenetics are important prognostic determinants in ALL. With appropriate study, up to 50% of adults with B-lineage ALL have the t(9;22) abnormality known as the Philadelphia chromosome (Ph[1]). A very poor prognosis, with few long-term survivors, is found with Ph[1]-positive ALL. Another poor prognostic marker is the t(4;11).

Prognosis in ALL is defined in part by the therapy given, with the currently used intensive multidrug regimens with CNS treatment being most effective (Table 5).

THERAPY
Chemotherapy

The treatment of ALL in adults entails intensive multiagent combination chemotherapy. A major advance has been reported from a German multicenter group that has employed a treatment schedule with an induction phase using eight drugs and a reinduction phase using an additional eight drugs [23]. CNS prophylaxis consisted of cranial irradiation with 24 GY and intrathecal methotrexate 10 mg/m^2 once weekly for 4 weeks during the second phase of treatment when complete remission had been achieved. This chemotherapy program was successful in achieving remissions in 74% of patients, with a median remission duration of 24.3 months and a probability of being in continuous complete remission at 5 years of 37%.

For those patients who relapse, second complete remissions can be obtained with rates of 10 to 75%, depending on the treatment regimen [12,24,25]. Regimens in current use include high-dose cytarabine combined with an anthracycline or amsacrine, high-dose methotrexate with folinic acid rescue, and teniposide and cytarabine. The durability of second remissions in ALL is poor and few patients are cured at this stage without further therapy. Younger patients have generally been considered for marrow transplantation to improve durability of remission.

Bone Marrow Transplantation
Allogeneic Bone Marrow Transplantation

Multiple centers reporting to the International Bone Marrow Transplant Registry continue to show promising results using allogeneic bone marrow transplantation (Table 6). Actuarial 5-year disease-free survival of 39% was seen in first complete remissions in adult patients and 26% in second remissions in adults and children. An analysis of adult patients with ALL who received allogeneic BMT in Seattle showed 5-year disease-free survival of 21% for first complete remissions, 15% for second or later complete remissions, and 12% for those transplanted in relapse [26].

Autologous Bone Marrow Transplantation

As in AML, autologous bone marrow transplant (ABMT) offers an alternative to allogeneic sources of marrow support for high-dose chemotherapy. The majority of trials have used either chemical or immunologic purging to remove residual tumor cells. The European Bone Marrow Transplant Group reported 20% disease-free survival in adult patients transplanted for high-risk first complete remission. A larger analysis, which included results from children, showed a disease-free survival rate of 44% and a relapse rate of 45%, with 39% of transplants unpurged [27]. There appeared to be an advantage to purging with adjusted-dose mafosfamide in first remission over purging with mAb (82% disease-free survival for the former compared to 40% for the latter at 20 mo), but there was no difference in outcome between purged and unpurged groups overall. Outcome was better for patients harvested and transplanted later than 3 months following remission.

ABMT for high-risk groups has not been sufficiently tested. Hoelzer defined high risk as time to complete remission greater than 4 weeks, patient age greater than 35 years, and leukocyte count greater than 30,000/µl [23]. Both the EBMT and the Minnesota groups demonstrated the lack of prognostic significance of a high initial leukocyte count on outcome following ABMT [27] although with allogeneic BMT this remains a significant predictor of relapse. A study by the Minnesota group of immunotoxin purging in T-cell ALL in

Table 4. Etiologic and Risk Factors in AML and ALL

AML	ALL
Chromosomal fragility syndromes	Chromosomal fragility
Bloom's syndrome	
Fanconi's anemia	
Mutations of suppressor oncogenes (p53)	Down's syndrome
Li–Fraumeni syndrome	
Age	Radiation exposure
Myelodysplasia	
Radiation or chemotherpy	

Table 5. Prognostic Factors in ALL

Factor	Good Prognosis	Poor Prognosis
Age	< 35 yr	> 35 yr
Sex	Female	Male
Time to complete remission	< 4 wk	> 4 wk
Cytogenetic finding	T-cell phenotype, Hyperdiploid cytogenetics	Philadelphia chromosome, t(9;22), t(4;11)
WBC	< 30,000/µl	> 30,000/µl

Table 6. Results of Bone Marrow Transplantation for Acute Leukemia*

	AML		ALL	
	Allogeneic (%)	Autologous (%)	Allogeneic (%)	Autologous (%)
CR1	60	60	40	40
CR2/3	40	50	25	20

*Results are average percentages of long-term disease-free survivors (at least 3 yr) for standard-risk patients.

remission showed worse than expected results, with residual leukemia in the marrow following purging, results of prognostic significance [28]. An improved outcome has been achieved with allogeneic transplantation in patients with Ph[1]-positive ALL. Whether ABMT can improve the outcome over chemotherapy alone remains to be seen.

A recent survey of ABMT of both adults and children with ALL beyond first relapse showed a disease-free survival rate of 32% and a relapse rate of 62% [27]. The Minnesota group has compared their experience with two consecutive series of patients, the first treated with CY/TBI and the second with TBI followed by cytosine arabinoside. There was no advantage to either regimen regarding toxicity or outcome. Survival and relapse rates were 29 and 63%, respectively, for the first regimen and 18 and 75%, respectively, for the second regimen in patients receiving autologous transplants [29]. No significant difference in outcome was demonstrated between children and adults in this study.

The majority of comparative trials of allogeneic and autologous transplantation include both adults and children with ALL. Autologous and allogeneic transplantation were compared after CY/TBI or high-dose cytosine arabinoside and TBI in high-risk patients, predominantly in second or third complete remissions, purging autologous marrow with cocktails of mAb [30]. There was no difference in outcome between children and adults. Relapse-free survival was similar in both groups with 27% of patients with allogeneic grafts alive and free of relapse at 4 years compared with 20% of those with autologous grafts. There was a trend to earlier deaths associated with GVH in the allogeneic group and later deaths in the autologous group associated with relapse. The relapse rates were significantly different with probabilities of relapse of 79% in the autologous group and 56% in the allogeneic group. Relapses occurred earlier in the autologous group. Furthermore, the probability of relapse in those developing acute or chronic GVH was only 37% compared with 75% in those who had none. Both observations argue strongly for a significant graft versus leukemia effect. Also, the similarity of relapse rates in patients with allogeneic grafts without GVHD and patients with autologous grafts suggests adequate purging methodology but inadequate anti-leukemic therapy. Benefits of ABMT included more rapid time to white cell engraftment, reduction in early mortality, and shorter duration of hospital stay for transplantation.

CHRONIC MYELOID LEUKEMIA

ETIOLOGY AND RISK FACTORS

Chronic myeloid leukemia (CML) has a slight male predominance and a peak incidence in the fifth and sixth decades. The only known risk factor for CML is prior radiation exposure.

CLASSIFICATION AND PROGNOSIS

CML usually presents with an elevated leukocyte count comprised of the entire spectrum of myeloid precursors and mature neutrophils. This is referred to as the chronic phase of CML. This phase is relatively benign and median survival is about 4 years. Most patients enter an accelerated phase where numerous signs and symptoms and laboratory findings indicate that the disease is becoming more aggressive. Finally, an acute phase is reached that is essentially analogous to acute leukemia. The characteristics of the blast cells at the time of blast crisis are usually myeloid, but in

20 to 30% of the cases the cells have features of the lymphoid lineage. Prognosis is extremely poor at the time of blast crisis. Therapy for acute leukemia can be administered with the expectation that only 25% of patients with myeloid blast crisis, and up to 60% of patients with lymphoid blast crisis, will achieve remission. Remissions are short-lived and long-term survival at this stage is essentially nil.

THERAPY

The treatment of CML during the first chronic phase has evolved from a single agent alkylator, such as busulfan, to a single agent such as hydroxyurea or interferon alpha. Initial treatment often uses hydroxyurea to lower the blast count if patients present with particularly high counts. When counts are stabilized, treatment with interferon alpha may be started, based on data showing up to 15% of patients treated with the drug daily achieving cytogenetic and hematologic remissions [30]. It has not yet been proven that progression to blast crisis has been delayed. Interferon alpha is administered subcutaneously daily with a dose of 5×10^6 U. Myelosuppression is expected, and the dose may need to be adjusted to maintain the leukocyte count between 2000 to 4000/μl.

An alternative form of therapy for patients with CML in the chronic phase is the use of allogeneic BMT. High-dose cyclophosphamide and total body irradiation or busulfan and cyclophosphamide combination are most commonly used as preparative regimens. Many groups have shown that HLA-identical sibling donor allogeneic BMT in patients in first chronic phase and who are under 55 years is curative in up to 60% of patients [31]. Younger patients have a better outcome. Matched unrelated donors are commonly sought for patients without HLA-identical siblings [32]. Long-term, disease-free survival in up to 30% of patients has been reported with these transplants, but the morbidity and mortality rates due to graft-versus-host disease are high.

Chronic myeloid leukemia in blast crisis can be approached in the same way as acute leukemia but the results are dismal. Marrow transplantation can be performed with long-term survival in about 10% of patients.

CHRONIC LYMPHOCYTIC LEUKEMIA

ETIOLOGY AND RISK FACTORS

Chronic lymphocytic leukemia (CLL) is the most common leukemia in the United States and occurs most often in patients over 60 years of age. There are no known predisposing factors, although familial clustering has been reported.

CLASSIFICATION AND PROGNOSIS

A classification system developed by Rai (Stages 0, I, II, III, and IV) has been used in the United States for many years. An alternative staging system (A, B, and C) has been proposed by Binet. Prognosis in CLL is linked to the stage of disease at presentation. Patients with lymphocytosis only (Rai Stage 0 or Binet Stage A) have a median survival of greater than 10 years from diagnosis. Patients presenting in more advanced stages have shorter survival expectancies (Rai Stage I or II—median survival 7 years; Rai Stage III or IV—median survival 4 years).

The information here is provided as guidance only. Prescribers should always consult the manufacturer's current prescribing information.

190

THERAPY

The treatment of symptomatic CLL has been the use of a single alkylator such as chlorambucil, often combined with prednisone, both administered orally either in a continuous (daily) or pulse (monthly) basis. When disease control becomes more difficult with alkylating agents, patients may be treated with the fluorinated analogue of adenine, fludarabine [33], or with the deoxyadenosine analogue, 2-chlorodeoxyadenosine [34]. These agents are relatively resistant to deamination by adenosine deaminase and lead to accumulation of metabolites that are toxic to lymphocytes. Patients with CLL refractory to alkylator therapy can achieve complete or partial remissions with the single agent fludarabine (Table 7). These remissions are usually not durable and relapse almost always occurs.

Table 7. Therapy for Chronic Lymphocytic Leukemia

Agent	Complete or Partial Response Rates (%)
Chlorambucil	70
2-Chlorodeoxyadenosine	50
Interferon alpha	67
Fludarabine (previous therapy)	57
Fludarabine (untreated)	79

HAIRY CELL LEUKEMIA

Hairy cell leukemia is most common in middle-aged males. There are no known predisposing factors.

Hairy cell leukemia is a chronic disease with a very good prognosis. There are no distinct stages recognized. Recent treatment results are very encouraging.

The treatment results of hairy cell leukemia have recently been improved by use of drugs such as 2-chlorodeoxyadenosine, pentastatin, and interferon alpha [35]. Complete remissions with excellent long-term survival in more than 90% of patients with newly diagnosed hairy cell leukemia have been reported with a single course of therapy with 2-chlorodeoxyadenosine [36] (Table 8).

Table 8. Therapy for Hairy Cell Leukemia

Agent	Complete or Partial Response Rates (%)
Pentastatin	> 95
2-Chlorodeoxyadenosine	> 95
Fludarabine	> 95

REFERENCES

1. Champlin R, Gale R: Acute myelogenous leukemia: Recent advances in therapy. *Blood* 1987, 69:1551–1562.
2. Wiernik PH, Banks PLC, Case DC Jr, *et al.*: Cytarabine plus idarubicin or daunorubicin as induction and consolidation therapy for previously untreated adult patients with acute myeloid leukemia. *Blood*, 1992, 79:313–319.
3. Berman E, Heller G, Santorsa J, *et al.*: Results of a randomized trial comparing idarubicin and cytosine arabinoside with daunorubicin and cytosine arabinoside in adult patients with newly diagnosed acute myelogenous leukemia. *Blood* 1991, 71:1666–1674.
4. Hiddemann W, Kreutzmann H, Straif K, *et al.*: High-dose cytosine arabinoside and mitoxantrone: A highly effective regimen in refractory acute myeloid leukemia. *Blood* 1987, 69:744–749.
5. Brown R, Herzig R, Wolff S, *et al.*: High dose etoposide and cyclophosphamide without bone marrow transplantation for resistant hematologic malignancy. *Blood* 1990, 76:473–479.
6. Phillips GL, Reece DE, Shepherd JD, *et al.*: High-dose cytarabine and daunorubicin induction and postremission chemotherapy for the treatment of acute myelogenous leukemia in adults. *Blood* 1991, 77:1429–1435.
7. Wolff S, Herzig R, Fay J, *et al.*: High-dose cytorabine and daunorubicin as consolidation therapy for acute myeloid leukemia in first remission: Long-term follow-up and results. *J Clin Oncol* 1989, 7:1260–1267.
8. Mayer R, Davis R, Schiffer C, *et al.*: Comparative evaluation of intensive post-remission therapy with different dose schedules of ara-C in adults with acute myeloid leukemia (AML): Initial results of a CALGB phase III study. *Proc ASCO* 1992, 11:261.
9. Vredenburgh J, McIntyre O, Cornwell GI, *et al.*: Mitoxantrone in relapsed or refractory acute nonlymphocytic leukemia. *Med Ped Oncol* 1988, 16:187–189.
10. Martinez JA, Martin G, Sanz GF, *et al.*: A phase II clinical trial of carboplatin infusion in high-risk nonlymphoblastic leukemia. *J Clin Oncol* 1991, 9:39–43.
11. Lazzarino M, Morra E, Alessandrino E, *et al.*: Mitoxantrone and etoposide: An effective regimen for refractory or relapsed acute myelogenous leukemia. *Eur J Haematol* 1989, 43:411–416.
12. Arlin Z, Ahmed T, Mittelman A, *et al.*: A new regimen of amsacrine with high-dose cytarabine is safe and effective therapy for acute leukemia. *J Clin Oncol* 1987, 5:371–375.
13. Capizzi RL, Davis R, Powell B, *et al.*: Synergy between high-dose cytarabine and asparaginase in the treatment of adults with refractory and relapsed acute myelogenous leukemia—A cancer and leukemia group B study. *J Clin Oncol* 1988, 6:499–508.
14. Estey E, Thall P, Kantarjian H, *et al.*: Treatment of newly diagnosed acute myelogenous leukemia with granulocyte-macrophage colony-stimulating factor (GM-CSF) before and during continuous-infusion high-dose ara-C + daunorubicin: Comparison to patients treated without GM-CSF. *Blood* 1992, 79:2246–2255.
15. Buchner T, Hiddemann W, Koenigsmann M, *et al.*: Recombinant human granulocyte-macrophage colony-stimulating factor after chemotherapy in patients with acute myeloid leukemia at higher age or after relapse. *Blood* 1991, 78:1190–1197.
16. Degos L: All-trans-retinoic acid in the treatment of acute promyelocytic leukaemia. *Presse Med* 1990, 19:1483–1484.
17. Warrell R, Frankel S, Miller W, *et al.*: Differentiation therapy of acute promyelocytic leukemia with tretinoin (all-trans-retinoic acid). *N Engl J Med* 1991, 324:1385–1393.
18. Clift R, Buckner C, Thomas E, *et al.*: Treatment of acute nonlymphoblastic leukemia by allogeneic marrow transplantation. *Bone Marrow Transplant* 1987, 2:243–258.

19. Copelan E, Biggs J, Thompson J, *et al.*: Treatment for acute myelocytic leukemia with allogeneic bone marrow transplantation following preparation with BuCy2. *Blood* 1991, 78:838–843.

20. Beatty P, Hansen J, Longton G, *et al.*: Marrow transplantation from HLA-matched unrelated donors for treatment of hematologic malignancies. *Transplantation* 1991, 51:443.

21. Yeager A, Kaizer H, Santos G, *et al.*: Autologous bone marrow transplantation in patients with acute nonlymphocytic leukemia using *ex vivo* marrow treatment with 4-hydroperoxycyclophosphamide. *N Engl J Med* 1986, 315:141–147.

22. Ball E, Mills L, Cornwell G, *et al.*: Autologous bone marrow transplantation for acute myeloid leukemia using monoclonal antibody-purged bone marrow. *Blood* 1990, 75:1199–1206.

23. Hoelzer D, Thiel E, Loffler H, *et al.*: Prognostic factors in a multicenter study for the treatment of acute lymphoblastic leukemia in adults. *Blood* 1988, 71:123–131.

24. Ochs J, Rivera G, Pollock B, *et al.*: Teniposide (VM-26) and continuous infusion cytosine arabinoside for initial induction failure in childhood acute lymphoblastic leukemia: A Pediatric Oncology Group pilot study. *Cancer* 1990, 66:1671–1677.

25. Capizzi RL, Poole M, Cooper MR, *et al.*: Treatment of poor risk acute leukemia with sequential high-dose ara-C and asparaginase. *Blood* 1994, 63:694–700.

26. Doney K, Fisher L, Appelbaum F, *et al.*: Treatment of adult acute lymphoblastic leukemia with allogeneic bone marrow transplantation. Multivariate analysis of factors affecting acute graft-versus-host disease, relapse, and relapse-free survival. *Bone Marrow Transplant* 1991, 7:453–459.

27. Gorin N: Autologous bone marrow transplantation in hematological malignancies. *Am J Clin Oncol* 1991, 14:S5–S14.

28. Uckun F, Kersey J, Vallera D, *et al.*: Autologous bone marrow transplantation in high-risk remission T-lineage acute lymphoblastic leukemia using immunotoxins plus 4-hydroperoxycyclophosphamide for marrow purging. *Blood* 1990, 76:1723–1733.

29. Woods W, Ramsay N, Weisdorf D, *et al.*: Bone marrow transplantation for acute lymphocytic leukemia utilizing total body irradiation followed by high doses of cytosine arabinoside: Lack of superiority over cyclophosphamide-containing regimens. *Bone Marrow Transplant* 1990, 6:9–16.

30. Talpaz M, Kantarjian H, Kurzrock R, *et al.*: Interferon-alpha produces sustained cytogenetic responses in chronic myelogenous leukemia—Philadelphia chromosome-positive patients. *Ann Intern Med* 1991, 114:532–538.

31. Clift RA, Buckner CD, Appelbaum FR, *et al.*: Allogeneic marrow transplantation in patients with chronic myeloid leukemia in the chronic phase—a randomized trial of two irradiation regimens. *Blood* 1991, 77:1660–1665.

32. McGlave P, Beatty P, Ash R, Hows J: Therapy of chronic myelogenous leukemia with unrelated donor bone marrow transplantation: Results in 102 cases. *Blood* 1990, 75:1728–1732.

33. Keating M, Kantarjian H, Talpaz M, *et al.*: Fludarabine: A new agent with major activity against chronic lymphocytic leukemia. *Blood* 1989, 74:19–25.

34. Piro L, Carrera C, Beutler E, Carson D: 2-Chlorodeoxyadenosine: An effective new agent for the treatment of chronic lymphocytic leukemia. *Blood* 1988, 72:1069–1075.

35. Saven A, Piro L: Treatment of hairy cell leukemia. *Blood* 1992, 79:1111–1120.

36. Piro L, Carrera C, Carson D, Beutler E: Lasting remissions in hairy-cell leukemia induced by a single infusion of 2-chlorodeoxyadenosine. *N Engl J Med* 1990, 322:1117–1121.

CYTOSINE ARABINOSIDE AND ANTHRACYCLINE

The combination of cytosine arabinoside and one of the anthracycline antibiotics has become the standard induction regimen for acute myeloid leukemia around the world.

Cytosine arabinoside is an antimetabolite that interferes with DNA synthesis after conversion to ara-CTP, which is a potent inhibitor of DNA polymerase. In addition, metabolites of ara-CTP accumulate in DNA, causing a defect in ligation of newly synthesized fragments of DNA. Cytarabine may be inactivated by two intracellular enzymes, cytidine deaminase and deoxycytidine deaminase.

The anthracycline antibiotics are a class of drug that mediate their effects by binding to DNA and intercalation. The anthracyclines enter cells through a passive transport process and can be pumped out of cells through the multidrug resistance protein MDR1 or P glycoprotein. The natural substance daunorubicin has been used in the treatment of leukemia for over 20 years. More recently, a synthetic anthracycline, idarubicin, appears to have greater activity than daunorubicin, largely because of the persistence of an active metabolite. Another synthetic compound, mitoxantrone, has been used in the treatment of acute leukemia and has the possible advantage of being less cardiotoxic.

DOSAGE AND SCHEDULING

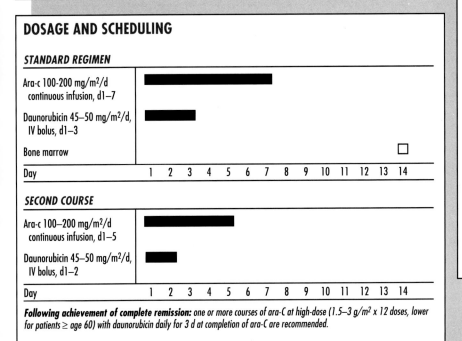

STANDARD REGIMEN

	Day	1	2	3	4	5	6	7	8	9	10	11	12	13	14
Ara-c 100-200 mg/m²/d continuous infusion, d1–7															
Daunorubicin 45–50 mg/m²/d, IV bolus, d1–3															
Bone marrow															

SECOND COURSE

	Day	1	2	3	4	5	6	7	8	9	10	11	12	13	14
Ara-c 100–200 mg/m²/d continuous infusion, d1–5															
Daunorubicin 45–50 mg/m²/d, IV bolus, d1–2															

Following achievement of complete remission: one or more courses of ara-C at high-dose (1.5–3 g/m² x 12 doses, lower for patients ≥ age 60) with daunorubicin daily for 3 d at completion of ara-C are recommended.

RECENT EXPERIENCE AND RESPONSE RATES
Most studies report complete remission rates of 60–70% (lower in patients over 60)

CANDIDATES FOR TREATMENT
Newly diagnosed patients with AML or relapsed AML (especially if first remission lasted 1 yr)

SPECIAL PRECAUTIONS
Rapid cell turnover and hyperuricemia with possible renal damage (start patients on allopurinol 300 mg/d if necessary)

ALTERNATIVE THERAPIES
None are standard

TOXICITIES
Drug combination: extremely myelotoxic, resulting in marrow aplasia with attendant pancytopenia; neutropenia 2–4 wk following induction; overwhelming sepsis possible (institute antibiotics); platelet transfusions if platelet count < 20,000/ml; mucositis, alopecia; **ara-C:** hepatotoxicity, with transaminasemia and/or jaundice in some patients; **Anthracyclines:** cardiotoxicity (monitored with MUGA scans)

DRUG INTERACTIONS
None noteworthy

NURSING INTERVENTIONS
Observe patients for any signs of infection; provide antimetics, particularly during the daunorubicin phase of the protocol; monitor blood counts and liver function tests daily; wash hands carefully

PATIENT INFORMATION
Patients undergoing induction therapy for AML are often quite ill prior to therapy. Considerable counseling and reassurance are necessary at this phase of the patient's disease. The patient needs to be informed rapidly about the various treatment options available once remission is achieved (consolidation with chemotherapy, BMT).

HIGH-DOSE CYTOSINE ARABINOSIDE

In an effort to increase the efficacy and durability of remissions, regimens containing cytosine arabinoside in high doses have been studied. High doses of ara-C give rise to higher levels of intracellular ara-C and increase the efficacy of the agent. As an induction regimen, high-dose ara-C is accompanied by an anthracycline antibiotic or l-asparaginase.

DOSAGE AND SCHEDULING

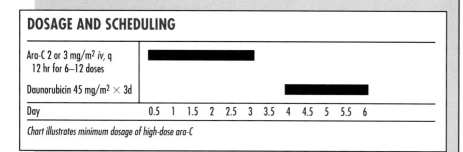

	0.5	1	1.5	2	2.5	3	3.5	4	4.5	5	5.5	6
Ara-C 2 or 3 mg/m² *iv*, q 12 hr for 6–12 doses												
Daunorubicin 45 mg/m² × 3d												
Day												

Chart illustrates minimum dosage of high-dose ara-C

RECENT EXPERIENCE AND RESPONSE RATES

Complete responses are seen in about 50% of patients tested in relapse

CANDIDATES FOR TREAMENT
AML in relapse

SPECIAL PRECAUTIONS
Tumor lysis syndrome with release of uric acid and phosphorus alkalinization of the urine should be induced and allopurinol, 300 mg/d, started immediately

ALTERNATIVE THERAPIES
Standard-dose ara-C; Carboplatin

TOXICITIES
Drug combination: neutropenia and thrombocytopenia; nausea, vomiting, diarrhea; elevated liver function tests; **High-dose ara-C:** cerebellar toxicity (slurred speech, ataxia), ototoxicity, conjunctivitis; extreme myelotoxicity resulting in narrow aplasia and pancytopenia

DRUG INTERACTIONS
None noteworthy

NURSING INTERVENTIONS
Observe patients for signs of infection; give antiemetic; monitor blood counts and liver function tests daily; wash hands carefully; watch for ataxia daily; manage conjunctivitis with glucocorticoid eyedrops every 6–8 hr

PATIENT INFORMATION
Patients should be informed that this regimen is quite myelotoxic and that prolonged myelosuppresion is expected.

MITOXANTRONE AND ETOPOSIDE

Both mitoxantrone and etoposide have shown activity as single agents in acute myeloid leukemia (AML). A combination of the two agents is a relatively effective therapy for patients with relapsed disease. The regimen is relatively well tolerated.

DOSAGE AND SCHEDULING

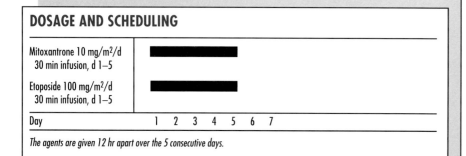

	1	2	3	4	5	6	7
Mitoxantrone 10 mg/m²/d 30 min infusion, d 1–5							
Etoposide 100 mg/m²/d 30 min infusion, d 1–5							
Day							

The agents are given 12 hr apart over the 5 consecutive days.

RECENT EXPERIENCE AND RESPONSE RATES

Complete response rate of 45–50%; as with most regimens used in relapse for AML, the duration of remission achieved is relatively brief. In a study by Lazzarino *et al.*, 61% of patients achieved complete remission including several patients with disease refractory to other therapy; the median CR duration was 5 mo with a range of 2 to 12 + mo [11].

CANDIDATES FOR TREATMENT
AML in relapse

SPECIAL PRECAUTIONS
Possibility of cardiotoxicity: obtain baseline MUGA scan

ALTERNATIVE THERAPIES
Ara-C and anthracycline, carboplatin, high-dose ara-C

TOXICITIES
Drug combination: myelosupression; severe oral mucositis; reactivation of herpes virus (administer acyclovir); mild nausea and vomiting, diarrhea, transaminasemia, alopecia

DRUG INTERACTIONS
None noteworthy

NURSING INTERVENTIONS
Parental hyperalimentation for grade 3 oral mucositis; monitor for myelosupression

PATIENT INFORMATION
Patients undergoing induction therapy for AML are often quite ill prior to therapy. Considerable counseling and reassurance are necessary at this phase of the patient's disease. The patient needs to be informed rapidly about the various treatment options available once remission is achieved (consolidation with chemotherapy, BMT).

BFM INTENSIFIED INDUCTION AND CONSOLIDATION THERAPY

A significant advance in the treatment of acute lymphocytic leukemia (ALL) in adults has come from a series of German multicenter studies, the BFM regimens (Berlin, Frankfurt, Munich). This intensive multiagent regimen has an induction phase with prednisone, vincristine, daunorubicin, and l-asparaginase followed by cyclophophamide, cytarabine, 6-mercaptopurine, and methotrexate given over a period of 52 days. Following this, a reinduction phase is begun using dexamethasone, vincristine, doxorubicin, cyclophosphamide, ara-C, and thioguanine over the next 42 days. Then a maintenance phase with 6-mercaptopurine and methotrexate is started for up to 130 weeks. Central nervous system (CNS) prophylaxis consists of cranial irradiation with 24 Gy and intrathecal methotrexate (10 mg/m^2, maximum single dose 15 mg), once weekly for 4 wk during phase 2 when complete remission is achieved after phase 1. If complete remission is delayed until after completion of phase 2, CNS prophylaxis is given immediately thereafter.

Several important prognostic factors were uncovered during this study. Favorable outcome was seen in patients who achieved complete remission in less than 4 wk, who were younger than 35 years, whose initial leukocyte count was less than 30,000, and whose immunophenotype was T-ALL. The absence of these good prognostic factors resulted in an adverse outcome; that is, the presence of two or three adverse factors was associated with a median remission duration of 9.6 mo, whereas the absence of these factors resulted in a better outcome.

CANDIDATES FOR TREATMENT
Patients with ALL at diagnosis

SPECIAL PRECAUTIONS
Patients should have urine alkalinized (place on allpurinol 300 mg/dl)

ALTERNATIVE THERAPIES
Bone marrow transplantation after induction

TOXICITY
Myelosuppression with attendant problems

DRUG INTERACTIONS
None noteworthy

NURSING INTERVENTIONS
Neutropenia is expected, therefore observe for any signs of infection; give antiemetics, particularly during daunorubicin phase of protocol; monitor blood counts and liver function tests daily; wash hands carefully

PATIENT INFORMATION
Patients undergoing induction therapy for ALL are often quite ill prior to therapy. Considerable counseling and reassurance are necessary at this phase of the patient's disease. The patient needs to be informed rapidly of the various treatment options available once remission is achieved (consolidation, BMT).

DOSAGE AND SCHEDULING

DRUG	DOSE AND DAYS
Induction	
Phase 1	
Prednisone	60 mg/m^2 d 1–28
Vincristine	1.5 mg/m^2 IV d 1,8,15,22
Daunorubicin	25 mg/m^2 IV d 1,8,15,22
l-Asparaginase	5000 U/m^2 IV d 1–14
Phase 2	
Cyclophosphamide	650 mg/m^2 IV d 29,43,57
ara-C	75 mg/m^2 IV d 31–34,38–41,45–48,52–55
6-Mercaptopurine	60 mg/m^2 PO d 29–57
Methotrexate	10 mg/m^2 IT d 31,38,45,52
Consolidation	
Phase 1	
Dexamethasone	10 mg/m^2 PO d 1–28
Vincristine	1.5 mg/m^2 IV* d 1,8,15,22
Doxorubicin	25 mg/m^2 IV d 1,8,15,22
Phase 2	
Cyclophosphamide	650 mg/m^2 IV d 29
ara-C	75 mg/m^2 IV d 31–34,38–41
Thioguanine	60 mg/m^2 PO d 29–42
Maintenance	
6-Mercaptopurine	60 mg/m^2 PO/d, weeks 10–18
Methotrexate	20 mg/m^2 PO/IV/wk and d 29–130

*Maximum dose of 2 mg/m^2.
CNS prophylaxis consisted of cranial irradiation with 24 Gy and intrathecal methotrexate, 10/mg^2 (maximum single dose, 15 mg/m^2), once weekly for 4 wk during phase II when complete remission was achieved.

RECENT EXPERIENCE AND RESPONSE RATES
Complete remission of 74%, with 34% of patients in continuous complete remission at 5 yr; median survival is 28 mo.

ECOG INTENSIFIED INDUCTION AND CONSOLIDATION THERAPY

Modifications of the BFM protocol have been used by cooperative groups such as the Cancer and Leukemia Group. The Eastern Cooperative Oncology Group (ECOG) is joining with MRC of the UK to examine the role of bone marrow transplantation in the first remission of ALL. Patients receive the following induction regimen and are then randomized to autologous BMT (or assigned to allogenic BMT if a donor is available). Both groups receive intensification before either transplantation or conventional consolidation/maintenance.

DOSAGE AND SCHEDULING

DRUG	DOSE AND DAYS
Induction	
Phase 1	
Daunorubicin	60 mg/m² IV push d 1,8,15,21
Vincristine	1.4 mg/m² IV push* d 1,8,15,21
Prednisolone	60 mg/m² PO qd d 1–28
l-Asparaginase	10,000 U IM or IV in 100 ml D5W over 30 min qd d 17–28
Methotrexate	12.5 mg IT d 15 *only*

If CNS leukemia is present at diagnosis, methotrexate IT or via an Ommaya reservoir is given weekly until blasts are absent. 24 Gy cranial irradiation and 12 Gy to the spinal cord are administered concurrent with Phase 2.

Phase 2 (weeks 5–8)	
Cyclophosphamide	650 mg/m² IV in 250 cc normal saline for 30 min, d 1,14,28
ara-C	75 mg/m² IV in 100 cc D5W for 30 min, d 1–4, 8–11, 15–18, 22–25
6-Mercaptopurine	60 mg/m² PO qd d 1–28
Methotrexate	12.5 mg IT d 1, 8, 15, 22

Postponed if total WBC count <3 x 10⁹/l

Intensification (weeks 13–16)	
HD Methotrexate	3 g/m² IV in NS 500 ml over 2 hr, d 1,8,22
l-Asparaginase	10,000 Iu/m² IV in 100 ml D5W over 30 min, d 2,9,23
Leucovorin rescue	10 mg/m² IV D5W 50 ml q 6 hr x 4 doses beginning 22–24 hr after completion of methotrexate; then 10 mg/m² PO q 6 hr x 72 hr

Begin 4 wk from d 28 of induction, Phase 2; postpone if WBC < 3 x 10⁹/l.
If randomized to autologous BMT or assigned to allogenic BMT, perform harvest (1–3 x 10⁸/kg nucleated cells) within 3–7 wk from start of intensification. Postpone harvest until marrow cellularity on biopsy ≥30%.

Day -6 to day -4: fractioned TBI total dose 1320 cGy; **For males only:** 400 cGy testicular boost; **Day -3:** etoposide 60 mg/kg IV; **Day 0:** allogeneic or autologous marrow infusion; **Day 0—+27:** GM-CSF 250 µg/m²/day over 4–6 hr IV

If randomized to chemotherapy, start conventional consolidation maintenance (beginning 1–2 mo after intensification).

Cycle I Consolidation	
ara-C	75 mg/m² IV in 500 cc D5W
Etoposide	100 mg/m² IV in 500 ml NS over 1 hr, d 1–5
Vincristine	1.4 mg/m²,* d 1, 8, 15, 22
Dexamethasone	10 mg/m² PO, d 1–28
Cycles II, IV Consolidation	
ara-C	75 mg/m² IV in 500 cc D5W over 30 min, d 1–5
Etoposide	100 mg/m² IV in 500 cc normal saline x 60 min, d 1–5

Begin 4 wk from day 1 of each cycle or when WBC count >3.0 x 10⁹/l, except Cycle IV which begins 2 mo from day 1 following Cycle III or when WBC count >3.0 x 10⁹/l.

Cycle III Consolidation	
Daunorubicin	25 mg/m² IV push, d 1, 8, 15, 22
Cyclophosphamide	650 mg/m² IV in 250 cc normal saline over 30 min, d 29
ara-C	75 mg/m² IV 100 cc D5W over 30 min, d 31–34, 38–41
6-Thioguanine	60 mg/m² PO, d 29–42

Begin 4 weeks from day 1 of Cycle II or when WBC count >3.0 x 10⁹/l.

Maintenance Therapy	
Vincristine	1.4 mg/m² IV* every 3 mo
Prednisolone	60 mg/m² PO x 5 d every 3 mo
6-Mercaptopurine	75 mg/m² PO/d
Methotrexate	20 mg/m² PO or IV/wk for 2.5 yr
Interferon alpha	3 MU SC 3 times/wk—Ph+ patients only

All drug doses are based on the lesser of the actual/corrected ideal body weight.
Maximum dose of 2 mg/m².

CANDIDATES FOR TREATMENT
ALL at diagnosis

SPECIAL PRECAUTIONS
Patients should have their urine alkalinized (place on allopurinol 300 mg/d)

ALTERNATIVE THERAPIES
Bone marrow transplant after induction

RECENT EXPERIENCE AND RESPONSE RATES
60% complete response rate

TOXICITY
Myelosuppression with attendant problems

DRUG INTERACTIONS
None noteworthy

NURSING INTERVENTIONS
Neutropenia is expected, therefore, observe for any signs of infection; give antiemetics, particularly during daunorubicin phase of the protocol; monitor blood counts and liver function tests daily; wash hands carefully

PATIENT INFORMATION
Patients undergoing induction therapy for ALL are often quite ill prior to therapy. Considerable counseling and reassurance are necessary at this phase of the patient's disease. The patient needs to be informed rapidly about the various treatment options available once remission is achieved (consolidation with chemotherapy, BMT).

CHAPTER 19: HODGKIN'S DISEASE
Jeffrey P. Letzer, Ellen R. Gaynor, and Richard I. Fisher

Hodgkin's lymphoma is a relatively rare disease accounting for only 14% of all newly diagnosed lymphomas. It occurs in a bimodal age distribution, with incidence rising sharply after age 10, peaking in the late twenties, and declining until age 45. After age 45 the incidence rises again steadily with age. Despite significant advances in the management of Hodgkin's disease, its etiology and its cell of origin remain unknown.

Diagnosis requires the examination of an adequate tissue sample, which in most cases involves excisional biopsy of an involved lymph node. On occasion, the initial biopsy may show only a hyperplastic process. If the clinical suspicion of Hodgkin's disease is strong, an additional deeper lymph node biopsy should be obtained because it may provide the diagnosis. Pathology material should always be reviewed by an experienced hematopathologist.

Pathologically, Hodgkin's disease is defined as a grouping of malignant lymphomas that share common clinical and histologic features. The diagnosis is based on the presence of bizarre-appearing tumor giant cells, called Sternberg-Reed cells, surrounded by a background of benign-appearing host-inflammatory cells. While Sternberg-Reed cells are necessary for the diagnosis, they are not specific to Hodgkin's disease and may be found in other neoplastic processes.

Several pathologic classification systems for Hodgkin's disease have been proposed over the years. The so-called Rye classification system is used extensively today (Table 1). Nodular sclerosis is the most common histologic subtype at the time of diagnosis in patients in developed countries. Because of the efficacy of treatment for Hodgkin's disease, histologic subtype is not an independent predictor of clinical outcome. With appropriate therapy, each of the histologic subtypes is potentially curable.

The majority of patients present with asymptomatic adenopathy most commonly located in the cervical lymph node chains. Under most circumstances, spread occurs in a nonrandom fashion to involve contiguous nodal groups; this orderly pattern of spread constitutes the basis for the prophylactic radiation therapy commonly given to contiguous uninvolved sites of disease. For reasons that are unknown, the disease most commonly involves axial lymph node groups (eg, cervical, axillary, mediastinal, para-aortic and inguinal nodes) with very distinct sparing of other lymph node groups (eg, mesenteric, epitrochlear, and popliteal).

As curative therapy, either radiation therapy or combination chemotherapy, became available for the treatment of Hodgkin's disease, various staging systems were developed, each being a further refinement of the one preceding it. The intent and ultimate value of any given staging system are its ability to improve selection of patients suitable for curative radiation therapy and those who are candidates for systemic therapy alone or in combination with radiation therapy.

A very commonly used staging system is the Cotswolds revision of the Ann Arbor Staging Classification system (Table 2), a four-stage system based on the extent of nodal and extranodal involvement. In addition to stage, patients are further classified according to the absence (A) or presence (B) of systemic symptoms. Symptoms that are of prognostic significance are fever, night sweats, and weight loss. Selected patients with extranodal disease contiguous to involved nodes are classified in the appropriate lymph node stage with the letter E. E patients have a more favorable prognosis than those patients with clearly disseminated extranodal disease.

Table 1. Rye Classification of Hodgkin's Disease

Lymphocyte predominance	Mixed cellularity
Nodular sclerosis	Lymphocyte depletion

Table 2. Cotswolds Revision of the Ann Arbor Staging Classification of Hodgkin's Disease

Stage I	Involvement of a single lymph node or lymphoid structure (eg, spleen, thymus, Waldeyers, ring) or involvement of a single extralymphatic site (IE)
Stage II	Involvement of two or more lymph node regions on the same side of the diaphragm (hilar nodes, when involved on both sides, constitute stage II disease; the mediastinum is a single site); localized contiguous involvement of only one extranodal organ or site and lymph node regions on the same side of the diaphragm (IIE); the number of anatomic sites involved should be indicated by a subscript (eg, II$_3$)
Stage III	Involvement of lymph node regions on both sides of the diaphragm (III), which may also be accompanied by involvement of the spleen (IIIS) or by localized contiguous involvement of only one extranodal organ site (IIIE) or both (IIISE) Stage III may be subdivided as: Stage III$_1$—with or without splenic hilar, celiac, or portal nodes Stage III$_2$—with para-aortic, iliac, mesenteric nodes
Stage IV	Diffuse or disseminated involvement of one or more extranodal organs or tissue, with or without associated lymph node involvement A = Asymptomatic B = Fever >38°C, night sweats, weight loss >10% of body weight in the previous 6 mo X = Bulky mediastinal disease

Adatped from Lister et al. [1]; with permission.

RADIATION THERAPY

Radiation therapy as a single modality treatment is curative in early stage Hodgkin's disease. The results quoted for efficacy of radiation therapy are frequently those obtained at large centers with extensive experience. It is important to appreciate that the quality of radiation therapy given in such centers may be considerably better than that given in centers with far less experience. Tumoricidal doses of radiation therapy are 35 to 44 Gy fractionated at a rate of 7.5 to 10 Gy per week. The dose of radiation therapy necessary to eradicate occult disease in contiguous nodal areas is unknown, but a minimum of 30 to 36 Gy is usually recommended.

CHEMOTHERAPY

Until the end of the 1960s, radiation therapy was the only successful therapeutic tool for the treatment of Hodgkin's disease. While available data may underestimate the efficacy of single-agent therapy because pilot studies are often conducted in heavily pretreated patients, single agents, in general, produce complete responses in less than or equal to 20% of patients, with a median duration of response of 3 to 6 months. Single-agent therapy is reserved for patients who are unable to tolerate combination therapy or who require salvage therapy. The vast majority of patients given systemic therapy today receive combination therapy.

The comparative efficacy of various chemotherapeutic regimens for advanced Hodgkin's disease has been defined in large randomized trials conducted by multicenter cooperative oncology groups. The four most important recent phase III trials are summarized in Table 3. Although follow-up is still limited in three of the cooperative group trials, several conclusions can be inferred from the data.

The ABVD and MOPP/ABVD (alternating) regimens appear to produce more frequent, and more durable, complete responses than MOPP alone. In the CALGB and Milan trials, patients treated with ABVD or MOPP/ABVD had higher rates of complete response, as well as higher rates of freedom from progression or failure-free survival. (See Bonadonna *et al.* for statistical analysis of the Milan trial [6].) Investigators at the National Cancer Institute, who are strong proponents of the MOPP regimen for the treatment of Hodgkin's disease, have criticized the randomized trials, suggesting that results obtained with MOPP were inferior because it was not given in these trials as it was in the NCI series [7].

In an Intergroup study of MOPP/ABV hybrid versus *sequential* MOPP/ABVD, the MOPP/ABV hybrid was superior with regard to failure-free survival and overall survival to sequential MOPP/ABVD. The Canadian NCI study of MOPP/ABV hybrid versus *alternating* MOPP/ABVD revealed no differences between the groups in terms of complete response, freedom from progression, or overall survival.

At the present time, it appears that MOPP/ABV hybrid and alternating MOPP/ABVD regimens are superior to MOPP alone, considering the number and durability of the complete response rates and the lower toxicity. ABVD may be equivalent to MOPP/ABVD although confirmatory data is needed. Because of the apparent equivalence of results, toxicity of the individual regimen becomes a major factor when choosing therapy for the individual patient with advanced Hodgkin's disease.

TREATMENT STRATEGIES

Whenever possible, eligible patients should be entered into clinical trials appropriate for their stage of disease. Table 4 summarizes the currently accepted standard of care, as well as expected outcome, for patients with Hodgkin's disease.

Table 3. Important Phase III Studies of Non-Hodgkin's Disease

Study	Dosage	Time	Evaluable Patients, *n*	CR(%)	FFP(%)	OS(%)
Santaro *et al.* [2]	MOPP x 12	10 yr	43	74	37	58
	MOPP/ABVD x 6/6		45	89	61	69
Glick *et al.* [3]	MOPP/ABV x 8	30 mo	737/2	81	80	90*
	MOPP ABVD x 6–8/3 (sequential)		—	76	67 FFS*	85*
			—			
Connors *et al.* [4]	MOPP/ABV x ≥8	4 yr	146	85	75	84
	MOPP/ABVD x ≥6/6 (alternating)		141	82	70	84
Canellos *et al.* [5]	MOPP x ≥6	5 yr	123	67	50 FFS	66
	MOPP/ABVD x 6/6		123	83*	65 FFS*	75
	ABVD x ≥6		115	82*	61 FFS	73

*Statistically significant (p<0.05).
†Statistical significance not reported [6].
‡22/287 = (8.4%) received involved-field radiation therapy to bulky sites.
CR—complete response; FFP—freedom from progression; FFS— failure-free survival; OS—overall survival.

Table 4. Standard Treatment and Reported Outcomes for Patients with Hodgkin's Disease

Stage	Standard Treatment*	FFP/R (%)	Overall Survival (%) (Includes Salvage)
I–II	Radiation therapy	67–86	79–95
III$_1$A	Radiation therapy	53–80	66–80+
III$_2$A, IIIB–IV	Chemotherapy	65–80	69+

*Any stage associated with bulky mediastinal disease requires combination chemotherapy followed by radiation therapy.
†Stage IIIA, patients with splenic involvement of greater than or equal to 5 nodules may be treated more optimally with chemotherapy alone.
FFP/R—freedom from progression/relapse.

Chemotherapy alone is currently the accepted treatment approach for Stage IIIA$_2$, IIIB, and IV Hodgkin's disease. Whether radiation therapy or chemotherapy represent optimal treatment for Stage IIIA$_1$ has not been determined. Investigators at Stanford suggest that the extent of splenic involvement is a useful discriminant in determining which patients with Stage IIIA disease are likely to attain durable complete response with radiation therapy alone. The standard of care for pathologically staged I and II Hodgkin's is extended-field radiation therapy.

There is interest in exploring the question of whether chemotherapy alone or some modified combination chemotherapy and radiation therapy program should replace standard radiation therapy alone in at least some subsets of early-stage disease [8,9]. Such an innovative approach would avoid the staging laparotomy with its attendant infectious and possible additional leukemogenic sequelae. It may also decrease the relapse rate from radiation therapy alone and thus possibly spare the increased toxicity from a combination of extensive radiation therapy and full chemotherapy [8]. A randomized study intending to explore the utility of short-course chemotherapy and limited radiation therapy in early-stage Hodgkin's disease has recently been initiated by the Southwest Oncology Group.

Patients with bulky mediastinal disease, regardless of stage, comprise one group for which there is general agreement that combined modality treatment (chemotherapy and mantle or involved-field–mediastinal radiation) is indicated. The definition of *bulky mediastinum* is a ratio greater than one third of the maximal mediastinal diameter over the internal transthoracic diameter at the level of T 5/6. If radiation therapy alone or chemotherapy alone is used to treat this group, the relapse rate is 46 to 74% with radiation therapy and 33 to 50% with chemotherapy. Although combined modality therapy has not been demonstrated to improve overall survival, it will maximize the complete response rate and minimize the relapse rate, the latter varying from 0 to 19% in the recent literature [7,10–12].

Due to the possible increased cardiopulmonary toxicities from the ABVD regimen in combination with mediastinal radiation therapy, some authors recommend either MOPP/ABVD (alternating) or MOPP/ABV hybrid in combination with mantle or involved-field radiation therapy for the treatment of Hodgkin's disease with bulky mediastinal disease [8,13].

SALVAGE THERAPY

Initial relapses in Hodgkin's disease tend to occur during the first 2 to 3 years after the completion of the first course of therapy. Patients relapsing after radiation therapy respond well to subsequent combination chemotherapy, with significant numbers achieving a durable complete response.

A variety of salvage regimens have been tried in patients relapsing after treatment with combination chemotherapy. In general, complete response rates are low but, more importantly, the remissions are not durable in most patients.

The success of high-dose therapy and bone marrow transplant in other malignancies prompted trials of this approach in patients with relapsed Hodgkin's disease. There are no prospective controlled trials of allogeneic versus autologous bone marrow transplant for relapsed Hodgkin's disease. Most of the studies that have been conducted have involved the use of autologous bone marrow support.

From pooled data, it appears that at the present time autologous bone marrow transplant offers the chance of cure to approximately one third of patients with recurrent Hodgkin's disease who undergo this treatment. Several retrospective analyses have suggested that patients most likely to benefit from this form of therapy are those who are transplanted after failing one or, at most, two prior chemotherapy regimens, those who have a good performance status, and those whose disease has been shown to be sensitive to chemotherapy given prior to the preparative regimen. Patients fulfilling these criteria should be considered for this form of salvage therapy.

EFFECTS OF TREATMENTS

Secondary Acute Myeloid Leukemia

The development of acute myeloid leukemia (AML) secondary to the treatment of Hodgkin's disease is a well recognized complication of the curative therapy of this disease. Thus one of the major goals in the development of combination chemotherapy regimens for Hodgkin's disease is to avoid agents known to be leukemogenic, without compromising the cure rate.

The risks for developing AML in patients who receive chemotherapy alone for advanced Hodgkin's disease are very low, especially when a limited number of cycles (eg, 6–8) are given. At the National Cancer Institute, nearly 400 patients have been treated with MOPP alone, and only one patient has developed AML. Although there have been reports of "actuarial risks" of secondary AML with MOPP as high as 11.5% at 15 years, such reports are frequently based on data with short follow-up and much longer duration of therapy than is presently considered standard. For example, Tucker *et al.* reported an actuarial risk of s-AML of 11.5% at 15 years based on 3 of 80 patients receiving chemotherapy only ("usually MOPP") [14]. However, two of the three patients were treated with MOPP for 22 and 24 cycles [15]. Thus when evaluation of the frequency of secondary AML is restricted to series in which a limited number of cycles of MOPP is given, results similar to those of the NCI are consistently seen. In a multicenter Italian study with a 9-year median follow-up, only 2 of 128 (1.5%) MOPP-treated patients developed s-AML, with a 19-year actuarial risk of 2.2%; the median number of cycles was 7.25 [16]. Thus MOPP alone given for 6 to 8 cycles appears to result in no more than a 2.2% risk of s-AML.

ABVD-containing regimens (whether ABVD, MOPP/ABVD, or MOPP/ABV hybrid) given without radiation appear to have an even lower risk of s-AML than MOPP alone. Bonadonna's group to date reports only one case of s-AML with ABVD alone [13], and the Vancouver group at 7 years' follow-up has not seen any s-AMLs associated with MOPP/ABV hybrid in 79 patients [10].

There is some agreement that the risk of s-AML is greatest in those patients who have received combined modality therapy. In the MOPP and radiation therapy group, actuarial risks for s-AML at greater than 10 years have been reported as low as 0.9% (in which MOPP comprised 83% of the chemotherapy) [17] to as high as 9.5% [18]; most reports are closer to the latter figure. Certain groups may be at even higher risk for s-AML: those who have received salvage MOPP after radiation therapy failure [18], those who have undergone splenectomy, and patients older than 40 years [19].

Combined modality therapy with ABVD-containing regimens and radiation therapy is associated with lower long-term risks for s-AML than is therapy with MOPP and radiation. Fifteen-year actuarial risks range from 0.7% [18] to only 5.4% [16]. The risks for s-AML in the groups with either alternating MOPP/ABVD or MOPP/ABV hybrid are not known.

Secondary Solid Tumors

Three large studies, including long-term follow-up of nearly 3800 patients with Hodgkin's disease who were treated with radiation therapy and/or chemotherapy (usually MOPP or ABVD), have reported 15 to 19–year actuarial risks for secondary solid tumors. The actuarial risks for the radiation therapy–only group ranged from 7 to 17%; for the chemotherapy-only group, 2 to 19%; and for the combined-modality therapy group, 4 to 14% [14,16,18]. The risk profile for developing secondary solid tumors after alternating MOPP/ABVD or MOPP/ABV hybrid remains to be determined.

The five most common noncutaneous cancers seen in patients receiving treatment for Hodgkin's disease are lung, gastrointestinal, soft tissue sarcoma, thyroid, and breast. The cancers are commonly, but not always, located in a previously irradiated bed.

Based on actuarial risks, up to 5% of Hodgkin's disease patients may develop aggressive non-Hodgkin's lymphoma with the exact risk groups not clearly delineated at present. The median time to the development of non-Hodgkin's lymphoma is approximately 12 years, similar to that for secondary solid tumors but twice as long as that for s-AML (6 years) [20].

Infertility

Infertility is a major problem with MOPP chemotherapy, especially in males. MOPP produces azoospermia in 95 to 100% of males, with a recovery of spermatogenesis in less than 20%. The recovery is usually only partial and may be delayed up to 10 years. Although MOPP causes amenorrhea in 40 to 50% of fertile women overall, this finding is very age-dependent. Whereas 85% of women older than 30 become amenorrheic, only 20% of women younger than 30 do [13]. Unlike the immediate occurrence of azoospermia in men, premature ovarian failure may be delayed as long as 10 years after chemotherapy in women.

ABVD, a major improvement over MOPP with respect to infertility, does not cause irreversible damage to spermatogenesis or ovarian function [21,22]. Based on the Milan experience including analysis of 64 patients, the MOPP/ABVD alternating regimen produces infertility in approximately 50% of males [13]. Another Italian report based on only 16 menstruating women indicated an infertility rate of only 6.2% [23]. Data on infertility due to MOPP/ABV hybrid are not available.

REFERENCES

1. Lister TA, Crowther D, Sutcliffe SB, *et al.*: Report of a committee convened to discuss the evaluation and staging of patients with Hodgkin's disease: Cotswold Meeting. *J Clin Oncol* 1989, 7:1630.

2. Santoro A, Bonfante V, Viviani S, *et al.*: Decrease in mortality rate by Hodgkin's disease after ABVD vs. MOPP: 10-year results. *Proc ASCO* 1991, 10:281.

3. Glick J, Tsiatis A, Schilsky R, *et al.*: A randomized phase III trial of MOPP/ABV hybrid vs. sequential MOPP/ABVD in advanced Hodgkin's disease: Preliminary results of the intergroup trial. *Proc ASCO* 1991, 10:271.

4. Connors JM, Klimo P, Adams G, *et al.*: MOPP/ABV hybrid versus alternating MOPP/ABVD for advanced Hodgkin's disease. *Proc ASCO* 1992, 11:317.

5. Canellos GP, Anderson JR, Propert KJ, *et al.*: Chemotherapy of advanced Hodgkin's disease with MOPP, ABVD, or MOPP alternating with ABVD. *New Engl J Med* 1992, 327:1478.

6. Bonadonna G, Valagussa P, Santoro A: Alternating non-cross-resistant combination chemotherapy or MOPP in Stage IV Hodgkin's disease: A report of 8-year results. *Ann Intern Med* 1986, 104:739–746.

7. Longo DL: The use of chemotherapy in the treatment of Hodgkin's disease. *Sem Oncol* 1990, 17:716–735.

8. Longo DL, Glatstein E, Duffey PL, *et al.*: Radiation therapy versus combination chemotherapy in the treatment of early-stage Hodgkin's disease: Seven-year results of a prospective randomized trial. *J Clin Oncol* 1991, 9:906–917.

9. Hoppe RT: Early-stage Hodgkin's disease: A choice of treatments or a treatment of choice? (Editorial). *J Clin Oncol* 1991, 9:897–900.

10. Klimo P, Connors JM: An update of the Vancouver experience in the management of advanced Hodgkin's disease treated with the MOPP/ABV hybrid program. *Sem Hematol* 1988, 25(suppl 2):34–40.

11. Hoppe RT: The management of bulky mediastinal Hodgkin's disease. *Hematol/Oncol Clin North Am* 1989, 3:265–276.

12. Levitt SH, Lee CKK, Aeppli D, *et al.*: The role of radiation therapy in Hodgkin's disease: Experience and controversy (the 54th Annual Janeway Lecture: 1989). *Cancer* 1992, 70:693–703.

13. Bonadonna G, Wiernik PH, Santoro A: Clinical treatment of Hodgkin's disease. pp. 701–727. In Wiernik PH, Canellos GP, Kyle RA, *et al.* (eds): Neoplastic Diseases of the Blood. New York: Churchill Livingstone, 1991.

14. Tucker MA, Coleman CN, Cox RS, *et al.*: Risk of second cancers after treatment for Hodgkin's disease. *New Engl J Med* 1988, 318:76–81.

15. Coleman CN, Kaplan HS, Cox R, *et al.*: Leukemias, non-Hodgkin's lymphoma and solid tumors in patients treated for Hodgkin's disease. *Cancer Surv* 1982, 1:733–744.

16. Cimino G, Papa G, Tura S, *et al.*: Second primary cancer following Hodgkin's disease: Updated results of an Italian multicentric study. *J Clin Oncol* 1991, 9:432–437.

17. Lavey RS, Eby NL, Prosnitz LR: Impact on second malignancy risk of the combined use of radiation and chemotherapy for lymphomas. *Cancer* 1990, 66:80–88.

18. Valagussa P, Santoro A, Fossati-Bellani F, *et al.*: Hodgkin's disease and second malignancies. *Proc ASCO* 1988, 7:227.

19. Urba WJ, Longo DL: Hodgkin's disease. *N Engl J Med* 1992, 326:678–687.

20. Dietrich PY, Henry-Amar M, Cosset JM, *et al.*: Characteristics and outcome of second cancers after Hodgkin's disease: A 25-year experience of the institut Gustave Roussy. *Proc ASCO* 1991, 10:277.

21. Viviani S, Santoro A, Ragni G, *et al.*: Pre- and post-treatment testicular dysfunction in Hodgkin's disease. *Proc ASCO* 1988, 7:227.

22. Bonadonna G, Valagussa P, Santoro A, *et al.*: Hodgkin's disease: The Milan Cancer Institute experience with MOPP and ABVD. *Rec Res Cancer Res* 1989, 117:169–174.

23. Brusamolino E, Lazzarino M, Morra E, *et al.*: Combination chemotherapy with alternating MOPP-ABVD in advanced Hodgkin's disease. *Haematologica* 1989, 74:173–179.

24. Longo DL, Young RC, Wesley M, *et al.*: Twenty years of MOPP therapy for Hodgkin's disease. *J Clin Oncol* 1986, 4:1295–1306.

25. Bonadonna G, Zucali R, Monfardini S, *et al.*: Combination chemotherapy of Hodgkin's disease with adriamycin, bleomycin, vinblastine, and imidazole carboxamide versus MOPP. *Cancer* 1975, 36:252.

MOPP
Mechlorethamine, Vincristine, Procarbazine, Prednisone

For 2.5 decades, MOPP has been the standard combination chemotherapy regimen for advanced Hodgkin's disease against which all other variations and new regimens have been compared. MOPP was one of the first chemotherapy regimens based on the premise that a combination of agents, each of which has single activity against a tumor yet has a different toxicity profile, may have additive efficacy with tolerable side effects.

MOPP includes a classic alkylating agent (*m*ustard); a vinca alkaloid, which is a spindle poison (vincristine, *O*ncovin®); a probable alkylating agent (*p*rocarbazine); and a glucocorticoid steroid (*p*rednisone).

DOSAGE AND SCHEDULING

	1	2	3	4	5	6	7	8	9	10	11	12	13	14
Nitrogen mustard 6 mg/m² IVP days 1,8	■							■						
Vincristine 1.4 mg/m² IVP days 1,8 (No "cap")	■							■						
Procarbazine 100 mg/m²/d po days 1–14	■■■■■■■■■■■■■■													
Prednisone 40 mg/m²/d po days 1–14	■■■■■■■■■■■■■■													
CBC with diff. days 1,8	□							□						
SMAC day 1	□													

Day

28-day cycle

DOSAGE MODIFICATIONS:

WBC	Platelets	Dose Adjustment [24]
>4000	>100,000	100% of all drugs
3000–3999		100% vincristine, prednisone
		75% nitrogen mustard, procarbazine
2000–2999		100% vincristine, prednisone
		50% nitrogen mustard, procarbazine
1000–1999	50,000–99,999	100% prednisone, 50% vincristine
		25% nitrogen mustard, procarbazine
<1000	<50,000	No drug given

It may be preferable to delay Day 1 treatment up to 1 week than to reduce significantly the dose of Day 1 drugs. Doses should not be reduced for cytopenias secondary to a myelophthisic bone marrow involvement.

RECENT EXPERIENCES AND RESPONSE RATES

Study	Evaluable Patients, n	CR(%)	FFS(%)	Cycle #/w Prednisone	Vincristine "Capped"
Longo, *et al.*, J Clin Oncol 1986, 4:1295–1306	188	84	54 (10 yr)	1,4	No
Longo, *et al.*, J Clin Oncol 1991, 9:1409	66	91	62* (8 yr)	Every	No
Santoro, *et al.*, Proc ASCO 1991, 10:281	43	74	—	1,4,7,10	No
Canellos, *et al.*, N Engl J Med 1992, 327:1478	123	67	50 (5 yr)	1,4	Yes

*Estimated from the data presented.
CR—complete response; FFS—failure-free survival; vincristine "capped" or not at 2 mg.

CANDIDATES FOR TREATMENT
Patients with Stages III2, IIIB, IV Hodgkin's disease

SPECIAL PRECAUTIONS
Patients with significantly elevated bilirubin
Elderly patients (severe constipation/obstipation)
Patients with peptic ulcer disease
Diabetic patients

ALTERNATIVE THERAPIES
MOPP/ABVD, MOPP/ABV, ?ABVD

TOXICITIES
Nitrogen mustard: severe nausea, metallic taste; infertility (83–100% males, 50% females); **Procarbazine**: flu-like symptoms (with initial exposure); peripheral neuropathy, psychosis, cerebellar dysfunction; **Vincristine**: peripheral neuropathy with loss of deep tendon reflexes, paresthesias, and motor deficit (*eg*, foot drop); constipation or ileus; alopecia (30%)

DRUG INTERACTIONS
Procarbazine: barbiturates, meperidine phenothiazines, antihistamines, sympathomimetics, tricyclic antidepressants, red wine and tyramine-rich foods, alcohol

NURSING INTERVENTIONS
Avoid extravasation of nitrogen mustard and vincristine (vesicants); if it occurs, consider local hyaluronidase injection as antidote for vincristine and local sodium thiosulfate for nitrogen mustard, with ice applied topically for the latter, heat for the former; monitor bowel function; provide prophylactic stool softeners or laxatives; give aggressive antiemetics pre-treatment; check CBC and Day 1 bilirubin prior to therapy

PATIENT INFORMATION
Patient should be informed that therapy may cause GI upset; taking dose with meals and an antiemetic may enhance tolerance (the procarbazine dose may be split); avoid drugs and food listed under drug interactions; call immediately if fever or prolonged bleeding develops; report development of paresthesias; offer sperm banking option to males

ABVD
Doxorubicin, Bleomycin, Vinblastine, and Dacarbazine

Once Bonadonna *et al.* demonstrated the efficacy of ABVD in a salvage setting, they moved the regimen into front-line therapy for advanced Hodgkin's disease. ABVD is an attractive alternative to MOPP therapy because it does not appear to cause sterility nor has it yet been associated with the development of secondary malignancies. Because it includes the drugs doxorubicin and bleomycin, cardiac and pulmonary toxicities can occur with the use of the regimen. In a randomized comparison of MOPP versus ABVD, early results suggest that ABVD is superior to MOPP therapy.

ABVD includes an anthracycline antibiotic (doxorubicin, *A*driamycin); an antibiotic inhibiting DNA replication by DNA polymerase via strand breaking (*b*leomycin); a vinca alkaloid, which is a spindle poison (*v*inblastine); and an alkylating agent (*d*acarbazine).

DOSAGE AND SCHEDULING

	1	2	3	4	5	6	7	8	9	10	11	12	13	14	15
Doxorubicin 25 mg/m² IVP days 1, 15	■														■
Bleomycin 10 U/m² IVP days 1, 15	■														■
Vinblastine 6 mg/m² IVP days 1, 15	■														■
Dacarbazine 375 mg/m² IVP days 1, 15	■														■
CBC with diff. days 1,15	□														□
SMAC day 1	□														
Day	1	2	3	4	5	6	7	8	9	10	11	12	13	14	15

28-day cycle. Pulmonary function tests with DLCO approximately q 2–3 cycles or sooner if new, noninfectious pulmonary signs or symptoms develop; PA and lateral CXR q 2 cycles.

DOSAGE MODIFICATIONS

WBC	Platelets	Dose Adjustment [25]
>4000	>130,000	100% of all drugs
3000–3999	100,000–129,000	50% doxorubicin, vinblastine, & dacarbazine
2000–2999	80,000–99,000	50% dacarbazine & 25% doxorubicin & vinblastine
1500–1999	50,000–79,000	25% dacarbazine & NO doxorubicin or vinblastine
<1500	<50,000	NO doxorubicin, vinblastine or dacarbazine

RECENT EXPERIENCES AND RESPONSE RATES

Study	Evaluable Patients, n	CR(%)	FFS(%)	FFP
Santoro, et al., Proc ASCO 1991, 10:281	35	71*/80†	—	73 (10 yr)†
Canellos, et al., N Engl J Med 1992, 327:1478	115	82	61 (5 yr)	—

*Prior to radiation therapy.
†Includes extensive radiation therapy.
CR—complete response; FFS—failure-free survival; FFP—freedom from progression.

CANDIDATES FOR TREATMENT
Patients with Stages III2, IIIB, IV Hodgkin's disease

SPECIAL PRECAUTIONS
Patients with less than normal left ventricular ejection fraction
Patients with significantly decreased baseline FEV_1 or DLCO (carbon monoxide diffusion capacity) or severe radiation pneumonitis
Patients with significantly elevated bilirubin

ALTERNATIVE THERAPIES
MOPP/ABVD, MOPP/ABV

TOXICITIES
Dacarbazine: severe nausea (doxorubicin is moderately emetic); **Vinblastine:** peripheral neuropathy with loss of deep tendon reflexes, paresthesias, motor deficit (*eg*, foot drop); constipation or ileus; **Bleomycin:** fevers, chills, anaphylaxis, skin reactions, pulmonary fibrosis (most significant; with pulmonary interstitial changes, DLCO<35% of baseline, or indication of pulmonary dysfunction, discontinue bleomycin at least temporarily; avoid cumulative doses greater than 400–450 U); **Doxorubicin:** cardiomyopathy (doses not to exceed 450 mg/m² with a history of mediastinal radiation or 550 mg/m² without; with decrease in LVEF >15% or absolute value <45%, discontinue the drug); pruritis; alopecia (60%, complete in 10%)

DRUG INTERACTION
Doxorubicin: heparin

NURSING INTERVENTIONS
Avoid extravasation of doxorubicin and vinblastine (vesicants), consider hyaluronidase as antidote and apply warm compresses; clinical phlebitis may develop even without extravasation, but is not an indication to stop the drug; decrease burning sensation from dacarbazine (irritant) by slowing infusion; reduce erythematous streaking of the vein ("flare") from pruritus and hives, with antihistamines or steroids; be prepared to treat anaphylaxis from bleomycin (keep epinephrine nearby), test dose should be given with first two doses

PATIENT INFORMATION
Patient should be informed that urine may turn red, complete hair loss can occur (2–4 weeks), mouth soreness with ulceration can occur (7–10 days); baking soda solutions can be applied; nausea can be controlled by avoiding food/fluid intake pretreatment

MOPP AND ABVD

The Goldie–Coldman hypothesis predicts that drug resistance in tumor cells may be overcome by the use of multiple drugs with different mechanisms of action introduced early in the course of treatment. Once they had demonstrated the activity of ABVD in MOPP-resistant disease, Bonadonna et al. developed the MOPP/ABVD regimen, in which monthly cycles of MOPP were alternated with ABVD. In a randomized study, Bonadonna et al. demonstrated that MOPP/ABVD was superior to MOPP alone in previously untreated patients with advanced disease [6]. Recently Canellos et al. in a randomized trial again demonstrated the superiority of MOPP/ABVD and ABVD alone over MOPP with respect to complete response rates and failure-free survival [5]. Whether these findings will translate into a survival advantage remains to be determined.

MOPP includes a classic alkylating agent (*m*ustard); a vinca alkaloid, which is a spindle poison (vincristine, *O*ncovin); a probable alkylating agent (*p*rocarbazine); and *p*rednisone. ABVD includes an anthracycline antibiotic (doxorubicin, *A*driamycin); an antibiotic inhibiting DNA replication by DNA polymerase via strand breaking (*b*leomycin); and a vinca alkaloid (*v*inblastine); and an akylating agent (*d*acarbazine).

CANDIDATES FOR TREATMENT
Patients with Stage III2, IIIB, IV Hodgkin's disease

ALTERNATIVE THERAPIES
MOPP/ABV, ?ABVD

For dosage modifications, special precautions, drug interactions, toxicities, nursing interventions, and patient information, see MOPP and ABVD protocols.

DOSAGE AND SCHEDULING

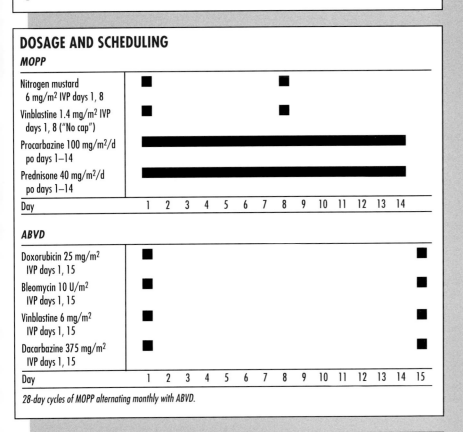

MOPP

Nitrogen mustard 6 mg/m² IVP days 1, 8

Vinblastine 1.4 mg/m² IVP days 1, 8 ("No cap")

Procarbazine 100 mg/m²/d po days 1–14

Prednisone 40 mg/m²/d po days 1–14

Day 1 2 3 4 5 6 7 8 9 10 11 12 13 14

ABVD

Doxorubicin 25 mg/m² IVP days 1, 15

Bleomycin 10 U/m² IVP days 1, 15

Vinblastine 6 mg/m² IVP days 1, 15

Dacarbazine 375 mg/m² IVP days 1, 15

Day 1 2 3 4 5 6 7 8 9 10 11 12 13 14 15

28-day cycles of MOPP alternating monthly with ABVD.

RECENT EXPERIENCES AND RESPONSE RATES

Study	Evaluable Patients, *n*	CR(%)	FFP(%)	FFS(%)
Santoro, et al., Proc ASCO 1991, 10:281	45	89	61 (10 yr)	—
Glick, et al., Proc ASCO 1991, 10:271*	737/2	76	—	67 (30 mo)
Connors, et al., Proc ASCO 1992, 11:317†	141	82	70 (4 yr)	—
Canellos, et al., N Engl J Med 1992, 327:1478	123	83	—	65 (5 yr)

*MOPP/ABVD given sequentially rather than alternating.
†Includes involved-field radiation for persistent nodal disease in initially bulky sites (only 8% of all patients).
CR—complete response; FFP—freedom from progression; FFS—failure-free survival.

MOPP/ABV HYBRID

To improve the efficacy of chemotherapy for advanced stage Hodgkin's disease (10–20% of patients are initially resistant to induction chemotherapy and up to one third of patients relapse after complete responses), Klimo and Connors in Vancouver developed the MOPP/ABV hybrid regimen [10]. They based their decision to use alternating, apparently non–cross-resistant agents on the Goldie–Coldman theory, which predicted that the efficacy of treatment would be improved by the earliest possible use of multiple active agents used in rapid alternation. The MOPP/ABV hybrid, in which the MOPP drugs are given Day 1 and the ABV drugs Day 8, has the theoretical advantage of maximally realizing the Goldie–Coldman theory compared with MOPP/ABVD, in which there is monthly alternation of MOPP only and ABVD only.

The efficacy of MOPP/ABV hybrid was first suggested by a single institution study at the University of British Columbia and then confirmed by two recent large trials comparing MOPP/ABV hybrid with MOPP/ABVD (either sequential in the American Intergroup study or alternating in the NCI of Canada study) [3,4]. Thus MOPP/ABV hybrid appears to be highly effective and perhaps more tolerable than MOPP or ABVD alone.

MOPP includes a classic alkylating agent (*m*ustard); a vinca alkaloid, which is a spindle poison (vinblastine, *O*ncovin); a probable alkylating agent (*p*rocarbazine); and *p*rednisone. ABV includes an anthracycline antibiotic (doxorubicin, *A*driamycin); an antibiotic inhibiting DNA replication by DNA polymerase via strand breaking (*b*leomycin); and a vinca alkaloid (*v*inblastine).

CANDIDATES FOR TREATMENT
Patients with Stage III2, IIIB, IV Hodgkin's disease

ALTERNATIVE THERAPIES
MOPP/ABVD, ?ABVD

For special precautions, drug interactions, toxicities, nursing interventions, and patient information, see MOPP and ABVD protocols.

DOSAGE AND SCHEDULING

	Day 1	Day 8
Nitrogen mustard 6 mg/m² IVP day 1	■	
Vincristine 1.4 mg/m² IVP day 1 (2.0 mg max.)	■	
Procarbazine 100 mg/m²/d po days 1–7	▬▬▬	
Prednisone 40 mg/m²/d po days 1–14	▬▬▬▬▬▬▬	
Doxorubicin 35 mg/m² IVP day 8		■
Bleomycin 10 U/m² IVP day 8		■
Vinblastine 6 mg/m² IVP day 8		■
CBC with diff. days 1,8	□	□
SMAC day 1	□	

Day: 1 2 3 4 5 6 7 8 9 10 11 12 13 14

28-day cycle. PFTs with DLCO q 4 cycles or immediately if new noninfectious pulmonary signs or symptoms develop; PA and lateral CXR q 2 cycles

RECENT EXPERIENCES AND RESPONSE RATES

Study	Evaluable Patients, *n*	CR(%)	FFP(%)	FFS(%)
Glick, *et al.*, Proc ASCO 1991, 10:271	737/2	81	—	80 (30 mo)
Conners, *et al.*, Proc ASCO 1992, 11:317*	146	85	75 (4 yr)	—

*Includes involved-field radiation for persistent nodal disease in originally bulky areas (only 8% of all patients).
CR—complete response; FFP—freedom from progression; FFS—failure-free survival.*

The non-Hodgkin's lymphomas are a group of monoclonal lymphoid malignancies defined by their characteristic lymph node pattern and cytology. Each pathologic entity has a distinctive clinical presentation, natural history, response to treatment, and survival pattern. Many histologic classifications have been proposed to encompass the diversity of non-Hodgkin's lymphomas. Currently, the Working Formulation proposed by the National Cancer Institute for classification of non-Hodgkin's lymphoma has been widely adopted in the United States [1]. This classification recognizes three prognostic groups of non-Hodgkin's lymphomas (low-, intermediate-, and high-grade categories), which are identified by the shape of survival curves generated from 1971 to 1975 clinical data.

The non-Hodgkin's lymphomas represent the seventh most common cause of death from cancer in the United States. The aggressive lymphomas, diffuse large cell lymphoma and, in particular, small, noncleaved cell lymphomas, are increasing in frequency with the AIDS epidemic.

ETIOLOGY AND RISK FACTORS

The cause of most non-Hodgkin's lymphomas is unknown. The rare entity HTLV-1–associated lymphoma is clearly linked to retroviral infection, but the specific molecular events leading to lymphomagenesis are not completely known. The risk of lymphoma is low among infected individuals and other host factors may play a role [2].

AIDS-associated lymphomas are also linked to retroviral infection, but in these cases the emergence of lymphoma is more likely secondary to virus-associated immunodeficiency rather than to a direct tumor-promoting effect of the HIV infection. Excessive B-cell proliferation, often stimulated by the Epstein–Barr virus, is thought to be the milieu necessary for lymphomagenesis [3]. The specific molecular events await definition. Whether similar mechanisms are pertinent to the etiology of other non-Hodgkin's lymphomas is speculative. Other established causes include genetic factors (such as x-linked lymphoproliferative syndrome in which genetically linked immunodeficiency results in B-cell lymphomas) and environmental exposures (Epstein–Barr virus and malaria in Burkitt's lymphoma; irradiation).

DIAGNOSIS

The diagnosis of a non-Hodgkin's lymphoma requires expert hematopathologic evaluation, often in conjunction with immuno-phenotypic, genotypic, and karyotypic studies (Table 1). The architectural pattern of diffuse or follicular involvement is evaluated on lymph node, not extranodal, material. Specialized studies often require fresh or frozen tissue and should be planned in advance of lymph node biopsy.

Demonstration of B-cell monoclonality can usually be performed on fixed tissue using immunoperoxidase methods. T-cell monoclonality requires molecular studies of fresh tissue (T-cell receptor gene rearrangement).

Some immunophenotypic patterns may identify specific disease entities, such as Ki-1 antigen in T-cell DLCL, or IgM immunophenotype with small lymphocytic lymphoma (Waldenström's macroglobulinemia). Chromosomal translocations may be associated with certain histologic patterns: t(2;5) in Ki-1 lymphomas; t(8;14) in Burkitt's lymphoma; t(11;14) in mantle zone lymphoma; and t(14;18) in follicular lymphomas. These chromosomal changes cannot be used in isolation to diagnose lymphoma. Rather, they add weight to a histologic diagnosis, and their specificity remains an area of current investigation.

Serum antibody studies of associated retroviral infection may be appropriate. HIV-associated lymphomas are those of intermediate and high-grade histologies, as are HTLV-1–associated lymphomas. Evidence of positive antibody titers with lymphadenopathy does not confer the diagnosis of lymphoma without histologic documentation.

STAGING

Once a diagnosis of non-Hodgkin's lymphoma is established, a full staging evaluation must be undertaken to plan treatment. Although the Ann Arbor staging classification for Hodgkin's disease is used in non-Hodgkin's lymphomas, it is not completely applicable. Recently, proposals for other staging systems have been made for low-grade, lymphoblastic, and small, noncleaved cell lymphomas to account for the high frequency of extranodal involvement and indicators of tumor bulk and cell proliferation. The standard staging studies for the lymphomas are provided in Table 2. In general, decisions regarding therapy may be based on full clinical staging with appropriate percutaneous biopsies.

Table 1. Diagnostic Studies in Non-Hodgkin's Lymphoma

1. Lymph node biopsy; extranodal site biopsies as indicated
2. Expert hematopathology using Working Formulation classification
3. Frozen tissue stored for special studies
4. Immunophenotyping by flow cytometry and/or immunoperoxidase of fixed or frozen tissue
5. Karotype performed on fresh tissue culture
6. Genotype performed on fresh tissue

Table 2. Studies Used for Staging Non-Hodgkin's Lymphomas

1. History
2. Blood work
   a. Complete blood count, platelets, review of smear
   b. Liver function tests
   c. Renal function tests
   d. Lactic dehydrogenase
3. Imaging
   a. Chest radiography
   b. CT scan of chest (if chest radiograph is positive), abdomen, and pelvis
   c. Lymphogram, if CT of abdomen or pelvis is negative
   d. Selected CNS, GI, bone studies depending on symptoms
   e. Gallium scan in intermediate-grade immunoblastic lymphoma and SNCL
4. Histology
   a. Lymph node biopsy
   b. Bone marrow biopsy (bilateral in low-grade histologies)
   c. CSF cytology in intermediate-grade and immunoblastic lymphoma with bone marrow
   d. Testicular disease, as well as in lymphoblastic lymphoma and SNCL

CT—computed tomography; CNS—central nervous system; CSF—cerebrospinal fluid; GI—gastrointestinal; LL—lymphoblastic lymphomas; SNCL—small noncleaved cell lymphomas.

LOW-GRADE LYMPHOMAS

According to the Working Formulation for classification of the non-Hodgkin's lymphomas, there are three histologic subtypes of low-grade lymphoma: small lymphocytic, follicular small cleaved, and follicular mixed small and large cell. A fourth subtype is often included within this category by many investigators, although it was not originally described in the Working Formulation. It is alternatively termed diffuse intermediate differentiation lymphoma, mantle zone lymphoma, or diffuse small cleaved cell lymphoma—centrocytic type.

The low-grade lymphomas are monoclonal B-cell diseases, presenting most often with generalized adenopathy with or without bone marrow involvement. Hepatosplenomegaly, other extranodal involvement (gastrointestinal tract, lung, skin, bone), and epidural or nerve compression may occur. Despite frequent bone marrow disease, meningeal involvement does not occur and central nervous system (CNS) prophylaxis is not required during therapy.

Approximately 10% of patients with low-grade lymphoma will be found to have clinical Stage I or II disease after complete clinical staging. These patients are often candidates for regional radiation therapy [4] (Table 3). Treatment outcome may be excellent with low morbidity. Prognostic factors include age, disease site, tumor bulk, and histology.

The majority of patients with low-grade lymphoma have advanced disease at presentation (intra-abdominal Stage II or Stage III or IV). There are many management options for such patients, and the criteria for selection among them remain controversial, because curative treatment is not established [5]. Despite high rates of complete response, relapse is usually noticed within 2 to 4 years of completing therapy [6]. Consolidative radiation therapy or maintenance with interferon may prolong disease-free intervals in some series.

The single-agent regimen pulse chlorambucil (16 mg/m² PO qd × 5 days) is well tolerated and effective in the palliative therapy of low-grade lymphoma. Objective responses are achieved in approximately 65% of patients, with median disease-free survival of 2 years [7]. Prompt tumor responses (in less than 3 mo) make this regimen more useful clinically than continuous daily chlorambucil. Hematologic toxicity is mild, although cumulative platelet depression may be encountered.

More recently, autologous stem cell transplantation (ASCT) has been used in patients with low-grade lymphoma. This intensive approach has been studied primarily in second or later remission and is limited to use in younger patients. Promising preliminary results have led to investigation of this modality in first remission [8,9]. Critical to ASCT is the collection of uninvolved normal hematopoi-etic stem cells. Technologies to purge tumor cells from involved marrow or to positively select normal stem cells are under investigation [10]. Bone marrow harvest and storage are often recommended in first remission; the value of ASCT in first remission remains to be determined.

INTERMEDIATE-GRADE LYMPHOMAS

The intermediate-grade lymphomas are a group of four diseases, the most prevalent being diffuse large cell lymphoma. Immunoblastic lymphoma, classified as a high-grade tumor, is usually managed as an intermediate-grade lesion and is often combined with diffuse large cell lymphoma in outcome data. These five malignancies share common clinical characteristics: slight male predominance, presentation in middle age, rapidly enlarging adenopathy with approximately one half of patients presenting with Stage I and II.

Masses may be bulky, particularly in the mediastinum (sometimes with associated superior vena cava obstruction or tracheobronchial compression) or abdomen. Involved extranodal sites are often symptomatic, such as ulcerated and/or hemorrhagic gastrointestinal tract disease or lytic bone lesions. Lymphomatous meningitis may be detected at diagnosis or may develop during treatment, particularly when there is involvement of the bone marrow. CNS prophylaxis lessens this risk and should be incorporated into most treatment protocols if bone marrow disease is identified. A curative treatment outcome is possible in approximately one half of patients with intermediate-grade lymphoma. Important prognostic factors include stage, performance status, disease bulk, number of extranodal sites, histology, response to treatment, and selection of treatment [11]. Patients with regional disease presentations (Stage I or II) require combination chemotherapy with or without regional radiation therapy because relapses are frequent with radiation alone [12]. Whether radiation therapy is an essential adjuvant to chemotherapy in early-stage disease is currently being studied prospectively. When radiation therapy is employed, it is often possible to shorten the period of chemotherapy.

There is no single standard chemotherapy regimen for intermediate-grade lymphomas [13–16] (Table 4). Many multiagent regimens are in use. A recent prospective clinical trial comparing four such regimens in patients with advanced disease revealed that complete response rates, and disease-free rates, and overall survival rates were similar for each chemotherapeutic protocol. These preliminary data establish a contemporary standard by which new regimens must be compared [17,18].

Table 3. Treatment Strategy for Low-Grade Lymphoma

1. Stages I and peripheral II: regional radiation therapy
2. Stages II (intra-abdominal), III and IV
   a. Patient's age ≤ 55 yr
      i. Consider intensive therapy protocols
      ii. Bone marrow harvest in patients with complete responses
      iii. Autologous stem cell transplantation in first or second remission (on protocol study)
   b. Patient's age ≥ 55 yr
      i. Consider observation
      ii. Palliative chemotherapy (chlorambucil or CVP) or regional irradiation

---

Table 4. Treatment Strategy for Intermediate-Grade Lymphoma

1. Stages I and peripheral II: combination chemotherapy with or without adjuvant radiation therapy
2. Stages II, III, and IV: combination chemotherapy
   a. CNS prophylaxis for patients with multiple sites of extranodal disease, bone, bone marrow, testicular, or paranasal sinus tumor
   b. Tumor lysis precautions with treatment initiation of bulky disease
   c. GI tract disease may require surgical resection
   d. Consider autologous stem cell transplantation for patients with histologically documented partial responses or in second remission

CNS—central nervous system; GI—gastrointestinal.

Intensification of initial treatment with high-dose chemotherapy plus cytokines (*ie*, G-CSF, GM-CSF) with or without ASCT is currently under investigation [19]. ASCT in patients in first complete remission is not recommended because only 20 to 30% of these patients relapse and prospectively randomized studies have not shown statistically increased rates of durable complete response or survival with ASCT in first remission [20].

In patients with initial partial remissions or in second remissions, ASCT is recommended. Histologic documentation of persistent or relapsed lymphoma is necessary because residual scar may make remission status uncertain. ASCT may be highly effective in those with responsive disease, good performance status, and few prior chemotherapy regimens [21].

HIGH-GRADE LYMPHOMAS

The Working Formulation recognizes three high-grade lymphomas, although one, immunoblastic lymphoma, is treated as an intermediate-grade lesion. Lymphoblastic lymphoma and the small, noncleaved cell lymphomas (Burkitt's and non-Burkitt's) are characterized by young age, male gender predominance, rapidly enlarging adenopathy that is often bulky, frequent bone marrow disease, and a high incidence of meningeal involvement if prophylaxis is not successfully carried out [22,23]. Almost all cases of lymphoblastic lymphoma are T-cell type, whereas small noncleaved cell lymphoma is B-cell phenotype.

Small, noncleaved cell lymphoma has been increasing in incidence during the past decade with the AIDS epidemic. This lymphoma is often seen in association with immunodeficiency states, and in this setting, sites of disease often may be unusual (gastrointestinal tract, parenchymal brain, soft tissue) [24].

Treatment of high-grade lymphomas is rapidly initiated, typically with high-dose, short-course combination chemotherapy, with CNS prophylaxis. Bulky disease may be associated with tumor lysis syndrome when rapid response occurs. Attention to hydration, alkalinization, prophylactic allopurinol, and monitoring of renal function, calcium, electrolytes, and phosphate balance is necessary.

In the setting of HIV infection, the use of intensive chemotherapy is controversial because treatment may be significantly complicated by opportunistic infections [25]. Nevertheless when the T-cell count is adequate, therapy may be well tolerated and excellent outcomes achieved.

HTLV-1–associated lymphomas are not identified separately in the Working Formulation. Most patients present clinically with a high-grade disease characterized by rapid onset, lytic bone lesions, subcutaneous nodules, hypercalcemia, and leukemic phase. Pathology is usually that of diffuse large cell lymphoma or immunoblastic lymphoma. In southern Japan, where HTLV-1 is endemic, a broader clinical spectrum is seen with indolent and aggressive clinical and histologic subtypes. Prognosis for patients with aggressive presentations is poor, with only transient responses to intensive regimens. Moreover, HTLV-1–infected patients are also at greater risk for opportunistic infection [2].

REFERENCES

1. National Cancer Institute: Summary and description of a working formulation for clinical usage. The non-Hodgkin lymphoma pathologic classification project. *Cancer* 1982, 49:2112–2135.

2. Shimoyama M: Diagnostic criteria and classification of clinical subtypes of adult T-cell leukemia-lymphoma. The Lymphoma Study Group. *Br J Haematol* 1991, 79:428–437.

3. Straus SE: Epstein–Barr virus infections: Biology, pathogenesis, and management. *Ann Intern Med* 1993, 118:45–58.

4. Paryani SB, Hoppe RT, Cox RS, *et al.*: Analysis of non-Hodgkin's lymphomas with nodular and favorable histologies, Stage I and II. *Cancer* 1983, 52:2300.

5. Portlock CS: Management of the low-grade non-Hodgkin's lymphomas. *Sem Oncol* 1990, 17:51–59.

6. Gribben JG, Freedman AS, Woo SD, *et al.*: All advanced stage non-Hodgkin's lymphomas with a polymerase chain reaction amplifiable breakpoint of bcl-2 have residual cells containing the bcl-2 rearrangement at evaluation and after treatment. *Blood* 1991, 78:3275–3280.

7. Portlock CS, Fischer DS, Cadman E, *et al.*: High dose pulse chlorambucil in advanced low-grade non-Hodgkin's lymphoma. *Cancer Treat Rep* 1987, 71:1029–1031.

8. Weisdorf DJ, Andersen JW, Glick JH, Oken MM: Survival after relapse of low grade non-Hodgkin's lymphoma: Implications for marrow transplantation. *J Clin Oncol* 1992, 10:942–947.

9. Freedman AS Ritz J, Nouberg D, *et al.*: Autologous bone marrow transplantation in 69 patients with a history of low-grade B cell non-Hodgkin's lymphoma. *Blood* 1991, 77:2524.

10. Gribben JG, Saporito L, Barber M, *et al.*: Bone marrows of non-Hodgkin's lymphoma patients with a bcl-2 translocation can be purged of polymerase chain reaction-detectable lymphoma cells using monoclonal antibodies and immunomagnetic bead depletion. *Blood* 1992, 80:1083–1089.

11. Shipp M, Harrington D, Anderson J, *et al.*: Predictive model for aggressive non-Hodgkin's lymphomas. The International NHL Prognostic Factor Project. *N Engl J Med* 1993, 329:987–992.

12. Yahalom J, Varsos G, Fuks Z, *et al.*: Adjuvant cyclophosphamide, doxorubicin, vincristine, and prednisone chemotherapy after radiation therapy in Stage I low-grade and intermediate-grade non-Hodgkin lymphoma: Results of a prospective randomized study. *Cancer* 1992, 71:2342–2350.

13. Mckelvey EM, Gottlieb JA, Wilson HE, *et al.*: Adriamycin combination chemotherapy in malignant lymphoma. *Cancer* 1976, 38:1494–1493.

14. Skarin AT, Canellos GP, Rosenthal DS, *et al.*: Improved prognosis of diffuse histiocytic and undifferentiated lymphoma by use of high dose methotrexate alternating with standard agent (M-BACOD). *J Clin Oncol* 1983, 1:91–98.

15. Klimo P, Conners JM: MACOP-B chemotherapy for the treatment of diffuse large-cell lymphoma. *Ann Int Med* 1985, 102:596–602.

16. Longo DL, Devita VT, Duffey PL, *et al.*: Superiority of ProMACE-CytaBOM over ProMACE-MOPP in the treatment of advanced diffuse aggressive lymphoma: Results of a prospective randomized trial. *J Clin Oncol* 1991, 9:25–38.

17. Miller TP, Dana BW, Weick JK, *et al.*: SWOG clinical trials for intermediate and high grade non-Hodgkin's lymphomas. *Sem Hematol* 1988, 25(Suppl 2):17–22.

18. Fisher RI, Gaynor E, Dahlberg S, *et al.*: Comparison of a standard regimen CHOP with three intensive chemotherapy regimens for advanced NHL. *N Engl J Med* 1993, 328:1002–1006.

19. Meyer RM, Hryniuk WM, Goodyear MD: The role of dose intensity in determining outcome in intermediate-grade non-Hodgkin's lymphoma. *J Clin Oncol* 1991, 9:339.

20. Haioun C, Lepage E, Gisselbrecht C, *et al.*: Autologous bone marrow transplantation (ABMT) versus sequential chemotherapy in first complete remission aggressive non-Hodgkin's lymphoma (NHL): First interim analysis on 370 patients (LNH87 protocol). *Proc ASCO* 1992, 11:316.

21. Gulati S, Yahalom J, Acaba L, *et al.*: Treatment of patients with relapsed and resistant non-Hodgkin's lymphoma using total body irradiation, etoposide, and cyclophosphamide and autologous bone marrow transplantation. *J Clin Oncol* 1992, 10:936–941.

22. Picozzi VJ, Coleman CN: Lymphoblastic lymphoma. *Sem Oncol* 1990, 17:96–103.

23. McMaster ML, Greer JP, Greco FA, *et al.*: Effective treatment of small-noncleaved-cell lymphoma with high intensity, brief duration chemotherapy. *J Clin Oncol* 1991, 9:941.

24. Knowles DM, Chamulak GA, Subar M, *et al.*: Lymphoid neoplasias associated with the acquired immunodeficiency syndrome (AIDS): The New York University Medical Center Experience with 105 patients (1981–1986). *Ann Intern Med* 1988, 108:744.

25. Kaplan LD, Kahn JO, Crowe S, *et al.*: Clinical and virologic effects of recombinant human granulocyte-macrophage colony stimulating factor in patients receiving chemotherapy for human immunodeficiency virus-associated non-Hodgkin's lymphoma: Results of a randomized trial. *J Clin Oncol* 1991, 9:929.

26. Luce JK, Gamble JF, Wilson HE, *et al.*: Combined cyclophosphamide, vincristine and prednisone therapy of malignant lymphoma. *Cancer* 1971, 28:306–317.

27. Armitage JO, Dick FR, Corder MP, *et al.*: Predicting therapeutic outcome in patients with diffuse histiocytic lymphoma treated with CHOP. *Cancer* 1982, 50:1695–1702.

CVP
Cyclophosphamide, Vincristine, Prednisone

CVP is a well-tolerated palliative regimen [26]. Monthly cycles are repeated to maximum response plus 2 cycles. Randomized studies have demonstrated no response or survival advantage with the use CVP over continuous daily alkylating agent therapy. Responses are more rapid with CVP (within 3 mo), but not more durable.

Toxicity is primarily hematologic with drug-induced neutropenia. Hemorrhagic cystitis may occur and hydration reduces its frequency. Vinca-associated neurologic toxicity is mild with a capped 2-mg dose. Corticosteroid toxicities are infrequent with monthly cycles.

DOSAGE AND SCHEDULING

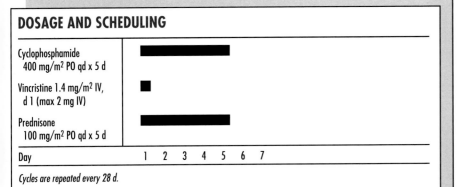

Cyclophosphamide 400 mg/m² PO qd x 5 d							
Vincristine 1.4 mg/m² IV, d 1 (max 2 mg IV)							
Prednisone 100 mg/m² PO qd x 5 d							
Day	1	2	3	4	5	6	7

Cycles are repeated every 28 d.

RECENT EXPERIENCES AND RESPONSE RATES

Study	Evaluable Patients, n	Complete Responses (%)	Median Survival (yr)
Hoppe RT, Blood 1981, 58:592	40	85	7.5
Anderson T, Cancer Treat Rep 1977, 61:1057	49	67	7

CANDIDATES FOR TREATMENT
Patients with low-grade non-Hodgkin's lymphoma

ALTERNATIVE THERAPIES
Single-agent chlorambucil or cyclophosphamide; CHOP

TOXICITIES
Prednisone: acne, thrush, thinning of the skin and striae; suppression of the adrenal–pituitary axis, hypokalemia, loss of muscle mass, increased appetite, myopathy, osteoporosis, cushingoid appearance, gastitis, peptic ulcer disease; euphoria, depression, psychosis, increased risk of infections and cataracts; **Cyclophosphamide:** myelosuppression with platelet sparing; nausea and vomiting, alopecia, darkening of skin and nails, mucositis (rare), hemorrhagic or sterile cystitis (5–10% of patients, usually reversible, but can lead to fibrosis and bladder cancer), immunosuppression, SIADH; infertility, **Vincristine:** severe local inflammation possible if extravasated, alopecia, peripheral neuropathies, ileus

DRUG INTERACTIONS
Cyclophosphamide: allopurinol, drugs that induce or block hepatic microsomal enzymes, sulfhydryl agents (*eg,* mesna); **Vincristine:** cisplatin, paclitaxel, and other drugs that affect peripheral nervous system

NURSING INTERVENTIONS
Give cyclophosphamide in the morning; administer vincristine as slow IV push to avoid extravasation; evaluate for neurologic deficit before each vincristine dose; maintain high fluid intake and encourage frequent voiding, stool softeners, and bulk diet

PATIENT INFORMATION
The most common side effects reported are leukopenia, hyperglycemia, weight gain, insomnia, alopecia, sensory neuropathy

CHOP
Cyclophosphamide, Hydroxydaunorubicin, Vincristine, Prednisone

CHOP is a potentially curative regimen in intermediate-grade lymphoma [12]. It is also used in low-grade lymphoma, particularly with evidence of histologic transformation. Responses are prompt (usually complete in less than 4 mo), and chemotherapy is continued for 2 cycles beyond maximal response or for a minimum of 6 cycles. Complete remission is achieved in 60 to 75% of patients [27].

Recent prospective comparison with more intensive, "second- and third-generation" regimens has shown no significant differences to date in response rates or survival outcome of patients with advanced intermediate-grade lymphomas. CHOP has, therefore, become the standard drug program in this setting [17].

Toxicity is moderate and reasonably well tolerated, even in the elderly. Total alopecia is the most distressing side effect to patients. Other adverse effects are similar to those outlined for CVP. Potential cardiac toxicity secondary to hydroxydaunorubicin (doxorubicin) should be monitored closely, and doses ≥ 450 mg/m^2 should be avoided whenever possible.

DOSAGE AND SCHEDULING

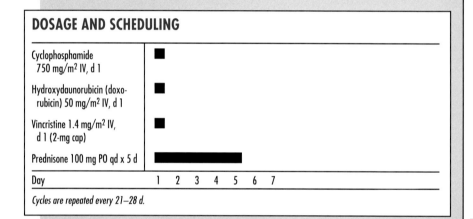

	Day	1	2	3	4	5	6	7
Cyclophosphamide 750 mg/m² IV, d 1		■						
Hydroxydaunorubicin (doxorubicin) 50 mg/m² IV, d 1		■						
Vincristine 1.4 mg/m² IV, d 1 (2-mg cap)		■						
Prednisone 100 mg PO qd x 5 d		■■■■■						

Cycles are repeated every 21–28 d.

RECENT EXPERIENCES AND RESPONSE RATES

Study	Evaluable Patients, n	Complete Responses (%)	Median Survival
Armitage JD, J Clin Oncol 1984, 2:898	75	51	31% at 4–9 yr
Gams RA, J Clin Oncol 1985, 3:1188	90	54	35% at 6 yr
Dixon DO, J Clin Oncol 1986, 5:197	412	53	30% at 12 yr

CANDIDATES FOR TREATMENT
Patients with low- or intermediate-grade non-Hodgkin's lymphoma

SPECIAL PRECAUTIONS
Patients with hepatic dysfunction
Patients with impaired cardiac function (contraindicated)

ALTERNATIVE THERAPIES
m-BACOD, MACOP-B, ProMACE-CytaBOM, COP-BLAM

TOXICITIES
Prednisone: acne, thrush, thinning of the skin and striae, suppression of the adrenal–pituitary axis, hypokalemia, loss of muscle mass, increased appetite, myopathy, osteoporosis, cushingoid appearance, gastitis, peptic ulcer disease, euphoria, depression, psychosis, increased risk of infections and cataracts; **Cyclophosphamide:** myelosuppression with platelet sparing, nausea and vomiting, alopecia, darkening of skin and nails, mucositis (rare), hemorrhagic or sterile cystitis, immunosuppression, SIADH, infertility; **Vincristine:** severe local inflammation possible if extravasated, alopecia, peripheral neuropathies, ileus; **Hydroxydoxorubicin:** myelosuppression (leukocytes and platelets, cumulative dose should not exceed 550 mg/m^2), nausea and vomiting; mucositis, alopecia, radiation recall, local tissue damage progressing to necrosis if extravasated, hyperpigmentation, phlebitis, irreversible congestive heart failure (dose-dependent), acute arrhythmias

DRUG INTERACTIONS
Cyclophosphamide: allopurinol, drugs that induce or block hepatic microsomal enzymes, sulfhydryl agents (*eg*, mesna); **Vincristine:** cisplatin, taxol, and other drugs that affect peripheral nervous system; **Hydroxydaunorubicin:** heparin, mediastinal radiation, interferon

NURSING INTERVENTIONS
Give cyclophosphamide in the morning; administer vincristine and hydroxydoxorubicin as slow IV push to avoid extravasation; evaluate for neurologic deficit before each vincristine dose; maintain high fluid intake and encourage frequent voiding, stool softeners, and bulk diet

PATIENT INFORMATION
The most common side effects reported are leukopenia, alopecia, nausea, vomiting, hyperglycemia, sensory neuropathy, insomnia

PROMACE-CYTABOM
Prednisone, Doxorubicin, Cyclophosphamide, Etoposide, Cytosine Arabinoside, Bleomycin, Vincristine, Methotrexate, Leucovorin

This third-generation drug regimen developed at the National Cancer Institute is well-suited to growth factor support and dose intensification [15]. Although the prospective Intergroup study revealed no statistically significant progression-free survival (45 vs 36%) or survival advantage for this regimen over CHOP, follow-up remains short and in younger patients this is often a highly effective regimen with low morbidity. Because mortality was greater with ProMACE-CytaBOM (4 vs 1%) than with CHOP, reflecting poor tolerance in the elderly, this program should only be used in young, otherwise well patients.

CANDIDATES FOR TREATMENT
Patients with intermediate-grade non-Hodgkin's lymphoma

SPECIAL PRECAUTIONS
Patients with renal dysfunction
Patients with impaired cardiac function (contraindicated)

ALTERNATIVE THERAPIES
CHOP, MACOP-B, m-BACOD

TOXICITIES
Cyclophosphamide, prednisone, vincristine, doxorubicin: see CHOP protocol for list of toxicities; **ara-C:** myelosuppression (leukopenia and thrombocytopenia), nausea and vomiting, stomatitis, flulike syndrome, transient transaminitis, infertility; **Bleomycin:** alopecia, stomatitis, nail bed thickening, hyperpigmentation and skin desquamation (common); acute anaphylaxis with ARDS, dose-related pneumonitis progressing to pulmonary fibrosis (max cumulative dose of 200 U/m^2); frequent severe fevers; **Methotrexate:** myelosuppression nausea and vomiting, severe mucositis with ulceration and bloody diarrhea, irreversible cirrhosis (rare), pneumonitis, alopecia, renal tubular necrosis; **Etoposide:** myelosuppression (leukopenia and thrombocytopenia), nausea and vomiting, alopecia, mucositis

DRUG INTERACTIONS
Cyclophosphamide, prednisone, vincristine, doxorubicin: see CHOP protocol list of interactions; **ara-C:** cisplatin, thiopurines, methotrexate, hydroxyurea; **Bleomycin:** radiation therapy, nephrotoxic drugs; **Etoposide:** ara-C, methotrexate, cisplatin, calcium antagonists, coumadin; **Methotrexate:** aspirin, NSAIDs, alcohol, 5-FU, l-asparaginase

NURSING INTERVENTIONS
See CHOP protocol for list of interventions; in addition, test dose of bleomycin (1 U IM) prior to first dose; use glass containers for infusion of bleomycin; administer etoposide over 1 hr to avoid hypotension and extravasation; monitor methotrexate levels if renal dysfunction develops; maintain leucovorin every 6 hr until methotrexate levels are nontherapeutic

PATIENT INFORMATION
The most common side effects reportd are alopecia, nausea, vomiting, weight gain, leukopenia, hyperglycemia, insomnia

DOSAGE AND SCHEDULING

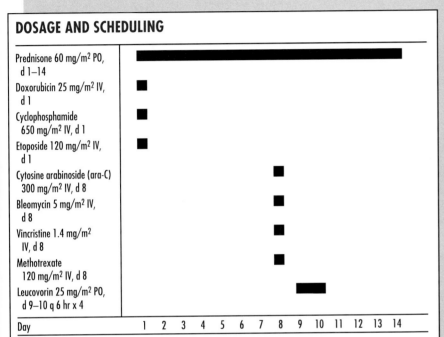

Day														

Prednisone 60 mg/m^2 PO, d 1–14

Doxorubicin 25 mg/m^2 IV, d 1

Cyclophosphamide 650 mg/m^2 IV, d 1

Etoposide 120 mg/m^2 IV, d 1

Cytosine arabinoside (ara-C) 300 mg/m^2 IV, d 8

Bleomycin 5 mg/m^2 IV, d 8

Vincristine 1.4 mg/m^2 IV, d 8

Methotrexate 120 mg/m^2 IV, d 8

Leucovorin 25 mg/m^2 PO, d 9–10 q 6 hr x 4

One double-strength co-trimoxazole is given BID throughout treatment. Cycles are repeated every 21 d until complete remission followed by 2 consolidation cycles (min 6 cycles).

DOSAGE MODIFICATIONS: *Reduce bleomycin if renal failure develops, withhold methotrexate if creatinine clearance ≤ 60 ml/min.*

RECENT EXPERIENCES AND RESPONSE RATES

Study	Evaluable Patients, *n*	Complete Responses (%)	Median Survival
Fisher RI, In Advances in Cancer Chemotherapy. Skarin AT, NY, 1986	37	80	Not reached
Miller TP, Sem Hematol 1988, 25 (suppl2):41	48	69	70% at 15 mo

STANFORD REGIMEN

Cyclophosphamide, Doxorubicin, Vincristine, Prednisone, l-Asparaginase, Methotrexate, Leucovorin, Radiation Therapy, Mercaptopurine

Many effective drug regimens have been developed for lymphoblastic lymphoma [21]. Key elements include high-dose steroids and alkylating agents, frequent administration of vincristine, CNS prophylaxis, and maintenance chemotherapy. All are complex drug programs, demanding attention to detail and specialized expertise. Lymphoblastic lymphoma is potentially curable in a high proportion of patients, but intensive, well-monitored therapy is critical to outcome. Good and poor risk groups may be identified according to prognostic features of stage, tumor bulk, disease sites, and age.

In addition to expected chemotherapy side-effects, one must be alert to possible tumor lysis syndrome with initiation of therapy. Hydration, alkalinization, allopurinol, and frequent monitoring of electrolytes, renal function, calcium, and phosphate balance are essential.

DOSAGE AND SCHEDULING

W	1	2	3	4	5	6	7	8	9	12	15	18	23	52
C	X			X					X	X	X	X		
D	X			X					X	X				
V	X	X	X	X	X	X			X	X	X	X		
P	X	X	X	X	†	†			X	X	X	X		
I				X	X	X	X	X						
M					X	X	X							
					X	X								
L					X	X	X							
					X	X								
X					X	X								
6													X—	x
m													X—	x

REGIMEN

C—cyclophosphamide 400 mg/m² PO x 3 d; D—doxorubicin 50 mg/m²; V—vincristine 1.4 mg/m² (2 mg maximum total); P—prednisone 40 mg/m²; I—l-asparaginase-6 kU/m² IM x 5; M—methotrexate 12 mg IT x 5 with L—leucovorin 10 mg/m² PO q 6 hr x 4; X—whole brain radiation 2400 cGy/12; 6—6-mercaptopurine 75 mg/m² PO daily; m—methotrexate 30 mg/m² PO weekly; †—taper.

Weeks 1–4 induction, 5–9 CNS prophylaxis, 10–22 consolidation, and 23–52 maintenance. Weeks 9– given for 5 d.

DOSAGE MODIFICATIONS: Reduce total dose of mercaptopurine by 25% if given with allopurinol; withhold methotrexate if creatinine ≤ 60 ml/min.

RECENT EXPERIENCE AND RESPONSE RATES

Study	Evaluable patients, n	Response rate (%)	Freedom from relapse
Coleman et al., J Clin Oncol 1986 11:1628–1637	44	100	70% at 3 yr

CANDIDATES FOR TREATMENT
Patients with lymphoblastic lymphoma

SPECIAL PRECAUTIONS
Patients with renal dysfunction
Patients with impaired cardiac function (contraindicated)

ALTERNATIVE THERAPIES
Acute lymphoblastic leukemia regimens

TOXICITIES
Cyclophosphamide, prednisone, vincristine, doxorubicin: see CHOP protocol for list of toxicities; **Methotrexate:** myelosuppression, nausea and vomiting, severe mucositis with ulceration and bloody diarrhea, irreversible cirrhosis (rare), pneumonitis, alopecia, renal tubular necrosis; **Mercaptopurine:** myelosuppression, hyperuricemia; **l-Asparaginase:** hypersensitivity reactions in 20–35% of patients (possibly life-threatening), fever, chills, nausea and vomiting (occasional), pancreatic dysfunction, lethargy, somnolence

DRUG INTERACTIONS
Cyclophosphamide, prednisone, vincristine, doxorubicin: see CHOP protocol for list of interactions; **Methotrexate:** aspirin, NSAIDs, alcohol, 5-FU, l-asparaginase; **l-Asparaginase:** prednisone

NURSING INTERVENTIONS
See CHOP protocol for list of interventions; in addition, mix intrathecal methotrexate with buffered nonbacteriostatic solution; monitor methotrexate levels if renal dysfunction develops; maintain leucovorin every 6 hr until methotrexate levels are nontherapeutic; administer l-asparaginase IV slow push over 30 min

PATIENT INFORMATION
The most common side effects reported are fever, leukopenia, headache, sensory neuropathy, seizures, alopecia, nausea and vomiting

VANDERBILT REGIMEN
Cyclophosphamide, Etoposide, Vincristine, Bleomycin, Methotrexate, Leucovorin, Prednisone

Small noncleaved cell lymphomas—Burkitt's and non-Burkitt's types—are rare high-grade lymphomas. When associated with HIV infection, this phenotype is one of the most common histologies, however. HIV-negative small, noncleaved cell lymphoma is a highly curable disease with high-dose, short-course therapy [22]. CNS prophylaxis is essential. As with lymphoblastic lymphoma, tumor lysis is a serious complication of effective initial therapy and must be anticipated with initiation of hydration, alkalinization, and allopurinol, and frequent monitoring of electrolytes, renal function, and calcium/phosphate balance.

Severe myelosuppression is to be expected with this drug protocol. Even with growth factor support, nadir fever should be anticipated, as well as the need for platelet support. Mucositis may occur in up to one half of all patients. Nevertheless, maintaining treatment schedule is important whenever possible to combat this rapidly growing neoplasm.

CANDIDATES FOR TREATMENT
Patients with high-grade non-Hodgkin's lymphoma

SPECIAL PRECAUTIONS
Patients with renal dysfunction

ALTERNATIVE THERAPIES
Stanford regimen using combined modality

TOXICITIES
Cyclophosphamide, prednisone, vincristine: see CVP protocol for list of toxicities; **Bleomycin:** alopecia, stomatitis, nail bed thickening, hyperpigmentation and skin desquamation (common), acute anaphylaxis with ARDS, dose-related pneumonitis progressing to pulmonary fibrosis (max cumulative dose of 200 U/m^2); frequently severe fever; **Methotrexate:** myelosuppression, nausea and vomiting, severe mucositis with ulceration and bloody diarrhea, irreversible cirrhosis (rare), pneumonitis, alopecia, renal tubular necrosis, **Etoposide:** myelosuppression (leukopenia and thrombocytopenia), nausea and vomiting, alopecia, mucositis

DRUG INTERACTIONS
Cyclophosphamide, prednisone, vincristine: see CVP protocol for list of interactions; **Bleomycin:** radiation therapy, nephrotoxic drugs; **Etoposide:** ara-C, methotrexate, cisplatin, calcium antagonists, coumadin; **Methotrexate:** aspirin, NSAIDs, alcohol, 5-FU, l-asparaginase

NURSING INTERVENTIONS
See CVP protocol for list of interventions; test dose of bleomycin (1 U IM) prior to first dose; use glass containers for infusion of bleomycin; administer etoposide over 1 hr to avoid hypotension and extravasation; mix intrathecal methotrexate with buffered nonbacteriostatic solution; monitor methotrexate levels if renal dysfunction develops and maintain leucovorin every 6 hr until methotrexate levels are nontherapeutic

PATIENT INFORMATION
These most common side effects reported are pancytopenia, infections, alopecia, bleeding, mucositis, peripheral neuropathy

DOSAGE AND SCHEDULING

Agent	Cycle 1						Cycle 2					
	Day 1	Day 2	Day 3	Day 8	Day 15	Day 22	Day 29	Day 30	Day 31	Day 36	Day 43	Day 50
CTX	X	X					X					
ETOP	X	X	X				X	X	X			
ADR							X	X				
VCR				X		X				X		X
BLEO				X		X				X		X
MTX					X						X	
LV			X		X						X	
PRED	X	X		X			X	X	X	X		

REGIMEN
In cycle 1, CTX—cyclophosamide 1500 mg/m^2; ETOP—etoposide 400 mg/m^2; VCR—vincristine 1.4 mg/m^2 (2 mg max), BLEO—bleomycin 10 U/m^2; MTX—methotrexate 200 mg/m^2; LV—leucovorin 15 mg/m^2 (q 6 hr x 6); PRED—prednisone 60 mg/m^2. In cycle 2, etoposide dose is reduced to 100 mg/m^2 and ADR (doxorubicin) is added at 45 mg/m^2. Allopurinol is routinely given. Patients with meningeal involvement at diagnosis receive methotrexate 12 mg/m^2 IT weekly x 5 and whole-brain radiation 2000 cGy in 10 fractions. Prophylactic intrathecal therapy is recommended.

DOSAGE MODIFICATIONS:
Cycle 2 can be delayed if ANC < 1000. Reduce bleomycin, if renal failure develops; withhold methotrexate if creatinine clearance ≤ 60 ml/min.

RECENT EXPERIENCE AND RESPONSE RATES

Study	Evaluable patients, n	Complete responses (%)	Disease-free survival
McMaster et al., J Clin Oncol 1991 9:941–946	20	85	65% at 29 mo

INCIDENCE AND ETIOLOGY

The incidence for multiple myeloma in the United States exceeds 3 people per 100,000 and appears to be increasing. Myeloma accounts for 1% of malignant disease and over 10% of hematologic malignancies. The occurrence of myeloma is more common in men than in women and more common in African-Americans than in Caucasians. It most commonly presents in the seventh decade, with fewer than 2% of patients under age 40.

The cause of multiple myeloma remains unknown. Monoclonal gammopathy of undetermined significance (MGUS) may offer a clue to its pathogenesis. More than 33% of patients with apparent benign monoclonal gammopathy will develop myeloma, another lympho-plasmacellular malignancy, or progression of their monoclonal gammopathy. The incidence of myeloma in patients with MGUS is 25% after 20 to 35 years of follow-up. These observations implicate MGUS as a premalignant clonal disorder that, on further transforming damage to the clone, can give rise to multiple myeloma.

Genetic predisposition, radiation exposure, chronic antigenic stimulation, and various environmental or occupational conditions have been observed as factors but account for only a small percentage of all myeloma. Recent reports demonstrate the importance of autocrine stimulation of the malignant clone by IL-6 and the apparent role of oncogene activation at various stages of the disease. These and other recently appreciated factors provide insight into the pathogenesis of myeloma, but their relationship to the original malignant event is not yet spelled out.

DIAGNOSIS AND STAGING

Diagnosis of myeloma is made by the presence of malignant plasma cells in the bone marrow (usually > 10%) or by biopsy proof of a plasmacytoma plus either protein evidence of myeloma with a monoclonal serum or urine protein or characteristic osteolytic lesions. For the past 18 years, the most commonly used staging system has been that proposed by Durie and Salmon (Table 1). It correlates tumor burden with the presence or absence of severe anemia, hypercalcemia, advanced skeletal disease, and the amount of monoclonal protein detected in serum or urine.

Clinical stage has proved to be predictive of survival in many series. Stage I patients generally survive over 5 years, whereas the median survival for Stage II patients is 3 to 4 years and for Stage III rarely more than 2 years. The presence of renal failure has an important negative prognostic significance in myeloma. More recent studies have demonstrated that elevated plasma ß-2 microglobulin and elevated plasma cell labeling index are also important adverse prognostic signs that may at times override the significance of clinical stage. The presence of both low plasma ß-2 microglobulin and elevated plasma cell labeling index appears to be a strong predictor of long survival in patients with myeloma.

PRIMARY DISEASE THERAPY

With the exception of bone marrow transplantation in relatively few cases, current methods of treatment for multiple myeloma are not intended to be curative. The goals of treatment are to extend survival several years, to produce objective disease regression with its attendant relief from pain and other disease symptoms, and to protect the patient's ability to lead an active life for as long as possible. For the past 25 years the standard treatment for multiple myeloma has been widely considered to be use of the single alkylating agent, melphalan,

or a combination of melphalan and prednisone (MP), which is usually given in a high-dose, intermittent, outpatient regimen (Fig. 1) [1]. When this treatment is used, objective responses, documented by a 50% or greater decrease in serum M-protein levels and control of other major manifestations of disease, are seen in 50% of patients. Unfortunately, response duration is generally less than 2 years and the median duration of survival is 24 to 30 months. Survival durations of up to 5 years are achieved in fewer than 20% of patients.

Numerous combination chemotherapy regimens have been developed in an attempt to improve on the results obtained from use of the MP regimen; most resemble either the vincristine, carmustine (BCNU), melphalan, cyclophosphamide, and prednisone (VBMCP) regimen or the VMCP/VBAP regimen, consisting of alternating cycles of vincristine plus prednisone combined with either melphalan plus cyclophosphamide or with BCNU plus doxorubicin. Because of promising preliminary results, several randomized clinical trials have been conducted to compare MP with more aggressive multidrug regimens. In an Eastern Cooperative Oncology Group (ECOG) trial, a 72% objective response rate with VBMCP was achieved, compared with only 51% for patients treated with MP [2]. Although the median survival duration and log-rank comparison of the survival curves were not significantly different, the response duration was superior with VBMCP (32 vs 18% at 3 years) as was the 5-year survival rate (26 vs 19%).

A Southwestern Oncology Group (SWOG) comparison of MP with VMCP/VBAP showed superior response, survival, and long-term survival rates with the more intensive multidrug regimen (5-year survival, 30 vs 19%) [3]. A comparative trial by the Medical Research Council (MRC) of Great Britain found a response and survival rate superiority with ABCM compared with melphalan [4]. The doxorubicin, BCNU, cyclophosphamide, and melphalan (ABCM) regimen resembles the VMCP/VBAP regimen, except that both vincristine and

Table 1. Clinical Staging System for Myeloma

Stage	Criteria	Myeloma Cell Mass (cells/m²)

I	All of the following:
	1. Hemoglobin > 10 g/dl
	2. Serum calcium value normal (≤ 12 mg/100 ml)
	3. On x-ray, normal bone structure or solitary bone plasmacytoma only
	4. Low M-component production rates
	  a. IgG value < 5 g/100 ml
	  b. IgA value < 3 g/100 ml
	  c. Urine light chain M-component on electrophoresis < 4 g/24 hr
		< 0.6 x 10¹² (low)

II	Fitting neither Stage I nor III	0.6–1.2 x 10¹² (intermediate)

III	One or more of the following:
	1. Hemoglobin < 8.5 g/100 ml
	2. Serum calcium value > 12 mg/100 ml
	3. Advanced lytic bone lesions
	4. High M-component production rates
	  a. IgG value > 7 g/100 ml
	  b. IgA value > 5 g/100 ml
	  c. Urine light chain M-component on electrophoresis > 12 g/24 hr
		1.2 x 10¹² (high)

Subclass		
A	Serum creatine < 2 mg/100 ml	
B	Serum creatine ≥ 2 mg/100 ml	

Modified from Durie, Salmon [9]; with permission.

prednisone are omitted. The 5-year survival rate is 24% when ABCM is used, compared with 17% with the use of melphalan alone. Combined, these three controlled trials representing 1301 patients have shown that the more intensive multidrug regimens produce 33% more responses and 5-year survival rates than do the MP or melphalan only regimens.

Some physicians assert that this 33% is not enough and point to the 17 reports of clinical trials comparing variations of VBMCP or VMCP/VBAP with MP in which there was no evidence of survival advantage and often no significant response difference to favor the multidrug regimens. In an attempt to resolve this discrepancy, a meta-analysis was carried out, which evaluated 18 published randomized trials involving 3814 patients [5]. The meta-analysis focused entirely on 2-year survival rates and, not surprisingly, found no difference between combination chemotherapy and MP. The meta-analysis itself is subject to criticism, however, because of its focus on 2-year survival (certainly not the primary goal of chemotherapy) and, on study selection, its omission of the MRC and ECOG studies (not published in manuscript form at that time) and inclusion of several studies of regimens clearly less dose intensive than either VBMCP or VMCP/VBAP.

It is not possible to compare diluted VBMCP or VMCP/VBAP–based regimens with MP and draw valid conclusions about the original regimen. Therefore, although the issue of single-agent versus combination chemotherapy is still open for debate, available data suggest that the VBMCP and VMCP/VBAP regimens offer most patients superior response rates and improved duration and quality of long-term survival compared with MP. One important

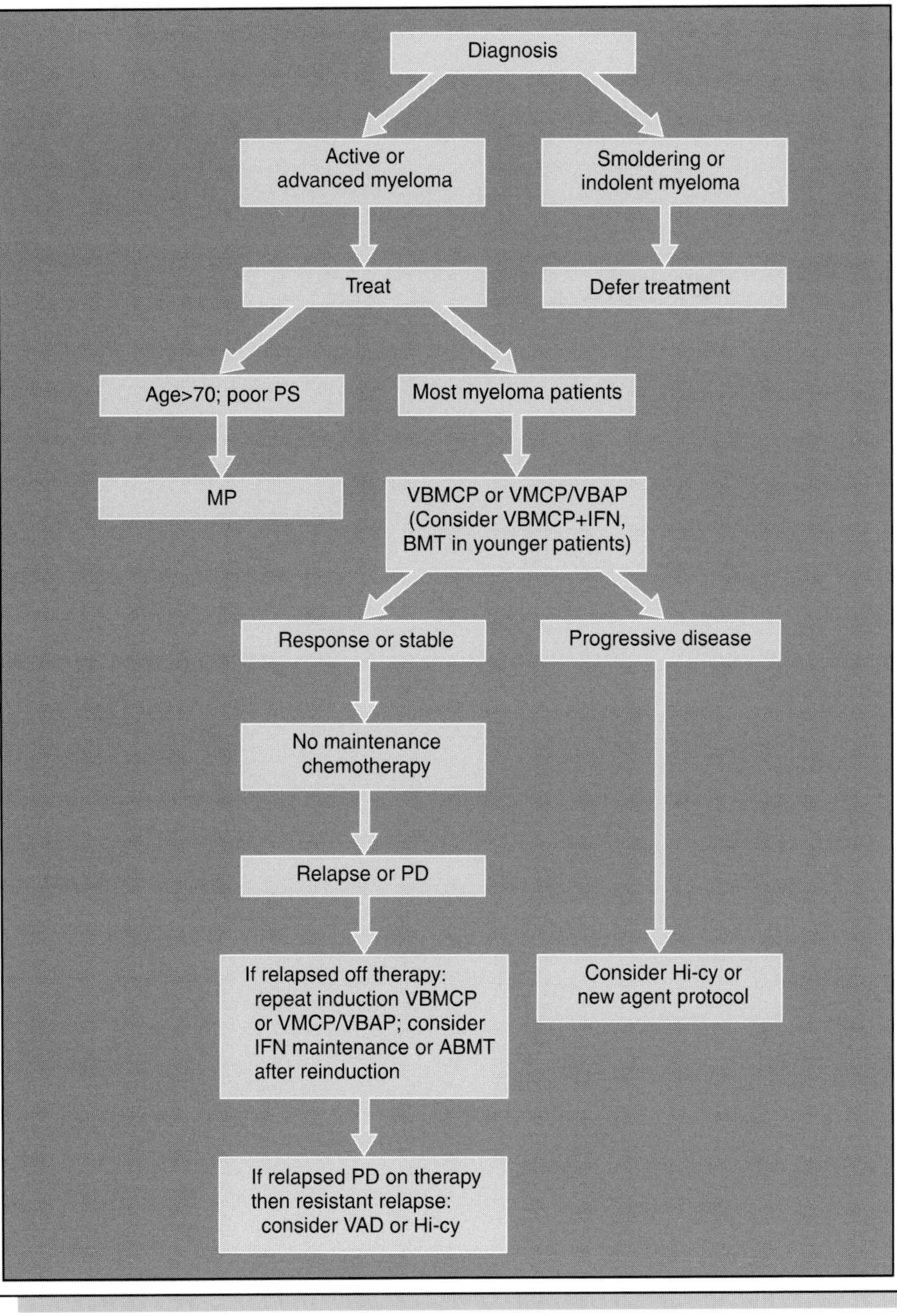

FIGURE 1

Treatment Strategy for Myeloma. Hi-cy—high-dose cyclophosphamide; PD—progressive disease; PS—poor survival rate.

exception found in the ECOG study is that elderly, bedridden patients cannot tolerate the VBMCP combination. Because of their unacceptably high rate of early infection and death when taking this regimen, it is advisable to treat them with the MP regimen instead. The other 80 to 90% of patients are likely to benefit from a more intensive regimen such as VBMCP, VMCP/VBAP, or ABCM.

Induction therapy is generally given for 1 to 2 years. Long-term maintenance therapy has been studied in three randomized clinical trials—using MP as the maintenance regimen. All three failed to show an increase in survival duration for patients randomly assigned to maintenance therapy compared with those who received no treatment. The role of intensification regimens or of maintenance therapy for selected subgroups of patients at risk for early relapse has yet to be conclusively evaluated.

Recently, much attention has been given to the possible role of interferon in treating myeloma. Most of this work has been done with r-interferon α-2 (rIFNα-2). This agent shows low but definite activity when used as a single agent in patients with refractory disease, yielding a 10 to 15% objective response rate and up to 30% symptomatic responses. The main interest has been in developing approaches that combine interferon with chemotherapy. An attempt to administer interferon simultaneously with MP as an induction regimen produced no improvement when compared with MP alone. Trials of interferon as maintenance therapy were initially promising after the report of an Italian group that the use of interferon nearly doubles the response duration compared with no maintenance therapy. More recent data from both the Italian Study and the Southwest Oncology Group show no prolongation of survival with interferon maintenance therapy [6]. A Swedish study is still under way, but at present there is no convincing role for interferon in maintenance therapy for multiple myeloma.

The ECOG developed a primary induction regimen that combines interferon with chemotherapy by alternating cycles of VBMCP with rIFNα-2. The results of a 54-patient phase II evaluation of this regimen showed an 80% objective response rate, including 30% complete remissions in which serum and urine M-protein concentrations disappeared and the bone marrow structure returned to normal [7]. The median response duration of 35 months and survival duration of 42 months are both about 12 months longer than is usually seen in this disease. A randomized trial comparing VBMCP with VBMCP plus rIFNα-2 is being conducted by the ECOG.

Studies are under way to evaluate the possible role of intensive therapy with autologous stem cell rescue (either from bone marrow or peripheral blood) as part of primary treatment of multiple myeloma. This aggressive approach remains an alternative for young patients with myeloma but is generally best considered an investigative therapy for most patients until the results of controlled studies can be evaluated.

THERAPY FOR RELAPSED OR REFRACTORY DISEASE

When patients with myeloma relapse during the no-maintenance phase, the best approach to salvage therapy appears to be to repeat the original induction regimen. The first retreatment with VBMCP has been reported to yield objective responses in 69%. However, remissions exceeding 1 year are the exception once relapse has occurred. For patients with resistant disease (relapse when receiving maintenance therapy or refractory to their most recent induction attempt) high-dose corticosteroid therapy with either dexamethasone or methylprednisolone produces responses in 20 to 25% but at the cost of substantial infection risk.

The vincristine, doxorubicin, and dexamethasone (VAD) regimen produces high response rates in patients who experience relapse, but this achievement may not be superior to the results that could be obtained by reinduction with the original regimen. In patients with resistant disease, the response rate is 30 to 40% and relapse generally occurs within 9 months. EDAP, an alternative infusion regimen combining etoposide, dexamethasone, cytarabine, and cisplatin, produces a similar response rate but at a prohibitively high risk for infection—perhaps with hematopoietic growth factor support this regimen will be better tolerated.

The regimen of high-dose intravenous cyclophosphamide (600 mg/m² days 1–4) produces up to 40% responses in patients with resistant myeloma and is relatively platelet sparing [8]. It is speculated that when granulocyte colony-stimulating factor (G-CSF) or prophylactic antibiotic support are used, this regimen might prove suitable for multiple cycles in patients with resistant disease. Without such support, the leukocyte nadir is predictably less than 500 cells/µl and the time to leukocyte recovery is 20 to 23 days.

NEW THERAPY APPROACHES

Several promising new treatment methods are under evaluation. These include the new drugs paclitaxel, all trans-retinoic acids (alone and in combination with interferon α), and topoisomerase inhibitors such as topotecan. One of the more intriguing biologic approaches involves the use of antibodies to IL-6. Investigation is still in the early stages, but these approaches hold the promise of new directions in the treatment of myeloma.

In summary, many regimens will produce responses in patients with resistant myeloma, but long-term disease control is uncommon. Intensive therapy with bone marrow transplantation or peripheral blood stem cell rescue may offer more durable disease control in carefully selected patients.

REFERENCES

1. Alexanian R, Haut A, Khan Au, et al.: Treatment of multiple myeloma: Combination chemotherapy with different melphalan dose regimens. JAMA 1969, 208:1680–1685.

2. Oken MM, Tsiatis A, Abramson N, et al.: Comparison of standard (MP) with intensive (VBMCP) therapy for the treatment of multiple myeloma. Proc ASCO 1984, 3:270.

3. Salmon SE, Tesh D, Crowley J, et al.: Chemotherapy is superior to sequential hemibody irradiation for remission consolidation in multiple myeloma: A Southwest Oncology Group Study. J Clin Oncol 1990, 8:1575–1584.

4. MacLennan ICM, Chapman C, Dunn J, et al.: Combined chemotherapy with ABCM vs melphalan for treatment of myelomatosis. Lancet 1993, 339:200–205.

5. Gregory WM, Richards MA, Malpas JS: Combination chemotherapy vs melphalan and prednisolone in the treatment of multiple myeloma: An overview of published trials. J Clin Oncol 1992, 10:334–342.

6. Salmon SE, Crowley J: Impact of glucocorticoids and interferon on outcome in multiple myeloma. Proc ASCO 1992, 11:316.

7. Oken MM, Kyle RA, Greipp PR, et al.: Alternating cycles of VBMCP with interferon in the treatment of multiple myeloma. Proc ASCO 1988, 7:225.

8. Lenhard RE Jr, Oken MM, Barnes JM, et al.: High-dose cyclophosphamide: An effective treatment for advanced refractory multiple myeloma. Cancer 1984, 53:1456–1460.

9. Durie BGM, Salmon SE: A clinical staging system for multiple myeloma. Cancer 1975, 36:842.

MP
Melphalan and Prednisone

First reported 23 years ago, melphalan and prednisone is the prototype regimen in the single-alkylating-agent therapy for multiple myeloma. The high-dose intermittent schedule has proved a simple, relatively safe way to administer melphalan. A 1972 study reported that prednisone doubled the response rate to melphalan and that it produced modest improvement in survival. MP became, and for some, remains, the standard chemotherapy for multiple myeloma. Treatment is generally administered in cycles of 3 to 6 weeks' duration and is continued for 1 to 2 years, although it sometimes has been continued it until disease progression.

An important problem with this protocol is the erratic absorption of oral melphalan, which sometimes leads to inadequate bioavailability in some patients who take apparently adequate oral doses.

CANDIDATES FOR TREATMENT
Patients with active or advanced myeloma, particularly those who are elderly and frail

SPECIAL PRECAUTIONS
Risk for infection greater during early cycles (use allopurinol to prevent hyperuricemia during early months); treatment-associated myelodysplastic syndrome and acute leukemia occur in some

ALTERNATIVE THERAPIES
Melphalan alone, VMCP/VBAP, ABCM

TOXICITIES
Melphalan: bone marrow suppression leading to neutropenia with increased risk for infection, thrombocytopenia with risk for bleeding, erythroid hypoplasia with risk for symptomatic anemia; long-term toxicity: testicular atrophy, amenorrhea, risk for treatment-induced acute leukemia; **Prednisone:** immunosuppression, infection, edema, exacerbation of diabetes, weight gain, menstrual abnormalities, mental status dysfunction (especially in elderly)

DRUG INTERACTIONS
None noteworthy

NURSING INTERVENTIONS
Instruct patient to seek medical attention if fever or other specific or subjective symptoms develop that could represent infection; monitor blood glucose if diabetic; antacid therapy may be used

PATIENT INFORMATION
Patient should take melphalan on empty stomach, prednisone after meals; anticipate possibility of mood and appetite changes or fluid retention; be alert to early signs of bleeding or infection

DOSAGE AND SCHEDULING

		1	2	3	4	5	6	7
Melphalan 8 mg/m^2 PO d 1–4	■■■■							
Prednisone 60 mg/m^2 PO d 1–4	■■■■							
CBC, serum creatine; cycle 1, 4, 7, etc. d 1	☐							
Day		1	2	3	4	5	6	7

Cycle duration, 4 weeks; treatment duration, 1 to 2 years.

DOSAGE MODIFICATIONS: *After first cycle, modify melphalan dose for depressed blood counts as follows: ANC 1000–2000/μl—give 75%; ANC 750–1000 or platelets 50,000–100,000/μl—give 50%; delay treatment for ANC < 750/μl or platelets < 50,000/μl.*

RECENT EXPERIENCES AND RESPONSE RATES

Study	Evaluable patients, n	Dosage and scheduling	Objective response (%)	Median survival (mo)
Alexanian, et al., Cancer 1972, 30:382–389.	77	Melphalan 0.25 mg/kg PO d 1–4 Prednisone 2 mg/kg PO d 1–4 Cycle duration, 6 wk	47*	24
Abramson, et al., Cancer Treat Rep 1982, 66:1273–1277.	72	Melphalan 8 mg/m^2 PO d 1–4 Prednisone 75 mg PO d 1–7 Cycle duration, 4 wk	43‡	25
Oken, et al., Proc ASCO 1987, 6:203	217	Melphalan 8 mg/m^2 PO d 1–4 Prednisone 60 mg/m^2 PO d 1–4	51†	30
Bergsagel, et al., N Engl J Med 1979, 301:743–748.	125	Melphalan 9 mg/m^2 PO d 1–4 Prednisone 100 mg PO d 1–4 Cycle duration, 4 wk	40*	28

Response requires ≥ 75% decrease in M-protein production.
†*Response requires ≥ 50% decrease in M-protein value.*
‡*Response evaluated at 6 months only.*

VBMCP
Vincristine, BCNU, Melphalan, Cyclophosphamide, Prednisone

VBMCP is a prototype combination chemotherapy regimen that is more intensive than standard MP. Initial reports of a markedly increased response rate in comparison with MP were confirmed in a large randomized trial. The regimen is one of multiple alkylating agents plus the vinca alkyloid, vincristine, and prednisone. Full-dose melphalan plus prednisone is part of the regimen but is administered at 5-week rather than 4-week intervals. Part of the increase in response rate may be attributed to the addition of three intravenous drugs to the sometimes erratically absorbed, orally administered melphalan.

BCNU, or carmustine, is a nitrosourea that is primarily an alkylating agent, as are both cyclophosphamide and melphalan. Vincristine is a vinca alkyloid and is cell cycle–specific for the M phase, interfering with the mitotic spindle formation.

CANDIDATES FOR TREATMENT
Patients with active myeloma unless they are elderly (> 70 years) and frail

SPECIAL PRECAUTIONS
Risk for infection greater during early cycles (use allopurinol to prevent hyperuricemia during early months); treatment-associated myelodysplastic syndrome and acute leukemia occur in some; VBMCP poorly tolerated by patients > 70 years of age and frail—MP is better choice

ALTERNATIVE THERAPIES
MP, VMCP/VBAP, ABCM, melphalan alone, VBMCP and interferon

DOSAGE AND SCHEDULING

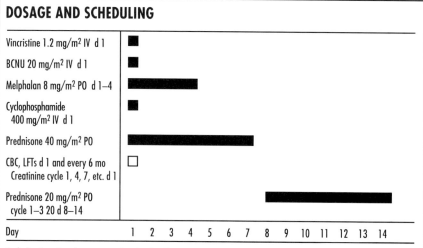

Vincristine 1.2 mg/m² IV d 1

BCNU 20 mg/m² IV d 1

Melphalan 8 mg/m² PO d 1–4

Cyclophosphamide 400 mg/m² IV d 1

Prednisone 40 mg/m² PO

CBC, LFTs d 1 and every 6 mo Creatinine cycle 1, 4, 7, etc. d 1

Prednisone 20 mg/m² PO cycle 1–3 20 d 8–14

Day 1 2 3 4 5 6 7 8 9 10 11 12 13 14

Cycle duration, 5 weeks; treatment duration, 1 to 2 years

DOSAGE MODIFICATIONS: *After first cycle, modify melphalan, BCNU, cyclophosphamide for depressed blood counts as follows: ANC 1000–2000/μl—give 75%; ANC 750–1000 or platelets 50,000–100,000/μl—give 50%; delay treatment for ANC < 750/μl or platelets < 50,000/μl; vincristine dose reduction required for hepatic insufficiency*

TOXICITIES
Drug combination: long-term toxicity: testicular atrophy, amenorrhea, risk for treatment-induced acute leukemia; **Melphalan:** bone marrow suppression leading to neutropenia with increased risk for infection, thrombocytopenia with increased risk for bleeding, erythroid hypoplasia with risk for symptomatic anemia; **Prednisone:** immunosuppression, infection, exacerbation of diabetes, weight gain, edema, mental status dysfunction—especially in elderly; **BCNU:** bone marrow suppression possibly longer than that with melphalan or cyclophosphamide, pain in injected extremity or at IV site, nausea, vomiting, liver or renal dysfunction; pulmonary fibrosis (rare); **Cyclophosphamide:** bone marrow suppression but relatively platelet sparing, nausea, vomiting, hemorrhagic cystitis, alopecia; rarely, pulmonary fibrosis, liver dysfunction; **Vincristine:** peripheral neuropathy, cranial nerve neuropathy, constipation, alopecia, vesicant if extravasated; SIADH (rare)

DRUG INTERACTIONS
Cyclophosphamide: barbiturates, phenytoin, chloral hydrate

NURSING INTERVENTIONS
Push fluids for 24 hours after cyclophosphamide to reduce risk for hemorrhagic cystitis; give antiemetic before administration; monitor blood glucose if diabetic; antacid therapy may be used

PATIENT INFORMATION
Maintain good fluid intake; take melphalan on empty stomach, prednisone after meals; anticipate possibility of mood and appetite changes or fluid retention; be alert to early signs of bleeding or infection; call physician for blood in urine; vincristine may cause severe constipation: monitor bowel pattern carefully, use mild laxatives, seek medical attention if persistent or severe

RECENT EXPERIENCES AND RESPONSE RATES

Study	Evaluable patients, *n*	Dosage and scheduling	Response (%)	Median survival (mo)	5-yr survival (%)
Case, *et al.*, Am J Med 1977, 63:897–903. Lee, *et al.*, In Wiernik (ed.) Controversies in Oncology 1982, pp 61–79.	81	Vincristine 0.03 mg/kg IV d 1 BCNU 0.5 mg/kg IV d 1 Melphalan 0.25 mg/kg PO d 1–4 Cyclophosphamide 10 mg/kg IV d 1 Prednisone 1 mg/kg PO d 1–7, then 0.5 mg/kg d 8–14, then taper	78*	38	—
Oken, *et al.*, Proc ASCO 1987, 6:203	214	Vincristine 1.2 mg/m² IV d 1 BCNU 20 mg/m² IV d 1 Melphalan 8 mg/m² PO d 1–4 Cyclophosphamide 400 mg/m² IV d 1 Prednisone 60 mg/m² PO d 1–7; (20 mg/m² PO d 8–14 cycle 1–13)	72*	31	26

*Response requires ≥ 50% decrease in M-protein value.

VBMCP PLUS IFN
Vincristine, BCNU, Melphalan, Cyclophosphamide, Prednisone and Interferon

The regimen of VBMCP plus interferon represents an attempt to combine an effective combination chemotherapy regimen with a biologic response modifier. The preparation used in this regimen is rIFN α-2. An alternating cycle strategy is used to avoid some of the synergistic myelotoxicity that may occur with simultaneous VBMCP and IFN administration.

Interferons suppress cell proliferation, alter cell differentiation, and stimulate several cell enzymes such as 2'5'-oligoadenylate synthetase. Their complex effects on the immune system include augmentation of natural killer cell activity and changes in T-cell subsets.

DOSAGE AND SCHEDULING*

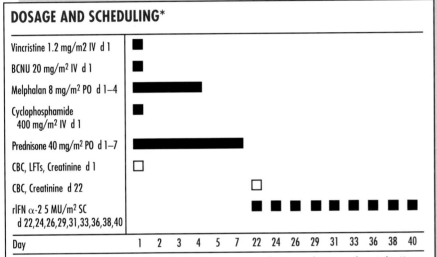

Vincristine 1.2 mg/m2 IV d 1
BCNU 20 mg/m² IV d 1
Melphalan 8 mg/m² PO d 1–4
Cyclophosphamide 400 mg/m² IV d 1
Prednisone 40 mg/m² PO d 1–7
CBC, LFTs, Creatinine d 1
CBC, Creatinine d 22
rIFN α-2 5 MU/m² SC d 22,24,26,29,31,33,36,38,40
Day: 1 2 3 4 5 7 22 24 26 29 31 33 36 38 40

*For cycle 1 of VBMCP, see VBMCP protocol; starting with cycle 2 and continuing for 2 years, administer as above. At day 43, give tenth dose of IFN and begin next cycle of VBMCP. Cycle duration, 6 weeks; treatment duration, 2 years.

DOSAGE MODIFICATIONS: After first cycle, modify melphalan, BCNU, cyclophosphamide for depressed blood counts as follows: ANC 1000–2000/µl—give 75%; ANC 750–1000 or platelets 50,000–100,000/µl—give 50%; delay treatment for ANC < 750/µl or platelets < 50,000/µl; when VBMCP dose is reduced because of cytopenias, next IFN cycle should be given at 25% dose reduction in relation to previous dose; interrupt IFN for severe performance status deterioration, ANC < 500/µl, platelets < 50,000/µL, elevated LFTs > 5 x normal, severe vomiting, diarrhea, or mental status changes; resume recovery at 50% dose; reduce vincristine dose for hepatic insufficiency

RECENT EXPERIENCES AND RESPONSE RATES

Study	Evaluable patients, n	Dosage and scheduling	Response (CR/PR%)	Median survival (mo)	5-yr survival (%)
Oken, et al., Proc ASCO 1990, 9:288	54	Vincristine 1.2 mg/m² IV d 1 BCNU 20 mg/m² IV d 1 Melphalan 8 mg/m² PO d 1–4 Cyclophosphamide 400 mg/m² IV d 1 Prednisone 60 mg/m² PO d 1–7; (20 mg/m² PO d 8–14, cycle 1) rIFN α-2 5 MU/m² sc d 22, 24, 26, 29, 31, 33, 36, 38, 40, 42†	30/50*	42	42

*Partial response requires ≥ 50% decrease in M-protein value; CR requires complete disappearance of M-protein from serum and urine and a normal bone marrow structure.
†The tenth and last dose of IFN α-2 is given on day 1 of the subsequent VBMCP portion of the cycle; six-week cycles are continued for 2 years.

CANDIDATES FOR TREATMENT
Patients with advanced, active myeloma and satisfactory performance status

SPECIAL PRECAUTIONS
Risk for infection greater during early cycles (use allopurinol to prevent hyperuricemia during early months); treatment-associated myelodysplastic syndrome and acute leukemia occur in some; VBMCP poorly tolerated by patients > 70 years of age and frail—MP is better choice for such patients; degree of myelosuppression increased with addition of IFN, particularly in elderly; avoid protocol in patients with active ischemic or congestive heart disease (exacerbated with IFN)

ALTERNATIVE THERAPIES
MP, mephalan alone, ABCM, VMCP/VBAP, VBMCP

DRUG INTERACTIONS
Cyclophosphamide: barbiturates, phenytoin, chloral hydrate; **IFN:** aspirin, NSAIDs, antihistamines, immunomodulators, theophyline, barbiturates

TOXICITIES
VBMCP: see VBMCP protocol for list of toxicities; **drug combination:** long-term toxicity: testicular atrophy, amenorrhea, risk for treatment-induced acute leukemia; **rIFN α-2:** fever, fatigue, flu-like symptoms (partially avoided with acetaminophen), pancytopenia, changes in consciousness, liver function abnormalities, blood pressure changes, numbness and tingling in fingers and toes; less frequently, convulsions, confusion, stupor, cardiac arrhythmias

NURSING INTERVENTIONS
Push fluids for 24 hours after cyclophosphamide to reduce risk for hemorrhagic cystitis; give antiemetic before administration; monitor blood glucose if diabetic, antacid therapy may be used; instruct patient in self-administration of IFN SC injections and recommend evening administration; give acetaminophen prior to IFN for flu-like syndrome associated with first few doses—may need to repeat as often as every 4 hours; assess patient performance and mental status; monitor weight, ensure adequate fluid, caloric, protein intake; use antidiarrheals and food supplements as needed

PATIENT INFORMATION
Patient should maintain good fluid intake; take melphalan on empty stomach, prednisone after meals; anticipate possibility of mood and appetite changes or fluid retention; be alert to early signs of bleeding or infection; seek medical attention for blood in urine; vincristine may cause severe constipation: monitor bowel pattern carefully, use mild laxatives, seek medical attention if persistent or severe; with IFN, may experience flu-like symptoms first few doses of cycle; tachyphylaxis will occur but does not produce fatigue

VMCP/VBAP AND ABCM

Vincristine, Melphalan, Cyclophosphamide, Prednisone/Vincristine, BCNU, Doxorubicin, Prednisone; and Doxorubicin, BCNU, Cyclophosphamide, Melphalan

This regimen consists of alternating cycles of vincristine plus prednisone combined with either melphalan plus cyclophosphamide or with BCNU plus doxorubicin. The strategy of rapid alternating cycles provides maximum early exposure to active combinations and theoretically could prevent or delay the emergence of resistant clones. An alternative strategy of giving three cycles of VMCP followed by three cycles of VBAP yielded essentially identical results in a SWOG study. Therefore, these results are pooled. A third variation on VMCP/VBAP, the ABCM regimen, eliminates vincristine and prednisone and yields similar results.

DOSAGE AND SCHEDULING

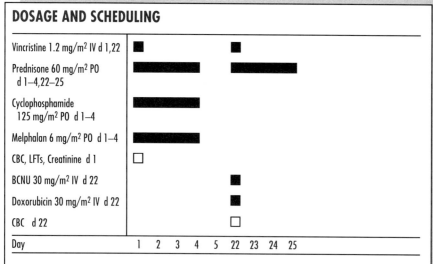

Vincristine 1.2 mg/m² IV d 1,22
Prednisone 60 mg/m² PO d 1–4,22–25
Cyclophosphamide 125 mg/m² PO d 1–4
Melphalan 6 mg/m² PO d 1–4
CBC, LFTs, Creatinine d 1
BCNU 30 mg/m² IV d 22
Doxorubicin 30 mg/m² IV d 22
CBC d 22

Day — 1 2 3 4 5 22 23 24 25

DOSAGE MODIFICATIONS: reduce dose of vincristine and doxorubicin for impaired liver function or significant treatment-induced cytopenias

RECENT EXPERIENCES AND RESPONSE RATES

Study	Evaluable patients, n	Dosage and scheduling	Response (%)	Median survival (mo)	5-yr survival (%)
VMCP/VBAP Durie, et al., J Clin Oncol 1986, 4:1227–1237; Salmon, et al., J Clin Oncol 1990, 8:1575—1584.	614	Vincristine 1.0 mg IV d 1, 22 Prednisone 60 mg/m² PO d 1–4, 22–25 Melphalan 6 mg/m² d 1–4 Cyclophosphamide 125 mg/m² PO d 1–4 BCNU 30 mg/m² IV d 22	38*	30	27
ABCM Maclennan, et al., Lancet 1992, 339:200–205.	314	Doxorubicin 30 mg/m² IV d 1 BCNU 30 mg/m² IV d 1 Cyclophosphamide 100 mg/m² PO d 22–25 Melphalan 6 mg/m² PO d 22–25	61†	32	25

*Response requires ≥ 75% decrease in M-protein production.
†Response = achievement of plateau phase.

CANDIDATES FOR TREATMENT
Patients with active myeloma who are elderly and frail (partially or totally bed-ridden)

SPECIAL PRECAUTIONS
Risk for infection greater during early cycles (use allopurinol to prevent hyperuricemia during early months); treatment-associated myelodysplastic syndrome and acute leukemia occur in some; do not use doxorubicin in patients with significant cardiac decompensation (ejection fraction < 45%, signs of consecutive heart failure [CHF], recent myocardial infarction [MI], or unstable angina); do not exceed cumulative doxorubicin dose of 450 mg/m²

ALTERNATIVE THERAPIES
MP, melphalan alone, VMCP/VBAP, ABCM

TOXICITIES
Melphalan: bone marrow suppression leading to neutropenia with increased risk for infection, thrombocytopenia with increased risk for bleeding, erythroid hypoplasia with risk for symptomatic anemia; **prednisone:** immunosuppression, infection, Cushing's syndrome, exacerbation of diabetes, weight gain, edema, mental status dysfunction—especially in elderly; **BCNU:** bone marrow suppression possibly longer than that with melphalan or cyclophosphamide, pain in injected extremity or at IV site, nausea, vomiting, liver or renal dysfunction; pulmonary fibrosis rare at this dose range; **cyclophosphamide:** bone marrow suppression but relatively platelet sparing, nausea, vomiting, alopecia, hemorrhagic cystitis, pulmonary fibrosis (rare), liver dysfunction (rare); **Vincristine:** peripheral neuropathy, cranial nerve neuropathy, constipation, alopecia, vesicant if extravasated; SIADH (rare); **Doxorubicin:** myelotoxicity, nausea, vomiting, alopecia, cardiotoxicity—generally at higher doses, vesicant if extravasated; **long-term toxicity:** testicular atrophy, amenorrhea, risk for treatment-induced acute leukemia

DRUG INTERACTIONS
Cyclophosphamide: barbiturates, phenytoin, chloral hydrate

NURSING INTERVENTIONS
Push fluids for 24 hours after cyclophosphamide to reduce risk for hemorrhagic cystitis; give antiemetic before administration; monitor blood glucose if diabetic; antacid therapy may be used

PATIENT INFORMATION
Patient should maintain good fluid intake; take melphalan on empty stomach, prednisone after meals; anticipate possibility of mood and appetite changes or fluid retention; be alert to early signs of bleeding or infection; seek medical attention for blood in urine; vincristine may cause severe constipation: monitor bowel pattern carefully, use mild laxatives, seek medical attention if persistent or severe

VAD
Vincristine, Doxorubicin, Dexamethasone

The VAD regimen combines vincristine and adriamycin by 4-day infusion with high-dose oral dexamethasone. It is primarily a salvage regimen in patients who have relapses but has gained an additional application as a treatment to be used prior to autologous bone marrow transplant harvest when alkylating agents are to be avoided. Responses to this regimen usually occur within 2 months, making VAD more rapid than MP or VMCP/VBAP and, possibly, VBMCP. The repeated cycles of high-dose corticosteroids are an important component in this regimen's effectiveness and may generate most of the activity in patients with refractory disease.

DOSAGE AND SCHEDULING

	Day 1 2 3 4 5 6 7 8 12 15 20
Vincristine 0.4 mg/m² IV continuous infusion d 1–4	▬▬
Doxorubicin 9 mg/m² IV continuous infusion d 1–4	▬▬
Dexamethasone 40 mg PO d 1–4	▬▬
CBC, LFTs, each cycle Creatinine every 3 cycles d 1	☐
Dexamethasone 40 mg PO (odd number cycles only) d 8–12,15–20	▬ ▬

Cycle duration, 4 weeks.
Trimethoprim/sulfamethoxazole 1 DS PO daily and clortrimazole troches, 10 mg 3x/d as prophylaxis while receiving therapy.

DOSAGE MODIFICATIONS: Reduce dose of vincristine and doxorubicin for impaired liver function; consider H₂ blocker or antacids for dexamethasone-associated dyspepsia; reduce dexamethasone for severe dyspepsia, edema refractory to diuretics, myopathy, severe hypertension, severe corticosteroid withdrawal symptoms or cushingoid changes, steroid psychosis or hallucinations; after first cycle, reduce doxorubicin for myelotoxicity: 75% if ANC is 1500–1000/mm³, 50% if ANC is 750–1000 or platelets are 50,000–100,000/μl

RECENT EXPERIENCES AND RESPONSE RATES

Study	Evaluable patients, n	Dosage and scheduling	Cycle duration (wk)	Objective response (%)
Alexanian, et al., Ann Intern Med 1986, 105:8–11.	39	Vincristine 0.4 mg/m² IV d 1–4 Doxorubicin 9 mg/m² IV d 1–4; both by continuous infusion Dexamethasone 40 mg PO d 1–4, 9–12, 17–20, 25–28	6	46†
Lokhorst, et al., Br J Haemotol 1989, 71:25—30.	31	Vincristine 0.4 mg/m² IV d 1–4 Doxorubicin 9 mg/m² IV d 1–4; both by continuous infusion Dexamethasone 40 mg PO d 1–4, 9–12, 17–20 (odd # cycles) Dexamethasone 40 mg PO d 1–4, (even # cycles)	4	60‡

*In previously treated patients
†Response requires ≥ 75% decrease in M-protein production.
‡Response requires ≥ 50% decrease in serum M-protein level.

CANDIDATES FOR TREATMENT
Alternative primary regimen for patients under consideration for stem cell harvest. Most often used in patients with relapsed myeloma.

SPECIAL PRECAUTIONS
Regimen is contraindicated in patients with poor liver function; prophylactic trimethoprim/sulfamethoxazole and clortrimazole troches advised during therapy; use allopurinol to prevent hyperuricemia during early months; doxorubicin is contraindicated in patients with significant cardiac decompensation (ejection fraction < 45%, signs of CHF, recent MI, or unstable angina); do not exceed cumulative doxorubicin dose of 450 mg/m².

TOXICITIES
Vincristine: peripheral neuropathy, cranial nerve neuropathy, constipation, alopecia, vesicant if extravasated; SIADH (rare); **Doxorubicin:** myelotoxicity, nausea, vomiting, alopecia, flare, cardiotoxicity (generally at higher doses), vesicant if extravasated; **Dexamethasone:** immunosuppression, infection, Cushing's syndrome, osteoporosis, exacerbation of diabetes, weight gain, hypertension, edema, mental status dysfunction—especially in elderly

DRUG INTERACTIONS
Doxorubicin and vincristine are compatible

NURSING INTERVENTIONS
Carefully place venous access catheter before initiating VAD; do not use a peripheral IV site—would expose patient to excessive risk for doxorubicin or vincristine extravasation injury; if right atrial catheter or central venous port is in place, administer doxorubicin and vincristine in an ambulatory outpatient setting with portable infusion pump; doxorubicin and vincristine may be mixed together; monitor regularly for hypertension, CHF, severe fluid retention, behavioral changes, symptoms of ulcer or dyspepsia, infections—including local Candida infections

PATIENT INFORMATION
Patient should anticipate possibility of mood and appetite changes or fluid retention; be alert to early signs of infection; vincristine may cause severe constipation: monitor bowel pattern carefully, use mild laxatives, seek medical attention if persistent or severe

Based on the National Cancer Institute's data, approximately 6500 children less than 15 years of age will be diagnosed with cancer in the next year. These 6500 children represent less than 1% of all new cancer patients in the United States. Nonetheless, cancer is the second leading cause of death in children under the age of 15 years and accounts for 3.6 deaths per 100,000 children each year. Fortunately, there have been dramatic improvements in therapy, and the prognosis for children diagnosed with cancer today is much better than it was even a few years ago.

There are many differences between childhood and adult malignancies. Most malignant neoplasms in children are of mesodermal origin, whereas those in adults are of epithelial origin. Carcinomas, for example, account for only 6.5% of the tumors in children under the age of 18 years, whereas in adults carcinomas are extremely common and account for 85% of tumors. Because readers of this chapter are more likely to be treating adolescent and young adult patients than young children, it is more useful to discuss malignancies occurring in children *older* than 12 years who might first be seen by an internist or family practitioner. Leukemia, central nervous system tumors, and lymphomas are the most common malignant diagnoses in children between 12 and 18 years of age (Table 1). These three diagnoses account for almost two-thirds of all neoplasms. Alternatively, neuroblastoma, GU tumors (such as Wilms'), and retinoblastoma, which are common in children, are extremely rare in children over the age of 12. Even when children between the ages of 15 and 18 years are analyzed, CNS tumors (33%), leukemia (15%), and lymphomas (15%) remain the most common malignant diagnoses, with carcinomas occurring in only 9% of the cases.

ACUTE LYMPHOBLASTIC LEUKEMIA

Leukemia is the most commonly occurring pediatric malignancy in the United States and is the most commonly diagnosed malignancy in adolescent patients. Acute lymphoblastic leukemia (ALL) is the most common type of leukemia in childhood and accounts for approximately 80% of the acute leukemia cases. Acute myeloblastic leukemia (AML) accounts for only approximately 20% of the acute leukemia cases. B-cell ALL (Burkitt's leukemia or FAB-L3) is very rare (< 1%) and is therefore not discussed in this chapter. The incidence of acute leukemia is almost 4 cases per 100,000 children each year, and this incidence results in approximately 1800 new cases of ALL and 370 new cases of AML each year in the United States.

ETIOLOGY AND RISK FACTORS

The incidence of ALL peaks between the ages of 3 and 5 years and thereafter declines, except for T-cell ALL, which appears to have its highest incidence in adolescent boys. The risk of ALL is greater in Caucasians than in African-Americans. Urbanization also appears to increase risk, with industrialized countries having a higher risk than nonindustrialized nations.

The risk of acute leukemia in siblings of children with ALL is four times higher (16 per 100,000 each year) than in the general population. The risk of ALL occurring in identical twins is 20-fold greater, and the younger the age at diagnosis, the higher the probability the disease will occur in the second twin. Genetic abnormalities that increase the incidence of ALL include Down's syndrome, Bloom syndrome, Klinefelter's syndrome, Wiskott–Aldrich syndrome, ataxia-telangiectasia, Fanconi's anemia, congenital agam-

maglobulinemia, and neurofibromatosis. Like the congenital immunodeficiency syndromes, immunosuppression by drugs, particularly in the setting of solid organ transplantation, increases the incidence of leukemia (particularly B-cell type).

Viral infections have been implicated as a cause of leukemia; however, they have not been closely linked except in the human T-cell lymphoma/leukemia virus infection (HTLV-1) and Epstein–Barr virus (EBV) infection in Burkitt's leukemia. Radiation therapy does increase the risk of leukemias (most often AML), and industrial chemicals have also been implicated.

PROGNOSIS AND PROGNOSTIC FACTORS

The cure rate of childhood ALL has dramatically improved over the past 20 years. From 95 to 98% of children with ALL achieve a complete remission and 65 to 75% are expected to be cured (Table 2). In older children, the disease tends to present with poor prognostic characteristics, and the cure rate is somewhat lower (approximately 50%) [1–3]. Table 2 details some of the largest and most effective clinical trials in childhood ALL. The first two trials listed are representative of the outcome in older patients with poor prognoses, whereas the others are most representative of patients with standard or good-risk ALL [4–8]. The outcome of therapy in young adults has been reviewed and demonstrates the effectiveness of modern therapy [9].

Because leukemia is a systemic disease it is not categorized by stages. The clinical presentation is usually that of a subacute illness with symptoms developing over weeks. Common presenting complaints, particularly in adolescents, are cough and lymphadenopathy. Other findings include fever, malaise, pallor, hemorrhage, organomegaly, pain (particularly in bone and joints), and anorexia. Central nervous system involvement may be evident by cranial nerve deficits or headache. Metabolic abnormalities as a result of the leukemic cell burden are usually evident, with decreased renal function, high lactate dehydrogenase (LDH), uric acid, potassium, phosphorus, and a low serum calcium. Children often present later in the course of their disease because of their ability to compensate.

Table 1. Relative Frequency of Malignancies in Children 12 Years of Age and Older

Diagnosis	Frequency (%)
Leukemias (all types)	20.5
Brain tumors (all histologic types)	20.0
Lymphomas	
Non-Hodgkin's lymphoma	12.0
Hodgkin's lymphoma	11.0
Sarcomas	
Ewing's and PNET	9.0
Osteosarcoma	5.5
Rhabdomyosarcoma and other soft tissue sarcomas	5.5
Carcinomas (all histologic types)	6.5
Others*	10.0

Data from University of Pittsburgh.
*Includes skin, teratomas, dysgerminomas, heptocellular, thyroid, and germ cell.
PNET—primitive neuroectodermal tumor.

The differential diagnoses at presentation include infectious mononucleosis, rheumatoid arthritis, idiopathic thrombocytopenic purpura, and aplastic anemia. Among the adolescents who present, lymphoma is often considered within the differential diagnosis; there is very little difference between a Stage IV lymphoma and leukemia, except for the degree of marrow involvement (ALL has ≥ 25% marrow blasts).

In childhood ALL, it is important to evaluate the prognostic features. With modern therapy, there is no difference in outcome between FAB-L1 and FAB-L2 morphology. However, FAB-L3 morphology (B-cell leukemia) has a poor prognosis unless intensively treated [10]. Among cases of ALL, B-lineage leukemia is most common; however, approximately 20% of ALL cases are of T-cell lineage, this type of ALL being very common in adolescence [3].

Chromosomal translocations are an important prognostic feature in childhood ALL. The overall frequency for specific translocations varies from very rare to approximately 6%. Nonrandom chromosomal translocations are extremely important because some have a very strong prognostic significance. For example, t(9;22), t(4;11), t(1;19), and t(8;14) indicate a poor prognosis [11–13]. Children with leukemic blasts that contain 52 or more chromosomes (hyperdiploidy) have a better response to therapy.

Large cooperative group clinical trials have made it possible to analyze the importance of prognostic variables (Table 3). The leukocyte count at diagnosis is the strongest prognostic variable in all large studies and correlates with the total amount of disease (organomegaly and lymphadenopathy). Patients over the age of 10 with ALL have a poor prognosis because they often present with multiple clinical features indicating poor prognosis, such as a mediastinal mass (T-cell disease) and a high leukocyte count. The correlation between presenting clinical and laboratory features and immunologic classification (Table 4) can be particularly helpful in predicting the response and planning therapy [16].

PRIMARY DISEASE THERAPY

Therapy is risk-directed. For example, girls with low leukocyte counts between the ages of 2 and 10 years without significant chromosomal abnormalities are treated less aggressively than adolescent boys presenting with T-cell disease, a high leukocyte count, central nervous system (CNS) involvement, and a mediastinal mass. Therapy should adhere to the prescribed protocol, usually entailing three phases of treatment.

Following the induction of complete remission, which occurs in approximately 95% of patients, there is a consolidation phase lasting 1 to 2 months, which incorporates CNS therapy (based on the risk or presence of CNS disease). The CNS is a sanctuary site in children and requires direct therapy. In low-risk patients intrathecal drugs may be adequate, whereas for older, high-risk patients the continued use of cranial radiation therapy is justified. Maintenance therapy continues for 2.5 to 3 years.

Protocols

For the small group of children who have ALL and an extremely good prognosis, therapy should be effective in producing cure in nearly 70% of cases. The induction phase includes vincristine, prednisone, and L-asparaginase. Following achievement of a complete remission, a consolidation phase with intensive intrathecal chemotherapy (usually methotrexate) should begin; often this is combined with vincristine, prednisone, oral methotrexate, and oral 6-mercaptopurine. Occasionally pulse therapy with cyclophosphamide or intravenous methotrexate is included in the consolidation phase. Cranial radiation therapy is not indicated in this group of patients because intrathecal therapy appears to be adequate CNS treatment. Delayed intensification or pulses during maintenance therapy have been shown to improve outcome. These pulses should include vincristine and prednisone and may also include cytosine arabinoside (ara-C), cyclophosphamide, and L-asparaginase. These intensive pulses can be given early in therapy or interspaced throughout the maintenance course. The backbone of maintenance therapy is oral 6-mercaptopurine and methotrexate.

BFM-Induction Therapy

Patients presenting with poor prognoses (ie, with features such as T-cell disease, high leukocyte count, mediastinal mass, adenopathy, and cytogenetic abnormalities) require more intensive therapy. Two general therapy plans have proven to be quite effective for these patients. First, the BFM-induction therapy includes prednisone, vincristine, daunomycin (4 doses), L-asparaginase, and intrathecal therapy [17]. Following remission, a consolidation phase is given that includes cyclophosphamide, 6-mercaptopurine, ara-C by intravenous push, intrathecal methotrexate, and craniospinal radiation therapy. Interim maintenance consists of 6-mercaptopurine and methotrexate, followed by delayed intensification, including a 4-week reinduction of dexamethasone, vincristine, doxorubicin, and L-asparaginase. A reconsolidation phase with cyclophosphamide, 6-thioguanine, and

Table 2. Clinical Trials in Childhood Acute Lymphoblastic Leukemia

Study	Children, n	Complete Remission Rate (%)	Analysis Time (yr)	Event-free Survival ± SE (%)
POG (T-cell ALL) (1981–1986) [4]	263	NA	4	50
SJCRH (high-risk X) (1979–1983) [5]	57	82	4	44 ± 10
POG (B-lineage) (1986–1990) [4]	1535	NA	4	72 ± 2.6
SJCRH XI (1984–1988) [6]	358	96	5	71 ± 4
BFM (1983–1986) [7]	653	98.3	5	64 ± 2
Dana–Farber 81-01 (1981–1985) [8]	289	96	7	72 ± 3

BFM—Berlin–Frankfurt–Münster; POG—Pediatric Oncology Group; SE—standard effort; SJCRH—St. Jude Children's Research Hospital.

ara-C with intrathecal methotrexate may be added following delayed intensification. Maintenance is then undertaken, which consists of vincristine and prednisone pulses superimposed on a background of 6-mercaptopurine and methotrexate.

New York Regimen

Alternatively, modifications of the New York regimen (or LSA2-L2) are also quite successful at producing cure in such children [18]. This treatment consists of induction that includes cyclophosphamide, daunomycin, weekly vincristine, and prednisone (28 days). Patients also receive L-asparaginase during induction and intrathecal methotrexate as CNS treatment or prophylaxis. For those achieving a complete remission, ara-C is given intravenously along with 6-thioguanine, intrathecal and intravenous methotrexate, L-asparaginase, and possibly cranial radiation therapy. The maintenance regimen includes intrathecal methotrexate and 6-thioguanine, cyclophosphamide, vincristine, prednisone, intravenous methotrexate, doxorubicin, ara-C, and 6-thioguanine. The BFM and New York regimens have been used extensively and modified by clinical investigators.

Table 3. Prognostic Significance of Clinical and Laboratory Features in Acute Lymphoblastic Leukemias

Study	Prognostic Variables	Poor Outcome
CCG [14]	WBC	$> 20 \times 10^9/l$
	Age	< 1 yr, ≥ 10 yr
	Sex	Male
	Med. mass	Present
	Splenomegaly	Below umbilicus
	Day-14 BM	$> 5\%$ blasts
	Hepatomegaly	Below umbilicus
	Platelet count	$< 50 \times 10^9/l$
	Lymph nodes	> 3 cm
	T-cell	Present
UKALL [15]	WBC	$> 10 \times 10^9/l$
	Age	< 1 yr, ≥ 10 yr
	Sex	Male
	Med. mass	Present
	Splenomegaly	Not defined
	Day-14 BM	$> 5\%$ blasts
	T-cell	Present
	Ph+ chromosome	Present
SJCRH [6]	WBC	$> 50 \times 10^9/l$
	Age	< 1 yr
	Day-14 BM	$> 5\%$ blasts
	T-cell	Present
	CD10	Absent
	DNA index	< 1.16
	CNS involvement	Present
	Ploidy	Pseudo- or hypodiploid

CCG—Children's Cancer Group; SJCRH—St. Jude Children's Research Hospital; UKALL—United Kingdom-ALL

Table 4. Correlation of the Presenting Clinical and Laboratory Findings of Childhood Acute Lymphoblastic Leukemia

Classification	Presenting Clinical Features	Laboratory Features at Diagnosis
T-cell ALL	Teenagers (median age, 10.3 yr) Male (M/F, 2.3:1) Mediastinal mass (60%)	WBC count $\geq 100 \times 10^9/l$ ($> 50\%$) Serum LDH > 1000 IU/l (60%) CNS leukemia (12.5%)
B-cell ALL	Abdominal mass (50%)	Low WBC count (median, $11 \times 10^9/l$) High serum LDH (median, 2000 IU/l) t(8;14)(q24;q32) t(2;8)(p11–12;q24) CNS leukemia at diagnosis (17%)
Ph+ ALL	Older age (median, 9.6 yr)	FAB-L2 morphology (50%) CNS leukemia at diagnosis (5%)
Pre-B ALL with (1;19)	Non-white race (40%)	High WBC count (median, $26.0 \times 10^9/l$) High serum LDH (median, 2000 IU/l)

ACUTE MYELOGENOUS LEUKEMIA

Acute myelogenous leukemia (AML) is a heterogeneous group of leukemias carrying a poor prognosis. AML can be divided into distinct clinical subgroups described by morphologic characteristics (FAB classification), surface antigen expression (immunophenotyping), and cytogenetic abnormalities [19,20]. Children with AML present with fever or signs and symptoms of pancytopenia. There is a higher incidence of the monomyelocytic and monocytic (AML-M4 and M5) subtypes of AML in pediatric series. However, the disease appears to be similar in adults and children because the immunophenotyping and cytogenetic abnormalities are similar. For further reference, the chapter on adult leukemia can be consulted.

ETIOLOGY AND RISK FACTORS

AML is associated with the same congenital syndromes known to increase the risk of ALL. In addition, one of the most important etiologic factors in the development of AML is previous treatment of malignancies with epipodophyllotoxins, alkylating agents, or radiation therapy. Patients who have received epipodophyllotoxins have an extremely high incidence of secondary AML, depending on the total dose and frequency with which these drugs were administered [21]. Such patients often have a cytogenetic abnormality involving chromosome 11 at band q23.

PROGNOSIS AND PROGNOSTIC FACTORS

The prognosis for pediatric patients with AML is slightly better than that for adults because children tolerate intensive therapy better. The complete remission rate in most pediatric series ranges from 72 to 85% [22,23]. When induction chemotherapy is increased, the risk of death from toxicity or pancytopenia increases, and when therapy is decreased, the complete remission rate is somewhat lower. After intensive consolidation and maintenance therapy, only about 30 to

45% of the initially diagnosed patients and about 45 to 50% of those who achieve a complete remission achieve long-term disease control [24,25]. The clinical and laboratory prognostic factors of two large pediatric series of AML are provided in Table 5 [19,26]. Because AML is a systemic disease, staging is not routinely performed.

Cytogenetic abnormalities have important prognostic implications in AML. Patients with monosomy 7 and 11q23 abnormalities have poor prognoses. Alternatively, the cytogenetic abnormalities t(8;21), t(15;17), and inversion(16) have been reported to portend good prognoses [20,27]. Patients with secondary AML following epipodophyllotoxins carry a poor prognosis; these patients often have 11q23 abnormalities. Approximately 60% of these patients achieve a complete remission but the vast majority relapse quickly.

PRIMARY DISEASE THERAPY

For the past two decades, the standard induction schedule (commonly referred to as *standard 7 + 3*) has been combination therapy of cytosine arabinoside (100–200 mg/m^2/d continuous IV infusion × 7 d) and daunorubicin (45 mg/m^2/d × 3 d). Attempts to improve the complete remission rate by increasing the dose or duration of ara-C have been unsuccessful. Combinations of ara-C with amsacrine or with mitoxantrone have also been shown to be effective remission induction therapies. The addition of drugs such as 6-thiaguanine, etoposide or the use of high-dose ara-C has not improved the remission induction rate except in a few small trials.

In a number of recent, large adult trials, idarubicin has been shown to be more effective than daunomycin for remission induction, particularly in younger adult patients [28]. Many planned pediatric trials will use idarubicin as a result of the data provided from the adult trials.

Induction Therapy for Patients with Therapy-Related AML

Patients who develop therapy-related AML following exposure to cytotoxic drugs generally have poorer prognoses because they have resistant disease. Therapy-related AML can be associated with cytogenetic abnormalities of chromosome 5 or 7. Patients who develop therapy-related AML following epipodophyllotoxins have developed FAB-M4 or FAB-M5 AML and have cytogenetic abnormalities of chromosome 11 at band q23. These patients generally have a short preleukemic phase and respond well to induction therapy. Although the complete remission rate for such patients is high, these patients have a poor disease-free survival rate. The best clinical management would appear to be allogeneic bone marrow transplantation during first remission.

POST-REMISSION CHEMOTHERAPY

The ideal number of maintenance courses and their durations remain controversial. The BFM childhood studies reported excellent results when children received protracted treatment for 2 years [22,25]. Alternatively, promising results were obtained in one nonrandomized study in which young patients were given daunorubicin and high-dose ara-C [29]. This study and others emphasize that intensive therapy with ara-C should be included in maintenance therapy.

Because of the low incidence of CNS involvement in patients with AML, CNS prophylactic therapy has not been a major component of

Table 5. Prognostic Factors Indicating Poor Outcome in Pediatric Acute Myeloblastic Leukemia

Characteristic	St. Jude (n = 251)			BFM-83 (n = 173)		
	Discriminator	CR	EFS	Discriminator	CR	EFS
Age	> 14 yr ≤ 14 yr	0.004	0.02		NS	NS
Spleen	≥ 6 cm < 6 cm	0.03	0.002	> 5 ≤ 5	NS	NS
Auer rods	+ −	NS	NS	+ −	NS	0.001
Coagulopathy	Present	< 0.001	0.001	Present	NS	NS
WBC count	≥ 10 < 10	0.05	0.002	< 20 20–100 > 100	0.01 0.001	0.04 0.05
FAB	M3	0.002	NS	M3	NA	NA
MPO		NA	NA	> 80% ≤ 80%	NS	0.001
Blasts—day 15		NA	NA	≥ 10% < 10%	0.002	0.001
BM eosinophils		NA	NA	≥ 3% < 3%	NS	0.01

P-value indicates significantly worse prognosis associated with that clinical or laboratory feature. Hemoglobin, platelet count, presence of CNS disease, and liver enlargement were not significant in either series.
CR—complete remission; EFS—event-free survival; NS—not significant.

most trials. However, patients with elevated leukocyte counts, monocytic or myelomonocytic leukemia, or chromosome 16 or t(8;21) abnormalities may have an increased risk of CNS disease. In the pediatric series of AML, where FAB-M4 and FAB-M5 morphologies are more common, CNS prophylactic therapy with intrathecal drugs has generally been administered without undue complications. Recently, the BFM investigators have analyzed their results of a clinical trial in which cranial radiation therapy was eliminated. The children who did not receive CNS prophylactic radiation had a statistically higher incidence of systemic relapse [30]. The relationship between the lack of CNS radiation therapy and the higher systemic relapse rate led these investigators to reinstitute CNS radiation therapy. Nonetheless, the role of CNS radiation therapy in AML therapy remains controversial, and the CNS is rarely the site of initial relapse.

Bone Marrow Transplantation in Post-Remission Therapy

A number of studies have compared intensive maintenance chemotherapy with either allogeneic or autologous bone marrow transplantation (BMT) for disease control [31]. Transplantation allows further intensification of effective chemotherapy. Additionally, in allogeneic BMT, graft versus leukemia has been shown to have significant antileukemic effects [32,33]. These benefits are partially offset by the problems associated with BMT, which include a higher mortality risk at the time of transplant and in allogeneic BMT the risk of graft-versus-host disease (GVHD). The International Bone Marrow Transplant Registry data indicate that allogeneic BMT in first remission results in a 5-year leukemia-free survival rate of about 50%. The actual relapse rate is approximately 20%. Outcome is related to age, with 50 to 60% event-free survival rates in patients under the age of 20 years versus 40% in those between the ages of 20 and 50 years.

The standard ablative or pretransplant therapy for allogeneic BMT has been cyclophosphamide and total-body radiation therapy or busulfan and cyclophosphamide. High-dose ara-C or etoposide has been incorporated into the pretransplant therapy with promising preliminary results. As yet, however, the use of additional drugs prior to allogeneic BMT has not demonstrated improved leukemia-free survival [24].

There remains considerable controversy as to whether patients with AML in first remission who have an HLA-identical sibling should receive BMT immediately, when they develop early relapse, or in second complete remission [34]. A number of ongoing trials in the cooperative pediatric groups are addressing this question. However, until results from randomized trials are available, BMT from sibling donors appears to be the treatment of choice for young patients (< 20 years of age) not being treated on protocols. BMT also appears to be the treatment of choice for high-risk patients (Table 5).

The alternative use of matched, unrelated donor (MUD) BMT is being explored for patients without a suitable sibling donor. Results demonstrate that successful transplants are possible but the risks of graft rejection and GVHD are considerably greater. Until further reports of MUD transplants are available, most clinicians feel they should be reserved for patients who relapse or are at extremely high risk for relapse.

Autologous Bone Marrow Transplantation
Autologous BMT carries a very low mortality rate when performed in children with AML. The significant limitation of this type of therapy is the likelihood of contamination of the cryopreserved marrow with leukemic cells.

Attempts to decrease the number of residual leukemic cells have lead most clinicians to purge the autologous marrow before cryopreservation [35]. Methods for purging autologous marrow of leukemic cells have included the use of drugs, monoclonal antibody and complement lysis, lecithin separation, monoclonal antibody positive selection, or long-term *in vitro* bone marrow culture. There is a large amount of laboratory evidence that purging can eliminate leukemic cells from the bone marrow. A number of studies have reported good results with purged marrows; however, other studies have demonstrated similar outcomes when purging was not used. No trials randomizing between purging and no purging have been undertaken.

Recently, evidence that relapse can occur from morphologically and cytogenetically normal marrow has been obtained using retroviral vectors to mark leukemic cells. This finding demonstrates that at least some relapses following autologous BMT have resulted from the infused marrow [36]. These studies *do not* determine whether purging is capable of eliminating the clonogenic leukemic cells or whether patients survive after purging because the cryopreserved marrows contained a lower number of viable leukemic cells. Purging may only be effective in a small group of patients with leukemic cells that are eliminated by the purging agent.

As noted previously, one advantage of allogeneic BMT over autologous BMT is that graft versus leukemia provides a significant improvement in leukemic control [33]. This beneficial effect of graft versus leukemia has resulted in a number of investigators attempting to induce graft versus leukemia in the autologous transplant setting. Most investigators are using interleukin-2 (IL-2) to activate T-cells after autologous BMT in an attempt to eliminate any residual leukemia.

Protocols

Currently both large pediatric cooperative groups (Childrens Cancer Group and The Pediatric Oncology Group) are running randomized protocols consisting of an intensive induction treatment period. Patients with an allogeneic sibling donor are encouraged to undergo allogeneic bone marrow transplant in first complete remission. Patients without a matched sibling donor are randomized between an autologous-purged transplantation or continued intensive chemotherapy. For further details on specific treatment, the section on AML in the chapter on leukemia should be consulted.

NON-HODGKIN'S LYMPHOMAS

There are major differences in the types of non-Hodgkin's lymphoma occurring in adolescent and adult populations. Most children have diffuse, high-grade lymphomas, which are comparatively uncommon in adults. The high-grade lymphomas that occur in children are categorized by histologic findings (Table 6). The histologic type is important in selecting therapy in advanced disease.

Approximately 700 new cases of non-Hodgkin's lymphoma are diagnosed in the United States annually. The risk of non-Hodgkin's lymphoma for males is 2.5 times greater than for females, and is 1.4 times higher in Caucasians than in African-Americans. Non-Hodgkin's lymphoma is rare in very young children, with the median age at diagnosis being 10 years. Clinical features at presentation are usually determined by the primary site, and the most frequent sites of involvement are the abdomen (approximately 31% of cases), the head and neck region (including Waldeyer's rings) (approximately 29% of cases), and the mediastinum (approximately 26% of cases). The

Table 6. Histologic Types of Non-Hodgkin's Lymphoma

Type	No.	Frequency (%)
Undifferentiated, SNCC	131	38.3
Lymphoblastic	101	29.9
Large cell	89	26.3
Other	17	5.0
Total	338	100

Data from Crist W, Personal communication, St. Jude Children's Research Hospital, 1962–1990.

Table 7. Staging of Non-Hodgkin's Lymphoma in Children

Stage	Criteria for Extent of Disease
I	A single tumor (extranodal) or single anatomic area (nodal)
II	A single tumor (extranodal with regional node involvement) Two or more nodal areas on the same side of the diaphragm Two single (extranodal) tumors, with or without regional node involvement, on the same side of the diaphragm A primary gastrointestinal tract tumor, grossly completely excised
III	Two single tumors (extranodal) on opposite sides of the diaphragm All primary intrathoracic tumors (mediastinal, pleural, thymic) All extensive unresectable primary intra-abdominal disease All paraspinal or epidural tumors
IV	CNS and/or bone marrow involvement

From Murphy SB et al. [37]; with permission.

disease may also arise in lymph nodes in other areas. There is a relationship between the primary site, histology, and age. For example, lymphoblastic lymphoma usually occurs in the mediastinum of adolescent boys, whereas Burkitt's lymphoma occurs in the abdomen of younger children.

ETIOLOGY AND RISK FACTORS

There is good evidence associating Epstein–Barr virus (EBV) infections with Burkitt's lymphoma. The HIV virus also results in an increased incidence of non-Hodgkin's lymphoma. Primary immunodeficiency, including syndromes such as Wiskott–Aldrich, ataxia-telangiectasia, common variable immunodeficiency, agammaglobulinemia, and X-linked lymphoproliferative disorder (Duncan's syndrome) all result in a higher incidence of lymphoma. Immunosuppression after solid organ transplantation increases the risk of B-cell lymphomas.

PROGNOSIS

The prognosis of patients with non-Hodgkin's lymphoma is dependent on the stage of the disease. Patients with Stage I and II disease of any histologic subtype have an excellent outcome [37]. Those with more advanced disease, particularly with Stage IV disease (involvement of the bone marrow or central nervous system), have a much poorer outcome. Therapy for patients with Stage III or IV non-Hodgkin's lymphoma is determined by the histologic type.

FIGURE 1

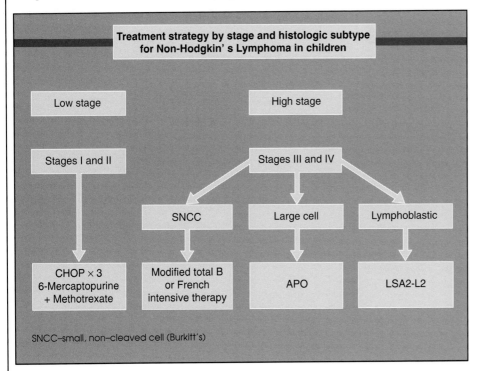

Treatment strategy by stage and histologic subtype for Non-Hodgkin's Lymphoma in children

SNCC–small, non-cleaved cell (Burkitt's)

STAGING

The Murphy system is most widely used for staging (Table 7). Approximately 40% of patients present with Stage I or II disease, 42% with Stage III, and 18% with Stage IV. Among patients with Stage IV disease, the marrow is the most common site of involvement, although as many as 17% of these children are classified as Stage IV based on CNS involvement only.

PRIMARY DISEASE THERAPY

The selection of therapy is based on stage and histology (Fig. 1). Surgery is seldom indicated and is primarily reserved for making the diagnosis.

For low-stage disease of any histologic type, the outcome is extremely good using cyclophosphamide, vincristine, high-dose methotrexate, and prednisone [37]. Six months of maintenance with 6-methylprednisolone and methotrexate appear to be indicated [37,38]. For Stage III and IV disease, therapy should be based on histologic type. For lymphoblastic lymphoma, intensive therapy has been very effective. The LSA2-L2 therapy (discussed earlier in this chapter) appears to be the treatment of choice [38].

For small, noncleaved-cell non-Hodgkin's lymphoma (Burkitt's), very short and very intensive therapy, such as the Pediatric Oncology Group's total B (including cyclophosphamide, doxorubicin, vincristine, high-dose ara-C, and high-dose methotrexate) or the French Cooperative Group's therapy, have produced outstanding results in patients with Stage III and IV B-cell, non-Hodgkin's lymphoma. These protocols are extremely intensive and require close attention to dosage and scheduling. For large cell lymphoma, the APO (vincristine, doxorubicin, prednisone, L-asparaginase, 6-mercaptopurine, and methotrexate) or similar regimens appear to be effective.

HODGKIN'S DISEASE

The presentation, diagnosis, staging, and therapy for Hodgkin's disease in children is similar to that in adults and can be found in the chapter on Hodgkin's disease in adults. Therefore, this discussion is limited to the unique characteristics of childhood Hodgkin's disease and its therapy.

ETIOLOGY AND RISK FACTORS

There is a binodal age peak in the incidence of Hodgkin's disease. In developing countries, the first incidence peak occurs before adolescence, but in industrialized nations, the first peak occurs in the mid-to-late 20s. Among adolescents in the United States, the disease is more common in Caucasians and the gender ratio is approximately equal. The incidence of Hodgkin's disease between the ages of 10 and 14 years is approximately 1.5 cases per 100,000 each year. This incidence increases between the ages of 15 to 19 years to approximately 3.9 per 100,000 Caucasians and 3.0 per 100,000 African-Americans.

The malignant cell in Hodgkin's disease is believed to be the Reed–Sternberg cell, but its normal counterpart is not known. The Reed–Sternberg cell apparently produces cytokines and these cytokines are responsible for the appearance of the histologic subtype. Recent research indicates a relationship between EBV infection and Hodgkin's disease, with molecular evidence for the EBV genome in Reed–Sternberg cells [39].

PROGNOSIS

The prognosis for Hodgkin's disease is directly correlated with the stage and the presence of systemic symptoms. With modern therapy, the histologic subtype is less important in predicting prognosis.

The prognosis for low-stage Hodgkin's disease (Stage IA and IIA) is excellent at 5 years. The disease-free survival rate in some groups treated with radiation therapy alone has been 40 to 65%, whereas groups receiving chemotherapy prior to radiation therapy have disease-free survival rates of 80 to 90%. However, the overall survival rates between these two groups are not dramatically different because patients who develop recurrent disease (particularly after radiation therapy alone) can usually be successfully retreated with chemotherapy. Relapses, when they occur, do so early; therefore some investigators chose to treat low-stage disease (Stage IA and IIA) with radiation therapy alone and reserve chemotherapy, with its concomitant side effects, for recurrent disease or higher-stage patients.

All patients with advanced Hodgkin's disease receive chemotherapy followed by radiation therapy (see below). Although the published series contain small numbers of patients, the 5-year event-free survival rates range from 54 to 86%.

STAGING

The usual clinical presentation is painless, supraclavicular cervical adenopathy. Two thirds of the patients who have cervical presentations will have some degree of mediastinal involvement. Primary disease presenting in the subdiaphragmatic site is rare (3% of cases). Hepatosplenomegaly and hepatomegaly often indicate advanced disease. The presence of systemic symptoms is extremely important and can portend a worse prognosis (Table 8).

PRIMARY DISEASE THERAPY

Because Hodgkin's disease is extremely sensitive to radiation, radiation therapy is generally considered the mainstay of therapy. Low-dose radiation therapy is considered to be approximately 2500 cGy, whereas full dose is 3500 to 4400 cGy. In children, the use of radia-

Table 8. Staging of Hodgkin's Disease in Children

Stage	Criteria
I	Involvement of a single lymph node region
I_E	Single extralymphatic organ or site
II	Involvement of two or more lymph node regions on the same side of the diaphragm
II_E	Localized involvement of an extralymphatic organ or site and one or more lymph node regions on the same side of the diaphragm
III	Involvement of lymph nodes on both sides of the diaphragm
III_S	Involvement of the spleen
III_E	Localized involvement of an extralymphatic organ or site
III_{SE}	Both spleen and extralymphatic organ sites involved
IV	Diffuse or disseminated involvement of one or more extralymphatic organs or tissues with or without associated lymph node involvement
Systemic symptoms (B)	Temperature > 38°C for > 3 consecutive days, unexplained weight loss of ≥ 10% in prior 6 mo, night sweats

tion therapy is limited by whether the patient has achieved full growth, because the long-term sequelae of full-dose radiation therapy on the growth of children can be severe.

The standard chemotherapeutic regimen used in Hodgkin's disease is MOPP (nitrogen mustard, vincristine, procarbazine, and prednisone) [40]. Alternatively, the apparently non–cross-resistant chemotherapeutic regimen of ABVD (doxorubicin, bleomycin, vinblastine, and dacarbazine) is an excellent option [41]. One of the long-term sequelae of MOPP is infertility; however, in general, ABVD is less favored in children because of the long-term sequelae of the anthracyclines and bleomycin (cardiac and pulmonary toxicity, respectively). Specific details of these two chemotherapy regimens can be found in the chapter on Hodgkin's disease.

In summary, patients with Stage IA or IIA disease who have obtained full growth may receive full-dose radiation therapy with a curative intent. Young patients who are still growing or who have bulky disease or extranodal lesions can receive three cycles of multiagent chemotherapy followed by low-dose radiation therapy [42]. Patients with Stage IIB and IIIA disease generally receive 6 cycles of chemotherapy. Often combinations of MOPP and ABVD (non–cross-resistant combinations) are used followed by low- or full-dose radiation therapy based on the age and growth of the child [43]. In the most advanced stages (Stage IIIB and IV), between 6 and 12 cycles of chemotherapy are administered and usually both combinations are used. However, some studies have shown excellent results using MOPP or ABVD exclusively, followed by radiation therapy, based on the extent of disease and age of the child.

CENTRAL NERVOUS SYSTEM TUMORS

CNS tumors are the second most common malignancy in children. During the first decade, there is a peak in the incidence of CNS tumors of 2.5 cases per 100,000 children each year. Tumors occurring in the first decade are usually embryonal neoplasms. During adolescence, the incidence of the typical adult supratentorial glial tumors increases (Table 9). Some other CNS tumors, including cerebellar astrocytomas, brain stem gliomas, medulloblastomas, and ependymomas usually occur in younger children. Thus, only astrocytomas of the cerebral hemisphere are discussed in detail.

Table 9. Relative Frequency of the Most Common Central Nervous System Tumors in Children

Tumor	Frequency (%)
Astrocytoma	
Supratentorial low-grade*	15–25
Supratentorial high-grade*	10–15
Cerebellar	10–20
Brain stem glioma	10–20
Medulloblastoma	10–20
Ependymoma	5–10
Others	15–20

More common in adolescents.

ETIOLOGY AND RISK FACTORS

Patients with neurofibromatosis have a marked increase in visual pathway gliomas, other glial tumors, and meningiomas. Tubular sclerosis is also associated with an increased incidence of glial tumors and ependymomas. There is an extremely high incidence of astrocytomas occurring in children with leukemia treated with CNS radiation therapy as prophylaxis for CNS disease. The incidence of meningiomas also appears to be increased in the long-term survivors of ALL. The presentation of these CNS tumors can occur as early as 2 years to as late as 24 years following the radiation therapy.

STAGING

Clinical presentation can be that of increased intracranial pressure, including headache that is present in the morning and associated with vomiting. Imaging studies are indispensable in CNS tumors, with magnetic resonance (MR) imaging being used more frequently because it provides greater resolution. Leptomeningeal spread may occur in children with aplastic gliomas. These patients should have their cerebrospinal fluid examined preoperatively if possible. In addition, MR imaging of the spine or myelography is necessary to fully evaluate the extent of disease in patients with these CNS neoplasms.

Astrocytomas of the Cerebral Hemisphere

Supratentorial astrocytic tumors comprise approximately 30 to 40% of childhood CNS tumors. One half of these are located in the cerebral hemisphere and the remainder occur in the deep midline structures including the thalamus, hypothalamus, third ventricle, and the basal ganglia. These tumors are more common in adolescent patients. In childhood, the male-to-female ratio is 2:1.

Astrocytomas are a diffuse group of neoplasms. Classification is generally low-grade (Kernohan grade I and II) versus high-grade (Kernohan grade III and IV, exemplified by anaplastic astrocytoma and glioblastoma multiforme).

Prognosis and Primary Disease Therapy

Prognostic features include the size of the tumor, histologic grade, and the extent of surgical excision. Among children, increasing age is associated with a worse prognosis.

The primary therapy is surgical resection. Complete excision improves survival regardless of the site. However, complete excision is often precluded because of the tumor's location. The beneficial effects of surgery are most evident in low-grade tumors where complete removal may lead to an 80% long-term survival rate. Patients with histologic grade III disease have about a 50% 3-year survival rate, whereas patients with grade IV disease have about a 15 to 20% 3-year survival rate.

The use of radiation in low-grade astrocytomas depends on the degree of resection. Patients with completely resected tumors have an excellent 5-year survival rate. Radiation therapy appears to improve the 5-year survival (35 to 70%) for incompletely resected tumors. Whole brain radiation is not necessary because these tumors usually recur locally.

Chemotherapy has an uncertain role in the adjuvant therapy of low-grade tumors. It should not be considered as initial treatment except in very young children. Patients who have a recurrence after prior radiation therapy are generally treated with the same chemotherapy regimens as that used for high-grade tumors.

Recent phase III chemotherapy trials in high-grade astrocytomas have not been very encouraging because they have not demonstrated an improved long-term outcome. Alkylating agents and nitosurea-based regimens have produced good response rates. The platinum drugs have produced disappointing response rates in the high-grade astrocytomas.

EWING'S SARCOMA AND PRIMITIVE NEUROECTODERMAL TUMORS

Ewing's sarcoma occurs most commonly in the second decade of life (64%) with very few cases occurring in the third decade (approximately 5%). The disease is more common in Caucasians than in African-Americans, and males are more often affected than females. Ewing's sarcoma of bone and soft tissue, as well as primitive neuroectodermal tumor (PNET), share a consistent nonrandom cytogenetic abnormality t(11;22). Recently, a second cytogenetic abnormality of chromosome 16 has been found in cases of Ewing's sarcoma.

The primary sites of Ewing's sarcoma are evenly split between the extremities and central axis. PNET is most commonly found in the central axis in or around the chest. There are no known environmental or genetic factors associated with Ewing's sarcoma.

PROGNOSIS

Workup should include evaluation of the primary site and a search for metastatic disease, which includes chest radiography and CT scan, bone scan, bone marrow aspirates and biopsies, and a serum LDH.

Approximately 20% of patients will present with identifiable metastatic disease. However, because failure has been very common in patients treated only with local therapy in the past, it is now believed that most patients have micrometastatic disease at diagnosis. Chemotherapy has dramatically improved the outcome for children with Ewing's sarcoma.

PRIMARY DISEASE THERAPY

Chemotherapy is extremely effective in the therapy of Ewing's sarcoma. In general, treatment with vincristine, actinomycin D, cyclophosphamide, and doxorubicin (VAC) has resulted in good-to-excellent 5-year disease-free survival rates of 55 to 70% for patients without evidence of metastatic disease. More recently, the combination of ifosfamide and etoposide has been shown to be extremely effective. The most recent Intergroup Ewing's Sarcoma Study demonstrated that the addition of ifosfamide and etoposide to VAC therapy improves event-free survival rates.

The 20 to 25% of patients who present with metastatic disease have a much poorer outcome. Generally, the progression-free survival rate at 3 years for patients with metastatic disease is around 30%, but the long-term disease-free survival is much poorer (5 to 10%). Such patients should receive intensive therapy, including etoposide and ifosfamide.

Primary disease control is achieved with surgery or radiation therapy. The control rate in distal extremity sites after combination radiation and chemotherapy is high. Large tumors and those in the axial sites are more often associated with local recurrence. In general, radiation therapy is favored where surgical excision would result in severe

dysfunction. Extremely high doses of radiation (4500–7000 cGy) are required for local disease control.

Protocols

The Intergroup protocol for Ewing's sarcoma has become the standard, consisting of vincristine, doxorubicin, and cyclophosphamide. Following a cumulative dose of 375 mg/m^2 of doxorubicin, actinomycin D is substituted. Therapy lasts for 54 weeks. Local disease control is instituted between weeks 9 and 12, at which time either surgery or radiation therapy to the local tumor is undertaken and doxorubicin interrupted.

For more advanced-stage disease, this protocol includes a more intensive arm that adds ifosfamide and etoposide to the treatment regimen, alternating courses of these two agents and the standard VAC. When the cumulative dose of doxorubicin reaches 375 mg/m^2, actinomycin D is substituted and treatment continues for a total of 1 year. Patients with metastatic disease receive similar therapy. However, doxorubicin is escalated in each course to 90 mg/m^2 (total dose of 450 mg/m^2). In addition, local therapy is delayed until week 12, and local therapy of metastatic disease is undertaken at a later time.

RHABDOMYOSARCOMA

Soft tissue sarcomas other than Ewing's sarcoma are a heterogeneous group of rare tumors. They are far more common in adults, and therefore much of the information about treatment comes from adult studies. In general, the prognosis for children with soft tissue sarcomas is better than that for adults. Soft tissue sarcomas that occur in adolescence, however, behave much like those found in adults. Thus, the management of soft tissue sarcomas in adolescent patients is similar to that in adults and can be found in detail in the chapter on sarcomas in adults.

Rhabdomyosarcoma is the most common soft tissue sarcoma occurring in patients under the age of 21 years and accounts for 5 to 8% of all cases of childhood cancer. The incidence rates are 8.4 cases per million Caucasian children each year, and 3.9 cases per million African-American children each year. Rhabdomyosarcoma can arise virtually at any site in the body and metastasizes to regional lymphatic tissues or more distant locations, usually the bone marrow and long bones.

ETIOLOGY

An increased incidence of rhabdomyosarcoma is found in families with Li-Fraumeni syndrome. The nonrandom cytogenetic abnormality t(2;13) has been identified in rhabdomyosarcoma, but there is no clear etiology of the disease.

PROGNOSIS

The prognosis for patients with rhabdomyosarcoma prior to the era of chemotherapy was extremely poor, with a 5-year survival rate of 14 to 36%. Currently, with intensive chemotherapy, the prognosis has improved. Patients with clinical group I disease have a 3-year survival rate of 88%; however, patients with metastatic disease at diagnosis have only about a 30% survival at 3 years [44]. Survival is also dependent on the primary site of disease; the highest survival occurs in patients with orbital or eyelid primaries (93%) and the lowest survival is in patients with retroperitoneal disease (46%).

There are four major pathologic subtypes of rhabdomyosarcoma. Table 10 provides the relative frequency, usual pathologic subtype, and patient age group for the different sites of presentation.

STAGING

Staging consists of assessing the extent of tumor and the presence of any distant metastases. Metastatic disease is usually found in the lymphatic system, lungs, and bones. Occasionally the liver and central nervous system may be involved (primarily in alveolar rhabdomyosarcoma).

Staging systems have been devised for clinical studies. The Intergroup Rhabdomyosarcoma Clinical Study has established a group rating system on which therapy is based (Table 11). Presently, the Intergroup Study is comparing this classification system to a modified TNM system for rhabdomyosarcoma staging.

Patients with no detectable metastases at diagnosis fare much better than those with metastatic disease. Patients who have their disease completely excised have a better disease-free survival rate than patients with microscopic or gross residual disease.

PRIMARY DISEASE THERAPY

The modalities of treatment are primarily surgical removal (if feasible), radiation therapy for control of any residual tumor, and systemic chemotherapy.

Table 10. Characteristics of Rhabdomyosarcoma

Site	Relative Frequency (%)	Usual Pathologic Subtype	Patient Age Group
Orbit	10	Embryonal	Young
Parameningeal	20	Embryonal	Young
Other head and neck	10	Embryonal	Young
Bladder, prostate	12	Botryoid/embryonal	Young
Vagina	2	Botryoid	Young
Paratesticular	6	Embryonal	Young
Extremities	20	Alveolar/undifferentiated	Adolescents
Trunk	10	Alveolar/undifferentiated	Adolescents
Other	10	Alveolar/undifferentiated	Adolescents

Table 11. Clinical Group Rating System for Rhabdomyosarcoma

Group	Criteria
IA	Localized, completely resected, confined to site of origin
IB	Localized, completely resected, infiltrated beyond site of origin
IIA	Localized, grossly resected, microscopic residual
IIB	Regional disease, involved lymph nodes, completely resected
IIC	Regional disease, involved lymph nodes, grossly resected with microscopic residual or histologic involvement of the most distal node sampled
IIIA	Local or regional grossly visible disease after biopsy only
IIIB	Gross residual tumor after > 50% resection of primary tumor
IV	Distant metastases present at diagnosis

Following attempts at surgical excision, radiation therapy will usually control primary disease. Clinical group I paratesticular and orbital or eyelid tumors receive no radiation therapy. However, higher clinical groups (ie, more advanced tumors) are generally treated with radiation therapy ranging from 4100 to 5440 cGy.

The vast majority of children with rhabdomyosarcoma are enrolled in the Intergroup Rhabdomyosarcoma Study, the details of which exceed the scope of this chapter. However, briefly, actinomycin D and vincristine are used for clinical group I paratesticular tumors or group I and II orbital primaries. For other clinical group I patients and for group II and III patients, the Intergroup Study is comparing vincristine, actinomycin D, and cyclophosphamide with 1) vincristine, actinomycin D, and ifosfamide or 2) vincristine, ifosfamide and etoposide. For clinical group IV patients, the combination of vincristine and melphalan is being compared with ifosfamide and etoposide at the start of treatment, with vincristine, actinomycin D, and cyclophosphamide added at week 13.

OSTEOSARCOMA

Osteosarcoma is the most common malignant bone tumor in the United States, and the annual incidence is 5.6 cases per million Caucasian children, with a lower rate among African-American children. Boys are more commonly affected than girls, and the peak incidence occurs in the second decade of life during the adolescent growth spurt.

Over the past two decades remarkable improvements in survival have resulted from more aggressive use of adjuvant chemotherapy [45]. Furthermore, advances in surgical techniques have improved the quality of life for survivors.

ETIOLOGY AND RISK FACTORS

Although the etiology of the disease is unknown, the relationship between bone growth and the development of osteosarcoma is clear. The most common site of disease is the distal femur, followed by the proximal tibia and the proximal humerus—all areas of rapid bone growth. In addition to radiation, alkylating agents appear to increase the risk.

Patients with hereditary retinoblastoma show a marked increase in the incidence of osteosarcoma, indicating a hereditary component. In addition, there is an increased incidence of osteosarcoma in patients with Li-Fraumeni syndrome.

PROGNOSIS

Prognosis for patients with osteosarcoma is related to the presence or absence of metastatic disease at diagnosis. The histologic subtype does not appear to make a difference, except in periosteal or justicortical osteosarcoma, which has a more indolent course and a lower rate of pulmonary metastases. Alternatively, multifocal osteosarcoma of bone at presentation is uniformly fatal and responds very poorly to therapy.

Studies using combinations of high-dose methotrexate, vincristine, adriamycin, bleomycin, cytoxan, actinomycin D, and cisplatin have reported relapse-free survival rates between 58 and 77% for patients without metastatic disease at diagnosis. For patients with metastatic disease at diagnosis the survival rate is poor.

Histologic grading of the degree of tumor necrosis following chemotherapy has been of prognostic significance [46]. The grading system for tumor necrosis runs from grade I (in which there is little to no effect identified on the tumor) to grade IV (in which there is no histologic evidence of viable tumor).

PRIMARY DISEASE THERAPY

In general, diagnosis is made based on radiographic and MR or CT studies of the involved bone. Biopsy for confirmation is generally performed and chemotherapy is administered preoperatively. Local disease control is achieved by surgery if possible because osteosarcoma is relatively radiation-resistant. Following surgery, chemotherapy is continued.

The disease has a propensity to metastasize to the lungs, as well as to the bone. Because radiation therapy is relatively ineffective at tolerated doses under 6000 cGy, most metastatic disease is treated by resection. Surgical resection of metastatic pulmonary disease provides long-term survival for a subset of patients [47].

Protocols

High-dose methotrexate has been the mainstay of chemotherapeutic regimens and has been shown to be extremely effective. In general, methotrexate is combined with either doxorubicin or cisplatin. Recently, ifosfamide has been incorporated into front-line studies. The combination of bleomycin, cyclophosphamide, and actinomycin D is also effective, particularly in patients who have been resistant to front-line combinations. More recently, a new agent, muramyl tripeptide (MTP-PE), has shown promising effects in pilot studies and is now being incorporated into phase III trials.

As yet, no specific chemotherapeutic regimen has been shown to be markedly superior to others in a randomized controlled trial. Clearly, the two best agents are high-dose methotrexate and adriamycin, and these drugs form the backbone of most modern chemotherapeutic regimens.

SUPPORTIVE CARE

Supportive care issues are extremely important in children and adolescents with cancer, as they are in adults. There are, however, differences in drug usage in children. Table 12 provides a list of the intravenous drugs used to treat infections in immunosuppressed patients, and Table 13 provides the usual pneumocystis prophylactic dose of trimethoprim and sulfamethotrexate for children.

Table 12. Intravenous Antibiotic Dosages for Children and Adolescents

Antibiotic	Dosage*
Acyclovir (VZV)	1500 mg/m^2/d ÷ q 8 hr
Acyclovir (HSV)	750 mg/m^2/d ÷ q 8 hr
Amikacin	27†
Amphotericin B	0.5–1.0 (single daily dose)
Amipicillin	150–300 (12 g)
Cefazolin	100 ÷ q 8 hr (6 g)
Cefoperazone	200 (12 g)
Cefotaxime	180 (12 g)
Cefoxitin	160 (12 g)
Ceftazidime	150 (6 g) ÷ q 8 hr
Ceftriaxone	80–100 (8 g) ÷ q 12 hr
Cefuroxime	150–240 (9 g) ÷ q 6 hr or q 8 hr
Chloramphenicol	75 (4 g)
Clindamycin	40 (4.8 g)
Erythromycin	40 (4 g)
Ganciclovir	10 ÷ q 12 hr
Imipenem	100 (4 g)
Metronidazole	30 (4 g)
Miconazole	50 ÷ q 8 hr
Nafcillin	150–200 (12 g)
Penicillin G	100–250,000 U/kg/d
Pentamidine	4 (single daily dose) IV or IM
Piperacillin	300 (24 g)
Ticarcillin	300 (18 g)
Ticarcillin and clav. acid	300 (18 g)
Tobramycin	8†
Trimethoprim/SMZ (RX for pneumocystis)	20 (TMP) ÷ q 6 hr
Vancomycin	40 (2 g)

*Intravenous dose in mg/kg/d (total max dose per day). All doses divided by q 6 hr unless otherwise indicated.
†Use ideal body weight to estimate starting dose.
HSV—herpes simplex; VZV—varicella.

Table 13. Trimethoprim and Sulfamethoxazole Prophylaxis for Children and Adolescents

Body Surface Area (m^2)	Tablet (regular strength)*	Liquid (ml)*
< 0.3	—	2.5
0.3–0.79	0.5	5.0
0.8–1.39	1	10.0
1.4—1.89	1.5	15.0
> 1.9	2	20.0

*Give dose BID on Monday, Wednesday, and Friday.

REFERENCES

1. Crist WM, Shuster JJ, Falletta J, *et al.*: Clinical features and outcome in childhood T-cell leukemia-lymphoma according to stage of thymocyte differentiation. A Pediatric Oncology Group Study. *Blood* 1988, 72:1891.

2. Falletta JM, Shuster JJ, Crist WM, *et al.*: Different patterns of relapse associated with three intensive treatment regimens for pediatric E-rosette positive T-cell leukemia. A Pediatric Oncology Group Study. *Leukemia* 1992, 6:541.

3. Steinherz PG, Siegel SE, Bleyer WA, *et al.*: Lymphomatous presentation of childhood acute lymphoblastic leukemia: A subgroup at high risk of early treatment failure. *Cancer* 1991, 68:751.

4. Crist W, Shuster J, Look T, *et al.*: Current results of studies of immunophenotype, age, and leukocyte-based therapy for children with acute lymphoblastic leukemia. *Leukemia* 1992, 6(suppl 2):162.

5. Dahl GV, Rivera GK, Look AT, *et al.*: Teniposide plus cytarabine improves prognosis in childhood acute lymphoblastic leukemia with a presenting leukocyte count ≥ 100 x 10⁹/L. *J Clin Oncol* 1987, 5:1015–1021.

6. Rivera GK, Raimondi SC, Hancock ML, *et al.*: Improved outcome in childhood acute lymphoblastic leukaemia with reinforced early treatment and rotational combination chemotherapy. *Lancet* 1991, 337:61–66.

7. Ritter J, Creutzig U, Reiter A, *et al.*: Childhood leukemia: Cooperative Berlin–Frankfurt–Münster trials in the Federal Republic of Germany. *J Cancer Res Clin Oncol* 1990, 116:100.

8. Niemeyer CM, Gelber RD, Tarbell NJ, *et al.*: Low-dose versus high-dose methotrexate during remission induction in childhood lymphoblastic leukemia (Protocol 81-01 Update). *Blood* 1991, 78:2514.

9. Nachman J, Sather HN, Buckley JD, *et al.*: Young adults 16–21 years of age at diagnosis entered on Childrens Cancer Group acute lymphoblastic leukemia and acute myeloblastic leukemia protocols. Results of treatment. *Cancer* 1993, 71(suppl 10):3377–3385.

10. Murphy SB, Bowman WP, Abromowitch M, *et al.*: Results of treatment of advanced-stage Burkitt's lymphoma and B cell (SIg+) acute leukemia with high-dose fractionated cyclophosphamide and coordinated high-dose methotrexate and cytarabine. *J Clin Oncol* 1986, 4:1732–1739.

11. Crist W, Carroll A, Shuster J, *et al.*: Philadelphia chromosome positive childhood acute lymphoblastic leukemia: Clinical and cytogenetic characteristics and treatment outcome. A Pediatric Oncology Group (POG) Study. *Blood* 1990, 76:489.

12. Raimondi SC, Behm FG, Roberson PK, *et al.*: Cytogenetics of pre-B cell acute lymphoblastic leukemia with emphasis on prognostic implications of the t(1;19). *J Clin Oncol* 1990, 8:1380.

13. Pui C-H, Frankel LS, Carroll AJ, *et al.*: Clinical characteristics and treatment outcome of childhood acute lymphoblastic leukemia with t(4;11)(q21;q23): A collaborative study of 40 cases. *Blood* 1991, 77:440.

14. Hammond D, Sather H, Nesbit M, *et al.*: Analysis of prognostic factors in acute lymphoblastic leukemia. *Med Ped Oncol* 1986, 14:124.

15. Eden OB, Lilleyman JS, Richards S, *et al.*: Results of Medical Research Council Childhood Leukemia Trial UKALL VIII (Report of the Medical Research Council on behalf of the Working Party on Leukemia in Childhood). *Br J Haematol* 1991, 78:187.

16. Chessells JM, Bailey C, Wheeler K, Richards SM: Bone marrow transplantation for high-risk childhood lymphoblastic leukaemia in first remission: Experience in MRC UKALL X. *Lancet* 1992, 340:565–568.

17. Riehm H, Gadner H, Henze G, *et al.*: Acute lymphoblastic leukemia: Treatment results in three BFM studies (1970–1981). In Murphy SE and Gilbert JR (eds): *Leukemic Research: Advances in Cell Biology and Treatment*. New York: Elsevier; 1983, pp 251–260.

18. Wollner N, Burchenal JH, Liebermann PH, *et al.*: Non-Hodgkin's lymphoma in children: A comparative study of two modalities of therapy. *Cancer* 1976, 37:123–134.

19. Creutzig U, Ritter J, Schellong G: Identification of two risk groups in childhood acute myelogenous leukemia after therapy intensification in study AML-BFM-78. *Blood* 1990, 75:1932–1940.

20. Kalwinsky DK, Raimondi S, Schell MJ, *et al.*: Prognostic importance of cytogenetic subgroups in *de novo* pediatric acute nonlymphocytic leukemia. *J Clin Oncol* 1990, 8:75–83.

21. Pui C-H, Ribeiro RC, Hancock ML, *et al.*: Acute myeloid leukemia in children treated with epipodophyllotoxins for acute lymphoblastic leukemia. *N Engl J Med* 1991, 325:1682.

22. Creutzig U, Ritter J, Riehm H, *et al.*: Improved treatment results in childhood acute myelogenous leukemia: A report of the German cooperative study AML-BFM-78. *Blood* 1985, 65:298–304.

23. Ravindranath Y, Steuber CP, Krischer J, *et al.*: High dose cytarabine for intensification of early therapy of childhood acute myeloid leukemia. A Pediatric Oncology Group Study. *J Clin Oncol* 1991, 9:572–580.

24. Gale RP, Butturini A, Horowitz MM: Does more intensive therapy increase cures in acute leukemia? *Sem Hematol* 1991, 28:93–94.

25. Ritter J, Creutzig U, Schellong G: Treatment results of three consecutive German childhood AML trials: BFM-78, -83, and -87. AML-BFM Group. *Leukemia* 1992, 6(suppl2):59–62.

26. Hurwitz CA, Schell MJ, Pui C-H, *et al.*: Adverse prognostic features in 251 consecutive children with acute myeloblastic leukemia. *Med Ped Oncol* 1993, 21:1–7.

27. Raimondi SC, Kalwinsky DK, Hayashi Y, *et al.*: The cytogenetics of childhood acute non-lymphocytic leukemia. *Cancer Genet Cytogenet* 1989, 40:13–27.

28. Vogler WR, Velez-Garcia E, Weiner RS, *et al.*: A phase III trial comparing idarubicin and daunorubicin in combination with cytarabine in acute myelogenous leukemia. A Southeastern Cancer Study Group Study. *J Clin Oncol* 1992, 10:1103–1111.

29. Wolff SN, Herzig RH, Fay JW, *et al.*: High dose cytarabine and daunorubicin as consolidation therapy for acute myeloid leukemia in first remission: Long-term follow up and results. *J Clin Oncol* 1989, 7:1260–1267.

30. Creutzig U, Ritter J, Zimmermann M, Schellong G: Does cranial irradiation reduce the risk for bone marrow relapse in acute myelogenous leukemia? Unexpected results of the Childhood Acute Myelogenous Leukemia Study BFM-87. *J Clin Oncol* 1993, 11:279–286.

31. Woods WG, Kobrinsky N, Buckley J, *et al.*: Intensively time induction therapy followed by autologous or allogeneic bone marrow transplantation for children with acute myeloid leukemia or myelodysplastic syndrome. A Childrens Cancer Group Pilot Study. *J Clin Oncol* 1993, 11:1448–1457.

32. Horowitz ME, Gale RP, Sondel PM, *et al.*: Graft-versus-leukemia reactions after bone marrow transplantation. *Blood* 1990, 75:555–562.

33. Sullivan KM, Weiden PL, Storb R, *et al.*: Influence of acute and chronic graft-versus-host disease on relapse and survival after bone marrow transplantation from HLA-identical siblings as treatment of acute and chronic leukemia. *Blood* 1989, 73:1720–1728.

34. Mayer RJ: Allogeneic transplantation versus intensive chemotherapy in first remission acute leukemia: Is there a "best choice?" *J Clin Oncol* 1988, 6:1532–1536.

35. Schiffman K, Clift R, Appelbaum FR, *et al.*: Consequences of cryopreserving first remission autologous marrow for use after relapse in patients with acute myeloid leukemia. *Bone Marrow Transplant* 1993, 11:227–232.

36. Brenner MK, Rill DR, Moen RC, *et al.*: Gene marking to trace origin of relapse after autologous bone marrow transplantation. *Lancet* 1993, 341:85–86.

37. Murphy SB, Fairclough DC, Hutchison R, *et al.*: Non-Hodgkin's lymphoma of childhood: An analysis of the histology, staging, and response to treatment of 338 cases at a single institution. *J Clin Oncol* 1989, 7:186–193.

38. Anderson JR, Jenkin RDT, Wilson JF, *et al.*: Long-term follow-up of patients treated with COMP or LSA2-L2 therapy for childhood non-Hodgkin's lymphoma. A report of CCG-551 from the Childrens Cancer Group. *J Clin Oncol* 1993, 11:1024–1032.

39. Weiss L, Movahed LA, Warnke RA, *et al.*: Detection of Epstein–Barr viral genomes in Reed–Sternberg cells of Hodgkin's disease. *N Engl J Med* 1989, 320:502–506.

40. DeVita VT Jr, Serpick A, Carbone PP: Combination chemotherapy in the treatment of advanced Hodgkin's disease. *Ann Intern Med* 1970, 73:881–895.

41. Bonadonna G, Valagussa P, Santoro A: Alternating non-cross-resistant combination chemotherapy or MOPP in stage IV Hodgkin's disease. *Ann Intern Med* 1986, 104:739–746.

42. Leventhal BG: Management of stage I-II Hodgkin's disease in children. *J Clin Oncol* 1990, 8:1123–1124.

43. Schellong G, Bramswig JH, Hornig-Franz I: Treatment of children with Hodgkin's disease–results of the German Pediatric Oncology Group. *Ann Oncol* 1992, 3(suppl 4):73–76.

44. Maurer HM, Gehan EA, Beltangady M, *et al.*: The Intergroup Rhabdomyosarcoma Study-II. *Cancer* 1993, 71:1904–1922.

45. Link MP, Goorin AM, Miser AW, *et al.*: The effect of adjuvant chemotherapy on relapse-free survival in patients with osteosarcoma of the extremity. *N Engl J Med* 1986, 314:1600–1606.

46. Rosen G, Caparros B, Huvos AG, *et al.*: Preoperative chemotherapy for osteogenic sarcoma: Selection of postoperative adjuvant chemotherapy based on the response of the primary tumor to preoperative chemotherapy. *Cancer* 1982, 49:1221–1230.

47. Goorin A, Delorey M, Lack E, *et al.*: Prognostic significance of complete surgical resection of pulmonary metastases in patients with osteogenic sarcoma: Analysis of 32 patients. *J Clin Oncol* 1984, 2:425–431.

CHAPTER 23: ACCESS DEVICES
Cheryl A. Steele and John H. Raaf

Intravenous access (and access to other body compartments) is an important part of the care of patients with cancer, particularly in patients being treated with chemotherapy [1,2]. Patients receiving cytotoxic drugs require blood sampling, intravenous drugs (such as analgesics, antibiotics, and antiemetics with blood components) and intravenous fluid support. Inadequate venous access may prevent optimal cancer treatment by delaying or preventing administration of adequate amounts of chemotherapy as defined by treatment protocols. Pre- and postchemotherapy hydration and parenteral nutrition support may also be needed.

To avoid the problems that develop in patients with cancer who do not have adequate access (Table 1), new techniques and devices have been developed over the past two decades (Table 2). Groeger states that in the United States alone 386,000 external hub and 134,000 subcutaneous port venous access devices are now implanted each year [4]. This technology, although initially costly, has resulted in greater comfort and a much improved quality of life for patients during therapy. The new methodology ensures safe delivery of cytotoxic drugs in patients who previously had to endure numerous painful (and often unsuccessful) attempts at peripheral and central venous cannulation.

Most chemotherapy is administered via a systemic intravenous route. This achieves a distribution of the blood throughout most tissues in the body, hopefully affecting even occult metastases. The timing of delivery may vary (continuous, bolus, or circadian-based) because different timing strategies have been devised to achieve maximal cytotoxic effect on tumor and minimal toxicity to normal tissues.

In regional chemotherapy, a cytotoxic drug is delivered to one organ or anatomic region to achieve a higher drug level there than elsewhere in the body (Table 3). Most regional chemotherapy approaches are still investigational and therefore are performed using investigational protocols. Regional approaches involve either administration of drug to a body cavity (intraventricular, intraperitoneal, intravesicular, intrapleural) or to a particular capillary bed by intra-arterial infusion. The use of the intra-arterial infusion approach is advantageous if the drug is taken up on the first pass through the capillary bed with high efficiency. This is the case for 5-fluorodeoxyuridine infusion into the liver, but it is not true for many other drugs or sites.

Of the intracavitary drug delivery systems, only intraventricular chemotherapy has become standard treatment, because this approach offers a way to deliver drugs into the cerebrospinal fluid and adjacent tissue, which lie beyond the blood-brain barrier. Intraperitoneal chemotherapy for ovarian cancer initially appeared innovative and promising, but results of numerous clinical trials indicate that this method is superior to systemic treatment only if there is minimal disease. In addition, it carries the serious risk for formation of extensive intraperitoneal adhesions that can lead to small bowel obstruction [5].

Venous access devices may be categorized according to whether they will be used short-term (up to 2–3 weeks) or long-term (from months to years). Short-term catheters are made of relatively stiff plastic (polyurethane or poly(vinyl chloride)), whereas long-term ones are made of Silastic, which is softer and minimizes endothelial trauma.

Short-term devices are simpler and less expensive to insert, whereas long-term devices provide a safer and more lasting route of access. Selection of patients to receive long-term access devices, and the type of device used, is still determined to a large degree by physician and patient preference, although data comparing the different devices are becoming available.

Table 1. Common Vascular Access Problems in Patients with Cancer

1. Many painful peripheral venipunctures are required for infusion of IV fluids and medications and for drawing of blood samples

2. Peripheral vein sclerosis ("exhaustion") by chemotherapeutic agents

3. Morbidity and mortality (especially in thrombocytopenic patients) of repeated attempts at percutaneous central line insertion, especially from pneumothorax and hemothorax

4. Infiltration and sometimes disastrous extravasation of cytotoxic drugs into soft tissue, with the loss of tendon, nerve, or hand/arm function

5. Prevention of optimal treatment by lack of venous access. Poor access can delay or prevent administration of adequate chemotherapy, as defined by treatment protocols; patients may not receive needed pre- and postchemotherapy hydration, blood products, or parenteral nutrition

Adapted from Raaf [3]; with permission.

Table 2. Venous Access Devices Available for Use in Patients with Cancer

I. Peripheral intravenous cannulas

II. Short-term central venous catheters
Single-lumen non-Silastic catheters
Triple-lumen non-Silastic catheters
Silastic noncuffed, nontunneled catheters

III. Long-term Silastic cuffed, tunneled catheters
Single lumen
Dual and triple lumen
Dual-lumen hemodialysis/infusion

IV. Subcutaneously implanted venous access ports

V. External and internal/implanted pumps

Table 3. Routes of Chemotherapy Administration

I. Systemic
Peripheral or central
Continuous, bolus, circadian-based

II. Regional
Intra-arterial (infusion, isolation-perfusion, tourniquet-infusion)
Intraventricular (intrathecal)
Intraperitoneal
Intrapleural
Intravesicular (urinary bladder)

REFERENCES

1. Raaf JH, Heil D, Rollins DL: Vascular access, pumps, and infusion. In McKenna RJ, Murphy GP (eds): *Cancer Surgery.* 19xx Philadelphia: JB Lippincott; 79–91.

2. Goodman MS, Wickham R: Venous access devices: An overview. *Oncol Nurs For* 1984, 11:16–23.

3. Raaf JH: Results from use of 826 vascular access devices in cancer patients. *Cancer* 1985, 55:1312–1321.

4. Groeger JS, Lucas AB, Coit D: Venous access in the cancer patient. *Principles & Practice of Oncology: PPO Updates* 1991, 5(3):1–14.

5. Markman M, Cleary S, Howell SB, Lucas WE: Complications of extensive adhesion formation after intraperitoneal chemotherapy. *Surg Gynecol Obstet* 1986, 162:445–448.

6. Broadwater JR, Henderson MA, Bell JL, et al.: Outpatient percutaneous central venous access in cancer patients. *Am J Surg* 1990, 160:676–680.

7. Broviac JW, Cole JJ, Scribner BH: A silicone rubber right atrial catheter for prolonged parenteral alimentation. *Surg Gynecol Obstet* 1973, 136:602–606.

8. Hickman RO, Buckner CD, Clift RA, et al.: A modified right atrial catheter for access to the venous system in marrow transplant recipients. *Surg Gynecol Obstet* 1979, 148:871–875.

9. Pasquale MD, Campbell JM, Magnant CM: Groshong versus Hickman catheters. *Surg Gynecol Obstet* 1992, 174:408–410.

10. Raaf JH: Vascular access, catheter technology and infusion pumps, In Moossa AR, Schimpff SC, Robson MC (eds): *Comprehensive Textbook of Oncology,* 2nd ed. 1991, Baltimore: Williams & Wilkins, pp. 583–589.

11. Dunn J, Nylander W, Richie R: Central venous dialysis access: Experience with a dual-lumen silicone rubber catheter. *Surgery* 1987, 102:784–788.

12. Bour ES, Weaver AS, Yang HC: Experience with the double lumen Silastic catheter for hemoaccess. *Surg Gynecol Obstet* 1990, 171:33–39.

13. Moss AH, McLaughlin MM, Lempert KD, et al.: Use of a silicone catheter with a Dacron cuff for dialysis short-term vascular access. *Am J Kidney Dis* 1988, 6:492–498.

14. Raaf JH, Heil D: Open insertion of right atrial catheters through the jugular veins. *Surg Gynecol Obstet* 1993, 177:295–298.

15. Cohen AM, Wood WC: Simplified technique for placement of long term central venous silicone catheters. *Surg Gynecol Obstet* 1982, 154:721–724.

16. Raaf JH: An atraumatic tunneling device for implantation of right atrial catheters and ports. *Surg Gynecol Obstet* 1989, 168:353–354.

17. Niederhuber JE, Ensminger W, Gyves JW, et al.: Totally implanted venous and arterial access system to replace external catheters in cancer treatment. *Surgery* 1982, 92:706–712.

18. Brothers TE, Von Moll LK, Niederhuber JE, et al.: Experience with subcutaneous infusion ports in three hundred patients. *Surg Gynecol Obstet* 1988, 166:295–301.

19. Ross MN, Haase GM, Poole MA, et al.: Comparison of totally implanted reservoirs with external catheters as venous access devices in pediatric oncologic patients. *Surg Gynecol Obstet* 1988, 167:141–144.

20. Mirro J Jr, Rao BN, Stokes DC, et al.: A prospective study of Hickman/Broviac catheters and implantable ports in pediatric oncology patients. *J Clin Oncol* 1989, 7:214–222.

21. Mueller BU, Skelton J, Callender DPE, et al.: A prospective randomized trial comparing the infectious and noninfectious complications of an externalized catheter versus a subcutaneously implanted device in cancer patients. *J Clin Oncol* 1992, 10:1943–1948.

22. Johnson S, Patt YZ: Caring for the patient on intraarterial chemotherapy...Are you ready? *Nursing 81* 1981, Nov: 108–112.

23. Lokich JJ: Hepatic artery infusion: Present status and future perspectives. *Sem Oncol* 1983, 10:249–250.

24. Reed ML, et al.: The practicality of chronic hepatic artery infusion therapy of primary and metastatic hepatic malignancies. *Cancer* 1981, 47:402–409

25. Oberfield RA: Intraarterial hepatic infusion chemotherapy in metastatic liver cancer. *Sem Oncol* 1983, 10:206–213.

26. Perri J, Erikson KA: Nursing issues for hepatic arterial infusion therapy. *Sem Oncol* 1983, 10:191–198.

27. Oncology Nursing Society: Module I—Catheters. In: *Access Device Guidelines: Recommendations for Nursing Education and Practice,* 1989.

28. Winters V: Implantable vascular access devices. *Oncol Nurs For* 1984, 11(6):25–30.

29. Oncology Nursing Society: Module II—Implanted Ports and Reservoirs. In: *Access Device Guidelines: Recommendations for Nursing Education and Practice,* 1989.

30. Myers C: The use of intraperitoneal chemotherapy in the treatment of ovarian cancer. *Semin Oncol* 1984, 11:275–284.

31. Malloy J: Administering intraperitoneal chemotherapy: A new approach. *Nursing 91* 1991, Jan:58–62.

32. Swenson KK, Eriksson JH: Nursing management of intraperitoneal chemotherapy. *Oncol Nurs For* 1986, 13:33–39.

33. Piccart MJ, et al.: Intraperitoneal chemotherapy: Technical experience at five institutions. *Sem Oncol* 1985, 12:90–96.

34. DeGraff PW, et al.: Complications of Tenckhoff catheter implantation in patients with multiple previous intraabdominal procedures for ovarian carcinoma. *Gynecol Oncol* 1988, 29:43–49.

35. Hoff ST: Concepts in intraperitoneal chemotherapy. *Sem Oncol Nurs* 1987, 3:112–117.

36. Jenkins J: Managing intraperitoneal chemotherapy: A medical, nursing, and personal challenge. *Sem Oncol* 1985, 12:97–100.

37. Howell SB: Intraperitoneal catheters for chemotherapy. *J Vasc Access Nurs* 1990, 1(1):8–10.

38. Almadrones L, Yerys C: Problems associated with the administration of intraperitoneal therapy using the Port-A-Cath system. *Oncol Nurs For* 1990, 17:75–80.

39. Davidson SA, et al.: Intraperitoneal chemotherapy: Analysis of complications with an implanted subcutaneous port and catheter system. *Gynecol Oncol* 1991, 41:101–106.

40. Sundaresan N, Suite ND: Optimal use of the Ommaya reservoir in clinical oncology. *Oncology* 1989, 3:15–20.

41. Esparza DM, Weyland JB: Nursing care for the patient with an Ommaya reservoir. *Oncol Nurs For* 1982, 9(4):17–20.

42. Hagle ME: Implantable devices for chemotherapy: Access and delivery. *Sem Oncol Nurs* 1987, 3:96–105.

43. Rahr V: Giving intrathecal drugs. *Am J Nurs* 1986, July:829–831.

44. Obbens E, Leavens ME, Beal JW, Lee YY: Ommaya reservoirs in 387 cancer patients: A 15-year experience. *Neurology* 1985, 35:1274–1278.

45. Barone RM, et al.: Intra-arterial chemotherapy using an implantable infusion pump and liver irradiation for the treatment of hepatic metastases. *Cancer* 1982, 50:850–862.

46. Von Roemeling R, MacDonald M, Langevin T, et al.: Chemotherapy via implanted infusion pump: New perspectives for delivery of long-term continuous treatment. *Oncol Nurs For* 1986, 13(2):17–24.

47. Keller JH, Ensminger WD: Stability of cancer chemotherapeutic agents in a totally implanted drug delivery system. *Am J Hosp Pharm* 1982, 39:1321–1323.

48. Niederhuber JE, Ensminger WD: Surgical considerations in the management of hepatic neoplasia. *Sem Oncol* 1983, 10:135–147.

49. Kemeny N, Daly J, Reichman B, *et al.*: Intrahepatic or systemic infusion of fluorodeoxyuridine in patients with liver metastases from colorectal carcinoma. *Ann Intern Med* 1987, 107:459–465.

50. Oncology Nursing Society: Module III—Pumps. In: *Access Device Guidelines: Recommendations for Nursing Education and Practice*, 1989.

SHORT-TERM CENTRAL VENOUS CATHETERS

Two decades ago, antineoplastic drugs were most often given intravenously to patients with cancer by peripheral cannulas placed in the veins of the hand or forearm. However, several complications were associated with this method, including cytotoxic drug extravasation into soft tissue, phlebitis, vein exhaustion, and patient discomfort. To reduce the degree of these complications, central venous catheters were introduced, and they are now the preferred method for short-term chemotherapeutic administration in many patients. A stiff, plastic (*eg*, polyurethane), 16-gauge central venous catheter provides a secure route of access. A triple-lumen polyurethane catheter with one 16-gauge and two 18-gauge lumens is commonly used for short-term chemotherapy administration in hospitalized patients. This temporary method is suitable for use over a period of 2 or 3 weeks at most.

PROCEDURE FOR IMPLANTATION

1. The external or internal jugular vein is preferred over the subclavian vein for catheter placement.
2. A J-wire is used to guide the catheter into place.
3. Catheter is sutured to skin to prevent dislodgment (sutures will erode eventually through skin and must be replaced) [6].

INDICATIONS
Patients requiring intravenous infusion of chemotherapy (bolus or continuous) as an inpatient over an interval of less than 2 weeks

ADVANTAGES
Preferred approach for patients requiring short-term infusions; catheters can be placed at bedside and replaced over a guide wire

DISADVANTAGES
Cannot be used with outpatients; stiff plastic catheter is more traumatic to vein endothelium; catheter must be sutured to skin

COMPLICATIONS
Pneumothorax or hemothorax with subclavian vein insertion; phlebitis, vein thrombosis, infection, dislodgment of catheter

GUIDELINES FOR CARE
Flush with heparinized saline daily and after each use; cleanse exit site and change dressing three times per week; watch for infection, occlusion, disconnection, leakage, vein thrombosis

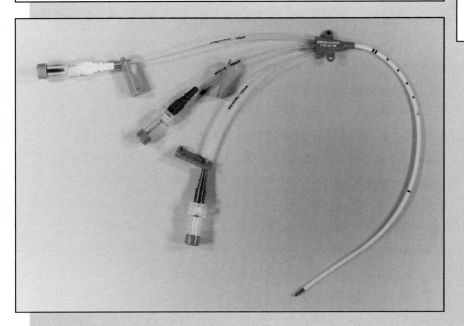

LONG-TERM RIGHT ATRIAL CATHETERS

Long-term right atrial catheters made of silicone come in several designs and may be used in many clinical situations. All such catheters are thick-walled, soft, cuffed, and tunneled and provide long-term access for hydration, hyperalimentation, or medications, including chemotherapy and antibiotics. Long-term venous access catheters have made safe continuous infusion of chemotherapeutic agents possible, offering the dual benefits over intermittent infusion of less toxicity with retained antineoplastic effect.

The Broviac [7] and Hickman [8] single-lumen Silastic catheters were the first long-term devices to become available. The Broviac catheter has a 1-mm internal diameter, the Hickman a 1.6-mm internal diameter. The Groshong catheter (single or dual lumen) is made of Silastic and has a Dacron cuff. A special feature is the slit valve near the closed distal tip designed to open only with pressure from injection, infusion, or aspiration. With the valve in its neutral, closed position, blood should not flow into the catheter, making flushing with heparinized solution unnecessary. Rather, the catheter is flushed with saline alone after each use or every 7 days [9].

Patients receiving multiagent chemotherapy or a bone marrow transplant may require intensive intravenous support through one or more routes of venous access. This need is met by a multilumen Silastic right atrial catheter, which allows simultaneous infusion of several, possibly incompatible, chemotherapeutic agents [10]. The dual-lumen, 2.2 mm and 3.2-mm lumen Silastic Raaf catheters may be inserted in the cephalic or external jugular vein in most patients. The Quinton-Raaf triple-lumen catheter is useful in bone marrow transplant recipients or in other patients requiring intensive intravenous support. This is a 12-French, cuffed, right atrial catheter that has two 1.0-mm and one 1.25-mm lumens. The different lumens are dedicated to infusion of antibiotics, blood products, parenteral nutrition, drugs for nausea or pain, or frequent sampling. It has been found that the complication rate of multilumen Silastic catheters is no greater than that for single-lumen catheters. The length of catheter function is the same. The PermCath is another useful and increasingly popular device in patients who need dialysis or plasmapheresis [11–13].

PROCEDURE FOR IMPLANTATION

1. Implantation is performed in the operating room by open [14] or closed technique [15].
2. In open technique, the external or internal jugular vein or cephalic vein is cut down and the catheter is placed into the central venous system.
3. Bleeding and discomfort are minimized during catheter threading by use of an atraumatic tunneling device [16].
4. Dacron cuff is placed in the tunnel at least 2 in. above the exit site to prevent extrusion of cuff or infection.
5. Intraoperative fluoroscopy confirms the catheter tip position in the right atrium and should demonstrate free flow of fluid in both directions through all lumens.

INDICATIONS
Patients requiring intravenous infusion of chemotherapy (bolus or continuous) as outpatient or inpatient; multilumen catheters are useful for intensive intravenous support

ADVANTAGES OVER POLYURETHANE SHORT-TERM CATHETERS
Eliminates multiple venipunctures; decreased risk of drug extravasation; larger lumen permits more rapid infusion; low incidence of phlebitis, vein thrombosis, and infection; Dacron cuff prevents dislodgment; lower rate of catheter thrombosis; multilumen catheters allow uninterrupted, simultaneous administration of parenteral nutrition, drugs, blood sampling, and other IV support in critically ill patients [1].

ADVANTAGES OVER IMPLANTED PORT
Easier to access; less expensive device and system; rapid infusion, especially of blood products; easier to remove at bedside or as outpatient procedure

DISADVANTAGES
External hub impedes daily activities and sports; less cosmetically acceptable than implanted port; time and expense required for maintenance; more easily damaged due to external components

COMPLICATIONS
Air embolism; arterial injury; cardiac arrhythmias; catheter damage; catheter malposition; catheter pinch-off; sepsis; catheter thrombosis; drug extravasation; endocardial wall damage; hemorrhage; needle or catheter dislodgment; one-way catheter

GUIDELINES FOR CARE
Flush catheter with heparinized saline; irrigation required daily; cover exit site with sterile dressing; change dressing three times per week; cleanse exit site with antiseptic during dressing changes

PATIENT AND FAMILY INFORMATION
Patient or family member should watch exit site for bleeding, inflammation, catheter damage (clamp should be made available); report to health care provider instances of fever or chills; change dressing and flush catheter with heparinized solution.

VENOUS PORTS

The use of implanted venous access ports is gaining popularity for patients with good performance status who are receiving chemotherapy. Ports consist of stainless-steel, titanium, or plastic chambers connected to a standard Broviac or Hickman Silastic long-term right atrial catheter [17–21].

PROCEDURE FOR IMPLANTATION

1. Catheters are introduced via the internal or external jugular or cephalic vein.
2. The port is implanted subcutaneously against the chest wall in an infraclavicular position.

To use the port, a needle is placed through the skin and septum into the port chamber. Drugs can be infused or blood samples withdrawn using this device. The Huber needle was designed to minimize coring of the Silastic septum, although a recent comparison of this side-hole design to that of a regular end-hole needle indicated that coring occurs with equal and rare frequency in both types of needle. Dual ports with two chambers attached to a dual-lumen catheter are also available, allowing two separate simultaneous infusions.

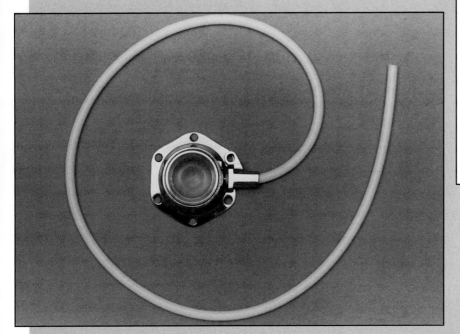

INDICATIONS

Patients requiring intravenous infusion of chemotherapy (bolus or continuous) mainly as an outpatient and when less intensive intravenous support is needed

ADVANTAGES OVER CATHETER WITH EXTERNAL HUB

Cosmetically preferable; lower rate of associated infection at "access site"; less easily damaged (no external components); less time and expense required for maintenance

DISADVANTAGES

More difficult to access than external hub, slower rate of infusion; Huber needles are costly and not always available; implant and device are 5 to 10 times more costly than external hub catheter; surgical procedure required to remove device

COMPLICATIONS

Extravasation of agents into the port pockets; catheter separation from the port; infection of the port pocket (may be virulent organisms such as *Pseudomonas*); port inversion

GUIDELINES FOR CARE

Flush with heparinized saline once a month; learn technique to access port using a Huber needle

PATIENT AND FAMILY INFORMATION

Patient or family members should observe port site for possible inflammation (drug extravasation or infection), skin erosion; report instances of fever or chills (due to sepsis) to health care provider

ARTERIAL CATHETERS

Arterial catheters with an external hub have been used for chemotherapy administration for many years and were popular until the very early 1980s. Arterial catheters are now used primarily with new implantable drug delivery systems for the infusion of chemotherapeutic drugs through a major artery directly into the tumor—usually a localized, inoperable tumor in the liver, head and neck, or bones [22]. This method of administration allows a high concentration of drug to be delivered to the tumor, in some cases with decreased systemic drug levels resulting in fewer systemic side effects [22–24]. In prolonged and continuous regional arterial infusion via external catheter, the catheter is attached to a portable infusion pump that continuously infuses the drug through the catheter around the clock for weeks or months in selected patients [25]. The largest reported experience with regional chemotherapy through an external arterial catheter (during the 1970s and early 1980s) has been in the treatment of colorectal cancer metastatic to the liver via hepatic arterial infusion. At the present time, however, external arterial catheters are infrequently used for long-term arterial infusions. Nevertheless, in some institutions, percutaneous radiographically inserted arterial catheters is sometimes used for bolus injections or short-term infusions of antineoplastic agents, with subsequent removal of the catheter at completion of infusion.

PROCEDURE FOR PLACEMENT

1. Hepatic arterial catheters are inserted by open surgical technique (requiring laparatomy) *or* percutaneously under fluoroscopy, depending on status of the patient [26].
2. In the surgically placed catheter, the gastroduodenal artery or inferior epigastric artery is used, and the catheter exits through a separate stab wound on the abdominal wall [22].
3. With percutaneous placement, a femoral or brachial-axillary insertion site is used, with pertinent anatomy visualized angiographically.
4. If infusion is to continue for more than 24 hr, the catheter can be sutured into place; the entire site is covered with a sterile occlusive dressing.
5. If catheter is to be placed in the femoral artery, the patient must be hospitalized and immobilized during chemotherapy infusion.

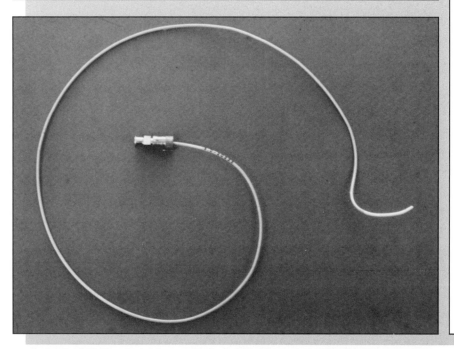

INDICATIONS

Patients requiring bolus injections or continuous infusions of antineoplastic agents regionally; patients whose disease is not widely metastasized; patients who can adapt to long-term arterial infusions and care for external catheter and pump

ADVANTAGES

Minimal systemic toxicity with maximal therapeutic response due to greater tumor exposure to high concentration of drug; long-term continuous infusion can be provided on outpatient basis; less costly than pump implantation

DISADVANTAGES

Continuous infusion imposes limitations on patient's activities (routine and sports); requires mastery of technical skills for proper home care; mandates regular visits to health care setting for monitoring and prevention of complications; mandates patient hospitalization and immobilization if infusion site is femoral artery

COMPLICATIONS

Infection at the site of catheter entry or sepsis; complete or partial arterial thrombosis; arterial occlusion; arterial stenosis; bleeding uncontrolled by pressure; catheter breakage in artery; catheter tip displacement/migration; cracked, leaking, or kinked catheter; catheter occlusion; diminished pulse (or loss) following percutaneous placement; tear and separation of intima from media of arterial wall; disconnection of catheter or tubing connectors during continuous infusions with blood backup; pump failure or malfunction; toxic effects of intra-arterially administered chemotherapeutic drugs or BRMs

GUIDELINES FOR CARE

Assess for and report to physician immediate postinsertion complications [27]: inflammation or infection; unusual resistance or catheter occlusion; unusual pain; bleeding at arterial catheter exit site; changes in length of exposed catheter; quality of pulse on the affected side monitored every 30 min for 6 hr—then hourly for next 6 hr; drug toxicity; **other considerations:** organize catheter care to minimize number of entries into system; administer short- and long-term infusions through positive pressure infusion pump to maintain patency of catheter and overcome hepatic arterial pressure; follow approved institutional procedures for accessing and flushing catheter, for exit site care and dressing change, for declotting the catheter if occlusion occurs

PATIENT AND FAMILY INFORMATION

Patient or family member should report infection at insertion site and changes in temperature, color, sensation, and movement of affected extremity (following percutaneous placement and upon discharge); care for exit site and change dressing (if continuous infusion at home); apply pressure to site if bleeding; clamp catheter if it breaks with hemostat and notify medical care provider immediately

ARTERIAL PORTS

The introduction of an implanted arterial port in the mid-1980s with an attached thick-walled soft catheter (which is better tolerated by arterial vessels) has been a major advance for intra-arterial chemotherapy. The maintenance of external arterial catheters for delivery of chemotherapy has historically been fraught with complications. The implanted arterial port is associated with fewer complications because it has no external component, the skin providing a protective barrier over the port. In addition, the attached silicone catheter is beaded and can be sutured to the artery itself, preventing migration or displacement. These catheters usually have a smaller lumen than those used with the venous port systems because arterial vessels are smaller.

The arterial port is placed for regional drug delivery (as discussed in the section on arterial catheters) and should be used for that purpose only, not for routine intravenous applications and medications [28]. Arterial ports also should not be used for laboratory sampling because the smaller lumen catheter is more likely to clot. Most of the experience with regional chemotherapy through an implanted arterial port and catheter system has been via hepatic arterial infusion in the treatment of colorectal cancer that has metastasized to the liver.

PROCEDURE FOR IMPLANTATION

1. Placement is done as an inpatient surgical procedure.
2. Arterial port is placed in a subcutaneous pocket, ideally overlying the anterior lower rib cage (to ensure stability); when implanted in the abdominal wall, it can be more difficult to access.
3. Catheter is inserted into the hepatic arterial system.

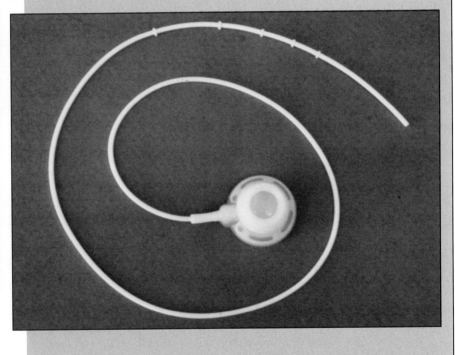

INDICATIONS

Patients requiring bolus injections or continuous infusion of antineoplastic agents regionally; patients whose disease is not widely metastasized

ADVANTAGES

Minimal systemic toxicity with maximal therapeutic response due to greater tumor exposure to high drug concentrations; can be used within 24 hr after implantation (unless postoperative edema and tenderness develop); can be used for intermittent or continuous infusion; long-term continuous infusion with ambulatory pump can be provided on outpatient basis; can be used for several months to years; limited patient responsibility and expense of maintenance (except with continuous infusion); dressing not required when off therapy; skin barrier protects against infection; little change in cosmetic appearance; nonrestricted patient activity

DISADVANTAGES

Requires surgical placement; needle accesses cause slight discomfort; excess adipose tissue over port can impede palpation and access; continuous infusion requires patient's mastery of technical skills and imposes limitations on activities; device must be removed surgically

COMPLICATIONS

Infection or sepsis; extrusion of port through skin; rotation of port; complete or partial arterial thrombosis; arterial occlusion; arterial stenosis; catheter tip displacement or migration, catheter occlusion; disconnection of tubing connectors during continuous infusion (with possible blood backup); pump failure or malfunction; dislodgment of needle from port (with subsequent port pocket extravasation); toxic effects of chemotherapeutic drugs; BRMs administered intra-arterially

GUIDELINES FOR CARE

Assess for and report to physician: immediate postoperative bleeding, draining hematoma, or excessive edema at the implant site; local or systemic symptoms of infection (normal parameters may be masked by depressed immune status); unusual resistance or port occlusion upon access; movement or erosion of implanted port; needle dislodgment with subsequent extravasation; unusual abdominal pain; drug toxicity [29]; **other considerations:** organize catheter care to minimize number of entries into system; use 90° noncoring needle to access port; follow approved institutional procedure for prepping skin prior to accessing port, for flushing port initially and after drug administration, for dressing and needle change during continuous infusion, for declotting port and catheter if occlusion occurs

PATIENT AND FAMILY INFORMATION

Patient or family members should assess implant site for infection or other complications; notify health care provider immediately of chills or fever; return *weekly* for routine flushing/heparinization; with continuous infusion at home, care for needle access site and ambulatory pump

INTRAPERITONEAL CATHETERS

Intraperitoneal catheters are used for the delivery of chemotherapeutic drugs directly into the peritoneal cavities of patients with intra-abdominal malignancies. Direct drug installation is intended to increase drug levels at the predominant site of disease, producing greater cytotoxicity than could be achieved by systemic drug administration [30]. The semipermeable peritoneal membrane enables prolonged malignant cell exposure to the chemotherapeutic drug. Most of the chemotherapeutic drugs delivered into the peritoneal cavity via catheter are absorbed by the portal venous system. Thus, the agents are partially detoxified and metabolized on the first pass through the liver, reducing systemic drug levels and the number of systemic side effects [31,32]. The use of intraperitoneal chemotherapy has been studied most extensively in ovarian cancer, a disease that remains confined to the peritoneal cavity virtually throughout its clinical course.

The Tenckhoff peritoneal dialysis catheter, a Silastic semipermanent device developed over 25 years ago, is the most frequently used intraperitoneal catheter. It allows chronic access to the peritoneal cavity [33]. The catheter has two Dacron cuffs to maintain its position within the abdominal cavity and to create a barrier against infection. The intra-abdominal portion of the catheter has many small holes, which facilitates drainage of peritoneal fluid after the treatment is completed [32].

PROCEDURE FOR PLACEMENT

1. Insertion is performed at the time of exploratory laparotomy, during the conclusion of a restaging procedure, *or* during a separate surgical procedure.
2. Catheter tip is placed in the abdominal cavity with one cuff positioned subcutaneously, the other just anterior to the peritoneum [34].
3. End of catheter is pulled through a subcutaneous tunnel and exits through a separate stab wound in the left or right lower abdominal quadrant [34].
4. Catheter site is completely healed approximately 2 weeks following insertion [32].

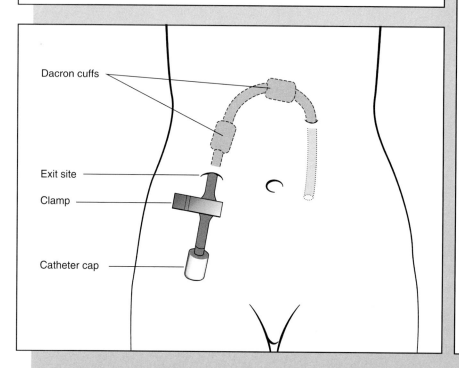

Dacron cuffs

Exit site

Clamp

Catheter cap

INDICATIONS

Patients with tumors confined to the peritoneal cavity; patients with small tumor volume (ideally, microscopic residual tumor for maximum efficacy) [30,32,35]

ADVANTAGES

Direct administration of chemotherapy to tumor exposes malignant cells to high concentration of chemotherapy (possibly 1000 times greater than that which can be safely given systemically) [31,32]; eliminates difficulty of access associated with implanted intraperitoneal ports in obese patient; infusion time of fluids (10–15 min) shorter than that with implanted intraperitoneal ports (30–45 min); catheter may be removed at bedside or as outpatient procedure

DISADVANTAGES

High maintenance (frequent care of dressings and catheter site); restricts water activities

COMPLICATIONS

Local or systemic infection; bacterial peritonitis; fluid leakage around catheter (1–7 d after catheter insertion) [36], one-way flow due to buildup on or around distal catheter [37], catheter inflow obstruction (inability to flush catheter); catheter outflow obstruction, abdominal pain; bowel perforation (associated with catheter implantation); paralytic ileus (related to catheter placement); toxic effects of chemotherapeutic drugs or BRMs administered intraperitoneally

GUIDELINES FOR CARE

Assess for and report to physician: immediate postoperative complications at catheter exit site; local or systemic symptoms of infection (normal parameters may be masked by depressed immune status); resistance or catheter occlusion [27]; abdominal pain; dislodgment of catheter; drug toxicity; **other considerations:** organize catheter care to minimize number of entries into the system [31]; use sterile technique during immediate postoperative period (days 1–14) in caring for the external portion of catheter, and exit site, and dressing changes [32]; follow approved institutional procedure for flushing catheter to maintain patency and for declotting occlusion of catheter

PATIENT AND FAMILY INFORMATION

Patient should inspect catheter site for signs of infection, notify health care provider immediately of chills, fever of 101°F or greater, abdominal pain or tenderness, persistent nausea or vomiting, persistent diarrhea or constipation; perform routine catheter care and dressing changes

INTRAPERITONEAL PORTS

Intraperitoneal implanted ports, like external Tenckhoff catheters, are used for the delivery of chemotherapeutic drugs directly into the peritoneal cavity of patients with intra-abdominal malignancies. The direct instillation is intended to maximize drug levels at the predominant site of disease, producing greater cytotoxicity than that achieved by systemic drug administration [30] (see discussion on intraperitoneal Tenckhoff catheters).

The intraperitoneal implanted port has two major components—a stainless steel port and a Silastic catheter designed like the Tenckhoff catheter. The port has a self-sealing silicone rubber septum that allows access into the port chamber by the insertion of a noncoring needle through the skin into the chamber [38]. There is a sidearm on the side of the port attached to the catheter. The catheter has two Dacron cuffs to maintain placement within the abdominal cavity. The intra-abdominal portion of the catheter has many small holes for drainage of peritoneal fluids after the treatment is completed [32]. The intraperitoneal port differs from venous and arterial ports by its much larger lumen size.

PROCEDURE FOR IMPLANTATION

1. Insertion is performed at the time of exploratory laparotomy, during the conclusion of a restaging procedure, *or* during a separate surgical procedure without exploratory laparotomy.
2. Catheter is passed through a subcutaneous tunnel to a position in the mid-abdomen (lateral to the umbilicus) where it is inserted into the peritoneal cavity [35,38,39].
3. Dacron cuffs should be located subcutaneously, just anterior to the peritoneum.
4. Port is placed subcutaneously in a pocket beneath the skin and affixed to the fascia of the muscles, overlying an anatomic area that provides support and stability (usually the lower rib cage) [35,38].

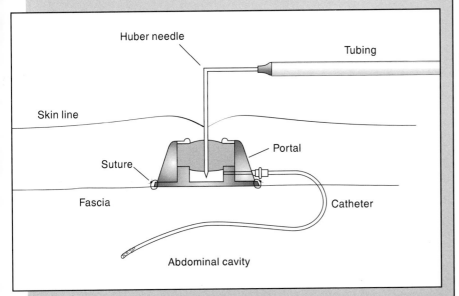

INDICATIONS
Patients with tumors that are confined to the peritoneal cavity; patients with small volume of tumor (ideally microscopic residual tumor confined to peritoneal cavity) [30,32,35]

ADVANTAGES
Administration of chemotherapy directly to the tumor exposing malignant cells to high concentration of drug (possibly 1000 times that given systemically) [31,32]; can be used immediately after placement; limited patient responsibility and expense of maintenance care; dressing is not required when off therapy; requires monthly flushing only for maintenance; skin barrier provides barrier against infection; little change in patient's cosmetic appearance; nonrestricted patient activity

DISADVANTAGES
Infusion time through port is nearly double that of Tenckhoff catheter [35]; can be difficult to drain, requiring suction; can be difficult to locate and access port if placed over abdomen [37]; needle accesses cause slight discomfort; requires surgical removal

COMPLICATIONS
Local or systemic infections; bacterial peritonitis; one-way flow due to buildup around the distal catheter; catheter inflow obstruction via the port; catheter outflow obstruction; extrusion of port; rotation of port; needle dislodgment and extravasation; abdominal pain and bowel perforation (associated with catheter implantation), paralytic ileus; toxic effects of chemotherapeutic drugs or BRMs administered intraperitoneally

GUIDELINES
Assess and report to physician [29]: immediate postoperative bleeding, draining hematoma, or excessive edema at the implant site; local or systemic infection (normal parameters may be masked by depressed immune status); unusual resistance or port occlusion; sudden pain or swelling at implant site; movement of port; erosion of port; needle dislodgment with subsequent pocket tissue extravasation; unusual abdominal pain; drug toxicity; **other considerations:** organize site access to minimize the number of entries into system; use noncoring needle to access port; maintain aseptic technique during access; follow approved institutional procedure for flushing system to maintain patency and for declotting for occlusion

PATIENT AND FAMILY INFORMATION
Patient or family member should assess the implant site for signs of complications; notify health care provider immediately of chills, fever of 101°F or greater, abdominal pain or tenderness, persistent nausea and vomiting, persistent diarrhea or constipation; avoid pressure or trauma at the implant site

INTRAVENTRICULAR RESERVOIRS

The first intraventricular implanted reservoir was devised by the neurosurgeon AK Ommaya in 1963. Since then, various subcutaneous reservoirs, that allow access to the cerebrol spinal fluid (CSF) via the lateral ventricles have been developed [40]. These intraventricular reservoirs or ventricular access devices are commonly referred to as *Ommaya reservoirs*. The reservoir is a mushroom-shaped, self-sealing, hollow silicone dome, approximately 3.4 cm in diameter, attached to a catheter measuring 7.25 cm in length [41,42]. The reservoir capacity is approximately 1.25 ml. A polypropylene needle guard at the base of the reservoir provides a surface that prevents penetration.

Intraventricular reservoirs are used primarily for the administration of chemotherapeutic drugs, particularly methotrexate and cytosine arabinoside to treat CNS carcinomatosis, lymphomatosis, and leukemic meningitis. Prophylactic administration of chemotherapy into the CSF is often performed in patients with leukemia to prevent leukemic spread into the spinal canal and cerebral ventricles. Intraventricular reservoirs are also used for the administration of antibiotics and analgesics. The reservoir offers access for measuring CSF pressure, although this application is rather limited. Finally, these reservoirs have been used for draining CSF to reduce intracranial pressure and for sampling CSF for analysis [41–43].

PROCEDURE FOR IMPLANTATION

1. Reservoir is implanted using local anesthesia with intravenous sedation, and ventricular size and location first evaluated by CT scan.
2. Following shaving and sterile prep, a curved incision is made in the right or left frontal region into the lateral ventricle.
3. Catheter tip is positioned at the foramen of Monro, with intraoperative radiography ensuring accurate placement [43].
4. Reservoir is inserted beneath the scalp flap and over the burr hole, leaving a bulge approximately 3.5 cm in diameter under suture line.
5. A pressure dressing covers the site for 24 hours; then a gauze dressing protects it until the sutures are removed (7–10 d) [41,43].

INDICATIONS

Patients with CNS leptomeningeal malignancies; prophylaxis of CNS involvement in acute lymphoblastic leukemia; direct installation of agents into the CNS tumor bed; monitoring of drug levels (to prevent toxicity); measuring of CNS pressures [40,41]

ADVANTAGES

Provides convenient, direct accessibility to ventricular CSF with predictable and consistent distribution of drug into the subarachnoid space and CNS; patient's discomfort and anxiety are reduced when tapped via a reservoir; allows approximately 200 punctures without danger of leakage [41–43]

DISADVANTAGES

Requires surgical placement; complications can be serious, mandating removal of device before completion of treatment; a small shaved area must be maintained on scalp

COMPLICATIONS

Infection due to repeated injections; displacement or migration of catheter; reservoir malfunction (possibly due to clogging of catheter) [40,41,43,44]; leukoencephalopathy [40,44]; toxic effects of intraventricularly administered chemotherapeutic drugs and BRMs

GUIDELINES FOR CARE

Assess for and report to physician: signs of infection at the implant site; change in patient's level of consciousness; fever; nausea and vomiting; headaches; dizziness; neck stiffness; reservoir malfunction or catheter displacement; drug toxicity; **other considerations:** collect specimens from the reservoir by gravity (Trendelenburg position); dilute drugs with nonbacteriostatic water, normal saline without preservative, or Elliot B's solution [29,41,43]

PATIENT AND FAMILY INFORMATION

Patient or family member should report headache, neck stiffness, or fevers; remain in flat position for 30 min following tap; recognize temporary side effects that may occur after tap; inform the health care provider of unusual signs or symptoms

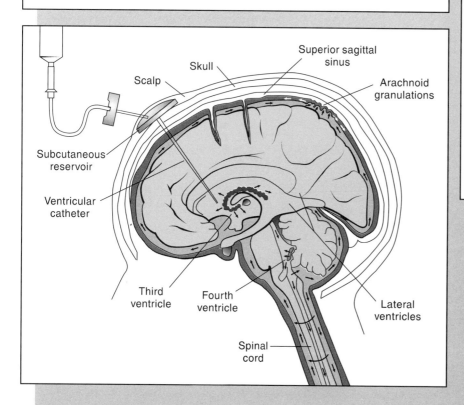

IMPLANTED PUMPS

Implanted pumps are used primarily for the continuous regional infusion of and, less frequently, for systemic infusion of chemotherapeutic drugs. For prolonged and continuous regional arterial delivery to a tumor-bearing organ, implanted pumps can deliver high concentrations of drug around-the-clock for periods of weeks to months [45,46]. Despite increased regional drug concentrations (up to 100 times greater than that with systemic infusion), minimal concentrations occur systemically because of the high first-pass extraction rate and dilution of the drug in the bloodstream after it has passed through the tumor-bearing organ [46]. Therefore, systemic toxicity may be decreased. The effectiveness and reliability of regional drug delivery depend on the stability and compatibility of the chemotherapeutic drugs used [47]. The chemotherapeutic drugs must not react with the pump components, each must have a viscosity that is sufficiently low to permit infusion, and each must be chemically stable at physiologic temperatures for periods of two to four weeks [47]. Most experience with regional chemotherapy delivered by an implantable infusion pump has been with hepatic arterial chemotherapy for colorectal cancer metastatic to the liver.

Both programmable and nonprogrammable implanted pumps are available. The most widely used model is calibrated and preset (nonprogrammable) to a specified rate of infusion—from 1.0 to 6.0 ml/d. The reservoir volume is 50 ml. An auxiliary self-sealing sideport, designed to bypass the central drug reservoir and the pumping mechanism, is used for bolus chemotherapy injections and diagnostic perfusion studies (pumps with dual sideports and catheters are also available). The catheter(s) is made of radiopaque silicone. The pump is a hollow titanium cylinder, divided into two chambers by accordion-like metal bellows. One chamber is the drug reservoir, which is refilled every 2 weeks by percutaneous injection using a special noncoring needle. The other chamber houses the fluorocarbon that expands at a constant rate, precipitating continuous infusion.

PROCEDURE FOR IMPLANTATION

1. For hepatic arterial chemotherapy, the catheter for drug delivery is placed in the common hepatic artery during laparotomy.
2. Preoperative angiograms must demonstrate that there will be sufficient perfusion of the tumorous regions of the liver [46,48].
3. Transverse incision is made through the skin and subcutaneous tissue, usually in the right abdominal wall, to create the pump pocket (never directly over the septum).
4. The pump is placed in the pocket and sutured to the underlying fascia [49].
5. For systemic chemotherapy, catheter tip is placed in superior vena cava or right atrium via a central vein [46].
6. Pump is placed in subcutaneous pocket in right or left subclavian fossa [46].

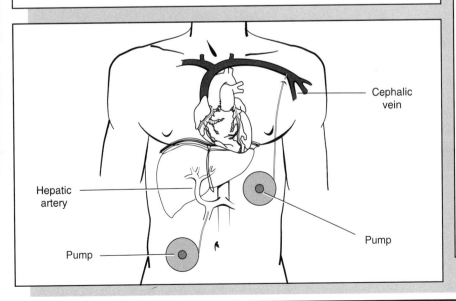

Cephalic vein

Hepatic artery

Pump

Pump

INDICATIONS
Patients requiring continuous infusion of chemotherapeutic drugs regionally (and in some instances systemically); patients with life expectancy of greater than a few months; patients without impaired ambulation or mobility; patients whose body size can accommodate pump bulk and weight; patients whose general status is satisfactory for undergoing major surgery; patients whose disease is not widely metastasized

ADVANTAGES
Improved quality of life; treatment provided on outpatient basis; no external tubings (and no restriction on activities); lower rate of catheter-related complications (compared to externally placed intra-arterial catheters); minimal systemic toxicity with maximal therapeutic response

DISADVANTAGES
Major surgery required for pump implantation; only FDA-approved drugs can be instilled into reservoir; pumps with batteries may develop component failure; pump and its surgical placement are costly; pump must be refilled by skilled health care provider *on schedule*; pump may have to remain in place despite treatment failure

COMPLICATIONS
Cessation of treatment due to battery depletion or component failure; pump pocket seroma (generally absorbed within weeks); pump pocket erosion; pump pocket infection; migration of the catheter auxiliary access port (in some models); rupture of the port connector at high injection pressures (in some models); complete or partial catheter occlusion; catheter migration or angulation; pump inversion; chemical irritation due to chemotherapy drug infusion; extravasation due to sideport needle displacement or pump malfunction; toxic effects of chemotherapeutic drugs or BRMs administered via sideport or reservoir

GUIDELINES FOR CARE
Assess for and report to physician [50]: immediate postoperative complications at the implant site; local or systemic infection; unusual resistance or catheter occlusion; variation in catheter placement; excess mobility of implantable pump under skin; improper increases or decreases in infusion rate; drug toxicities; noncompliance of patient; **other considerations:** obtain and use special refill kit and refer to manufacturer's guidelines for maintenance and refilling of pump; drain and measure medication remaining in reservoir prior to refilling

PATIENT AND FAMILY INFORMATION
Monitor temperature daily for first week following discharge and notify health care provider of 2° increase; report inflammation or swelling over pump site or unusual signs or symptoms; avoid activity that may raise body temperature; avoid rough physical activity and sports; inform health care provider of air travel

The organ most frequently affected by anticancer therapy (radiation, chemotherapy, and biologic response modifiers) is the bone marrow, and one of the most serious therapy-related toxicities is myelosuppression (Table 1). Although anticancer therapy has a selectivity for cancer cells over normal ones because of the higher growth fraction of tumor cells, the hematopoietic system, which by nature is a highly proliferative organ, is readily susceptible to similar therapy-related damage. The amount of damage sustained by the hematopoietic system from anticancer therapy is dependent upon a number of factors, including the ability of the marrow to tolerate the assault of therapy and the exposure time to the anticancer agent [1–3] (Table 2).

PATHOPHYSIOLOGY

To appreciate the hematopoietic system's tolerance to therapy-related injury, it helps to have an understanding of its anatomy and physiology. The bone marrow is comprised of a hierarchy of undifferentiated cells that give rise to differentiated mature peripheral blood cells. These cells ultimately manifest the damage inflicted on the bone marrow by the therapy. The most immature cells in the bone marrow are the totipotential stem cells, which, through the capability of self-renewal, maintain a constant stem cell compartment (regardless of the peripheral demand). They are also able to differentiate to daughter progenitor cells, which are committed to the various marrow cell types and are responsible for replenishing depleted peripheral blood cells. The two earliest "uncommitted" progenitors derived from the stem cell are the lymphoid and the multipotential, mixed (granulocyte/erythroid/monocyte/megakaryocyte) progenitors, which can differentiate later to "committed" progenitors of one or two cell types (ie, erythroid, granulocyte/monocyte, or megakaryocyte, etc.). The more immature the progenitor when damaged, the greater the scope of its effect. The microenvironment, comprised of monocyte/macrophages, fibroblasts, fat cells, and endothelial cells, provides the foundation and proper milieu for maintaining normal hematopoiesis.

A group of biologic agents—proteins and glycoproteins—produced by the microenvironment and the hematopoietic cells themselves are responsible for controlling self-renewal of the stem cells, proliferation and differentiation of progenitors, and functional activation of the mature effector cells. These agents are known as hematopoietic growth factors, including granulocyte and granulocyte–macrophage colony-stimulating factors and cytokines and lymphokines, including tumor necrosis factor, the interferons, and interleukins. Recently these agents have been produced by recombinant DNA technology and are undergoing clinical trials to have their specific activities defined.

In addition to the ancestral hierarchy of the bone marrow, the different cell types can be defined by their kinetic characteristics. These physiologic characteristics also help to determine a cell's sensitivity to a particular type of therapy, as well as the severity and rapidity of the development of blood count depression. There are stem cells that have left the cell cycle and reside in G_0, a resting state. These cells can be called back into cycle as needed to undergo self-renewal and to replenish peripheral supplies of blood cells. There are also cells continuously in cell cycle and those that have left the cell cycle as terminally differentiated, mature blood cells, such as erythrocytes and granulocytes. Damage to stem cells frequently produces delayed peripheral blood count nadir and recovery because these cells probably reenter the cell cycle for self-renewal before undergoing differentiation to more mature forms. When damage occurs at the level of the multipotential, uncommitted progenitor, leukopenia is frequently the first manifestation followed by thrombocytopenia, because the terminal half-life in neutrophils is shorter than that in platelets (6–8 hours vs 5–7 days, respectively). Anemia is less frequently a problem because of the much longer half-life of erythrocytes (120 days), except when cisplatin is used or complete myeloblation is accomplished.

CAUSES

The major types of anticancer therapy that produce hematologic toxicity are chemotherapy, biologic therapy, and radiation therapy. The timing and duration of the toxicity are somewhat different for these three modalities as discussed below.

Chemotherapy

The pathophysiology by which chemotherapy produces hematologic toxicity is the same as the drug's mechanism of action on a tumor and, like its effect on a tumor, is dependent upon the extent of damage the drug inflicts and the cell's ability to repair the damage. First the drug must be delivered to the tissue. Because peripheral blood circulates through the bone marrow, the bone marrow is continuously exposed to blood levels of the drug (or a metabolite of the drug that has been activated elsewhere). The agent crosses the membrane of the cells by one of two mechanisms—passive diffusion or carrier-mediated transport. The former process is dependent upon the size and lipid solubility of the drug; the latter involves transport by receptors specific for each type of drug. In many cases, the drug is taken up by the cell because of its resemblance to a natural compound with which it may compete. Once inside, the drug may be activated by either a chemical or enzymatic process, if activation has not occurred elsewhere. The four most common targets of chemotherapeutic agents are enzymes, nucleic acids, microtubules, and receptors (Table 3).

Table 1. Types of Myelosuppression

Neutropenia: deficiency in the number of functional neutrophil granulocytes
Thrombocytopenia: shortage of functional platelets
Anemia: abnormally low concentration of erythrocytes and hemoglobin
Leukopenia: deficiency in the number of circulating leukocytes
Lymphopenia: deficiency in the number of circulating lymphocytes

Table 2. Factors Determining Severity of Hemotologic Toxicity from Anticancer Agents

Bone marrow reserves
 Age of patient
 History of radiation therapy or chemotherapy
 Bone marrow involvement with cancer
 Patient's nutritional status
Patient's ability to metabolize drugs normally
Type of radiation or chemotherapy used
Dose, schedule, and method of administration of the anticancer agent

Table 3. Targets of Chemotherapeutic Agents

Agent	Target	Activity
Antimetabolites	Enzymes: purine and pyrimidine biosynthetic pathways; polymerases involved in nucleic acid synthesis	Depends on concentration and binding affinity for enzyme and degree of natural product competition
Alkylating agents	Nucleic acids: bind covalently to nucleotide bases of DNA	Results in inhibition of additional nucleic acid synthesis
Antitumor antibiotics	Nucleic acids: insert covalently between nucleotide bases of DNA	Results in inhibition of additional nucleic acid synthesis
Vinca alkaloids	Microtubules: influence assembly and stabilization of microtubules	Most active during mitosis
Hormonal agents	Receptors: compete with true hormones for cell membrane receptors	Interferes with the signals normally induced by true hormones

The types of hematopoietic cells most frequently affected by commonly used chemotherapeutic agents are noted in Table 4. The antimetabolites such as antifolates, antipurine, and antipyrimidines can cause significant erythrocytic changes, though not as dramatic as those observed with true vitamin B12 and folate deficiencies. The mechanism of action and the site of activity of a particular drug in the cell cycle are frequently useful in predicting the rapidity of development and duration of hematologic toxicity. Cycle-active agents that are phase-specific, especially those affecting the S and M phases (such as the antimetabolites and the vinca alkaloids, respectively) produce neutropenia and thrombocytopenia more rapidly. Intermediate effects are observed with the anthracyclines. Prolonged and delayed nadirs frequently develop with the nitrosoureas and mitomycin C. Bleomycin, vincristine, and 1-asparaginase do not generally cause myelosuppression in the absence of a metabolic defect.

Biologic Therapy

Neutropenia is the primary dose-limiting toxicity of interferon α. The toxicity is associated with doses greater than 3×10^6 U/m² 3 times weekly for prolonged periods. Interferon-induced neutropenia is almost always self-limiting and reversible, usually clearing within

Table 4. Drug-induced Myelosuppression

	Route of administration	Degree of supression*	Time to nadir (wk)*	Time to recovery (wk)*	Affected cell type
Alkylating agents					
Busulfan	PO	Moderate—marked	2–4	6–8	G,P
Chlorambucil	PO	Moderate	2–3	4–8	L,G
Cyclophosphamide	IV	Moderate	1–2	2–4	G
Melphalan	PO	Moderate	2–3	4–7	G,P
Thiotepa	IV	Moderate—marked	2–3	4–6	P,G
Antibiotics					
Daunorubicin	IV	Marked	2	3–4	G,P
Doxorubicin	IV	Marked	2	3–4	G,P
Idarubicin	IV	Marked	2	3–4	G,P
Mitoxantrone	IV	Marked	1–2	3	G,P
Mitomycin	IV	Moderate	Up to 8	Up to 10	G,P
Antimetabolites					
Cytosine arabinoside	IV	Moderate—marked	2	3	G,P
Fluorouracil	IV	Mild—moderate	1–2	2–3	G,P
Mercaptopurine	PO	Moderate	1–2	3–4	G,L,P
Methotrexate	IV	Moderate—marked	1–2	2–3	G,P
Vinca alkaloids/ Epipodophyllotoxins					
Etoposide	IV	Mild—moderate	1–2	3	G,P
Vinblastine	IV	Moderate	1–2	2–3	G
Vincristine	IV	—	—	—	—
Miscellaneous					
Cisplatin	IV	Moderate	2–3	4–6	G,P,E
Carboplatin	IV	Moderate	2–3	4–6	G,P,E
Dacarbazine	IV	Mild	2–3	4–5	G,P
Hydroxurea	PO	Moderate—marked	1	2–3	G,P
Procarbazine	PO	Moderate	3–4	4–6	P,G

*Somewhat dependent on dose, administration, and scheduling.
E—erythrocytes; G—granulocytes; L—leukocytes; P—platelets.

48 hours of discontinuing therapy. Rarely, an immune-induced neutropenia occurs that may not be reversible.

Although interleukin-2 (IL-2) therapy may also cause leukopenia, more frequently it causes thrombocytopenia that can be dose-limiting. Platelet transfusions for platelet counts less than 25,000 can sometimes allow additional doses of IL-2. Thrombocytopenia usually reverses within 24 to 48 hours of concluding therapy. Life-threatening hemorrhage thought to be due to this problem is exceedingly rare. There is a weak positive association between response to treatment and thrombocyte nadir.

Radiation Therapy

Most therapeutic radiation is ionizing and is comprised of the higher energy portion of the electromagnetic spectrum and particulate radiation. As high-energy radiation interacts with matter, electrons are removed from their orbits. X-rays are emitted when an electron strikes a target and it is slowed by the nuclei, releasing energy. Gamma radiation is produced by an unstable nucleus decaying to a more stable form. Electrons themselves can be accelerated by linear accelerators (in a linear path) or betatrons (circular path) to generate higher energy x-rays that have greater penetration and are sparing of the skin. Other atomic constituents (protons, α particles, neutrons, etc.) can be used to produce ionization, but are not used routinely for radiation therapy. The more densely ionizing the radiation (ie, the greater the penetration), the greater the hematologic toxicity.

There are two types of radiation effects on mammalian cells: direct and indirect. In the former, the radiation particle interacts directly with a biologic molecule in the cell. In the latter, damage is produced in the cell by a secondary agent, such as a free radical generated by the interaction of the ionizing particle with a water molecule. Both normal and malignant tissues that proliferate are most sensitive to radiation damage, and those with the highest rate of proliferation will demonstrate the effects most rapidly. Like chemotherapy, the susceptibility of cells to radiation damage is dependent upon the cell's status in the cell cycle. The most sensitive cells are those in the G_0 phase, followed by those in M and G_2 phases. Cells in late G_1 and S phases are the most resistant. In the bone marrow, the most radiosensitive cells are the stem cells. Because the bone marrow is one of the most proliferative organs in the body, it is also one of the most radiosensitive. The dose of radiation and the size of the exposed area, in addition to bone marrow reserve, determine the extent of damage. Even a few hundred rads to the total body, and thus the entire hematopoietic system, may result in hematopoietic failure and death within a few weeks. Regional radiation for tumor therapy, which includes a limited area of active bone marrow, may result in a transient decrease in peripheral blood counts, as well as destruction of stroma supporting hematopoiesis, with long-term or permanent loss of hematopoietic activity in that area.

DIAGNOSIS

Bone Marrow

The simplest method of assessing bone marrow composition and function is by aspiration and biopsy. While peripheral blood smears may assist in the diagnosis of a hematologic abnormality, bone marrow samples can determine whether the abnormality is, for example, due to toxicity from the therapy or due to replacement by tumor. The safest areas for bone marrow aspiration and biopsy are the anterior and posterior iliac crests. Aspirates may be performed cautiously at the level of the second intercostal space on the sternum only when conditions preclude adequate sampling from the pelvis. The bone marrow in the pelvis is usually inadequate if radiation therapy has been administered to this region. Biopsies are especially important when aspirates are inadequate (ie, a "dry" tap or inadequate spicules) or when tumor or fibrosis is suspected. The method of assessing cellularity is by bone marrow biopsy.

Peripheral Blood

Evaluation of the peripheral blood is carried out by obtaining a complete blood count, including leukocytes, hemoglobin, and hematocrit, platelets, and reticulocytes. A manual differential of the leukocytes, or analysis on one of the more technologically advanced cell analyzers, is usually preferred in order to assess the presence of immature and mature forms of eosinophils, basophils, and neutrophils. Erythrocyte morphology, including cell size, shape, and hemoglobin, may also be obtained from the peripheral blood smear. Platelet size may be assessed and counts made directly from the slide (erythrocyte machine count $\times$ number of platelets/5 fields at $100\times$ = platelet count/mm^3).

HEMATOPOIETIC TOXICITIES

Neutropenia

Neutropenia is a deficiency in the number of functional neutrophil granulocytes (Table 5). The accepted "normal" number of neutrophils varies somewhat among different ethnic groups with, for example, African-Americans and some Jewish sects normally demonstrating neutrophil counts of 1000/µl or less. These neutrophils function normally, and the patients are usually without sequelae. A second group of patients, such as those with myelodysplastic syndrome or acute leukemia, may demonstrate adequate numbers of neutrophils but because these cells frequently do not function normally, they are considered functionally neutropenic. For the general population, however, criteria for neutropenia are

Neutropenia: absolute neutrophil count (ANC) of < 1000/µl
ANC = leukocytes $\times$ (% segmented + band-form neutrophils)

Neutrophils play an important role in host defense against infection. They function by migrating out of the bone marrow into the circulation where their life span is approximately 5 to 7 hours. Under the influence of chemotactic factors, they move into infected tissue to act as phagocytes by a variety of intracellular mechanisms that destroy the bacteria causing the infection. Although a neutrophil nadir of $\geq$ 1000/µl produces little risk of serious infection, several studies have demonstrated an increasing incidence of such infections with higher grades of neutropenia [4]. Furthermore, the duration of the neutropenia contributes to the severity and types of infections. Fungal infections, for example, are uncommon in patients who experience neutropenia even as high as grade 4 for short periods of time, but become more common as the duration of neutropenia increases.

Table 5. Characteristics of Treatment-related Neutropenia

Pattern of temporal occurrence concurrent with treatment cycles

Recovery to normal count between cycles of therapy

Pretreatment, peripheral blood and/or bone marrow is normal

Patients who have a reduced bone marrow reserve secondary to previous toxic exposure or bone marrow involvement with tumor may manifest more severe neutropenia and/or neutropenia of longer duration than expected following exposure to anticancer therapy. The recent emphasis on dose intensification and bone marrow transplantation has increased the frequency, severity, and duration of such neutropenic nadirs.

Fevers in the setting of neutropenia mandate treatment with broad-spectrum antibiotics. The antibiotic combination often includes an aminoglycoside plus an antipseudomonal penicillin, with or without a cephalosporin, and vancomycin, with the specific regimen dictated by the infections characteristic of the particular hospital. Amphotericin may be added when the patient remains febrile and neutropenic after 48 to 72 hours of adequate antibacterial therapy in the setting of a long nadir. Because of the short half-life of neutrophils and the potentially severe side effects of leukocyte transfusions, the use of such transfusion is nearly obsolete.

In 1991, two recombinant hematopoietic growth factors, granulocyte–colony-stimulating factor (G-CSF) and granulocyte–macrophage–colony-stimulating factor (GM-CSF), were approved by the FDA for use in preventing the complications of chemotherapeutic myelosuppression, specifically neutropenia [5]. Early studies of these agents following myelosuppressive chemotherapy (G-CSF) and chemotherapy/radiation therapy with bone marrow transplantation (GM-CSF) have demonstrated fewer days of neutropenia, a generally lower incidence of serious infections, and fewer days of antibiotic requirements in cycles of therapy with growth factors than in cycles of therapy without growth factors. The use of these agents in the setting of radiation-induced myelosuppression is still under investigation.

Thrombocytopenia

Thrombocytopenia is a shortage of functional platelets, which may place the patient at risk of hemorrhage. Like neutropenia, a *quantitative* deficiency may be due to decreased production, increased consumption, or splenic pooling. *Qualitative* thrombocytopenia is used to describe a lack of functioning platelets regardless of the absolute numbers.

Combinations of cancer therapy and other etiologies may exacerbate the condition, producing more severe and prolonged thrombocytopenia than expected from a particular therapy. The normal platelet count ranges from 150,000 to 450,000/μl. However, on a functional basis, individuals with more than 1,000,000 platelets may even demonstrate signs of a bleeding disorder in the setting of some myeloproliferative syndromes. Although thrombocytopenia is a less frequent complication of standard chemotherapy than neutropenia, it has increased in incidence with dose-intensified therapy.

Evaluation of thrombocytopenia is made by assessing the number of circulating platelets by complete blood count analysis or peripheral blood smear. An increase in the size of the platelets on the smear suggests early release of platelets from the bone marrow, as in peripheral consumption or in bone marrow involvement with malignancy. Bone marrow aspiration and/or biopsy is frequently required to assess the cause of thrombocytopenia, especially quantitative thrombocytopenia. The functional status of platelets is usually assessed by a bleeding time (if the platelet count is adequate, ie, > 80,000/μl) and platelet aggregation studies.

Significant thrombocytopenia is managed with transfusion of donated platelets. Recently, the threshold level at which prophylactic transfusions are administered has become somewhat controversial.

Because the risk of spontaneous hemorrhage increases dramatically as the platelet count decreases, prophylactic transfusion is recommended when the count reaches 20,000/μl in patients at risk for other coagulation abnormalities or those with significant medical problems. A lower platelet count threshold may be used in low-risk, otherwise healthy patients. At the present time, hematopoietic growth factors (such as IL-1, IL-3, and IL-6) to enhance platelet counts are still under clinical investigation.

Anemia

Anemia is defined as an abnormally low concentration of erythrocytes and hemoglobin. Generally, a normal hemoglobin for an adult woman is 12 to 14 g/dl and for an adult man, 14 to 16 g/dl. Patients with cancer, especially those receiving antineoplastic therapy, frequently develop anemia, most often without concomitant neutropenia and thrombocytopenia. The potential risks and sequelae of anemia are usually less serious than those of neutropenia and thrombocytopenia. Anemia in the cancer patient may be caused by either a deficiency in production or an increase in consumption.

Although severe anemia is not considered a significant problem with conventional cancer therapy, dose-intensified regimens of chemotherapy, radiation therapy, or combination therapy and the increased use of bone marrow transplantation have added to the incidence and severity of anemia. Transfusion continues to be the mainstay of erythrocyte support. Erythropoietin, the growth factor for erythrocyte precursors, has been approved for treatment of patients with anemia associated with zidovidine therapy, patients with chronic renal insufficiency, and, most recently, patients with anemia associated with cancer chemotherapy.

STEM CELLS

Bone marrow transplantation has been used for many years as a means of abrogating hematologic toxicity caused by very high doses of chemotherapy, radiation therapy, or the combination of these modalities [6]. The effective use of bone marrow transplantation is dependent upon two factors: 1) a dose response effect of the chemotherapy on the cancer under treatment (*eg*, lymphoma), and 2) the use of therapeutic agents whose dose-limiting toxicity is primarily bone marrow suppression. Commonly used chemotherapeutic agents include nitrosoureas, alkylating agents, more recently, etoposide, and in some cases radiation therapy. Hematopoietic stem cells are obtained from the patient (autologous) or from an HLA-matched donor (allogeneic) under general anesthesia by repeated aspiration of the pelvic bones and sternum. The cells may be manipulated *in vitro* to destroy residual tumor cells (autologous) or to eliminate cells associated with graft-versus-host disease (allogeneic).

An alternative method of obtaining autologous hematopoietic stem cells for bone marrow reconstitution following myeloblative therapy is by apheresis of peripheral blood progenitors [7]. Although the concentration of stem cells in the bone marrow is normally more than 100 times greater than that in peripheral blood, methods are being explored for successfully increasing the peripheral blood population of such cells. These techniques include repeated leukophereses during the recovery phase of chemotherapy, administration of hematopoietic growth factors prior to chemotherapy to induce release of stem cells from the marrow into the peripheral circulation (still considered investigational), and use of hematopoietic growth factors following chemotherapy to enhance the yield and quality of stem cells released during recovery from chemotherapy alone. The ability to use peripheral stem cells in place of autologous bone marrow may obviate the need for general anesthesia used for harvesting and has made transplantation available to patients who could not otherwise undergo bone marrow harvest because of bone involvement by tumor or prior pelvic irradiation. Although reconstitution has been reported in many studies [8], the adequate number of mononuclear cells needed to accomplish reconstitution has been difficult to assess with the few data available on long-term engraftment.

Hematopoietic Growth Factors Following ABMT

The early studies of autologous bone marrow transplantation (ABMT) reported successful reconstitution of hematopoiesis following reinfusion of the bone marrow and maximum supportive care. More recent studies have shown that the use of the hematopoietic growth factors (G-CSF and GM-CSF) following reinfusion of marrow further reduces the hematologic toxicity of therapy. Shorter time to myeloid engraftment with variable results for platelets, a shorter duration of infectious episodes, and reduced duration of hospitalization have all been reported following the use of ABMT

and growth factor. (Only GM-CSF has thus far been approved for use in the setting of ABMT for lymphoid malignancies.) Because the stem cells need to mature to be susceptible to the effects of hematopoietic growth factors, a period of neutropenia still exists. Clinical studies using growth factors that are active at the stem cell phase are presently under investigation and may further reduce the period of cytopenia.

As with bone marrow reinfusions, hematopoietic growth factors have also recently been used following reinfusion of stem cells from peripheral blood (PBSC) to further accelerate recovery; in some studies bone marrow and PBSC with and without hematopoietic growth factors have been combined. Areas still under investigation include content of tumor cells, comparison of quality of stem cells derived from bone marrow versus peripheral blood versus with and without hematopoietic growth factor, method for determining optimum timing of peripheral stem cell harvest, minimal number of cells required for reconstitution, *ex vivo* expansion of stem cells to be used for reconstitution, and the feasibility of carrying out bone marrow transplantation on an outpatient basis as a result of reduced hematologic toxicity.

REFERENCES

1. Jandl J (ed): *Blood—Textbook of Hematology*. 1987, Boston: Little, Brown.

2. Perry MC (ed): *The Chemotherapy Source Book*. 1992, Baltimore: Williams & Wilkins.

3. Perez BL (ed): *Principles and Practice of Radiation Oncology*. 1992, Philadelphia: JB Lippincott.

4. Bodey GP, Buckley M, Sathe YS, *et al.*: Quantitative relationships between circulating leukocytes and infection in patients with acute leukemia. *Ann Int Med* 1966, 64:328–340.

5. Metcalf D, Morstyn G: Colony-stimulating factors: General biology. In DeVita V, Hellman, Rosenberg (eds): *Biologic Therapy of Cancer*. 1991, Philadelphia: JB Lippincott.

6. Armitage J, Antman K (eds): *High-Dose Cancer Therapy*. 1992, Baltimore: Williams & Wilkins.

7. Kessinger A, Armitage JO: The evolving role of autologous peripheral stem cell transplantation following high dose therapy for malignancies. *Blood* 1991, 77:211–213.

8. Kessinger A: Reestablishing hematopoiesis after dose-intensive therapy with peripheral stem cells. In Armitage J, Antman K (eds): *High-Dose Cancer Therapy*. 1992, Baltimore: Williams & Wilkins; 182–194.

9. American College of Physicians: *Ann Int Med* 1992, 116:403–406.

10. American Association of Blood Banks: Circular of information for the use of human blood and blood components. February 1991.

NEUTROPENIA

Neutropenia is defined as a deficiency in the number of functional neutrophil granulocytes. The criterion for neutropenia is an absolute neutrophil count less than 1000/μl. Patients with neutropenia are at greater risk of developing infections, particularly if they are undergoing dose-intensified or prolonged chemotherapy.

CAUSATIVE FACTORS

Primary: benign; chronic—severe, congenital, cyclic, idiopathic; **secondary:** neoplastic—hematologic malignancy, metastatic tumor; nonneoplastic—autoimmune, drug-related (chemotherapy, antibiotics, anticonvulsants, antidepressants); infection (bacterial, viral, mycobacterial); radiation; hematologic disease (aplastic anemia, myelofibrosis, paroxysmal nocturnal hemoglobinuria, T-gamma syndrome), organomegaly, nutritional deficiency

PATHOLOGIC PROCESS

Many unknown, possibly overproduction of cytokine suppressors or loss of growth factor receptors on progenitors, inhibition of nucleic acid and protein syntheses, maturation arrest, overproduction of hematopoietic inhibitors, antibody-induced destruction, drug-induced destruction, replacement of bone marrow by tumor or fibrosis, defective folate metabolism

DIFFERENTIAL DIAGNOSES

See list of causative factors

PATIENT ASSESSMENT

Leukocyte count and differential, review of smear for morphology, bone marrow aspiration and biopsy, karyotype, culture bone marrow, special bone marrow stains, including reticulin and acid-fast bacilli; serum B_{12} and folate levels, analysis for T-cell receptor gene rearrangement

INTERVENTIONS

1. Prevention
   a. Avoid concurrent myelosuppressive agents and radiation therapy
   b. Chemotherapy dose reduction, if appropriate, maintaining schedule
   c. Delay interval between treatment cycles until neutrophil recovery
   d. Interrupt radiation therapy until neutrophil recovery
   e. Hematopoietic growth factor support (G-CSF, GM-CSF, see below)
   f. Nutritional support
2. Prevention and treatment of sequelae
   a. Avoid exposure to infection/reverse isolation
   b. Meticulous personal hygiene
   c. Early antimicrobial treatment for associated fevers (broad-spectrum antibiotics, with staphylococcal and gram-negative coverage; biliary tree-enteric anaerobe; bowel-enteric anaerobe)
   d. Transfusion of neutrophils

GRANULOCYTE–COLONY-STIMULATING FACTOR (G-CSF) OR FILGRASTIM

1. **Indications:** Patients with nonmyeloid malignancies receiving myelosuppressive anticancer drugs associated with a significant incidence of severe neutropenia and fever (contraindicated in patients with known hypersensitivity to *E. coli*-derived proteins)
2. **Dose and administration:** 5 μg/kg/d SC or IV to begin ≥ 24 hr after chemotherapy; continue administration for up to 2 wk until ANC ≥ 10,000/mm^3 following neutrophil nadir
3. **Lab monitoring:** Baseline CBC and platelet counts, biweekly thereafter
4. **Adverse reactions:** medullary bone pain, increased uric acid, alkaline phosphatase, LDH, transient decreased blood pressure (rare)

GRANULOCYTE-MACROPHAGE–COLONY-STIMULATING FACTOR (GM-CSF) OR SARGRAMOSTIM

1. **Indications:** Patients with non-Hodgkin's lymphoma, ALL and Hodgkin's disease undergoing ABMT (contraindicated in patients with excessive leukemia myeloid blasts in bone marrow or peripheral blood or those with known hypersensitivity to GM-CSF, yeast-derived products or any component of the product)
2. **Dose and administration:** 250 μg/m^2/d for 21 d by 2-hr IV infusion beginning 2–4 hr after ABMT; discontinue therapy when neutrophil count is > 20,000/mm^3
3. **Lab monitoring:** If blast cells appear, discontinue therapy; biweekly monitoring of renal and hepatic function and CBC with differential
4. **Adverse reactions:** > 5% incidence over placebo; diarrhea, exacerbation of preexisting asthma, renal or hepatic dysfunction, rash, exacerbation of arrhythmia, malaise, fever, headache, bone pain, hives, myalgia, dyspnea, peripheral edema

TOXICITY GRADING

	0	1	2	3	4
WBC x 10^3	> 4.5	3.0– < 4.5	2.0– < 3.0	1.0– < 2.0	< 1.0
Neutrophil x 10^3	> 1.9	1.5– < 1.9	1.0– < 1.5	0.5– < 1.0	< 0.5

THROMBOCYTOPENIA

Thrombocytopenia is a shortage of functional platelets due to decreased production, increased consumption, defective function, or splenic pooling. The condition is often exacerbated by cancer therapy and can place the patient at risk of hemorrhage.

INTERVENTIONS

1. Prevention
   a. Avoid antiplatelet agents (*eg*, ASA)
   b. Chemotherapy dose adjustment, maintaining schedule
2. Prevention and treatment of sequelae
   a. Avoid invasive procedures
   b. Use progesterones to prevent menses
   c. GI tract prophylaxis (*ie*, antacids, stool softeners)
   d. Platelet transfusion (see below)

PLATELET TRANSFUSION

1. **Indications:** Prophylaxis for patients with platelet counts < 10,000–20,000/mm^3, prophylaxis for surgery if counts < 50,000/mm^3, treatment of hemorrhage if < 50,000–100,000/mm^3; signs and symptoms indicating need for transfusion: easy bruisability, petechiae, mucous membrane bleeding
2. **Preparations:** All are ABO compatible and may be leukocyte-depleted at the bedside; from whole blood (random donor), $\geq 5.5 \times 10^{10}$/bag; apheresis (single donor), $> 3 \times 10^{11}$/bag; leukocyte-poor and single donor delay development of alloimmunization; HLA matched—for patients already alloimmunized
3. **Dose and administration:** 6 U (random donor) or 1 bag (single donor) IV infusion. Count should increase 5,000–10,000/μl/random donor bag. A poor response in platelet increment may be due to splenomegaly, fever, sepsis, disseminated intravascular coagulation (DIC), alloimmunization (1-hr increment < 50% of expected suggests alloimmunization)
4. **Risks and adverse reactions:** *immune*—fever, allergic reaction, graft-versus-host reaction; *nonimmune*—volume overload, transmission of infection

CAUSATIVE FACTORS

Quantitative: *decreased production*—congenital, acquired: alcoholism, drug-related (chemotherapy/radiation, diuretics, H2 blockers), infections (viral), nutritional deficiency, tumor involvement of bone marrow, myelofibrosis, primary hematologic disorder; *increased consumption*—autoimmune (ITP, TTP, hematologic malignancy), DIC, drug-related (heparin, antibiotics, infection); **qualitative:** *drug-related*—nonsteroidal anti-inflammatory agents, antimicrobials, psychiatric drugs, alcohol; *concomitant illness*—uremia, chronic liver disease, myeloproliferative disorders

PATHOLOGIC PROCESS

Clot formation, antibody-induced destruction, inhibition of nucleic acid synthesis, bone marrow replacement with tumor or fibrosis, sequestration in enlarged spleen, defective maturation, drug-induced acetylation of platelet cyclooxygenase

DIFFERENTIAL DIAGNOSES

See list of causative factors above

PATIENT ASSESSMENT

CBC, peripheral blood smear, mean platelet volume, bone marrow aspiration or biopsy, karyotype, platelet aggregation studies, bleeding time (if platelet count adequate)

TOXICITY GRADING

	0	1	2	3	4
Platelet					
x 10^3	> 130	90– < 130	50– < 90	25– < 50	< 25

ANEMIA

The patient with anemia has an abnormally low concentration of erythrocytes and hemoglobin. The potential risks of anemia are less serious than those of neutropenia and thrombocytopenia; however, with the trend toward intensified therapy doses and BMT, the incidence and severity of anemia are increasing. Transfusion continues to be the conventional method of support.

INTERVENTIONS

1. Prevention—erythropoietin support (see below)
2. Prevention and treatment of sequelae
   a. Transfusion of erythrocytes (see below)
   b. Management of fatigue

TRANSFUSION OF ERYTHROCYTES

1. **Indications:** Patients with symptomatic anemia requiring increased red cell mass and improved oxygen-carrying capacity. Symptoms may include tachycardia, dyspnea, angina, decreased mentation, transient ischemic attacks, syncope, postural hypotension, inability to maintain reasonable level of daily activity (contraindicated in asymptomatic patients with vitamin-responsive anemia, Fe-responsive anemia, erythropoietin-responsive anemias)
2. **Preparations:** *All ABO-compatible and cross-matched* —PRBC is blood component of choice, majority of plasma removed, 50–75 ml remain in each unit; preservative solution added; Hct = 70–80%; 1 U increases Hb in 70 kg adult by 1–1.5 g/dl; *leukocyte-poor erythrocytes*—used to prevent febrile transfusion reactions and alloimmunization to leukocyte, antigen and platelet transfusion; *washed erythrocytes*—for patients with history of transfusion-related allergic reactions (usually due to plasma proteins), Hct = 50–70%
3. **Dosage and administration:** Dose based on severity. In otherwise healthy patients, transfuse to Hb ≥ 8 g/dl. In patients with cardiac disease, etc., frequently transfuse to Hb ≥ 10 g/dl. Infuse over 4 hr via IV catheter with normal saline for flushing
4. **Risks and adverse reactions:** *Nonimmune*—volume overload, Fe overload, transmission of infections: hepatitis (1–2:100 transfusions), cytomegalovirus, HIV, HTLV-1, Epstein–Barr virus, bacterial infections (rare), Lyme disease, babesiosis, Chagas' disease, brucella, malaria, ?TB; *immune*—acute or delayed hemolysis, fever (most common reaction with transfusion), allergic (urticaria, wheezing, angioedema), graft-versus-host (prevented by radiation therapy of blood product with 1500–3000 cGy)

ERYTHROPOIETIN (EPO)

1. **Indications:** Patients with chronic renal failure (CRF), patients with anemia due to chemotherapy (contraindicated in patients with uncontrolled hypertension or with hypersensitivity to mammalian cell–derived products of human albumin)
2. **Dose and administration:** *CRF*—50–100 U/kg IV tiw, reduce dose if target Hct is reached or if Hct increases > 4% in 2 wk; increase dose if target not reached or no increase of 5–6% in 8 wk; maintenance dose is individualized; *chemotherapy*—150 U/kg SC tiw; can be increased to 300 U/kg tiw after 8 wk; decrease if hematocrit > 40%
3. **Lab monitoring:** blood pressure, Hct 1–2 x wk during dose adjustment, Fe and Fe-binding capacity
4. **Adverse reactions:** *CRF patients*—hypertension, thrombotic events, headache, shortness of breath, tachycardia, hypercalcemia, nausea and vomiting, diarrhea (most frequent); flu-like symptoms, rash, urticaria, and ?seizures (rare); *patients receiving chemotherapy*: diarrhea, edema; fever, shortness of breath, paresthesia, URI (less frequent)

CAUSATIVE FACTORS

Blood loss, chemotherapy/radiation, chronic disease: tumor, infection, drug-related (zidovidine, etc.), hemolysis: autoimmune—tumor (CLL, lymphoma, etc.), drug-related; mechanical—chemotherapy (mitomycin C), DIC (tumor- or infection-related); nutritional deficiency: poor nutrition, postsurgery of gastrointestinal tract; bone marrow involvement: hematologic malignancy, metastatic tumor, myelofibrosis; concomitant illness: renal insufficiency, endocrine deficiencies

PATHOLOGIC PROCESS

Defective hemoglobin production, defective glucolysis, defective DNA synthesis, defective iron and B_{12} absorption, defective purine/pyrimidine synthesis, blockade in folate metabolism, erythrocyte parasites, bacterial toxins, antibody-induced destruction, erythropoietin deficiency, production of cytokines that inhibit hematopoiesis, replacement of bone marrow by tumor or fibrosis

DIFFERENTIAL DIAGNOSES

See list of causative factors

PATIENT ASSESSMENT

Erythrocyte count, hemoglobin concentration, hematocrit, mean corpuscular hemoglobin, mean corpuscular volume, mean corpuscular hemoglobin concentration, reticulocyte count, erythrocyte morphology, additional tests based on clinical evaluation: total and fractionated bilirubin, serum iron, total iron binding capacity, stool hematocrit, serum vitamin B_{12}, red cell folate, hemoglobin electrophoresis, direct and indirect Coombs' test, bone marrow aspiration and biopsy, thyroid function tests

TOXICITY GRADING

	0	1	2	3
Hbg g%,	> 11,	9.5–10.9,	< 9.5,	Transfusion required
Hct%	> 32	28–31.9	< 28	Transfusion required

CHAPTER 25: GASTROINTESTINAL TOXICITIES
Barry C. Lembersky and Mitchell C. Posner

The gastrointestinal tract is a very common site of treatment-related toxicity, which may contribute to profound patient morbidity and limit the dose or intensity of cancer therapy. Gastrointestinal dysfunction may cause pain, the inability to eat or properly digest food with progressive malnutrition, nausea and vomiting, perforation, and bleeding and may lead to serious infection. This chapter describes the side effects of systemic cancer therapy on the gastrointestinal tract and outlines current methods of prevention and management.

MUCOSITIS

It is estimated that approximately one million Americans are diagnosed with cancer each year, and 400,000 of these patients develop oral complications associated with cancer treatment [1]. Oral complications of chemotherapy occur through two interrelated pathophysiologic mechanisms. Because cells of the upper digestive tract undergo turnover on a 7- to 14-day cycle, they are susceptible to chemotherapy-induced *direct stomatotoxicity*. The resultant mucosal atrophy may lead to stomatitis, cheilosis, glossitis, and esophagitis. *Indirect stomatotoxicity* results from chemotherapy-induced myelosuppression and infections from the bacterial, fungal, and viral potential pathogens that colonize the oral cavity. The greater the degree and duration of neutropenia, the greater the risk of infection. In addition, the direct cytotoxic effect of chemotherapy may disrupt the protective barrier of the oral epithelium and further enhance the predisposition to secondary infection. Importantly, the mouth has been identified as the source of sepsis in 25 to 54% of neutropenic patients [2].

Assessment and Diagnosis

The frequency and severity of mucositis depend on the particular antineoplastic drug and its dose, schedule, and regimen (ie, given alone or in combination with other cytotoxic agents or radiation therapy). However, patients differ markedly in their ability to tolerate a given chemotherapeutic regimen. Patients who develop oral toxicity with the first course of therapy will invariably show similar side effects during subsequent courses unless the doses are decreased or the drugs changed. The state of oral health, performance status, and age are critical factors for the risk of complications. Young patients are reported to experience more toxicity than older patients. This may be related to a high incidence of hematologic malignancies and intent to deliver the most intensive therapies to young patients [3].

Pre-existing oral disease unrelated to the cancer increases the risk of oral complications. At the National Institute of Health Consensus Development Conference, it was strongly recommended that all patients receiving chemotherapy undergo pretreatment dental evaluation with the following objectives: 1) establish baseline data with which all subsequent examinations can be compared, 2) identify risk factors for the development of oral complications, 3) develop strategies to avoid treatment-related complications, and 4) perform necessary dental treatment to reduce the likelihood of oral complications induced by cancer therapy. Invasive prophylactic dental procedures should be performed well before the onset of chemotherapy-induced neutropenia and thrombocytopenia. Bacterial and fungal surveillance cultures are not necessary, but suspicious lesions should be cultured.

Patients suffering from mucositis often describe a burning sensation in the mouth within 3 to 10 days of the initiation of chemotherapy. This frequently precedes objective signs and should alert the clinician to the problem. Any of the mucosal surfaces may then develop erythema and progress to erosion and ulceration over the next 3 to 5 days. Intense pain, inability to handle secretions, and severe reduction in oral intake may ensue. The damage is usually reversible, with self-healing occurring over the 1- to 2-week period following cessation of therapy.

Oral infections often follow mucositis but may also occur in the absence of direct stomatotoxicity (Table 1). The most common sites of oral candidiasis are the sides and top of the tongue, the buccal, gingival, and palatal mucosa, and the commissures of the lips. The infection is manifest as painless, white, raised, curdlike strands or patches that tend to coalesce and adhere to the underlying mucosa. Forceful removal of the plaque reveals an erythematous or ulcerated mucosal surface. Diagnosis should be made by microscopic evaluation using a KOH preparation and tissue cultures. Herpes simplex virus and varicella zoster are the two most common viral pathogens causing oral infection in immunocompromised patients. The characteristic vesicular lesions usually rupture within a day, resulting in diffuse ulceration that eventually crusts over. Diagnosis rests with viral cultures or the demonstration of characteristic intranuclear inclusions in the epithelial cells of stained smears. With oral bacterial infections, the mucosa often has a necrotic appearance along with red painful ulcerations. Patients with chronic periodontal disease may develop acute periodontal or gingival bacterial infections that are edematous and painful, although in myelosuppressed patients the signs of inflammation are often absent. Fever is common in patients suffering from oral bacterial infections, and cultures from affected intraoral locales and blood may be positive.

Management

A program of routine oral hygiene should be instituted at the outset of chemotherapy. Patient and family education, as well as continued guidance and motivational support, are important to the success of preventative treatment. Components of a comprehensive oral care regimen include daily brushing and flossing, mouthwashing with saline, hydrogen peroxide, or sodium bicarbonate solution, and lip lubrication with petrolatum or K-Y jelly. Flossing is contraindicated during periods of severe thrombocytopenia, but brushing should continue unless significant bleeding occurs. Ongoing oral care will depend on the severity of symptoms that develop and patient tolerance.

A variety of topical agents and oral rinses are used to prevent or minimize mucositis in patients receiving chemotherapy (Table 2). Chlorhexidine, a broad-spectrum topical antimicrobial agent has been studied in several randomized, placebo-controlled, double blind, prophylactic trials producing varying results. Interpretation of

Table 1. Oral Infections in Patients with Cancer

Fungal	Bacterial
Candida albicans	Pseudomonas
	Klebsiella
Viral	*Escherichia coli*
Herpes simplex	Serratia
Varicella zoster	Proteus
	Enterobacter
	Staphylococcus
	Streptococcus

these studies is difficult due to differences in the concentration and dosage schedules of chlorhexidine and the patient populations. However, a number of trials in patients undergoing induction chemotherapy for acute leukemia or bone marrow transplantations for hematologic malignancies have shown that chlorhexidine (0.12%) mouth rinses significantly reduce the incidence and severity of mucositis and candidiasis [4]. It should be considered for prophylactic use in patients undergoing intensive chemotherapy. Although both nystatin oral suspension and clotrimazole troches are commonly used for antifungal prophylaxis in patients with leukemia and bone marrow transplantations, the clinical results have in general been disappointing. In contrast, retrospective studies have shown a 50 to 80% incidence of severe herpes simplex (HSV) oral infection in severely myelosuppressed patients who are seropositive for the HSV antibody. Thus, patients undergoing induction treatment for acute leukemia or bone marrow transplantation should be tested for the presence of HSV antibody. Such patients are likely to benefit from prophylactic treatment with acyclovir [5]. Other agents that have been investigated for prophylaxis include allopurinol, benzydamine hydrochloride, beta-carotene, sucralfate, and vitamin E. Evidence of efficacy is lacking, so none can be recommended for routine use.

Prophylactic oral cryotherapy is increasingly being used in clinical practice. Quite simply, patients are instructed to suck on ice chips for 30 minutes, 5 minutes prior to each dose of 5-fluorouracil (5-FU). A randomized study of 95 patients receiving 5-FU plus leucovorin demonstrated that oral cryotherapy resulted in a significant reduction in mucositis, as judged by physician and patient [6]. The low cost and ease of administration make oral cryotherapy an attractive preventative measure. One recent trial suggests that the administration of granulocyte–colony-stimulating factor (G-CSF) results in decreased mucositis in patients being treated with methotrexate, vinblastine, doxorubicin, and cisplatin in combination for bladder cancer [7]. However, confirmation by studies with other chemotherapy regimens or other growth factors have not yet been reported.

The management of overt mucositis is palliative and expectant. The frequency of general oral care procedures should be increased if possible. A variety of topical anesthetics exist, all of which result in significant amelioration of pain, albeit for a limited period of time (Table 2). Solutions or suspensions are generally appropriate for diffuse mucositis, whereas anesthetic topical films with bioadhesive materials are effective in reducing discomfort when applied over discrete mucosal ulcerations [8]. These intraoral bandages should not be used when there is concurrent oral infection. Pain relief is essential and systemic analgesics (morphine) are indicated when local therapy is inadequate. Early diagnostic and therapeutic intervention for infection may improve outcome. Bacterial and significant viral infections usually require systemic antibiotics. Although oral candidiasis may be treated with topical antifungal agents, fluconozole or amphotericin B may be necessary for refractory or disseminated infection.

DIARRHEA

Chemotherapy-induced diarrhea results from a direct toxic effect on the rapidly proliferating mucosal cells of the small and large intestine. The antimetabolites are the most common class of drugs causing diarrhea, although it may be the clinical manifestation of any of the drugs implicated in direct stomatotoxicity. Between 25 and 65% of patients with metastatic colon cancer experience some degree of diarrhea associated with 5-FU therapy. There appears to be no significant difference in the incidence or severity of 5-FU–induced diarrhea between bolus or infusional administration of comparable dose. However, the addition of leucovorin or other biomodulators to 5-FU resulted in increased frequency and severity of diarrhea in a number of randomized trials. It is important to note that chemotherapy-induced diarrhea may be extremely severe and the cause of fatal toxicity, especially in elderly patients.

Assessment and Diagnosis

Diarrhea occurring in patients receiving chemotherapy is usually the result of the direct effect of treatment, but may also be related to gastrointestinal infection, malabsorption, mechanical obstruction, or ancillary drug therapy, particularly antibiotics. It is extremely important that patients be evaluated promptly and the severity of symptoms and volume status assessed. With weekly boluses of 5-FU, the onset of diarrhea is usually after the fourth week of therapy; when administered as a 5-day bolus, symptoms may commence toward the conclusion of a treatment or anytime thereafter.

Management

Mild-to-moderate diarrhea may be treated symptomatically with strict attention to adequate fluid intake to prevent dehydration. It is recommended that patients with severe watery or bloody diarrhea, crampy abdominal pain, fever, or overt dehydration be admitted to the hospital for intravenous fluids, antibiotics, and antidiarrheal medications. All chemotherapy should be stopped immediately and further treatment at a reduced dose delayed until complete resolution of symptoms.

Table 2. Topical Agents for Prevention and Treatment of Mucositis

Class	Agent	Dose/Schedule	Guidelines and Comments
Broad-spectrum antibiotic	Chlorhexidine gluconate 0.12%	Mouth rinse BID (do not swallow)	Clinical trials do not consistently show benefit
Antifungal	Nystatin oral suspension or lozenge	200,000 U QID	Preventative use unproven; effective for treatment of established oral candidiasis
Antifungal	Clotrimazole troche	10 mg QID	Preventative use unproven; effective for treatment of established oral candidiasis
Topical anesthetic	Viscous xylocaine 2%	15 cc q 4 hr, swish	Limited duration of effect
Topical anesthetic	Dyclonine hydrochloride 0.5%	15 cc q 4 hr, swish	Limited duration of effect
Topical anesthetic	Diphenhydramine and kaolin	15 cc q 4 hr, swish	
General cleaning	Hydrogen peroxide and saline 1:2	15 cc QID, swish	Following toothbrushing
General cleaning	Sodium bicarbonate and water—1 tsp in 500 cc	15 cc QID, swish	Following toothbrushing

A number of drugs that slow peristalsis are available for the management of drug-induced diarrhea (Table 3). These should be started at the onset of diarrhea and given only when other causes have been reasonably excluded. There has been one provocative report of the effectiveness of somatostatin analogue for the treatment of 5-FU–induced severe diarrhea [9], but confirmatory studies are needed.

CONSTIPATION

The differential diagnosis of constipation in patients with cancer is quite diverse. Subacute constipation may be multifactorial, resulting from alteration in diet, decreased fluid intake, physical inactivity, and use of narcotic analgesics or drugs with anticholinergic action (antidepressives). The onset of new constipation may be the harbinger of serious complications of the underlying cancer, such as hypercalcemia, uremia, intestinal obstruction, or spinal cord compression.

Among the chemotherapeutic agents, only vincristine and vinblastine cause drug-induced autonomic nerve dysfunction with resultant reduction in gastrointestinal peristalsis. The clinical manifestations include constipation, obstipation, colicky abdominal pain, and adynamic ileus. This presentation may be particularly difficult to differentiate from acute intestinal obstruction or other causes of a surgical abdomen. Symptoms generally appear a few days after drug administration. Geriatric patients or those taking significant doses of narcotic analgesics are most susceptible. Treated conservatively this condition usually resolves over a 1- to 2-week period. However, great care should be taken to avoid constipation with the judicious use of mild laxatives and stool softeners in all patients receiving vinca alkaloids.

NAUSEA AND VOMITING

Cancer patients identify nausea and vomiting as one of the most distressing and feared side effects of their illness and therapy. Complications of nausea and vomiting include weight loss, dehydration, electrolyte abnormalities, esophageal tears and gastrointestinal bleeding, aspiration pneumonia, psychologic distress, diminished quality of life, and reduced patient compliance with anticancer therapy.

The pathophysiology of chemotherapy-induced nausea and vomiting is the result of a complex neuronal reflex arch. Two anatomically distinct regions of the brain are involved: the chemoreceptor trigger zone, a richly vascularized area located on the caudal margin of the fourth ventricle and the vomiting center in the medulla oblongata. Located outside the blood–brain barrier, the chemoreceptor trigger zone may be stimulated directly by chemotherapeutic agents, their metabolites, or other humoral factors and indirectly by afferent nerve impulses arising in the gastrointestinal tract. The vomiting center is the final coordinating center and receives input from the trigger zone, limbic system, cerebrum, vestibular system, and visceral afferent fibers from the gastrointestinal tract. The connections to the limbic system and cerebral cortex have been postulated as one explanation for the conditioned response of anticipatory vomiting. Through efferent neuronal pathways in the vagus nerve the vomiting center mediates the autonomic and somatic reflexes culminating in nausea and vomiting, such as vasoconstriction, tachycardia, diaphoresis, diaphragmatic and abdominal muscle contraction, and intestinal retroperistalsis.

The chemoreceptor trigger zone is rich in dopamine, cholinergic, and histamine receptors, and antagonism of these receptors forms the basis of action of many of the effective antiemetics currently used [10]. Recent extensive studies have demonstrated a high concentration of serotonin receptors in the trigger zone of animals [11] and serotonin appears to be a principal neurotransmitter in the emetic reflex in humans [12]. A current working hypothesis suggests that chemotherapy and radiation treatment induce cellular changes in the gastrointestinal tract. Damaged enterochromaffin cells of the upper gastrointestinal tract release serotonin locally, resulting in activation of receptors on visceral afferent fibers in the vagus nerve. These visceral afferents activate serotonin receptors in the trigger zone and vomiting center, thus initiating the emetic reflex arch.

Assessment and Diagnosis

Although chemotherapy is the most frequent cause of nausea and vomiting in patients with cancer, other causes are sufficiently common to warrant consideration in the differential diagnosis. Careful evaluation, including physical examination, measurement of serum electrolytes, and liver and renal function tests, is mandatory. Radiographic studies to evaluate the gastrointestinal tract or a CT scan of the brain may be necessary. The emetogenic properties of chemotherapeutic agents vary greatly and are influenced by dose, schedule, concomitant drugs, and radiation therapy (Table 4).

Table 3. Medical Therapy for Chemotherapy-Induced Diarrhea

Agent	Dose/Schedule	Guidelines and Comments
Kaolin and pectin	30–45 cc after each loose bowel movement	Acts as an intestinal absorbant, useful for mild diarrhea
Diphenoxylate with atropine	2.5 mg, 1–2 tablets after each loose bowel movement	Not to exceed 12 tablets in 24 hr; useful for mild-to-moderate diarrhea
Loperamide	2 mg, 1–2 tablets after each loose bowel movement	Not to exceed 12 tablets in 24 hr; useful for mild-to-moderate diarrhea
Camphorated opium tincture	5–10 cc QID	Acute toxicity may be CNS depression
Tincture of opium	0.6 cc QID	Contains 25 times more morphine than Paregoric; do not confuse preparations
Somatostatin analogue	150 µg/hr by continuous venous infusion	Effective for 5-FU–induced diarrhea

Table 4. Emetic Potential of Common Cytotoxic Agents

High (< 90%)	Moderately high (60–90%)	Moderate (30–60%)	Low (10–30%)
Cisplatin	Cyclophosphamide	Carboplatin	Bleomycin
Dacarbazine	Cytosine arabinoside	5-Fluorouracil	Etoposide
Nitrogen mustard	Ifosfamide	Doxorubicin	Vincristine
Streptozotocin	Hexamethylmelamine	Danuorubicin	Vinblastine
	BCNU	Mitomycin C	Melphalan
	CCNU	Procarbazine	Mitoxantrone

GASTROINTESTINAL TOXICITIES

Typically, nausea or vomiting begins 6 to 8 hours after the intravenous administration of an alkylating agent and may persist for up to 36 hours. Cisplatinum and dacarbazine elicit nausea and vomiting in virtually every patient, with symptoms usually commencing very shortly after drug administration. Symptoms usually resolve within 24 hours but occasionally may persist for days.

There is wide variation in patient tolerance to the emetic potential of chemotherapeutic agents. Certain characteristics influence the frequency and severity of symptoms, and recognition of these individualized factors may help to identify patients who require more or less rigorous attention to the control of side effects. A history of heavy alcohol intake, for instance, decreases the risk of nausea and vomiting. Patients with poor previous emetic control are at especially high risk of subsequent anticipatory nausea and vomiting, which underscores the importance of adequate prevention during the initial chemotherapy treatment.

Management

The clinical management of chemotherapy-induced nausea and vomiting requires a comprehensive strategy of pharmacologic intervention, patient and family support, and psychologic and behavioral adjustment. A major principle in management is the prophylactic administration of antiemetic drugs (Table 5). Knowledge of the mechanisms of action, routes of administration, and adverse reactions of the various classes of currently available antiemetics is mandatory for effective therapy.

Phenothiazines

Prochlorperazine and thiethylperazine are the most commonly prescribed antiemetic agents and are adequate when given with chemotherapy of mild emetic potential. Both appear to be marginally more effective than chlorpromazine and may be administered orally or rectally. When either is given intravenously, hypotension is a dose-limiting side effect. The mechanism of action is blockade of dopamine receptors in the chemoreceptor trigger zone; hence extrapyramidal side effects, especially in young patients, are common.

Butyrophenones

Haloperidol and droperidol are structurally related to the phenothiazines. They are useful agents for the prevention and treatment of mild-to-moderate emetogenic chemotherapy. Although some studies have demonstrated the efficacy of butyrophenones in cisplatinum-induced chemotherapy, they have been replaced by more effective antiemetics for this application. One disadvantage of droperidol is that it is only available as an intravenous formulation. Side effects include sedation, occasional dystonic reactions, and other extrapyramidal events.

Metoclopramide

Although metoclopramide, a substituted benzamide, is ineffective in low doses, at high doses it prevents and reduces cisplatinum-induced nausea and vomiting in approximately 50% of patients. It is also beneficial when used with other highly emetogenic agents. Although metoclopramide was originally thought to be a dopamine antagonist, recent evidence suggests that, at its effective high-dose range, it acts principally through blockade of serotonin receptors. Adverse reactions to metoclopramide include sedation, diarrhea, and akathisia (restlessness). Parkinsonian-like symptoms such as tremor and rigidity are more likely to occur in the elderly, whereas major dystonic reactions occur most frequently in patients under 30 years of age. These neurologic side effects can be quite distressing and are to a

Table 5. Frequently Used Antiemetic Agents

Class/Action	Agent	Dose/Schedule	Side Effects
Phenothiazines—dopamine antagonist	Prochloperazine	10–20 mg PO q 4–6 hr 25 mg PR q 4–6 hr 10 mg IV q 4–6 hr	Dystonic reaction
	Thiethylperazine	10 mg PO or PR, q 6–8 hr	
	Chlorpromazine	10–25 mg PO q 4–6 hr 10–25 mg IV q 3–4 hr	
	Promethazine	25 mg PO, PR, IM q 4–6 hr	
Butyrophenones—dopamine antagonist	Haloperidol	1–3 mg IV q 2–4 hr	Dystonic reaction
	Droperidol	1–2.5 mg IV q 4 hr	Sedation
Substitued benzamides—serotonin antagonist	Metoclopramide	1–3 mg/kg IV q 2 hr × 2–3 10 mg PO before meals	Dystonic reaction Sedation Diarrhea
Cannabinoids—unknown	Dronabinol	5–10 mg PO q 3–6 hr	Dysphoria Sedation Dry mouth
Serotonin receptor—antagonist	Ondansetron	0.15 mg/kg IV q 2–4 hr × 3 32 mg IV × 1 8 mg PO q 8 hr	Headache Diarrhea
	Granisetron	10 mcg/kg	
Adjunctive agents	Dexamethasone	10–20 mg IV × 1	
	Lorazepam	1–2 mg IV × 1	
	Diphenhydramine	25–50 mg IV or PO q 4 hr	

great extent preventable with concomitant administration of diphenhydramine or a benzodiazepine.

Serotonin Receptor Antagonists

Elucidation of the role of serotonin receptors in the pathophysiology of chemotherapy-induced emesis has led to the development of a new class of agents, selective serotonin receptor antagonists. Ondansetron and Granisetron are commercially available, but many other similar compounds are under active clinical investigation. These agents probably act competitively to block serotonin receptors in the vagal afferent nerves of the gastrointestinal tract and centrally in the trigger zone. Randomized, blind studies using a variety of doses and schedules have shown ondansetron to be significantly more effective than high-dose metoclopramide for the prevention of cisplatinum-induced nausea and vomiting [13,14]. Approximately 65 to 75% of patients obtain significant acute emetic control with ondansetron. Ondansetron treatment results in a longer time to first emetic episode, fewer side effects, decreased need for salvage antiemetics, and substantial patient preference over metoclopramide. However, clinical evidence suggests that ondansetron is no more effective than metoclopramide in controlling delayed emesis occurring beyond 24 hours of cisplatinum administration. Similar advantages to ondansetron have been seen in the prevention of acute emesis due to noncisplatinum-containing regimens [15].

Serotonin antagonists are well tolerated. Unlike most other classes of antiemetics, they are devoid of dopamine receptor antagonism and therefore extrapyramidal symptoms are virtually nonexistent. The most common side effects are headache, diarrhea, and rarely transient elevations of transaminase levels.

The recommended intravenous dosage of ondansetron is 0.15 mg/kg every 4 hours for three doses. The results of a recent randomized, double-blind study suggest that a single intravenous dose of ondansetron, 32 mg, given 30 minutes prior to cisplatinum it equally as effective in controlling acute emesis as the standard multiple-dose regimen [16]. If confirmed, the safety, efficacy, and simplicity of single, high-dose ondansetron will be beneficial in decreasing nursing and pharmacy costs and facilitating the administration of cisplatinum on an outpatient basis. In addition, in selected instances ondansetron may be effective when taken orally. A recently reported placebo-controlled trial in 673 patients receiving moderately emetogenic, noncisplatinum combination chemotherapy showed that oral ondansetron, 8 mg three times daily for 3 days, is superior to placebo in preventing nausea and maintaining food intake and resulted in complete emetic control in 66% of patients [17].

Cannabinoids

The active constituent of dronabinol is delta-9-tetrahydrocannabinol, the principal psychoactive substance in marijuana. Dronabinol has mild-to-moderate antiemetic properties, although the mechanism of action is unknown. It is currently indicated for the treatment of chemotherapy-associated nausea and vomiting in patients who fail to respond adequately to other antiemetic regimens. Toxicities include euphoria and dysphoria, mild sedation, dry mouth, and dizziness. The elderly are at greater risk for these unpleasant side effects and the drug should generally be reserved for younger patients.

Adjunctive Agents

Lorazepam, the most studied benzodiazepine, has only minimal activity as an antiemetic. However, its anxiolytic and amnestic properties serve both to diminish anticipatory nausea and to reduce the memory of unpleasant emetic episodes. Steroids have mild antiemetic activity as single agents, although the mechanism is not well defined. Side effects of single-dose or short-course steroid treatment are negligible. Both benzodiazapines and steroids are commonly used in multidrug antiemetic regimens.

Combination Antiemetic Therapy

Because of the biochemical complexity of the pathophysiology of nausea and vomiting, the combination of antiemetics with differing mechanisms of action and side effects may enhance efficacy and tolerance. Previous clinical studies have shown that dexamethasone added to phenothiazines, butyrophenones, and high-dose metoclopramide is more effective than the single agents. In a recently reported randomized crossover trial of 102 patients receiving moderate- to high-dose cisplatinum, 91% of patients had complete antiemetic control in the group treated with dexamethasone plus ondansetron compared with 64% receiving standard-dose ondansetron alone [18]. Similar improvements in effectiveness have been reported when lorazepam is added to a variety of antiemetic agents. Several commonly used combination antiemetic regimens are presented in Table 6.

HEPATIC TOXICITY

Surprisingly, hepatotoxicity is an unusual complication for most chemotherapeutic agents used singly or in standard-dose combinations. The hepatotoxic reaction most commonly seen is an incidental elevation of transaminases, although cholestasis, frank hepatic necrosis, and fibrosis may occur. In addition, hepatic veno-oclusive disease has been reported rarely with some chemotherapeutic agents at conventional doses and much more frequently at the higher doses used in allogeneic or autologous bone marrow transplantation.

Assessment and Diagnosis

Among chemotherapeutic agents currently available, mithramycin (plicamycin) is the most hepatotoxic. In past decades, mithramycin was used for the treatment of a variety of malignancies, and elevations of transaminases, often to very high levels, occurred in virtually 100% of patients. With the advent of less toxic and more efficacious chemotherapeutic agents, mithramycin is currently used only for the treatment of hypercalcemia of malignancy in which lower doses are partially effective. In this clinical setting, the drug produces an approximately 15% incidence of mild reversible hepatic dysfunction.

Other chemotherapeutic agents that cause elevations of hepatic enzymes include the nitrosoureas (BCNU, CCNU, streptozotocin) cytosine arabinoside, and methotrexate. The hepatic dysfunction is usually mild, reversible, and clinically insignificant. Chronic oral

Table 6. Combination Regimens for Highly Emetogenic Chemotherapy

1. Metoclopromide 2 mg/kg IV q 2 hr × 3 + Diphenhydramine 25 mg IV q 4 hr × 2 **or** + Dexamethasone 10 mg IV × 1	2. Odansetron 0.1 mg/kg IV q 8 hr or Ondansetron 30 mg IV × 1 + Lorazepam 1–2 mg IV × 1 + Dexamethasone 10 mg IV × 1

methotrexate, as used for nonmalignant conditions such as psoriasis and rheumatoid arthritis, may result in hepatic fibrosis, which tends to remain stable or regress when therapy is discontinued. Frank cirrhosis, a much more serious complication, may also occur. A high cumulative dose, rather than the duration of therapy, is most clearly associated with this toxicity. 5-Fluorouracil, though largely catabolized by the liver, does not result in hepatotoxicity. In contrast, however, when fluorodeoxyuridine (FUDR) is given as an intra-arterial hepatic infusion, clinical hepatitis and sclerosis of the intra- and extrahepatic ducts may be seen. The hepatitis is almost always reversible with temporary cessation of the intra-arterial therapy, whereas sclerosis of intra- and extrahepatic bile ducts accompanied by cholestatic jaundice is often irreversible and mandates discontinuation of treatment.

Management

As a general rule, liver function tests should be evaluated prior to each cycle of chemotherapy. Drugs that are extensively metabolized by the liver or are excreted into the bile should be used with great caution in the presence of hepatic dysfunction due to the likelihood of altered drug pharmacokinetics and resultant increased toxicity. Although based in large part on empirical data, guidelines for dose modifications of chemotherapeutic agents have recently been summarized [19]. When the serum bilirubin is between 1.5 and 3.0 mg/dl, the dose of doxorubicin, vinblastine, vincristine, and etoposide should be reduced by 50%. At serum bilirubin levels between 3.1 and 5.0 mg/dl, the dose of doxorubicin should be reduced by 75%, cyclophosphamide and methotrexate should be reduced by 25%, and the vinca alkaloids and etoposide should be withheld. At serum bilirubin levels above 5.0 mg/dl, excessive clinical toxicity is likely to be encountered with all of these drugs and they should not be used. However, prudent clinical judgment is required in this clinical setting. Use of the drug may be warranted if the hepatic dysfunction is due primarily to direct effects of the underlying malignancy, and a rapid antitumor effect may be expected by the administration of some or all of these drugs, as in certain hematologic and lymphoid malignancies.

GASTROINTESTINAL BLEEDING

Gastrointestinal bleeding is a frequent clinical problem in cancer patients. Upper gastrointestinal bleeding due to esophagitis or gastric and duodenal ulceration may be induced or exacerbated by cytotoxic agents, steroids, and nonsteroidal anti-inflammatory drugs commonly prescribed for patients with cancer. Primary tumors of the esophagus, stomach, and colon may be the source of both massive and subacute gastrointestinal hemorrhage. Among nongastrointestinal cancers, melanoma that has metastasized to the bowel wall is the most common cause of bleeding. Bleeding may accompany gastrointestinal infections, such as candidal or herpetic esophagitis, and is common in severe graft-versus-host disease. Chemotherapy-induced severe thrombocytopenia and coagulation defects will of course complicate any gastrointestinal bleeding.

Assessment and Diagnosis

Initial evaluation requires rapid assessment of the magnitude of the bleeding and the status of the circulatory system. Impending or frank hypovolemic shock due to massive bleeding must be treated with immediate volume replacement. Transfusions of packed red blood cells are necessary to maintain the serum hematocrit at approximately 30%. Platelet transfusion is indicated for clinically significant bleeding when the platelet count is less than 50,000. Fresh frozen plasma

should be given to correct abnormalities of the partial thromboplastin or prothrombin time.

The appropriate choice of invasive diagnostic procedures should be based on the history and physical examination. Hematemesis almost always indicates upper gastrointestinal blood loss and can be easily confirmed by nasogastric tube aspiration. This procedure also enables therapeutic gastric lavage with saline solution for ongoing bleeding. Bright red blood per rectum indicates bleeding from the sigmoid colon or rectum and can be assessed by sigmoidoscopy. Maroon-colored stools are suggestive of bleeding from the lower small bowel or right colon. Fiberoptic endoscopy of the upper or lower gastrointestinal tract is the most useful and accurate diagnostic procedure in most cases of gastrointestinal bleeding. Technetium-labeled red cell scans and angiography may be diagnostic when the source of the bleeding is out of the reach of endoscopic procedures and the rate of bleeding is approximately 1.0 cc/minute.

Management

Acute diffuse upper gastrointestinal bleeding is often initially managed conservatively with intravenous administration of H_2 blockers. Fastidious patient monitoring of volume status and appropriate blood replacement are mandatory. If bleeding does not stop, an intravenous infusion of vasopressin may be added. However, caution and experience are needed with this approach because serious side effects such as acidosis, hypertension, and visceral ischemia may ensue.

A variety of specifically directed therapeutic interventions may be employed, depending on the nature of the lesion. Sclerotherapy is frequently effective in the treatment of bleeding esophageal varices. Single or multiple bleeding sites that are accessible are often controlled by therapeutic endoscopy, including electrocoagulation and laser photocoagulation. Such procedures are frequently useful for bleeding tumors of the esophagus and stomach and may obviate the need for surgery. External beam radiation therapy may also be palliative in this setting. Arterial lesions demonstrated by angiography may be suitable candidates for selective radiologic embolization. This therapy is reserved for bleeding sites in the upper gastrointestinal tract because embolization of the colon is accompanied by an unacceptable incidence of bowel infarction and perforation. Surgery is only indicated when nonoperative treatment has failed to control the bleeding and when a discrete source has been identified that is amenable to a limited surgical procedure. In general, cancer patients with active gastrointestinal hemorrhage are poor operative candidates due to significant comorbidity; consideration of surgery must be individualized.

GASTROINTESTINAL TOXICITY OF BIOLOGIC AGENTS

Interferon Alpha

Interferon alpha, which is currently approved only for the treatment of hairy cell leukemia and AIDS-related Kaposi's sarcoma, has also shown activity in myeloproliferative syndromes, indolent lymphomas, myeloma, renal cell cancer, and melanoma. Toxicity is generally restricted to a transient flu-like syndrome seen in virtually all patients consisting of fever, myalgias, chills, and anorexia. Nausea is occasionally a significant problem. Some patients complain of a metallic taste, especially when therapy is initiated. Infrequently, high-dose regimens of interferon have been associated with profound watery diarrhea. Dose-related, reversible, mild-to-moderate elevations in hepatic transaminase levels occur in approximately 30% of patients and are more common in patients with preexisting abnormalities of liver function tests [20]. In patients with preexisting hyperbilirubinemia, cases of cholestatic jaundice and hepatic failure with death have been observed very rarely.

Interleukins

Interleukin-2 (IL-2), a human recombinant glycoprotein cytokine, is approved for the treatment of metastatic renal cell cancer and has activity in the treatment of advanced melanoma. At its recommended high-dose bolus schedule significant nausea, vomiting, and diarrhea occur in approximately 75% of treated patients and stomatitis in 30% [21,22]. The incidence appears to be dependent on dose and schedule, as lower dose and continuous infusion regimens are associated with nausea, diarrhea, and stomatitis in only 25% of patients [23]. Elevation of serum bilirubin levels above 5.0 mg/dl occur in approximately 20% of patients and is usually associated with modest increases in hepatic transaminase levels. Studies suggest that this is due to reversible cholestasis and is usually not dose limiting [24]. The standard antiemetics and antidiarrheals used to treat these toxicities are of variable efficacy and are often required in combination [24].

Bowel perforation is an unusual complication with high-dose IL-2, and in one large series was seen in 4 of 315 treated patients [25]. The exact pathophysiology remains unknown. Interruption of IL-2 treatment and surgical intervention are required for treatment.

Interleukin-4 (IL-4), a lymphokine that modulates the proliferation of activated T-cells, has recently been studied in early clinical trials. In phase I testing, 12 of 84 treatment courses were complicated by significant gastroduodenal erosion or ulceration, associated with abdominal pain and occasional gastrointestinal bleeding. The authors suggest that the pathophysiology may result from IL-4–induced alterations in prostaglandin synthesis in the gastric mucosa. In contrast, upper gastrointestinal ulceration due to IL-2 is distinctly uncommon [26].

REFERENCES

1. Consensus Development Conference on Oral Complications of Cancer Therapies: *Diagnosis, Prevention, and Treatment.* National Cancer Institute Monograph, Vol. 9. 1990, Bethesda, MD; 1–10.

2. Peterson DE: Toxicity of chemotherapy induced oral lesions. In Perry MC, Yarbro SW (eds): *Toxicity of Chemotherapy.* 1984, New York: Grune & Stratton. 155–180.

3. Sonis S, Clark J: Prevention and management of oral mucositis induced by antineoplastic therapy. *Oncology* 1991, 5:11–18.

4. Peterson DE: Oral toxicity of chemotherapeutic agents. *Sem Oncol* 1992, 19:478–491.

5. Redding SW: Role of herpes simplex virus reactivation in chemotherapy-induced oral mucositis. National Cancer Institute Monograph, Vol. 9. 1990, Bethesda, MD; 103–105.

6. Mahood DJ, Dose AM, Loprinzi CL, *et al.*: Inhibition of fluorouracil-induced stomatitis by oral cryotherapy. *J Clin Oncol* 1991, 9:449–452.

7. Gabrilove JL, Jakubowski A, Scher H, *et al.*: Effect of G-CSF on neutropenia and associated morbidity due to chemotherapy for transitional cell carcinoma of the urethelium. *N Engl J Med* 1988, 318:1414–1422.

8. LeVeque FG, Parzuchowski JB, Farinacci GC, *et al.*: Clinical evaluation of MGI 209, an anesthetic, film-forming agent for relief from painful oral ulcers associated with chemotherapy. *J Clin Oncol* 1992, 10:1963–1968.

9. Petrelli N, Rodriquez-Bigos M, Creaven P, *et al.*: Efficacy of somatostatin analogue for treatment of chemotherapy induced diarrhea in colorectal cancer. *Proc ASCO* 1992, 493 (abstract).

10. Mitchell EP: Gastrointestinal toxicity of chemotherapeutic agents. *Sem Oncol* 1992, 19:566–579.

11. Higgins GA, Kilpatrick GJ, Brencie KT, *et al.*: 5-HT3 receptor antagonists injected into the area postrema inhibit cisplatin-induced emesis in the ferret. *Br J Clin Pharmacol* 1989, 97:247–255.

12. Cobbedu LX, Hoffman IS, Fuenmayor NT, *et al.*: Efficacy of ondansetron and the role of serotonin in cisplatin induced nausea and vomiting. *N Engl J Med* 1990, 322:810–816.

13. Marty M, Pouillart P, Scholl S, *et al.*: Comparison of the 5-hydroxytyptamine 3 (serotonin) antagonist ondansetron with high dose metoclopramide in the control of cisplatin-induced emesis. *N Engl J Med* 1990, 322:816–821.

14. Hainsworth J, Harvey W, Pendegrass K, *et al.*: A single blind comparison of intravenous ondansetron, a selective serotonin antagonist, with intravenous metoclopramide in the prevention of nausea and vomiting associated with high dose cisplatin chemotherapy. *J Clin Oncol* 1991, 9:721–728.

15. Bonneterre J, Chevalber B, Mety R, *et al.*: A randomized double-blind comparison of ondansetron and metoclopramide in the prophylaxis of emesis induced by cyclophosphamide, fluorouracil, and doxorubicin or epirubicin chemotherapy. *J Clin Oncol* 1990, 8:1063–1069.

16. Beck TM, Heketh PJ, Madajewicz S, *et al.*: Stratified, randomized double-blind comparison of intravenous ondansetron administered as a multiple-dose regimen versus two single dose regimens in the prevention of cisplatin-induced nausea and vomiting. *J Clin Oncol* 1992, 10:1969–1975.

17. Beck TM: Efficacy of ondansetron tablets in the management of chemotherapy-induced emesis: Review of clinical trials. *Sem Oncol* 1992, 19(suppl 15):20–25.

18. Roila F, Tonato M, Cognetti F, *et al.*: Prevention of cisplatin-induced emesis: A double blind multicenter randomized crossover study comparing ondansetron and ondansetron plus dexamethasone. *J Clin Oncol* 1991, 9:675–678.

19. Perry MC: Hepatoxicity of chemotherapeutic agents. In Perry MC (ed): *The Chemotherapy Source Book.* 1992, Baltimore: Williams & Wilkins; 635–647.

20. Quesada JR, Talpaz M, Rios A: Clinical toxicity of interferons in cancer patients: A review. *J Clin Oncol* 1986, 4:234–243.

21. Lotze MT, Matory MD, Raynor AA, *et al.*: Clinical effects and toxicity of interleukin-2 in patients with cancer. *Cancer* 1986, 58:2764–2772.

22. Margolin KA, Rayner AA, Hawkins MJ, *et al.*: Interleukin-2 and lymphokine activated killer cell therapy of solid tumors: Analysis of toxicity and management guidelines. *J Clin Oncol* 1989, 7:486–498.

23. West WH, Tauer KW, Yannelli JR, *et al.*: Constant-infusion recombinant interleukin-2 in adoptive immunotherapy of advanced cancer. *N Engl J Med* 1987, 316:898–905.

24. Lotze MT, Rosenberg SA: Interleukin-2: Clinical applications. In DeVita VT, Hellman S, Rosenberg SA (eds): *Biologic Therapy of Cancer.* 1991, Philadelphia: JB Lippincott.

25. Schwartzentruber D, Lotze MT, Rosenberg SA: Colonic perforation: An unusual complication of therapy with high-dose interleukin-2. *Cancer* 1988, 62:2350–2353.

26. Rubin JT, Lotze MT: Acute gastric mucosal injury associated with the systemic administration of interleukin-4. *Surgery* 1992, 111:274–280.

MUCOSITIS

Mucositis is a common side effect of chemotherapy and radiation therapy and may result in significant pain, dehydration, malnutrition, poor quality of life, limitation in cancer therapy, and secondary systemic infection. Radiation and certain chemotherapeutic agents cause direct damage to the oral mucosa, the severity of which depends on dose intensity, schedule, and concomitant treatment. In addition, chemotherapy-induced myelosuppression increases the risk for serious intraoral infections.

Effective management requires thorough pretreatment assessment, correction of preexisting oral pathology, a comprehensive preventative oral hygiene program, treatment of infection, and attention to pain control.

CAUSATIVE AGENTS

Alkylating agents: nitrogen mustard, cyclophosphamide, ifosfamide, procarbazine; **antimetabolites:** methotrexate, fluorouracil, cytosine arabinoside, mercaptopurine, hydroxyurea; **antibiotics:** bleomycin, doxorubicin, daunomycin, mithramycin, mitomycin; **vinca alkaloids:** vincristine, vinblastine; **biologics:** IL-2, IFN-α

PATHOLOGIC PROCESS

Direct stomatotoxicity due to high rate of turnover of cells of the upper digestive tract, resulting in mucosal atrophy that may lead to stomatitis, cheilosis, glossitis, and esophagitis, and indirect stomatotoxicity due to chemotherapy or biologic induced myelosuppression and infections from bacterial, fungal, and viral colonizing pathogens

PATIENT ASSESSMENT

Baseline data on oral health, identify risk factors (performance status, patient age, agent given); clinical examination, CBCs, culture of oral cavity, microscopic evaluation of tissue cultures

PREVENTION AND MANAGEMENT

1. Pretreatment preventative measures
   a. Complete oral and dental evaluation
   b. Correction of underlying pathology
2. Routine oral hygiene
   a. Daily brushing with soft brush and fluoride toothpaste
   b. Flossing
   c. Mouthwash four times daily
   d. Lip lubrication
   e. Severely myelosuppressed or HSV antibody-positive patients should receive oral acyclovir, 200 mg 5 × d
   f. Oral cryotherapy (ice chips 5 × d) for 5-FU-induced mucositis
3. Management of mild-to-severe mucositis
   a. Culture oral cavity
   b. Obtain complete blood counts
   c. Patient should be on bland diet and perform hygienic measures every 2 hr
   d. Administer topical anesthetics (xylocaine, dyclonine, diphenhydramine)
   e. Administer topical or systemic antibiotics based on findings
   f. Give systemic analgesics as needed

TOXICITY GRADING

0	1	2	3	4
No symptoms	Painless erythema	Painful erythema	Painful erythema	Requires parenteral or enteral support
	Ulcers	Edema or ulcers	Edema or ulcers	
	Mild soreness	Can eat	Cannot eat	

DIARRHEA

Diarrhea results from a direct toxic effect on the gastrointestinal mucosa. It is most frequently seen with antimetabolites and is related to dose and intensity of drug administration. There is considerable interpatient variability. Symptoms may range from mild to severe. All chemotherapy should be stopped at the first signs of significant diarrhea, although symptoms may continue to progress for a few days. Appropriate management requires strict attention to hydration and the institution of antidiarrheals and antibiotics if the diarrhea is severe or bloody or there is concomitant fever. For patients experiencing severe diarrhea all subsequent chemotherapy should be given with great caution and at reduced dose intensity.

MANAGEMENT AND INTERVENTION

1. Mild-to-moderate diarrhea
   a. Maintain adequate fluid intake
   b. Provide appropriate antidiarrheal medication (see Table 3)
2. Severe diarrhea
   a. Stop chemotherapy until resolution
   b. Admittance to hospital if watery or bloody stools, crampy abdomen, fever, or overt dehydration
   c. Provide intravenous fluids, antibiotics, and antidiarrheal medication
   d. Proceed cautiously with subsequent chemotherapy

CAUSATIVE AGENTS

Antimetabolites, particularly 5-FU, methotrexate, cytosine arabinoside

PATHOLOGIC PROCESS

Direct toxic effect on rapidly proliferating mucosal cells of the small and large intestine

DIFFERENTIAL DIAGNOSES

Direct toxic effect of chemotherapeutic agent; gastrointestinal infection—*Clostridium dificile*, gram negative enteritis, viral enteritis, parasitic infection; other drugs—especially antibiotics; malabsorption, obstruction, dumping syndrome

PATIENT ASSESSMENT

Evaluation of volume status; complete blood counts, electrolytes, liver function tests; abdominal radiographic studies; blood cultures; stool leukocytes; stool cultures for enteric pathogens, ova, parasites, *C. dificile*; stool *C. dificile* toxin titer

TOXICITY GRADING

0	1	2	3	4
None	Increase of 2–3 stools per day over pretreatment	Increase of 4–6 stools per day, nocturnal stools, or moderate cramping	Increase of 7–9 stools per day, incontinence, or severe cramping	Increased of ≥ 10 stools per day, grossly bloody stools, or need parenteral support

NAUSEA AND VOMITING

Nausea and vomiting are some of the most distressing and feared side effects of cancer treatment. Recent research has helped elucidate the role of a variety of neurotransmitters in the pathophysiology of chemotherapy-induced nausea and vomiting and greatly enhanced prevention and treatment. Chemotherapeutic agents differ markedly in their emetic potential and symptoms depend on dose, schedule, and concomitant medications. There is also considerable interpatient variability. Effective management requires patient and family education and early prophylactic treatment. Combinations of antiemetics with differing mechanisms of actions and side effects are more effective than single agents alone.

MANAGEMENT AND INTERVENTION

1. Prophylactic administration of antiemetic drugs (see Table 5)
2. Provide patient support and guidelines for psychologic and behavioral adjustments
3. Provide adjuvant agents (*eg*, benzadiazapines and steroids)
4. Consider combination antiemetic therapy to evaluate efficacy against highly emetogenic chemotherapy

TOXICITY GRADING

	0	1	2	3	4
Nausea	None	Able to eat, reasonable intake	Intakes significantly decreased but can eat	No significant intake	—
Vomiting	None	1 episode in 24 hr	2–5 episodes in 24 hr	6–10 episodes in 24 hr	> 10 episodes in 24 hr or requiring parenteral support

CAUSATIVE AGENTS AND FACTORS

High potential: cisplatin, dacarbazine, nitrogen mustard, streptozotocin; **moderately high potential:** cyclophosphamide, cytosine arabinoside, ifosfamide, hexamethylmelamine, BCNU, CCNU (all dependent on dose, schedule, concomitant drugs, radiation therapy); **patient characteristics:** poor emetic control with other agents, history of nervous stomach or motion sickness, anticipatory symptoms (seen more in younger patients)

PATHOLOGIC PROCESS

Neuronal reflex arch; stimulation of serotonergic and dopaminergic receptors in the chemoreceptor trigger zone. After further coordination by the vomiting center, efferent neuronal pathways mediate actonomic and somatic responses that result in nausea and vomiting.

DIFFERENTIAL DIAGNOSES

Chemotherapy; radiation to brain, abdomen, chest, spine; brain metastasis; gastrointestinal or biliary tract obstruction; hypercalcemia; hyponatremia; uremia; narcotics

PATIENT ASSESSMENT

Physical examination, measurement of serum electrolytes, liver and renal function tests; abdominal radiograph and brain CT scan, if necessary

RENAL AND UROLOGIC COMPLICATIONS

Urologic complications of cancer constitute a major source of morbidity and oftentimes mortality in patients with neoplastic disorders [1,2]. It is imperative that total or near-total urinary tract obstruction, once recognized, receive early therapeutic intervention for preservation of renal function. Major urinary tract obstruction may cause significant functional and structural changes within the kidney, pelvis, and ureter, predisposing the patient to urinary tract infection. In the most extreme cases, acute and chronic renal failure can ensue from an obstructed urinary tract. While primary cancers may cause urinary tract obstruction, cancer therapy may also produce renal and urothelial damage [3]. Likewise, impaired urinary tract function can occur secondary to effects of cancer treatment such as tumor cell lysis, a condition in which the kidney is overwhelmed by breakdown products of rapid cellular dissolution.

URINARY TRACT OBSTRUCTION

Retroperitoneal tumors causing ureteral obstruction can occur with any solid neoplasm. Urologic and gynecologic cancers, together with lymphomas, are the most common causes of obstruction. Anatomically, retroperitoneal lymph nodes, which are often the drainage sites for many urologic and gynecologic cancers or the sites of lymphomatous infiltration, are located along the para-aortic, para-caval, and periureteral locations in the retroperitoneal space. Lymphadenopathy of mild-to-moderate size occurring strategically along the course of the ureter can result in unilateral hydronephrosis in a relatively short period of time. Retroperitoneal lymph node metastases and primary retroperitoneal tumors can attain a large size without causing ureteral obstruction because of their location with respect to the ureter. Prostate cancer more often causes distal urinary tract obstruction due to obstruction at the bladder neck. This is also true of advanced cervical cancer, which may infiltrate the retroperitoneal surfaces and obstruct ureters as well. Testicular cancer, especially seminoma, can invade the retroperitoneal space, obstructing both ureters simultaneously. Metastatic neoplasms from many sources can invade the retroperitoneal areolar tissues, forming a plaquelike sheet of tumor that can involve and obstruct the ureters. Adenopathy may not be evident on imaging studies, making diagnosis difficult. Metastatic breast cancer, for example, may result in a desmoplastic reaction that may mimic primary retroperitoneal fibrosis. Regardless of the cause of urinary tract obstruction, prompt diagnosis and treatment are imperative, because the ability to deliver potentially nephrotoxic drugs that are curative (such as cisplatin) will be compromised if there is irreparable renal damage.

Whether obstruction is caused by a gynecologic, urologic, or hematopoietic neoplasm, the clinical manifestations are usually similar. Acute obstruction of a ureter is generally defined by excruciating pain, related to distention of the renal capsule and collecting system. Pain is usually the presenting symptom and may be related to the rapidity of ureteral and pelvic dilation proximal to the obstruction. The pain is probably not a result of hyperperistalsis of the ureter in attempts to overcome an obstructed segment. However, equally important is the asymptomatic patient who is discovered by routine serum chemistries, abdominal computer tomographic (CT) scan, or radionuclide excretion on bone scanning undertaken to monitor a neoplasm [4]. Often, obstructions in individuals with prostatic carcinoma, cervical carcinoma, and lymphoma are first noticed by these routine examinations. These patients usually have obstruction that progresses gradually, making their clinical presentation more subtle than that of individuals with a rapidly developing obstruction.

Bladder neck obstruction secondary to prostate cancer, the most common cause of urinary obstruction in males, predominantly causes urinary symptomatology, such as frequency, hesitancy, nocturia, and dysuria. In a gradually developing obstruction, some patients may have periods of oliguria alternating with periods of polyuria.

Diagnostic Approaches

The urinalysis and routine chemistries, although usually not specific, may reveal isosthenuria or an elevation of the serum creatinine or BUN. Proteinuria may be present in both acute and chronic obstructions. A variety of sophisticated evaluations that look at the fractional excretion of sodium may be helpful in determining the duration of obstruction. For example, a fractional excretion of sodium (FEna) of less than 1% may suggest partial obstruction of short duration, whereas a FEna of greater than 1% would be more consistent with prolonged obstruction.

The mainstay for the diagnosis of obstruction is imaging procedures. Ultrasonography is a rapid and readily available noninvasive method used to identify obstruction; it has become the preferred method to determine the anatomy of the upper urinary tracts. Radionuclide studies are also very helpful and relatively noninvasive. Technetium concentration in the course of bone scans may lead to definitive studies that can quantify renal blood flow. On occasion, retrograde and antegrade pyelography may still be needed for diagnosis. Interventional approaches, such as cystoscopic evaluation, are usually performed as a staging study for patients with various gynecologic and urologic neoplasms.

The complications of urinary obstruction secondary to neoplasm include infection, urinary lithiasis, and polycythemia, as well as loss of renal function. Hypertension may also occur with chronic bilateral obstruction, caused by abnormalities of the renin–angiotensin system.

Management

It is imperative to establish the histologic diagnosis of the underlying neoplasm in the patient initially presenting with ureteral obstruction, because the therapeutic strategies for testicular cancer, retroperitoneal lymphoma, carcinoma of the uterine cervix, metastatic breast cancer, and prostate cancer are different. Once the underlying primary disease is known, appropriate therapeutic modalities can be introduced. In prostate cancer, for example, bilateral ureteral obstruction with hydronephrosis and impending renal failure due to bladder neck obstruction is best treated by urethral catheterization or suprapubic cystostomy. Bilateral orchiectomy is the most rapid method to achieve androgen deprivation, but it may not be necessary if obstruction can be relieved by alternate means, allowing other endocrine therapeutic approaches to be considered. In cases in which one or both ureters are obstructed by retroperitoneal metastases or lymphoma producing loss of renal function, percutaneous nephrotomy(ies) with placement of antegrade or retrograde ureteral stents should be considered immediately if the neoplasm has not been therapeutically controlled. Localized radiation therapy can be effective in relieving isolated metastases obstructing the ureter in a wide spectrum of radiosensitive tumors.

The use of systemic chemotherapy in patients with testicular cancer who present with bilateral hydronephrosis and azotemia is of critical importance. Because cisplatin is nephrotoxic and brisk diuresis is necessary to diminish tubular contact with excreted drug, the presence of renal function abnormalities mandates consideration of temporary percutaneous nephrostomies. In the absence of renal function abnormalities, it is reasonable to inaugurate chemotherapy without bypass procedures because resolution of tumor masses can be anticipated in 48 to 72 hours. Likewise, lymphomas causing retroperitoneal obstruction (without hindering renal function) can be treated with either radiation therapy or combination chemotherapy, depending upon the underlying histology, without invasive procedures for bypass. Fortunately, these diseases are exquisitely radiosensitive and chemosensitive. Patients often have relief of their urinary symptomatology with localized or systemic treatments. It is also imperative to inhibit xanthine oxidase with allopurinol to prevent a surge of uric acid, which could compromise renal function.

Surgical relief of obstruction is usually contemplated if systemic therapy is likely or if renal function is already compromised. Viability of the remaining function of the obstructed kidney(s) needs to be addressed rapidly. There are multiple surgical approaches to relieve obstruction. Selection is predominantly dependent on the anatomical location of the obstruction and the ability of the patient to withstand the surgical procedure. Urethral catheterization, suprapubic percutaneous cystostomy, and percutaneous unilateral or bilateral nephrotomies with later placement of ureteral stents are substantially less traumatic than open surgical procedures and are thus preferred when they can be utilized.

It is imperative to address problems of infection associated with urinary obstruction and to minimize the likelihood of infectious complications during manipulation of the obstructed urinary tract. In addition, postobstructive diuresis and natriuresis can be major medical challenges, requiring intensive metabolic monitoring. Following the relief of bilateral obstruction, postobstructive diuresis usually occurs secondary to volume expansion and the circulation of natriuretic factors. Urinary flow as high as 3 to 4 l/hr has been recorded with associated natriuresis. Metabolic abnormalities in sodium, potassium, chloride, bicarbonate, and other ions demand appropriate monitoring. Volume status and attention to blood pressure changes require hospitalization and very detailed investigations during the first week following the relief of long-standing obstruction.

Ethical issues relating to relief of urinary tract obstruction should always be fully discussed with the patient and family in the case of refractory terminal cancer. A sincere and forthright discussion among physicians, family, and patient must ensue before a surgical procedure is undertaken to relieve urinary obstruction, particularly if there is no hope of prolongation of life.

GENITOURINARY HEMORRHAGE

One of the most dramatic clinical events in cancer management is the development of uncontrolled urinary tract hemorrhage. In the past this was often due to bleeding from the bladder (hemorrhagic cystitis) secondary to radiation therapy and/or treatment with cyclophosphamide or ifosfamide treatment. Forunately, today, it is an uncommon event because the use of mesna with ifosfamide has greatly reduced the extent of urethelial damage caused by this alkalating agent. Bleeding diathesis superimposed on urothelial damage from toxic drugs or their metabolites in the urine is most often the etiology of urinary tract hemorrhage. An additional list of agents that have been implicated in urinary tract hemorrhage include l-asparaginase, dactinomycin, mitomycin C, mithramycin, and 6-mercaptopurine. Additionally, in patients with cancer on anticoagulants who receive antibiotics that can have a synergistic effect, the urinary tract is placed at increased risk for bleeding.

The management of hemorrhagic cystitis resulting from treatment with cyclophosphamide or ifosfamide requires the combined efforts of urologist and oncologist alike. Catheter drainage and continuous irrigation, intravesical cautery, and intravesical therapy with formalin all have been used with reported success. For refractory bleeding, surgical approaches, including cystotomy with installation of phenol and ligation of the bladder vessels, have been required. In the most severe instances, urinary diversion and removal of the organ to stop life-threatening bleeding has been necessary.

UROLOGIC COMPLICATIONS SECONDARY TO CANCER THERAPY

The most common and perplexing issues that face oncologists are abnormalities in renal function caused by anticancer therapies. In recent years, chemotherapies have become intensive, drugs are given at higher doses, and combinations of chemotherapeutic agents and biologic response modifiers are increasingly used in the overall management of cancer patients. Nephrotoxicity has been associated with commonly used cancer therapies; alterations in dosing of potentially nephrotoxic chemotherapeutic agents can help reduce risk. Nephrotoxicity is typically defined as a doubling in the serum creatinine from a normal baseline and a blood urea nitrogen (BUN) concentration greater than 40 mg/dl. Table 1 lists the salient features of potential nephrotoxic agents, whereas Table 2 suggests modifications of chemotherapeutic agents when renal failure presents [5].

Cisplatin

Cisplatin is one of the most commonly used antineoplastic agents having a wide spectrum of activity. The agent is primarily excreted through the kidneys and tends to accumulate in the renal tubular cells selectively. Pathologic changes of the kidney include interstitial edema and tubular dilatation with relative sparing of glomeruli. Platinum resorption in the tubule leads to enzyme inhibition, alkylation of specific molecules, and general cellular injury from proximal tubular binding.

The appropriate administration of cisplatin requires vigorous hydration with a high concentration of chloride. Chloride favors the persistence of cisplatin rather than the formation of the aquated dihydroxydiammino platinum, which is the active chemotherapeutic species. Urine output in excess of 200 ml/hr should be maintained before and for at least 18 hours after cisplatin therapy. This volume level is achieved with adequate saline administration with or without a diuretic to minimize renal side effects. Most nephrotoxicity is traceable to underhydration and inattentive supervision of urinary volumes on a continuing basis. Carboplatin, a congener of cisplatin, has virtually no nephrotoxicity.

Cyclophosphamide

Cyclophosphamide produces a wide range of urologic effects, including hemorrhagic cystitis (as discussed above). The most commonly described defect of renal function is impaired water excretion, most commonly seen with high-dose cyclophosphamide (> 50 mg/kg) used for bone marrow transplantation [6]. Clinical manifestations of impaired water excretion include hyponatremia, decreased serum osmolality, and elevated urinary sodium, with normal serum vasopressin levels. This condition probably results from a direct toxic effect of cyclophosphamide metabolites on distal tubules and collecting ducts. Hypotonic solutions and solutions that induce hyponatremia should be avoided when effecting the diuresis needed to prevent hemorrhagic cystitis.

Streptozotocin

Renal damage is common following streptozotocin therapy, and may present as tubular dysfunction with phosphate wasting or as complete Fanconi syndrome with aminoaciduria, proteinuria leading to renal insufficiency. Careful and diligent monitoring of renal function must occur following administration.

Semustine (CCNU)

Nitrosoureas are excreted primarily in the urine. Renal dysfunction is associated with cumulative semustine doses of greater than 1500 mg/m^2. The onset of renal dysfunction may be delayed for years following completion of therapy. Pathologic lesions demonstrate the development of fibrosis and glomerular sclerosis, as well as interstitial fibrosis [7].

Methotrexate

Methotrexate has become one of the most frequently used antineoplastic agents in cancer chemotherapy today; it is given alone or in combination, in a variety of dosage schedules, and often in doses in excess of what is known to be toxic, together with "rescue" doses of leucovorin. Methotrexate competitively binds to dihydrofolate reductase, the enzyme responsible for converting folic acid to reduced folate cofactors. Reduced folates are essential for the metabolic transfer of one carbon unit, essential reactions in the *de novo* biosynthesis of thymidylic acid and the *de novo* synthesis of purine precursors.

When methotrexate is used in relatively high doses, drug-induced nephrotoxicity can become a prominent feature. Although the exact mechanism of damage is unclear, there are presently three hypotheses that have been suggested. The first relates to methotrexate (or its metabolites) precipitation in the renal tubules causing an obstructive nephropathy. Methotrexate also may have a direct effect on renal tubular cells, altering regeneration of epithelial cells and ion secretory channels and other metabolic processes with a secondary feedback decrease in glomular filtration rate (GFR). A third possibility may be a direct effect on glomular perfusion, causing a decrease in GFR.

There are two basic treatment programs for the systemic use of methotrexate, including conventional low-dose methotrexate (5–60 mg/m^2) and high-dose methotrexate (200 mg–30g/m^2) with various rescue programs. There is a definite relationship between renal toxicity and increasing methotrexate dose; in some early studies, renal failure was implicated in 20% of toxic deaths associated with high-dose methotrexate administration.

Table 1. Potentially Nephrotoxic Chemotherapeutic Agents by Class

Drug	Risk			Type		Specific tubular damage	Type	
	High	Int	Low	Acute	Chronic		Immed	Delayed
Alkylating agents								
Cisplatin	X			X	X	X	X	X
Cyclophosphamide			X			X		X
Streptozotocin*	X			X	X	X		X
Semustine		X			X			X
Carmustine			X		X			X
Lomustine			X		X			X
Antimetabolites								
Methotrexate†	X			X			X	
Cytosine arabinoside			X	X			X	
5-Fluorouracil‡			X	X	X		X	
5-Azacytidine			X	X			X	
6-Thioguanine			X	X			X	
Antitumor antibiotics								
Mitomycin§			X		X		X	X
Mithramycin¶	X			X			X	
Doxorubicin			X	X		X		
Biologic agents								
Interferon alpha			X	X			X	
Interferon gamma		X		X			X	
Corynebacterium parvum			X	X			X	
Interleukin-2		X		X			X	

From Weber et al. [11]; with permission.
*Fanconi's syndrome as the most severe manifestation.
†Only seen with intermediate- to high-dose regimens.
‡Only seen when given in combination with mitomycin C.
§Hemolytic–uremic syndrome as the most severe manifestation.
¶Frequent with antineoplastic doses, rare in doses used for hypercalcemia.

A number of investigations have reported differences in the solubility of methotrexate relative to pH in the clinical setting. In general, methotrexate is 2 to 10 times more soluble at a pH of 6.9 or greater than at a pH of 5.7. Thus, the solubility of methotrexate as a function of pH may be an important and critical factor in the pathogenesis of renal dysfunction.

In clinical studies in which methotrexate was given in high doses, without prior urinary alkalinization or vigorous hydration, a substantial incidence of nephrotoxicity occurred. However, this high incidence (47%) fell dramatically when urinary alkalinization and hydration became part of the treatment program. This improvement was attributable to the prevention of methotrexate precipitation in the renal tubules. In contrast to adults, pediatric patients seem to experience less severe nephrotoxicity even without alkalinization, although these children have often received very vigorous hydration as part of their methotrexate protocol.

The use of hydration has a profound effect on diminishing the nephrotoxicity associated with high-dose methotrexate therapy. Urinary alkalinization, with either acetazolamide or sodium bicarbonate, has likewise diminished the incidence of nephrotoxicity. Methotrexate metabolites are also thought to be nephrotoxic. Among them are 7-hydroxymethotrexate, which is less soluble than methotrexate, particularly in acid urine, and may be more susceptible to tubular precipitation. Deglutamated methotrexate, 4-amino-4-deoxy-N^{10}-methylpteroic acid has been implicated as a less soluble metabolite that may precipitate under adverse conditions. Regardless of the actual toxic moiety, acute renal failure as a consequence of renal tubular precipitation is a feature of high-dose methotrexate administration. A wide spectrum of rescue agents, including leucovorin, thymidine, carboxypeptidase, and dihydrofolate reductase, have been used to prevent and treat methotrexate-induced renal failure.

Mitomycin C

Mitomycin C, an antitumor antibiotic isolated from the broth of *Streptomyces caespitosis*, is primarily used in the treatment of gastrointestinal and breast cancers. Nephrotoxicity is dose related and cumulative. Clinically, rising BUN, creatinine, and proteinuria are the most common features. Although the mechanism of injury is not known, one study in which electron microscopy was used demonstrated IgG precipitation of the tubular epithelium with fibrin deposits in the glomular and interstitial vessels. Clinically, this patient had associated microangiopathic hemolytic anemia. In the compendium of patients with cancer-associated hemolytic uremic syndrome, mitomycin C

featured prominently as the therapeutic modality given to these patients, usually in combination with 5-fluorouracil.

Mithramycin

Mithramycin, a rarely used antineoplastic agent, is frequently administered, however, in the management of cancer-related hypercalcemia. The doses required for hypercalcemia are much lower than the antitumor dose; thus, renal toxicity, in this setting, is rarely observed. However, when used as a therapeutic, nephrotoxicity, presenting as proteinuria and diminution in creatine clearances, was reported in up to 40% of patients receiving doses in the range of 125 to 250 µg/kg. The dose for hypercalcemia is generally 25 µg/kg. On rare occasions, a hemolytic uremic syndrome may also occur with mithramycin.

Biologic Response Modifiers

Biologic response modifiers including interferon alpha and gamma, *Corynebacterium parvum*, interleukin-2 and the newly introduced colony-stimulating factors, G-CSF and GM-CSF, have all been associated with nephrotoxicity [9]. The most prominent offender is the administration of interleukin-2, with or without associated LAK cell therapy. Early studies with IL-2 reported a nearly 50% incidence of oliguria and azotemia. In one study of adoptive immunotherapy with IL-2, 10 of 20 patients developed creatinine elevations between 2.1 and 10 mg/dl during the course of therapy, although these elevations were usually transient and reversible on drug cessation. Renal physiology studies with IL-2 administration have demonstrated universal diminution in GFR and reduction in FEna, similar to that seen in endotoxic shock. With more recent alterations in dosing schedules, IL-2–induced nephrotoxicity has been diminished, although not eliminated. In one recent study of weekly, low-dose IL-2, reversible nephrotoxicity occurred in 2 of 23 patients.

RENAL AND METABOLIC COMPLICATIONS

HYPERCALCEMIA

Hypercalcemia is the most common metabolic complication of cancer. It occurs with a frequency of 10% (squamous cell lung cancer) to 50% (multiple myeloma) (Table 3). The histology of the tumor, and not the presence or absence of bone metastases, is the main determinant of the development of this complication. The underly-

Table 2. Dose Modifications of Chemotherapeutic Agents with Renal Failure

75% of usual dose*	50% of usual dose†	Contraindicated‡
Bleomycin	Cyclophosphamide	Methotrexate
Melphalan		Streptozotocin
6-Mercaptopurine		Cisplatin

From Weber et al. [11]; with permission.
Renal failure—creatinine clearance < 25 cc/min.
*Partial renal excretion—nonnephrotoxic.
†Renal excretion—minimal nephrotoxicity.
‡Renal excretion—significant nephrotoxicity.

Table 3. Tumors Associated with Hypercalcemia

Tumor	Postulated mechanism
Solid tumors	
Breast carcinoma	PGE, other growth factors acting locally
Squamous cell lung cancer	Parathyroid hormone–related peptide
Renal cell carcinoma	released by tumor
Hematologic malignancies	
Multiple myeloma	Activation of local osteoclasts by cytokines including lymphotoxin
Lymphoma	Similar to multiple myeloma, possible increased levels of 1,25- dihydroxy-vitamin D3

ing malignancy is usually clinically obvious, although hypercalcemia can rarely precede the development of the tumor. The therapy of tumor-induced hypercalcemia is provided in Table 4.

TUMOR LYSIS SYNDROME

Tumor lysis syndrome is characterized by hyperkalemia, hyperuricemia, hyperphosphatemia, and hypercalcemia caused by rapid release of intracellular contents. It occurs as a complication of chemotherapy or radiation therapy of highly drug-sensitive tumors, especially in patients with large tumor burdens. The tumors commonly associated with tumor lysis are Burkitt's lymphoma, acute lymphoblastic leukemia, aggressive lymphomas, and small cell lung cancer.

Tumors susceptible to this complication are generally identifiable in advance. Intravenous hydration should be initiated 24 to 48 hours prior to initiation of chemotherapy. Electrolytes should be monitored frequently and corrected when necessary. Allopurinol, an inhibitor of xanthine oxidase, should be started at 300 to 600 mg/d to prevent hyperuricemia. If renal function worsens, dialysis is effective if started early.

HYPONATREMIA AND SIADH

The syndrome of inappropriate antidiuretic hormone secretion (SIADH) and consequent hyponatremia are caused by tumor release of ADH or arginine vasopressin (AVP). This condition occurs most commonly with small cell lung cancer (about 10%), but may rarely accompany other tumors.

In the pathologic setting, ADH acts on the renal tubule to increase absorption of water. When this occurs "inappropriately" (ie, in the setting of a patient who is normovolemic), SIADH is the consequence. The urine osmolality is consistently higher than the serum osmolality, and urinary sodium is high despite serum hyponatremia.

Hyponatremia due to SIADH needs to be distinguished from that due to cardiac, hepatic, renal, or adrenal dysfunction, and diuretic use. The diagnosis of SIADH is made based on the following criteria: serum hyposmolality (is greater than 280 mOsm/kg), urine osmolality is greater than serum osmolality, urine sodium is greater than 20 mEq/l, there has been no recent or concomitant diuretic use, the patient is clinically normovolemic, and renal, adrenal, and thyroid functions are normal.

In mild cases of SIADH, fluid restriction is effective management. If severe and symptomatic hyponatremia occurs, careful correction of serum sodium at a rate not to exceed 1 mEq/hr can be carried out with hypertonic saline (3%) with or without furosemide. Correction should be stopped when half the deficit of sodium has been replaced or when the serum sodium approaches 125 mEq/l. Such measures should generally be attempted in the intensive care unit with frequent monitoring of serum electrolytes.

URIC ACID NEPHROPATHY

Acute uric acid nephropathy may often occur in a patient with cancer when there is rapid turnover of cellular contents, usually secondary to lysis of tumors sensitive to chemotherapy or radiation therapy. Elevated plasma levels of urate due to nucleic acid breakdown overwhelm the renal system's capacity to clear these metabolites. In response to hyperuricemia, the kidney increases the secretion of urate at the tubular level. Because of the mechanisms of acidification within the distal tubule, the potential for uric acid precipitation and tubular obstruction develops.

Uric acid nephropathy most often occurs in association with chemotherapy-responsive tumors such as leukemias and lymphomas, especially Burkitt's lymphoma. The most important clinical goal is to anticipate the development of this complication prior to the initiation of therapy. Vigorous hydration, prophylactic use of allopurinol before, during, and following antineoplastic therapy, and meticulous attention to serum electrolytes, especially potassium and phosphate, are crucial in the overall management of patients undergoing cytoreductive therapy.

Allopurinol, a structural analogue of hypoxanthine, is a potent inhibitor of xanthine oxidase. Allopurinol therapy facilitates urinary excretion of three end products of purine metabolism—xanthine,

Table 4. Therapy for tumor-induced hypercalcemia

Agent	Dose	Postulated mechanism	Toxicity	Comment
Normal saline hydration and diuresis	Achieve normovolemia; then add furosemide if needed	Counteracts increased renal absorbtion of Ca due to dehydration Ca and Na absorption; diuresis therefore increases renal Ca clearance	Fluid overload, congestive heart failure, electrolyte imbalance	Correction of underlying dehydration is cornerstone of therapy; however, saline diuresis alone is not effective treatment and other measures should be initiated
Calcitonin	4–8 U/kg SC or IM every 6 hr	Increased renal clearance of Ca; inhibits bone resorption	Rare hypersensitivity reactions	Rapid onset of action; effective even when patient is dehydrated; effects are short-lived (≤ 48 hr)
Biphosphonates (etidronate)	Max 7.5 mg/kg/d for 3–5 days by slow IV infusion	Inhibits bone resorption directly	Nephrotoxicity, local irritation at injection site	Moderately effective; patient should be euvolemic before administration
Mithramycin	25 µg/kg by slow IV bolus	Directly kills osteoclasts leading to decreased bone resorption	Thrombocytopenia, nausea, hepatotoxicity	Delayed onset of action (24–48 hr)
Corticosteroids (prednisone)	20–100 mg/d	Inhibits osteoclasts and bone resorption; decreases GI Ca absorption; acts on underlying tumor	Hyperglycemia, hypertension, other usual complications with steroids	Usually effective in hematologic malignancies and some breast cancer
Gallium nitrate	100–200 mg/m²/d continuous IV infusion for up to 5 days	Inhibits bone resorption	Nephrotoxicity (dose-limiting but not usually a problem at recommended doses)	More effective than biphosphonates in randomized studies; delayed onset of action (over several days); adequate hydration (urine output > 2 l/d) is critical

hypoxanthine, and uric acid. Because the solubility of uric acid in urine is a critical factor in hyperuricemic nephropathy, allopurinol has become an extremely effective agent in the management of this problem. Following the administration of allopurinol, there is usually a prompt decrease in plasma and urinary uric acid levels. The maximum effect on uric acid levels is usually achieved by day five of therapy but occasionally may take up to two weeks.

It is important to emphasize that not all patients undergoing cytoreductive therapy need to be placed on allopurinol. Individuals undergoing cytoreductive therapy for rapidly dividing cancer, such as Burkitt's lymphoma, non-Hodgkin's lymphoma, Hodgkin's disease, leukemias, and some testicular cancers, are the best candidates for allopurinol treatment. Once cytoreduction has been achieved, it is imperative to discontinue allopurinol therapy, allowing for uric acid to rise to normal levels. Although rare, both xanthine nephropathy and hyperphosphatemic nephropathy may occur as a part of acute tumor lysis syndrome [10].

RADIATION NEPHROPATHY

Although uncommon today, in the past, radiation damage to the kidney was a major complication of curative therapy of large abdominal and retroperitoneal neoplasms in which both kidneys were included in the radiation therapy port. With radiation damage, alterations in GFR, renal plasma flow, and tubular excretory capacity occur following delivery of 400 cGy to the bulk of both kidneys. Clinically, radiation nephropathy can be described as an acute syndrome in which signs and symptoms of renal and cardiovascular dysfunction occur following therapeutic radiation therapy to the kidneys. These changes usually occur over 6 to 12 months following the delivery of greater than 2300 cGy to both kidneys during a 4 to 5 week period.

Acute radiation nephropathy presents with signs and symptoms similar to cardiovascular compromise secondary to hypertension. Chronic radiation nephropathy may be insidious, occurring as late as 10 years following radiation therapy. Patients may present with asymptomatic renal failure and a clinical syndrome suggestive of chronic glomerulonephritis.

Today, the most effective treatment for radiation nephropathy is prevention through careful localization of the kidneys during treatment field planning and limitation of dosage and volume. It appears that the delivery of 200 cGy in 10 fractions over a 10-week period is a reasonably safe treatment plan for large abdominal tumors that will encompass both kidneys. There is also some potential for synergistic radiation nephropathy to occur in association with nephrotoxic agents such as dactinomycin.

REFERENCES

1. Garnick MB: Urologic and renal complications of cancer and its treatment. In Holland JF, Frei E III (eds): *Cancer Medicine*, 3rd ed. 1993, Philadelphia: Lea & Febiger.

2. Abelson HT, Garnick MB: Renal failure induced by cancer chemotherapy. In Rieselbach RE, Garnick MB (eds): *Cancer and the Kidney*. 1982, Philadelphia: Lea & Febiger; 769–813.

3. Garnick MB, Mayer RJ, Abelson HT: Acute renal failure associated with cancer treatment. In Brenner BM, Lazarus JM (eds): *Acute Renal Failure*, 2nd ed. 1988, New York: Churchill Livingstone; 621–657.

4. D'Orsi CJ, Kaplan WD: The radiologic and radionuclide evaluation of the kidney. In Rieselbach RE, Garnick MB (eds): Cancer and the Kidney. 1982, Philadelphia: Lea & Febiger; 56–102.

5. Rieselbach RE, Garnick MB: Renal diseases induced by antineoplastic agents. In Schrier RW, Gottschalk CE (eds). *Diseases of the Kidney*, 4th ed. 1988, Boston: Little, Brown; 863–892.

6. DeFronzo RA, Colvin OM, Braine H, *et al.*: Cyclophosphamide and the kidney. *Cancer* 1973, 33:483–491.

7. Harmon WE, Cohen HT, Schneeberger E, *et al.*: Chronic renal failure in children treated with methyl CCNU. *N Engl J Med* 1979, 300:1200–1203.

8. Price TM, Murgo AJ, Keveney JJ, *et al.*: Renal failure and hemolytic anemia associated with mitomycin C. *Cancer* 1989, 55:51–56.

9. Averbuch SD, Austin H, Sherwin S, *et al.*: Acute interstitial nephritis with the nephrotic syndrome following recombinant leukocyte A interferon therapy for mycosis fungoides. *N Engl J Med* 1984, 310:32–35.

10. Cadman E, Lundberg W, Bertino J: Hyperphosphatemia and hypocalcemia accompanying rapid cell lysis in a patient with Burkitt's lymphoma and Burkitt cell leukemia. *Am J Med* 1977, 62:283.

11. Weber B, Garnick MB, Rieselbach R: Nephropathies due to antineoplastic agents. In Massry SG, Glassock RJ (eds): *Textbook of Nephrology*, 2nd ed. 1989, Baltimore: Williams & Wilkins; 818–822.

URINARY TRACT OBSTRUCTION

Retroperitoneal tumors causing ureteral obstruction can occur with any solid neoplasm. Urologic and gynecologic cancers, together with lymphomas, are the most common causes of obstruction. The effects of obstruction on kidney function result in an early inability to concentrate the urine maximally. Renal blood flow is also markedly diminished, particularly in the setting of unilateral obstruction. Regardless of the precipitating neoplasm, the presenting clinical manifestation is usually excruciating pain.

MANAGEMENT OR INTERVENTION

1. Establish histologic diagnosis of the underlying neoplasm
2. Introduce appropriate therapeutic modalities based on primary disease and obstruction:
   a. For prostate cancer causing bilateral obstruction, consider urethral catheterization, suprapubic cystostomy, immediate bilateral orchiectomy, or other endocrine therapeutic approaches
   b. For lymphomas causing retroperitoneal obstruction, radiation therapy or combination chemotherapy can be employed
   c. For isolated metastases, localized radiation therapy can be effective
   d. For retroperitoneal metastases or lymphoma with loss of renal function, immediate percutaneous nephrotomy(ies) with placement of antegrade or retrograde stents in the immediate future, if the neoplasm has not been controlled, should be considered
   e. For sensitive neoplasms and testicular cancer, the presence of renal function abnormalities mandates consideration of temporary percutaneous nephrostomies
3. Inhibit xanthine oxidase with allopurinol to prevent a surge of uric acid, which could compromise renal function during systemic treatment
4. Minimize likelihood of infectious complications during manipulation of the obstructed urinary tract
5. Carefully manage postobstructive diuresis and natriuresis with intensive metabolic monitoring

CAUSATIVE FACTORS

Retroperitoneal tumors; urologic cancers, gynecologic cancers, and lymphomas causing lymphadenopathy in the para-aortic, paracaval, and periureteral locations; prostate and advanced cervical cancers commonly causing distal urinary tract obstruction; testicular cancers, especially seminoma, capable of obstructing both ureters simultaneously; metastatic neoplasms forming a plaquelike sheet of tumor

PATHOLOGIC PROCESS

Dilatation of proximal anatomic regions due to obstruction; kidney increases in weight and size and gradually atrophies; inability to concentrate urine maximally and marked diminution of renal blood flow

DIFFERENTIAL DIAGNOSES

Retroperitoneal fibrosis, ureteral metastases, bladder neck obstruction, lymphadenopathy, kidney stones

PATIENT ASSESSMENT

Ultrasonography (method of choice); radionuclide studies; bone scans with technetium concentration to quantify renal blood flow; on occasion, retrograde and antegrade pyelography; cystoscopy and other interventional approaches for staging purposes; FEna to determine duration of obstruction

TOXICITY GRADING

	0	1	2	3	4
BUN or serum creatinine	$\leq 1.25 \times N$	$1.26–2.5 \times N$	$2.6–5 \times N$	$5.1–10 \times N$	$> 10 \times N$
Proteinuria	No change	1+ < 0.3 g% < 3 g/l	2–3+ 0.3–1.0 g% 3–10 g/l	4+ > 1.0 g% > 10 g/l	Nephrotic syndrome
Hematuria	No change	Microscopic	Gross	Gross + clots	Obstructive uropathy

N—upper limit of normal value of population under study.

GENITOURINARY HEMORRHAGE

Hemorrhage into the genitourinary tract is a problem often seen with certain malignancies. It requires vigilant anticipation and specialized care. Specific anti-neoplastic agents, such as cyclophosphamide and ifosfamide, are associated with this complication. Management differs according to the site of the process, tumor involvement, and status of the patient.

MANAGEMENT OR INTERVENTION

1. Hemorrhagic cystitis
   Catheter drainage and continuous irrigation
   Intravesical cautery
   Intravesical therapy with formalin
2. Refractory bleeding
   Cystotomy with instillation of phenol and ligation of the bladder vessels
   In severe cases, urinary diversion and removal of the organ to stop life-threatening bleeding are necessary.

CAUSATIVE AGENTS

Cyclophosphamide, ifosfamide, l-asparaginase, actin-omycin D, mitomycin C, mithramycin, 6-mercap-topurine, anticoagulants

PATHOLOGIC PROCESS

Toxic metabolites of certain chemotherapeutic agents have direct effect on urethral surface; high concentrations of these metabolites can cause erosion of the bladder mucosal system, leading to microscopic and gross bladder hemorrhage

DIFFERENTIAL DIAGNOSES

Chemotherapeutic agents, tumor involvement, prostate disorders

PATIENT ASSESSMENT

Clinical examination, urinalysis, cystoscopy, urinary irrigation and drainage

TOXICITIY GRADING

	0	1	2	3	4
Hematuria	No change	Microscopic	Gross	Gross + clots	Obstructive uropathy

CYTOTOXIC DRUG-INDUCED PULMONARY TOXICITY

When the patient with cancer presents with respiratory symptoms and radiographic signs of a diffuse lung infiltrate, the ensuing search for a cause and appropriate treatment may prove frustrating and fruitless. A specific cause cannot be found in 15 to 30% of patients, despite the use of bronchoalveolar lavage and transbronchial or open lung biopsy [1]. Even at autopsy a definitive diagnosis is not made in up to 15% of such patients [2]. The possible cause of a diffuse pulmonary infiltrate in the setting of malignancy includes 1) recurrence or progression of the underlying malignancy, 2) opportunistic infection in an immunocompromised host (immunocompromise secondary to corticosteroid therapy, chemotherapy-induced bone-marrow suppression, radiation therapy, malnutrition, or mucosal disruption), 3) drug-induced pulmonary disease, 4) radiation-induced pulmonary disease, 5) idiopathic pulmonary fibrosis, 6) unrelated lung disease (e.g., cardiogenic pulmonary edema, aspiration pneumonia in a debilitated patient), or 7) an unusual complication of cancer or its treatment (e.g., pulmonary alveolar proteinosis in hematologic malignancy [3], fat embolization in the immunocompromised host [4], or veno-occlusive disease secondary to the administration of bleomycin, nitrosoureas, or high-dose chemotherapy [1,5]). The difficulty in identifying a specific cause occurs because often several of these factors coexist, each of which is capable of producing an indistinguishable clinicopathologic picture. Performance of a lung biopsy or bronchoalveolar lavage is frequently necessary to eliminate potentially reversible factors, such as infection and malignancy, even if another cause is strongly suspected. Reported mortality rates in patients with a diffuse pulmonary infiltrate range from less than 5% up to 90%, depending on the underlying disease, the severity of respiratory dysfunction, and the degree of impairment of the host's defenses [1].

The diagnosis of chemotherapy-related pulmonary toxicity is very difficult to make because there are generally no specific markers, histologic findings, or diagnostic clinical features of drug-induced lung injury. Three typical patterns of damage may occur: 1) chronic pneumonitis or fibrosis, 2) acute hypersensitivity pneumonitis, and 3) noncardiogenic pulmonary edema. Rarely, chest pain may occur during drug therapy.

CHRONIC PNEUMONITIS OR FIBROSIS

Almost all cytotoxic drugs that cause pulmonary damage (with the exception of procarbazine) are associated with this pattern of presentation. Patients commonly present with progressive dyspnea, dry cough, fatigue, and malaise, which develop over several weeks to months [6]. Hemoptysis may occasionally occur, but when present should alert the attending physician to consider other causes. Fine bibasal crackles become more coarse with time, and later are accompanied by cyanosis. The most common chest radiographic abnormality is a diffuse reticulonodular pattern, which progresses to pulmonary fibrosis. Pleural effusions seldom occur, but may do so in association with mitomycin C, busulfan, or bleomycin therapy [6].

Chemotherapeutic agents induce three characteristic histopathologic abnormalities. First, type II pneumocytes (progenitor cells) proliferate in response to degeneration and desquamation of type I pneumocytes (alveolar lining cells, particularly vulnerable to damage). Alterations in nucleic acid metabolism caused by the drug produce atypical type II pneumocytes that exhibit a wide variation in size, giant cell formation, and prominent nucleoli. Second, a chronic inflammatory cell infiltrate occurs. Finally, a variable degree of fibroblastic proliferation and fibrosis is seen [7]. Vascular endothelial cells may become swollen with exudation of fluid into interstitial and intra-alveolar spaces, but the extent to which this contributes to fibrosis is unclear [8].

Details of the mechanisms of drug-induced pulmonary fibrosis are generally not known. A number of pulmonary homeostatic mechanisms are important in maintaining the integrity of the lung microenvironment and may be altered by cytotoxic agents. An individual drug may affect one or more of these systems or act through pathways yet to be determined. Some agents may act to alter the balance between oxidants and antioxidants in pulmonary tissues. Highly reactive oxygen-free radicals are able to induce lipid peroxidation, leading to damage to cellular membranes, or cause other inflammatory reactions within the lung. Certain chemotherapeutic agents have shown the ability to increase free-radical production directly (e.g., bleomycin, cyclophosphamide), or reduce antioxidant defenses (e.g., carmustine, cyclophosphamide), thus shifting the balance in favor of an excess of oxidants. Similarly, imbalances may be induced in other homeostatic systems, including matrix repair (favoring collagenesis by stimulating fibroblast growth, such as with bleomycin), proteolysis (enhancing the effect of proteolytic enzymes directly or indirectly by inactivating antiproteolytic enzymes [such as alpha-1-antitrypsin]), and the immunologic tolerance of the lung. This last system is usually required to prevent overreactions to inhaled substances that may cause tissue damage. Some drugs may alter suppressor–effector cell balance such that the drug is recognized as a foreign antigen, thereby inducing an inflammatory reaction [6].

The presence of certain risk factors reduces pulmonary tolerance to different cytotoxic agents. For instance, the cumulative dose of drug administered is important in the development of fibrosis caused by bleomycin and busulfan administration, but there is no clear dose-response relationship with other antineoplastic drugs [9]. Other factors that influence the toxicity of more than one drug include increasing age [9], concurrent or sequential radiation therapy [6], oxygen therapy [10], and the use of multiple drug regimens [6]. Factors important in individual drug usage are mentioned further on in this chapter.

Unfortunately, there is no simple way to determine which patients will develop clinically significant chemotherapy-induced pulmonary toxicity. Chest radiographic changes do not reliably predict the onset of clinical toxicity and may follow the onset of basal crackles [11]. Although computed tomographic (CT) scan of the chest has allowed appreciation of subtle changes in the lungs not visible on radiographs, these abnormalities may not correlate with changes in pulmonary function tests [12], and their presence may in fact create diagnostic difficulties in patients in whom metastatic lesions are suspected. Gallium-67 scanning reveals abnormalities in some patients with bleomycin toxicity, but it is unclear in what proportion of patients this occurs [12]. Further studies are required to determine the sensitivity of this technique.

The most widely used method of assessment for chemotherapy-induced lung toxicity is serial pulmonary function tests (PFTs). Serious limitations exist, however, regarding the ability of the characteristic changes of a reduction in diffusing capacity (DLCO) and lung volumes to predict the onset of clinically important pulmonary fibrosis [13]. The interpretation of such changes may be difficult due to the presence of confounding factors. Patients receiving chemotherapy often develop anemia, which is well recognized as able to affect the DLCO. The presence of pulmonary metastases may directly influence PFTs and have been reported to progress and regress parallel to serial changes in the PFTs [14]. More general problems, such as pain, weakness, the use of analgesics, and recent surgery, may alter the reliability of PFTs. One report suggests that as many as 23% of PFTs are unevaluable due to the presence of these factors [14]. Even if these factors could be taken into account, there is no clear evidence that pulmonary toxicity could be effectively avoided by using a serial assessment of PFTs. Indeed, abnormalities may develop abruptly only at the onset of clinical symptoms [11]. Despite these limitations, clinicians often adminster PFTs in patients at risk, and therapy with the potentially offending agent is usually ceased in patients who develop significant reduction in DLCO or lung volumes.

In general, the treatment for pulmonary toxicity is supportive. Drug therapy should be discontinued immediately, and often a trial of corticosteroids is beneficial. However, the response to these measures is unpredictable, and depends in large part on the offending agent and underlying disease.

Pulmonary fibrosis caused by the cytotoxic antibiotic, *bleomycin*, manifests as a subacute or chronic pneumonitis that is complicated in its later stages by progressive interstitial fibrosis, hypoxia, and death. The pathogenesis of this lung injury is poorly understood. Although substantial evidence points to the generation of oxygen-free radicals as an important mechanism [15], bleomycin also stimulates collagen synthesis [16] and induces an immune response in the lungs—observed in bronchoalveolar lavage specimens as accumulation of tissue macrophages and neutrophils and alteration in the helper–suppressor lymphocyte ratio [15]. Whether vascular endothelial cells or type I pneumocytes, which exhibit early morphologic changes, are the most sensitive to the effects of bleomycin is also controversial. The sensitivity of the lung to bleomycin may be explained by the observation that bleomycin is concentrated in the lung and inactivated by a hydrolase enzyme, which is relatively deficient in the lung compared with other tissues, such as liver [6].

Pulmonary fibrosis is reported in 2 to 40% of patients who receive bleomycin [11]. There appears to be a critical cumulative dose, 400 to 450 U, above which the risk for interstitial fibrosis rises dramatically and a dose-toxicity relationship becomes evident. However, the incidence of pulmonary damage at doses below this threshold is 2 to 6%, and fatal cases have been documented at total doses of as little as 50 U [17]. Other factors associated with increased bleomycin toxicity include increasing age, sequential or concurrent radiation therapy, treatment with high inspired oxygen therapy during or after bleomycin administration, use of multidrug regimens (especially cyclophosphamide), renal dysfunction, and administration by bolus injections versus continuous infusion [11].

The course of disease in patients who develop pulmonary fibrosis varies. Overall, mortality in all patients receiving bleomycin has been estimated at 1 to 2%, but is reported as between 10 and 83% in patients with established toxicity [11]. For those who develop mild toxicity, cessation of bleomycin therapy may lead to quick clinical recovery, often with a delay in resolution in radiologic abnormalities. A response may occur to corticosteroid therapy; however, no controlled studies have examined this approach systematically. Relapse of symptoms or development of infiltrates has been associated with the tapering of steroid therapy after an initial response [11].

Mitomycin and *neocarzinostatin* are other cytotoxic antibiotics implicated in pulmonary fibrosis. Mitomycin causes a syndrome similar to that produced by bleomycin; however, associated risk factors are much less well documented. Oxygen therapy, previous radiation treatment, and the use of multidrug regimens may increase the incidence of mitomycin toxicity. The reported frequency of pulmonary toxic effects associated with mitomycin is 3 to 12%, with a mortality approaching 50%. Prompt recognition of the syndrome is important because there are no established successful interventions, although corticosteroid therapy may be of benefit [6].

Several alkylating agents have been associated with pulmonary toxicity. *Busulfan* lung injury occurs in approximately 4% of patients [9], although up to 46% have subclinical damage as determined at autopsy [6]. The mechanism by which busulfan acts has not been elucidated. The interval between initiation of treatment and onset of symptoms is generally longer than for other cytotoxic agents and can be as much as 10 years [6]. Although a strict dose-toxicity relationship does not exist, there appears to be a threshold cumulative dose of busulfan, 500 mg, above which pulmonary fibrosis may occur, and below which the risk is minimal unless other potentially toxic modalities, such as chemotherapeutic drugs or radiation, have also been used [18]. Pulmonary injury is also more likely the longer therapy is continued [9]. This toxicity carries a grave prognosis, with a mean survival after diagnosis of 5 months and a 50% overall mortality rate [6].

There is some evidence that *cyclophosphamide* inflicts damage to the lungs either directly via generation of oxygen-free radicals or indirectly via a stimulatory effect on T lymphocytes, although these data mostly come from animal studies [18]. Multidrug regimens and, possibly, radiation therapy enhance the toxicity of cyclophosphamide, but no definite relationship has been established with age, duration of treatment, or dose. In fact, cases have been reported after administration of as little as 150 milligrams of cyclophosphamide, and the delay from institution of treatment to development of symptoms has varied from 2 weeks to 13 years [6]. Unlike with most other cytotoxic agents, fever is often striking [6]. Withdrawal of corticosteroid therapy that is part of a treatment regimen can precipitate symptoms. This illness also carries a poor prognosis—the mortality rate being approximately 50% [18].

Chlorambucil and *melphalan* produce interstitial pneumonitis and fibrosis similar in nature and prognosis to other alkylating agent–induced damage.

Carmustine (BCNU) was the first nitrosourea to be associated with pulmonary toxicity. In a rat model, granulomatous lung disease was seen in addition to fibrosis, changes that were accompanied by an elevation in the serum levels of angiotensin-converting enzyme [19]. Reductions in levels of the antioxidant, glutathione, have also been observed, which may predispose the lung to oxidant injury [18]. In humans, histologic changes similar to those produced by other cytotoxic agents are observed, except for the absence of an inflammatory cell infiltrate [6]. The likelihood of developing pulmonary toxicity increases linearly with the cumulative dose administered, rising sharply after 1500 mg/m^2 has been administered [20]. The duration of treatment is probably unimportant [20]. Younger patients are reported to be at greater risk, but this may be due to increased tolerance to a higher dose of drug [20]. Pre-existing lung disease, a history of tobacco use, and concurrent use of cyclophosphamide therapy may also increase the risk for pulmonary fibrosis, but this does not appear to be so for radiation therapy [20]. The prognosis for patients with this complication of BCNU therapy is extremely poor, with the overall mortality rate estimated to be greater than 90%, despite cessation of the drug therapy and the use of corticosteroids [6]. The majority of disease progression occurs over several months, but death within 2 to 3 days has been reported [6].

Other nitrosoureas implicated in pulmonary fibrosis are *lomustine (CCNU)* and *semustine (methyl-CCNU)*. Toxicity has occurred mostly in patients who had received unusually high cumulative doses of drug, but there have been reports of cases after the use of low-dose lomustine [18].

Patients who develop *methotrexate*-associated pulmonary toxicity usually present with the clinical picture of a hypersensitivity pneumonitis, or, less commonly, acute pleuritis or noncardiogenic pulmonary edema. These effects generally carry a good prognosis; however, about 10% of patients will develop pulmonary fibrosis [6].

When combined with mitomycin, the vinca alkaloids, *vinblastine* and *vindesine*, have been associated with acute respiratory failure, with or without pulmonary infiltrates. They may also rarely cause lung injury when used alone. Occasionally, fibrosis also occurs. The prognosis is poor if pulmonary infiltrates develop, and the use of corticosteroids may help reduce symptoms [21].

ACUTE HYPERSENSITIVITY PNEUMONITIS

An acute syndrome, consisting of malaise, fatigue, myalgias, fevers, chills, headache, dyspnea, and cough, may develop within weeks of commencement of *bleomycin, methotrexate,* or *procarbazine* therapy. Symptoms occur over hours to days and may be precipitated by withdrawal of corticosteroid therapy as part of a multidrug regimen. The syndrome is characterized by pulmonary or peripheral eosinophilia and pulmonary infiltrates. The prognosis is generally good—complete resolution occurs after cessation of the offending drug therapy [6].

The mechanism by which *methotrexate* produces this clinical picture is not straightforward. The fact that symptoms do not always recur upon rechallenge of the drug implies that hypersensitivity is not the sole mechanism for the action, and a direct toxic effect may be involved [18]. Hypersensitivity pneumonitis occurs in about 8% of patients receiving the drug, and there are no clear precipitating causes for the syndrome [22]. The frequency of administration may be important because patients receiving methotrexate daily and weekly appear to be more likely to develop pulmonary injury than do those receiving it two to four times weekly [9]. In addition to the clinical features outlined previously, methotrexate toxicity is often associated with skin eruptions and acute pleuritic chest pain [22]. Chest radiographs usually reveal a diffuse pulmonary infiltrate, and a pleural effusion may accompany this or occur alone; these changes tend to clear with resolution of symptoms [22]. Lung biopsy specimens reveal an extensive mononuclear cell inflammatory infiltrate, and, on occasion, granulomata [22]. This syndrome carries a mortality rate of approximately 1%, and about 10% of patients develop pulmonary fibrosis. Even though in a few cases symptoms and radiographic abnormalities have surprisingly cleared despite continuation of drug therapy, withholding of further therapy with methotrexate is usually recommended [22]. The efficacy of corticosteroids has not been proved, but anecdotal reports have described a rapid response to these agents in some patients [6].

Procarbazine-induced hypersensitivity pneumonitis is rare, and, in all reported cases, other chemotherapeutic agents have been used. Fibrosis is generally not a feature of lung toxicity as a result of use of this drug (there is a single reported case) [18].

NONCARDIOGENIC PULMONARY EDEMA

This form of pulmonary edema is a rare acute complication seen in association with *cytosine arabinoside, teniposide, methotrexate,* and *cyclophosphamide* administration. It may occur after oral, intravenous, or intrathecal (methotrexate) administration. Patients present with symptoms and signs identical to those seen as a result of any other cause of pulmonary edema. The mechanism by which this syndrome occurs is unknown, but in some instances it may be through central nervous system effects on pulmonary capillary permeability [6].

RADIATION-INDUCED PULMONARY TOXICITY

Damage to the lung after radiation therapy to the chest may be expressed as either an acute pneumonitis or chronic fibrosis. The former is most likely an immunologic reaction [23], whereas fibrosis is the result of direct damage to pulmonary parenchyma and indirect damage as a result of microvascular insult [24].

It is usually not possible to avoid radiation fibrosis by means of limiting the total dose of radiation if a sufficient dose is to be given to the tumor. After 30 Gy is administered in 2-Gy fractions to a partial lung volume of 100 cm², 5% of patients develop pulmonary injury, whereas after 60 Gy, fibrosis is universal. It is therefore necessary to alter other factors that influence the degree of normal tissue damage to avoid clinically significant chronic lung injury. By far the most important radiobiologic measures that can be taken are limitation of the treatment volume, minimization of the dose per fraction, preferential use of electrons, gamma, or x-rays over other particle beams, and reduction of the dose rate of delivery of the radiation (to a practical minimum). The total time over which the radiation is delivered is unimportant in the development of fibrosis [24].

MECHANISM OF LUNG INJURY

The mechanism by which radiation causes cellular injury is by ionization of DNA. Ionization is either a consequence of interaction with electrons scattered by the passing radiation particles, or with oxygen-free radicals formed after collision of scattered electrons with nearby water molecules. The result is base damage, protein cross-linking, and strand breakages [25].

The cellular mechanisms by which the acute changes in the lung occur are unclear. Changes occur within 6 to 12 weeks and are thought to be a result of direct damage to the lung. However, an increase in lymphocytes recovered from bronchoalveolar lavage specimens has been reported in both irradiated and nonirradiated lung in patients with radiation pneumonitis. This evidence suggests a role for an immunologically mediated mechanism, such as hypersensitivity, either in response to or because of direct lung injury in the treatment field [23].

There is great debate in the literature regarding which population of cells is the primary target of radiation damage. It is likely that the stromal and microvascular endothelial cells of the parenchymal connective tissue all contribute to the sequence of changes that lead to the late effects of radiation.

HISTOPATHOLOGY

In lung the immediate effects of radiation are on type II pneumocytes, with early release of surfactant, although this is usually subclinical. After about 3 months, alveolar cells slough and there is accumulation of protein-rich fluid in the interstitium and alveoli due to changes in capillary permeability, as evidenced by swelling of endothelial cells. After 6 months there is sclerosis of alveolar walls and interstitial fibrosis. With further time there may be progressive loss of lung volume and pleural thickening, the severity of which is determined by the degree of radiation damage [26].

CLINICAL FEATURES AND DIAGNOSIS

Acute radiation pneumonitis develops in 5 to 15% of patients receiving thoracic radiation therapy. It is characterized by the insidious onset of exertional dyspnea and a nonproductive cough 6 to 12 weeks after radiation therapy. A low-grade fever is common, but it may be high and spiking in severe cases. Pleuritic chest pain may occur from rib fractures or pleural injury. A reticulonodular infiltrate is usually seen in the treatment field on a chest radiograph but, not infrequently, also in the contralateral lung. PFTs typically show reduced lung volumes, impaired gas exchange, hypoxia, and compensatory hypocapnia, and there is an increase in lymphocytes in bronchoalveolar lavage fluid. In severe cases there is progression of clinical symptoms and signs and radiologic abnormalities [26].

If lung volumes and patients' treatment factors are carefully selected, radiation fibrosis is mostly subclinical. It is present radiographically by about 1 year, and can usually be distinguished from other forms of pulmonary infiltrate by the sharp boundaries of the

changes (coincident to the radiation field), and because the abnormalities do not correspond to anatomic lung boundaries [27].

RISK FACTORS

Respiratory compromise after radiation therapy is more likely to occur in patients with preexisting lung disease and treatment at any stage with bleomycin, cyclophosphamide, vincristine, dactinomycin, busulfan, mitomycin, or doxorubicin [6,27]. Acute pneumonitis is predisposed to by previous radiation therapy and may be precipitated by withdrawal of corticosteroid therapy during treatment. Other contributing factors include underlying infection and manipulation of the lung during surgery [27].

MANAGEMENT

High-dose corticosteroids (e.g., prednisolone, 100 mg/d) may produce an objective response in moderate to severe acute pneumonitis, but the use of these agents has not been established prospectively. If a response is achieved, the dose should be maintained for several weeks, then tapered slowly. In mild cases, treatment should be supportive, with the use of cough suppressants, antipyretics, and analgesics. Anticoagulants and antibiotics have been used, but no benefit from use of these agents has been observed [27].

Supportive care is also the mainstay of symptomatic pulmonary fibrosis. Oxygen should be used for marked hypoxemia, and if right heart failure develops, it should be treated aggressively.

REFERENCES

1. Rosenow EC: Diffuse pulmonary infiltrates in the immunocompromised patient. *Clin Chest Med* 1990, 11:55–64.

2. Rosenow EC, Wilson WR, Cockerill FR: Pulmonary disease in the immunocompromised host (first of two parts). *Mayo Clin Proc* 1985, 60:473–487.

3. Bedrossian CWM, Luna MA, Conklin RH, *et al.*: Alveolar proteinosis as a consequence of immunosuppression: A hypothesis based on clinical and pathologic observations. *Hum Pathol* 1980, 11:527–535.

4. Rosen JM, Braman SS, Hasan FM, *et al.*: Nontraumatic fat embolism. *Am Rev Respir Dis* 1986, 134:805–808.

5. Lombard CM, Churg A, Winokur S: Pulmonary veno-occlusive disease following therapy for malignant neoplasms. *Chest* 1987, 92:871–876.

6. Cooper JAD, White DA, Matthay RA: Drug-induced pulmonary disease: Part 1. Cytotoxic drugs. *Am Rev Respir Dis* 1986, 133:321–340.

7. Walker-Smith GJ: The histopathology of pulmonary reactions to drugs. *Clin Chest Med* 1990, 11:95–117.

8. Jordana M, Richards C, Irving LB, *et al.*: Spontaneous *in vitro* release of alveolar macrophage cytokines after intrathecal installation of bleomycin in rats: Characterization and kinetic studies. *Am Rev Respir Dis* 1988, 137:1135–1140.

9. Ginsberg SJ, Comis RL: The pulmonary toxicity of antineoplastic agents. *Sem Oncol* 1982, 9:34–51.

10. Hakkinen PJ, Whitely JW, Witschi HR: Hyperoxia, not thoracic x-irradiation, potentiates bleomycin and cyclophosphamide-induced lung damage in mice. *Am Rev Respir Dis* 1982, 126:281–285.

11. Jules-Elysee K, White DA: Bleomycin-induced pulmonary toxicity. *Clin Chest Med* 1990, 11:1–20.

12. Bellamy EA, Husband EA, Blaquiere RM, *et al.*: Bleomycin-related lung damage: CT evidence. *Radiology* 1985, 156:155–158.

13. Luuresma PB, Star-Kroeson MA, van der Mark THW, *et al.*: Bleomycin-induced changes in the carbon monoxide transfer factor of the lung and its components. *Am Rev Respir Dis* 1983, 128:880–883.

14. White DA, Stiver DE, Smith G, *et al.*: Serial pulmonary function studies during bleomycin therapy. *Am Rev Respir Dis* 1987, 135(suppl):A39.

15. Chandler DB: Possible mechanisms of bleomycin-induced fibrosis. *Clin Chest Med* 1990, 11:21–30.

16. Muggia FM: Pulmonary toxicity of antitumor agents. *Cancer Treat Rev* 1983, 10:221–243.

17. Blauer KA, Skarin AT, Balikial JP, *et al.*: Pulmonary complications associated with combination chemotherapy programs containing bleomycin. *Am J Med* 1983, 74:557–563.

18. Twohig KJ, Matthay RA: Pulmonary effects of cytotoxic agents other than bleomycin. *Clin Chest Med* 1990, 11:31–54.

19. Smith AC, Boyd MR: Effects of bischloronitrosourea (BCNU) on pulmonary and serum angiotensin-converting enzyme activity in rats. *Biochem Pharmacol* 1984, 32:3719–3722.

20. Aronin PA, Mahaley MS, Rudnick SA, *et al.*: Prediction of BCNU toxicity in patients with malignant gliomas: An assessment of risk factors. *N Engl J Med* 1980, 303:183–188.

21. Luedke D, McLaughline TT, Daughaday C, *et al.*: Mitomycin C and vindesine associated with pulmonary toxicity with variable clinical expression. *Cancer* 1985, 55:542–545.

22. Sostman HD, Matthay RA, Putman CE: Methotrexate-induced pneumonitis. *Medicine* 1976, 55:371–388.

23. Gibson PG, Bryant DH, Morgan GW, *et al.*: Radiation-induced lung injury: A hypersensitivity pneumonitis? *Ann Intern Med* 1988, 109:288–291.

24. Peters LJ, Brock WA, Travis EL: Radiation biology at clinically relevant fractions. In DeVita VT, Hellman S, Rosenberg SA (eds): *Important Advances in Oncology.* 1990, Philadelphia: JB Lippincott; 65–82.

25. Hall EJH: The physics and chemistry of radiation absorption. In *Radiobiology for the Radiologist*, 3rd ed. 1987, Philadelphia: JB Lippincott.

26. Gross NJ: Pulmonary effects of radiation therapy. *Ann Intern Med* 1977, 86:81–92.

27. Rosiello RA, Merrill WW: Radiation-induced lung injury. *Clin Chest Med* 1990, 11:65–71.

CHRONIC PNEUMONITIS OR FIBROSIS

All chemotherapeutic agents with the potential for pulmonary toxicity (with the exception of procarbazine) may cause chronic pulmonary fibrosis. Patients typically present with progressive dyspnea, dry cough, fatigue, and malaise weeks to months after completion of chemotherapy. Chest radiographs usually show a widespread, fine reticulonodular pattern. Pleural effusions are uncommon but may occur after therapy with mitomycin, busulfan, or bleomycin. Risk factors for fibrosis have been identified for various drugs. None of the currently used methods for monitoring patients, including pulmonary function tests, can reliably predict the onset of fibrosis. Treatment consists of excluding other, treatable causes of a diffuse pulmonary infiltrate, and supportive measures. The prognosis is highly variable, but symptoms may progress, leading to chronic debility or even to death—from respiratory failure.

CAUSATIVE AGENTS

Antibiotics: bleomycin, mitomycin, neocarzinostatin; **alkylating agents:** busulfan, cyclophosphamide, chlorambucil, melphalan; **nitrosoureas:** carmustine (BCNU), lomustine (CCNU), semustine (methyl-CCNU), **antimetabolites:** methotrexate, cytosine arabinoside, mercaptopurine; **villa vincas:** vinblastine, vindesine

PATHOLOGIC PROCESS

Unknown—possibly due to imbalance in one or more of the following: oxidant–antioxidant system, matrix repair, proteolysis, pulmonary immunologic tolerance

DIFFERENTIAL DIAGNOSES

Recurrent or progressive malignancy, opportunistic infection, radiation-induced pulmonary disease, idiopathic pulmonary fibrosis, unrelated (e.g., cardiogenic pulmonary edema, aspiration), unusual complication (e.g., alveolar proteinosis, fat embolism)

PATIENT ASSESSMENT

Baseline assessment: clinical history and examination, chest radiograph, PFT (if risk factors), bronchoscopy—may help exclude other causes ± implicate cytotoxic agent; **identify risk factors:** cumulative dose (bleomycin, busulfan, carmustine), age > 70 yr (bleomycin), concurrent or prior radiation therapy (bleomycin, busulfan, mitomycin), other cytotoxic therapy (carmustine, cyclophosphamide, mitomycin, bleomycin, methotrexate), oxygen therapy (bleomycin, cyclophosphamide, mitomycin), preexisting lung disease (carmustine), renal insufficiency (bleomycin), route of administration (bleomycin: bolus IV), duration of treatment (busulfan); **monitoring** (role in avoiding clinically significant toxicity not defined): clinical assessment, PFT—cease drug if significant decrease in DLCO or vital capacity, chest radiograph, CT scan of chest

MANAGEMENT OR INTERVENTION

1. Prevention
   a. Identify risk factors
   b. Monitor—role undefined
   c. Limit dose—bleomycin 450 U, busulfan 500 mg, carmustine 1500 mg/m^2
2. Treatment
   a. Cease drug therapy
   b. Corticosteroids of no proven benefit (may alleviate symptoms)
   c. Recommence therapy if symptoms precipitated by withdrawal
3. Supportive care
   a. Oxygen
   b. Cough suppressants, antipyretics
   c. Treat right heart failure: manage aggravating factors (sepsis, electrolytes, renal failure, anemia) and reduce afterload (*ie*, ACE inhibitor), restrict fluid, and prescribe bed rest

TOXICITY GRADING

0	1	2	3	4
No symptoms	Asymptomatic, with abnormality in PFT	Dyspnea on significant exertion	Dyspnea at normal level of activity	Dyspnea at rest

ACUTE HYPERSENSITIVITY PNEUMONITIS

An acute syndrome, consisting of malaise, fatigue, myalgias, fevers, chills, headache, dyspnea, and cough, may develop within weeks of commencement of therapy with the offending drug. Symptoms occur over hours to days and may be precipitated by withdrawal of corticosteroid therapy as part of a multidrug regimen. The syndrome is characterized by pulmonary or peripheral eosinophilia and pulmonary infiltrates. The prognosis is generally good; complete resolution occurs after cessation of the offending drug therapy.

MANAGEMENT OR INTERVENTION

1. Treat sepsis (may need a course of antibiotics to exclude infection)
2. Withdraw cytotoxic drug therapy
3. Administer corticosteroids (prednisolone, 100 mg/d), taper slowly
4. Prescribe supportive care (e.g., oxygen)

TOXICITY GRADING

0	1	2	3	4
No symptoms	Asymptomatic, with abnormality in PFTs	Dyspnea on significant exertion	Dyspnea at normal level of activity	Dyspnea at rest

CAUSATIVE AGENTS
Bleomycin, methotrexate, procarbazine

PATHOLOGIC PROCESS
Unknown

DIFFERENTIAL DIAGNOSES
Recurrent or progressive malignancy, opportunistic infection, unrelated (e.g., cardiogenic pulmonary edema, aspiration)

PATIENT ASSESSMENT
Clinical history and examination, chest radiograph, full blood examination—peripheral eosinophilia (10–20% eosinophils), septic workup—sputum and blood cultures, bronchoscopy—may show pulmonary eosinophilia

NONCARDIOGENIC PULMONARY EDEMA

This is a rare, acute complication seen in association with cytosine arabinoside, VM-26, methotrexate, and cyclophosphamide administration. It may occur after oral, intravenous, or intrathecal (methotrexate) administration. Patients present with symptoms and signs identical to those seen from any other cause of pulmonary edema.

MANAGEMENT OR INTERVENTION

1. Administer diuretics
2. Reduce afterload
3. Prescribe oxygen therapy if hypoxemia is a problem
4. Recommend bed rest

TOXICITY GRADING

0	1	2	3	4
No symptoms	Asymptomatic, with abnormality in PFTs	Dyspnea on signifcant exertion	Dyspnea at normal level of activity	Dyspnea at rest

CAUSATIVE AGENTS
Cytosine arabinoside, teniposide, methotrexate, cyclophosphamide

PATHOLOGIC PROCESS
Unknown, but sometimes may be through central nervous system effects on pulmonary capillary permeability

DIFFERENTIAL DIAGNOSES
Cardiac failure, lymphangitic carcinomatosis, fibrosis, inflammatory disease, drug overdose (heroin, morphine, dextropropoxyphene)

PATIENT ASSESSMENT
Clinical history and examination, full blood examination, BUN, chest radiography, EKG, cardiac enzymes, bronchoscopy (may exclude other causes)

RADIATION-INDUCED PULMONARY TOXICITY

Damage to the lung after radiation therapy to the chest may be expressed as either an acute pneumonitis or chronic fibrosis. Acute radiation pneumonitis is characterized by the insidious onset of fever, exertional dyspnea, and a nonproductive cough 6 to 12 weeks after radiation therapy. A reticulonodular infiltrate is usually seen in the treatment field on a chest radiograph but, not infrequently, also in the contralateral lung. PFTs typically show reduced lung volumes, impaired gas exchange, hypoxia, and compensatory hypocapnia. Progression may occur in severe cases. High-dose corticosteroid use may induce a clinical response.

Radiation fibrosis is mostly subclinical if lung volumes and patients' treatment factors are carefully selected. It is present radiographically by about 1 year.

MANAGEMENT OR INTERVENTION

1. Prevention
   a. Identify patients at risk
   b. Limit treatment volumes and total dose during radiation therapy
2. Treatment
   a. Administer corticosteroids (prednisolone, 100 mg/d), taper slowly
   b. Prescribe supportive care (give oxygen, cough suppressants, analgesics, antipyretics)
   c. Treat right heart failure

TOXICITY GRADING

0	1	2	3	4
No symptoms	Asymptomatic, with abnormality in PFTs	Dyspnea on significant exertion	Dyspnea at normal level of activity	Dyspnea at rest

CAUSATIVE FACTOR
Radiation therapy

PATHOLOGIC PROCESS
Ionization of cellular DNA—direct or indirect—resulting in damage to pneumocytes, stromal cells, capillary endothelium; damage to primary target cells unknown

DIFFERENTIAL DIAGNOSES
Recurrent or progressive malignancy, opportunistic infection, chemotherapy-induced pulmonary disease, idiopathic pulmonary fibrosis, unrelated (e.g., cardiogenic pulmonary edema, aspiration)

PATIENT ASSESSMENT
Baseline assessment: clinical history and examination, chest radiograph, PFT (if risk factors), bronchoscopy (may help exclude other causes ± implicate cytotoxic agent, **identify risk factors:** radiation therapy treatment volume and total dose, preexisting lung disease, cytotoxic drug administration (past, present, or future)—bleomycin, cyclophosphamide, vincristine, dactinomycin, busulfan, mitomycin, doxorubicin, prior radiation therapy to the chest, underlying infection, prior thoracic surgery, withdrawal of corticosteroid therapy

When a patient with cancer develops symptoms of cardiovascular disease, the treating physician is often presented with a diagnostic and therapeutic dilemma. The cardiac manifestations of neoplasia may be the result of 1) direct or indirect effects of malignancy, 2) exacerbation of preexisting, underlying cardiovascular disease, 3) direct toxicity related to treatment with either cytotoxic drugs or radiation therapy, or 4) indirect complications of chemotherapy (eg, anemia, hypokalemia, sepsis, fluid overload). Careful clinical evaluation and the use of sophisticated noninvasive (and occasionally invasive) investigations allow the physician to evaluate accurately changes in the structure and function of the heart. However, difficulty may arise in interpreting the interplay between these factors and, therefore, in evaluating the underlying cause of the clinical presentation. Hypertension and atherosclerotic vascular or valvular disease occurs more frequently with increasing age, as does cancer. In addition, many common cancers (eg, lung, bladder, head and neck) and cardiovascular disease share smoking as a common etiologic factor. The challenge for the physician, therefore, is to identify and treat the contributing factors appropriately while at the same time not subjecting often very ill patients to unnecessary investigations that may have limited potential for therapeutic benefit.

Cardiotoxicity due to anticancer drugs may manifest itself in a number of ways. The most common direct toxicity is a cardiomyopathy, usually chronic, but occasionally acute. Pericarditis, electrocardiographic (EKG) changes, arrhythmias, or exacerbation of ischemic heart disease (including infarction) can also occur. Hypotension is a particular feature of biologic response modifiers.

CARDIOMYOPATHY

The use of *anthracyclines* is the major cause of chemotherapy-induced cardiac complications, and these agents exhibit a cardiotoxicity that is unique in terms of pathology and mechanism. Although delivery of a single dose is limited by bone marrow suppression and mucositis, chronic administration is limited by a cardiomyopathy that is dependent on the cumulative dose. The earliest pathologic change is focal and consists of single degenerate myocytes surrounded by normal myocardium. Later lesions show more widespread injury and replacement by fibrosis. Specific anthracycline-induced changes can be identified on endocardial biopsy specimens and have been graded by Billingham *et al.* [1]. Morphologic change is almost universally present in cardiac biopsy specimens from patients who have received cumulative doxorubicin doses of more than 240 mg/m². Although structural changes are initially subclinical, abnormalities can be detected by a decline in cardiac contractility as assessed by serial echocardiograms or nuclear gated blood pool scans. Clinical congestive heart failure (CHF) develops in less than 5% of patients who have received a cumulative doxorubicin dose of 450 mg/m², in 15% who have had 600 mg/m², and in 20% of those given 700 mg/m² [2]. Most oncologists discontinue therapy at a lifetime cumulative dose of 450 to 550 mg/m², even if, as is not infrequently the case, the patient's tumor is still responsive to the drug. These figures are modified by the presence of certain risk factors that reduce patient tolerance to anthracyclines, including preexisting hypertension or heart disease, prior megavoltage therapy to the heart, and age [2,3]. Young children (especially those less than 4 years old) appear to be susceptible to an anthracycline cardiotoxicity that may, on occasion, manifest itself years later [4]. Although conflicting reports exist, cyclophosphamide probably does not augment doxorubicin-induced cardiac damage [5].

Other manifestations of anthracycline cardiotoxicity can be detected prior to clinical manifestations of CHF by echocardiography (fractional shortening), radionuclide gated blood pool scan (left ventricular ejection fraction [LVEF]) with or without stress, cardiac catheterization, endomyocardial biopsy, and, arguably, by EKG changes (nonspecific ST-T changes and flattening of the QRS complex). A suggested monitoring regimen is to assess the LVEF serially [6]. For those patients with a normal baseline LVEF (≥ 50%), a second determination should be performed after a cumulative doxorubicin dose of 500 mg/m² has been administered. For those patients with any risk factors the LVEF should be measured after between 350 and 400 mg/m² of doxorubicin has been administered. A second measurement should be made only if further doxorubicin therapy or potentially cardiotoxic treatment (eg, mediastinal radiation therapy for Hodgkin's disease or small cell lung cancer) is to be prescribed. If further doxorubicin is to be given, the LVEF should be measured prior to each subsequent dose. A decrease in the LVEF of 10% or more or decline to 50% or less should lead to cessation of treatment. If a decision to treat has been made in a patient with a baseline LVEF of 30 to 50%, reassessment should occur after each dose has been given and therapy should be discontinued if the LVEF falls by 10% or more or to 30% or less.

When clinical CHF occurs, it usually develops 30 to 60 days after the last dose of anthracycline has been administered; however, it may occur during treatment or years later. It has been traditionally ascribed a poor prognosis and high mortality rate, but with close monitoring, identification of aggravating factors (ie, sepsis, hypokalemia, renal failure, anemia), and aggressive treatment with afterload-reducing agents, fluid restriction, and bed rest, many patients experience improvement in symptoms and cardiac function. Maximum benefit following these measures may not be seen for up to 1 year.

The risk for cardiac failure can be lessened by several methods. Less cardiotoxic analogues of doxorubicin are available (eg, epirubicin, idarubicin) that provide an increased therapeutic ratio; however, their use is similarly limited by cardiac damage. Lowering of the cardiac risk also results from 96-hour infusion [7] or weekly scheduling [5] of doxorubicin therapy, implying that toxicity is related to peak dose rather than the area under the curve. That these regimens have not been widely adopted is probably due to the need for prolonged infusions to be delivered via a central venous catheter, increased risk for mucositis with a 96-hour infusion and extravasation, the cost of weekly visits, and the relative lack of data on the antitumor activity of such regimens.

The most effective means of abrogating cardiotoxicity is by the addition of the cardioprotectant, dexrazoxane, to anthracycline therapy [8]. This agent is a strong intracellular iron chelator. Its development follows the observation that the most likely mechanism of myocardial damage is lipid peroxidation of myocyte mitochondrial membrane that is mediated by an anthracycline-Fe^{3+} complex that either initiates an iron-dependent free-radical cascade or acts itself as an oxidant. It is thought that these reactions overwhelm the heart's limited antioxidant mechanisms [9]. Dexrazoxane acts to limit the availability of iron to behave as an oxidant or participate in free-radical generation. More importantly, it has been shown to reduce anthracycline cardiotoxicity significantly in several randomized clinical trials, with nearly all studies showing no alteration in antitumor activity of doxorubicin [10,11].

A rare, idiosyncratic, acute illness can occur with anthracycline administration, often at low cumulative doses. The pericarditis–myocarditis syndrome occurs 1 to 23 days after administration of the last dose, and patients present with fever, pericarditis, and CHF. It is often fatal and death occurs secondary to CHF.

The anthracenedione, *mitoxantrone*, was developed in the search for anthracycline analogues. Although it causes less alopecia, nausea, and vomiting, is less cardiotoxic, and does not produce an extravasation injury, it has a limited spectrum of activity, and its use is largely restricted to the treatment of lymphoma, leukemia, and breast cancer. CHF occurs in less than 5% of patients but is seen more often in those who have had prior anthracycline exposure, chest radiation therapy, or underlying heart disease. There is no obvious dose limitation [12].

The dose-limiting toxicity of *high-dose cyclophosphamide* used in bone marrow transplantation is cardiac toxicity. It may occur at doses of 100 mg/kg given over 48 hours but is most frequent after doses of 200 mg/kg or more. There is no cumulative damage with repeated administration of low doses. Clinically, high-dose cyclophosphamide therapy produces a fulminant illness, with CHF and pericarditis developing in 10 to 14 days. Age greater than 50 years and prior anthracycline exposure put patients at higher risk [13].

CHF has been reported in association with *amsacrine* therapy in less than 1% of treated patients, but most, if not all, have previously received an anthracycline [14]. *Mitomycin C* administration is associated with CHF in approximately 5% of patients, with increasing incidence above cumulative doses of 300 mg/m^2 [15].

PERICARDITIS

Anthracyclines and *high-dose cyclophosphamide* are both associated with an acute pericarditis–myocarditis syndrome, as mentioned previously. The pericarditis that occurs after the administration of granulocyte-macrophage colony-stimulating factor (GM-CSF) is a self-limiting illness that is part of a more general serositis [16].

EXACERBATION OF ISCHEMIC HEART DISEASE

Ischemic chest pain occurs in up to 1.5% of patients receiving 5-fluorouracil (5-FU), although the incidence has been reported to be as high as 4.5% in patients with previous ischemic heart disease [17]. Cardiac arrest or sudden death has been reported. Symptoms may recur upon further challenge with the drug and are often accompanied by EKG and cardiac enzyme changes consistent with ischemia or infarction. Coronary artery spasm is the most likely mechanism. The pain often occurs after the third or fourth day of treatment (whether by continuous IV or daily bolus) in patients with underlying coronary artery disease or a history of chest radiation treatment. This spasm is best treated with nitrates and calcium blockers. Doses of 5-FU should be scheduled weekly if more is to be given after an episode of ischemic chest pain.

Other agents with which ischemic episodes have been associated include the *anthracyclines* (doxorubicin and daunorubicin), *vinca alkaloids* (vinblastine, vincristine, and vindesine) and *interleukin-2* (in about 4% of patients). There are isolated reports of myocardial infarction with the use of *etoposide*, *amsacrine*, and *interferon alpha*.

ARRHYTHMIAS

The most frequent EKG abnormalities observed during *anthracycline* treatment are nonspecific ST-T wave changes, reduction in QRS voltages, sinus tachycardia, supraventricular tachycardias, premature atrial and ventricular contractions, T-wave abnormalities, and prolonged QT interval [2]. The incidence of such changes is related to the frequency of monitoring. These changes are usually self-limiting, resolve within 1 week, and are only rarely accompanied by life-threatening arrhythmias. *Amsacrine* is reported to be associated with life-threatening arrhythmias, but in less than 1% of treated patients. *Paclitaxel* is associated with a diverse spectrum of disturbances, including ventricular arrhythmias (premature ventricular contractions and ventricular tachycardia), asymptomatic bradycardia (in up to 20%), and varying degrees of heart block [3]. Nonfatal supraventricular tachyarrhythmias have been reported after the administration of *interferons* and *interleukin-2*. In the case of *interferon alpha*, these tachyarrhythmias occur with increasing age, prior cardiac disease, prior treatment with anthracyclines, and high doses.

HYPOTENSION

The agents most commonly associated with hypotension are the biologic response modifiers. The cause of this effect is thought to be an increase in vascular permeability, leading to both a decrease in intravascular volume and a reduction in systemic vascular resistance. Up to almost 70% of patients receiving *interleukin-2*, with or without LAK cells, require vasopressor support, which appears to be dose related. Capillary leak syndromes and resultant hypotension have been observed after the administration of *interferon alpha*, *beta*, or *gamma*, and GM-CSF [18]. A hypersensitivity reaction to polyoxyethylated castor oil, the vehicle of *paclitaxel*, also results in hypotension.

REFERENCES

1. Billingham ME, Mason GW, Bristow MR, *et al*.: Anthracycline cardiomyopathy monitored by morphological changes. *Cancer Treat Rep* 1978, 62:865–872.

2. Praga C, Beretta G, Vigo PL, *et al*.: Adriamycin cardiotoxicity: A survey of 1273 patients. *Cancer Treat Rep* 1979, 62:931–934.

3. Allen A: The cardiotoxicity of chemotherapeutic drugs. *Sem Oncol* 1992, 19:529–542.

4. Lipschultz SE, Colan SD, Gelber RD, *et al*.: Late effects for doxorubicin therapy for acute lymphoblastic leukemia in childhood. *N Engl J Med* 1991, 324:808–815.

5. Torti FM, Bristow, Howes AE, *et al*.: Reduced cardiotoxicity of doxorubicin delivered on a weekly schedule: Assessment by endomyocardial biopsy. *Ann Intern Med* 1983, 99:745–749.

6. Schwartz RG, McKenzie WB, Alexander J, *et al*.: Congestive heart failure and left ventricular dysfunction complicating doxorubicin therapy: Seven year experience using radionuclide angiocardiography. *Am J Med* 1987, 82:1109–1118.

7. Legha SS, Benjamin RS, Mackay B, *et al*.: Reduction of doxorubicin toxicity by prolonged continuous intravenous infusion. *Ann Intern Med* 1982, 96:133–139.

8. Koning J, Palmer P, Franks CR, *et al.*: Cardioxane-ICRF-187: Towards anticancer drug specificity through selective toxicity reduction. *Cancer Treat Rev* 1991, 18:1–19.

9. Olsen RD, Mushin PS: Doxorubicin cardiotoxicity: Analysis of prevailing hypotheses. *FASEB J* 1990, 47:359–370.

10. Speyer JL, Green MD, Kramer E, *et al.*: Protective effect of the bispiperazinedione ICRF-187 against doxorubicin-induced cardiac toxicity in women with advanced breast cancer. *N Engl J Med* 1988, 319:745–752.

11. Basser RL, Green MD: Strategies for the prevention of anthracycline cardiotoxicity. *Cancer Treat Rev* 1993, 19:57–77.

12. Shenkenberg TD, Von Hoff DD: Mitoxantrone: A new anticancer drug with significant clinical activity. *Ann Intern Med* 1986, 105:67–81.

13. Steinherz LJ, Steinherz PG: Cyclophosphamide cardiotoxicity. *Cancer Bull* 1985, 37:231.

14. Weiss RB, Grillo-Lopez AJ, Marsoni S, *et al.*: Amsacrine-associated cardiotoxicity: An analysis of 82 patients. *J Clin Oncol* 1986, 4:918–928.

15. Verweij J, Funke-Kupper AJ, Teule GJJ, *et al.*: A prospective study on the dose dependency of cardiotoxicity induced by mitomycin-C. *Med Oncol Tumor Pharmacother* 1988, 5:159–163.

16. Leischke GJ, Maher D, Cebon J, *et al.*: Effect of bacterially synthesized recombinant human granulocyte-macrophage colony stimulating factor in patients with advanced malignancy. *Ann Intern Med* 1989, 110:57–64.

17. LaBianca R, Beratta G, Cleric M, *et al.*: Cardiac toxicity of 5-fluorouracil: A study of 1083 patients. *Tumori* 1982, 68:505–510.

18. Hawkins MJ, Sznol M: The cardiovascular effects of human recombinant cytokines. In Muggia FM, Green MD, Speyer JL (eds): *Cancer Treatment and the Heart.* 1992, Baltimore: Johns Hopkins University Press; 296–328.

CARDIOMYOPATHY

Chemotherapy-induced cardiomyopathy is most frequently caused by the *anthracyclines*. The degree of myocardial damage is related to the cumulative dose of drug a patient has received. The clinical syndrome is one of chronic, low-output cardiac failure, which usually occurs 30 to 60 days after the last dose, although it may occur during treatment or years later. Ideally, this situation should be avoided by preemptive measures: therapy for cardiac failure should include afterload reduction and bed rest. Improvement of symptoms can occur for up to 1 year later; however, some patients experience an inexorable downhill course.

Both *anthracyclines* and *high-dose cyclophosphamide* are rarely associated with an often fatal acute pericarditis–myocarditis syndrome.

MANAGEMENT OR INTERVENTION

1. Prevention
   a. Identify and monitor patients at risk
   b. Administer by prolonged infusion (rather than bolus) every 3–4 weeks
   c. Use less cardiotoxic analogues—*eg*, epirubicin
   d. Cease therapy once predetermined dose reached, beyond which there is an unacceptable risk for CHF (doxorubicin: 500 mg/m^2 [5% chance CHF], epirubicin: 900 mg/m^2 [5% chance CHF])
   e. Coadminister cardioprotective agent—dexrazoxane IV 30 min prior to doxorubicin; ratio of dexrazoxane to doxorubicin should be 10–20:1 (*eg*, dexrazoxane 500–1000 mg/m^2 with standard doxorubicin 50 mg/m^2)
2. Treat cardiac failure
   a. Treat aggravating factors (sepsis, electrolytes, renal failure, anemia, arrhythmias)
   b. Reduce afterload (*eg*, ACE inhibitor)
   c. Restrict fluid intake
   d. Recommend bed rest

TOXICITY GRADING

0	1	2	3	4
None	Asymptomatic, decline of resting ejection fraction by < 20% of baseline value	Asymptomatic, decline of resting ejection fraction by < 20% of baseline value	Mild CHF, responsive to therapy	Severe or refractory CHF

CAUSATIVE AGENTS
Anthracyclines: daunorubicin, doxorubicin, epirubicin, idarubicin; **anthracenediones:** mitoxantrone; **others:** high-dose cyclophosphamide, amsacrine, mitomycin C, interleukin-2 ± LAK cells

PATHOLOGIC PROCESS
Anthracycline-Fe^{3+} complex initiates oxygen–free radical formation, leading to lipid peroxidation of mitochondrial membrane and sarcoplasmic reticulum with resultant myocyte degeneration and fibrosis; or the anthracycline-Fe^{3+} complex itself may act as an oxidant

DIFFERENTIAL DIAGNOSES
Preexisting cardiac disease, pulmonary embolism, infective heart disease in immunosuppressed patients (endocarditis/myocarditis), radiation-induced cardiomyopathy

PATIENT ASSESSMENT
Baseline assessment: clinical history and examination, chest x-ray, EKG, LVEF—radionuclide-gated cardiac scan; **identify risk factors:** pre-existing heart disease, peripheral vascular disease, smoker, family history, hypertension, prior thoracic radiation, potential future thoracic radiation (*eg*, Hodgkin's disease), small cell lung cancer, prior anthracyclines, age—especially children < 4 yr; **monitoring** (for doxorubicin, but same general policy holds for other anthracyclines): serial cardiac scans; if baseline LVEF ≥ 50%, determine again only if further anthracycline or potentially cardiotoxic treatment (*eg*, thoracic radiation) planned—if no risk factors, repeat after 500 mg/m^2, if risk factors, repeat after 350–400 mg/m^2, repeat after each subsequent dose, cease if LVEF changes by ≥ 10% or < 50%; if baseline LVEF is 30–50%, repeat LVEF after each dose, consider stress testing to assess for cardiac reserve; if **cardiac failure:** assess severity grade according to New York Heart Association or World Health Organization (WHO), check for aggravating factors (sepsis, urea and electrolytes, BUN, hemoglobin)

EXACERBATION OF ISCHEMIC HEART DISEASE

Up to 1.5% of patients receiving 5-FU experience ischemic chest pain or myocardial infarction (or even cardiac arrest), although a number of up to 4.5% has been reported in patients with underlying ischemic heart disease or in those who have previous exposure to anthracyclines. The most likely mechanism is coronary artery spasm.

MANAGEMENT OR INTERVENTION

1. Prescribe nitrates
2. Administer calcium blockers
3. Alter schedule to weekly administration

TOXICITY GRADING

0	1	2	3	4
None	Nonspecific T-wave flattening	Asymptomatic, ST- and T-wave changes suggesting ischemia	Angina without evidence for infarction	Acute myocardial infarction

CAUSATIVE AGENTS

5-FU; anthracyclines; vincristine, vinblastine, vindesine; interleukin-2, interferons alpha and gamma; amsacrine, etoposide

PATHOLOGIC PROCESS

Coronary artery spasm, ?hypotension (biologic response modifiers)

DIFFERENTIAL DIAGNOSES

Underlying heart disease—atheroma, valvular; pericarditis; pleuritic pain—tumor, pulmonary embolism, musculoskeletal; esophageal pain—esophagitis, spasm; anxiety; other

PATIENT ASSESSMENT

Baseline assessment: clinical history and examination, chest x-ray, EKG, LVEF—radionuclide-gated cardiac scan; **identify risk factors**: pre-existing heart disease, peripheral vascular disease, smoker, family history, hypertension, prior thoracic radiation, potential future thoracic radiation (*eg*, Hodgkin's disease), small cell lung cancer, prior anthracyclines, age—especially children < 4 yr, check for aggravating factors (sepsis, urea and electrolytes, BUN, hemoglobin)

Many cancer treatments are associated with neurotoxicity. The more common drugs and agents producing neurotoxic effects are listed in Table 1. In many instances, neurotoxicity has become the dose-limiting toxicity. The incidence of chemotherapy-associated neurotoxicity is increasing. This is due to several factors that paradoxically are the consequence of improvements in the treatments of patients with cancer.

Improvements in supportive care permit the use of higher doses of chemotherapy, thereby increasing the exposure of drug to the nervous system. For example, the use of colony-stimulating factors, such as G-CSF and GM-CSF, has allowed a marked escalation in the doses used for several chemotherapy agents while reducing the severity of leukopenia. The dose-limiting toxicity of taxol is no longer myelosuppression; instead, with the use of colony-stimulating factors, peripheral neuropathy has become the major toxicity [1].

Increasing lengths of survival with improvements in treatment of systemic malignancy allow toxicity with a long latency to become manifest. Methotrexate-induced leukoencephalopathy, noted months to years after prophylactic treatment of the central nervous system of children with acute lymphocytic leukemia, was first seen when the development of new treatment regimens induced long-term remissions and cures [2,3].

Development of new therapeutic agents that cross the blood–brain and blood–nerve barriers increases exposure of the nervous system to the drug. Spiromustine, an experimental agent, is specifically designed to treat tumors in the brain. The drug is a combination of a phenytoin moiety, which readily crosses the blood–brain barrier, and a nitrogen mustard. Preclinical testing was promising, but initial clinical testing was stopped because of development of severe encephalopathy, a result of the rapid penetration of the drug into the brain [4].

NEUROLOGIC SYNDROMES ASSOCIATED WITH CHEMOTHERAPY

Cognitive Dysfunction (Dementia)

Dementia and encephalopathy are common neurotoxic effects of chemotherapy. However, there are many other treatable causes that

Table 1. Neurotoxic Effects of Chemotherapeutic Agents

Agent	Class	Neurotoxicity	Comments
Methotrexate	Antimetabolite	Acute somnolence, chronic leukoencephalopathy, mineralizing microangiopathy, myelopathy from intrathecal injection	Acute syndrome may be helped with folinic acid; CSF elevated during early stages of myelopathy
Cytosine arabinoside	Antimetabolite	Irreversible cerebellar syndrome, chronic leukoencephalopathy, myelopathy with intrathecal injection	Purkinje cell destruction seen with cerebellar dysfunction; synergy with methotrexate in myelopathy
Cisplatin	Nonclassic alkylating agent	Predominantly large fiber sensory polyneuropathy; hearing loss, tinnitus; possible optic neuropathy, retinal cone dysfunction	New agents (Org 2766, WR2721) may help prevent neuropathy; hearing loss generally irreversible
Vincristine	Vinca alkaloid, microtubule depolymerizer	Sensorimotor polyneuropathy, autonomic neuropathy, cranial neuropathy, SIADH, possible encephalopathy, myositis	Toxicity worse with underlying neuropathy; GI dysmotility after treatment indicates severe toxicity (no more vincristine should be given)
5-Fluorouracil	Antimetabolite	Cerebellar dysfunction, transient confusion and disorientation, Wernicke–Korsakoff-like syndrome, optic neuropathy, parkinsonism (rare)	Cerebellar signs partially reversible; confusion and other toxicity possibly related to effect on normal thiamine metabolism
Cyclophosphamide	Alkylating agent	SIADH	SIADH seen with large-dose treatment
Ifosfamide	Alkylating agent	Reversible encephalopathy; extrapyramidal signs: athetosis, myoclonus, opisthotonic posturing	Frequent (20% of patients); low serum albumin, elevated creatinine, pelvic tumor, and prior cisplatin treatment are risk factors
L-Asparaginase	Antimetabolite	Organic brain syndrome with psychosis, depression, intracranial hemorrhage and thrombosis, seizures, hyperglycemia	Organic brain syndrome may result from reduced L-asparagine and L-glutamine, altering clotting mechanisms; controversial treatment; fresh frozen plasma (FFP) vs FFP + heparin vs FFP + antithrombin III
BCNU, CCNU	Nitrosoureas, alkylating agents	Necrotizing encephalopathy with intra-arterial injection, retinal toxicity with common carotid injection	Focal brain necrosis probably secondary to streaming phenomenon; minimal neurotoxicity with IV injection
Procarbazine	Alkylating agent	Peripheral neuropathy, encephalopathy with large dose	Penetrates blood-brain barrier; has monoamine oxidase properties
Interferon	Biologic response modifier	Encephalopathy, progressive vegetative state with intraventricular injection, parkinsonism with intraventricular injection, hearing loss	May cause diffuse cerebral edema; some patients have persistent cognitive deficits after systemic treatment
Paclitaxel	Tubulin polymerizer	Peripheral neuropathy, autonomic neuropathy, seizures (rare)	Neuropathy is predominantly sensory with rapid onset
Misonidazole, metronidazole	Radiosensitizers	Peripheral neuropathy	Dose-limiting neuropathy

From Gilbert, Freimer [38]; with permission.

must be considered first in patients with cancer. Metabolic derangements are by far the most common causes of altered mental status in cancer patients [5]. Hepatic and renal dysfunction, electrolyte imbalance, seizures, and hypoxia are among the treatable causes. Furthermore, both systemic and central nervous system infections (encephalitis, meningitis) can result in encephalopathy. In all patients with acute or subacute onset of encephalopathy, a complete evaluation must be undertaken before the diagnosis of chemotherapy-induced neurotoxicity is made.

Chronic dementia is a common consequence of both intrathecal chemotherapy and cranial radiotherapy. The combination of both treatment modalities, particularly if the chemotherapy succeeds the radiotherapy, markedly increases the risk of toxicity. Patients usually begin to exhibit loss of cognitive function 1 to 2 years after completion of treatment [2,3,6,7]. There is often a progressive loss of function and some patients develop intractable seizures or coma. Microvascular changes and large areas of demyelination are the pathologic hallmarks of this toxicity; hence the name leukoencephalopathy has been given to this syndrome [8–10]. Methotrexate, cytosine arabinoside, thiotepa, and intra-arterial carmustine can cause leukoencephalopathy, an irreversible, progressive dementia [11–14]. Although high-dose systemic administration of methotrexate, cytosine arabinoside, and thiotepa can cause leukoencephalopathy, intrathecal administration of these agents is more likely to cause this toxicity. Leukoencephalopathy has also been reported with high-dose intravenous treatment, intra-arterial (cranial arteries) administration, and biologic response modifiers.

Methotrexate in high-dose intravenous administration can cause a transient, reversible encephalopathy [15]. In addition, transient encephalopathy that develops in close temporal relationship to chemotherapy administration has been reported with L-asparaginase, levamisole, vincristine, ifosfamide, procarbazine, interferon, and interleukin [16–19]. These reactions are generally thought to be idiosyncratic, although caution should be used if retreatment is considered.

Encephalopathy can also result from chemotherapy-induced metabolic abnormalities, such as hyperglycemia associated with corticosteroids, L-asparaginase, or streptozocin; hyponatremia from vincristine or cyclophosphamide treatment (inappropriate antidiuretic hormone secretion); or hyponatremia from a salt-wasting nephropathy from cisplatin. The treatment of these "secondary" effects of chemotherapy is focused on correcting the underlying problem. Future treatment with the same drugs is often possible, but reoccurrence of the metabolic derangement is likely.

Seizures

The differential diagnosis of seizures in patients with cancer is extensive. Structural lesions such as brain metastases, carcinomatous meningitis, infectious meningitis, dural metastases, and cerebrovascular events commonly cause seizures. Metabolic abnormalities, such as hypoxia, hyponatremia, hypomagnesemia, and hypoglycemia can also result in seizures.

Generalized tonic-clonic seizures suggest a global process, particularly when associated with encephalopathy. Hypoglycemia, however, may present with focal neurologic deficits, which rapidly clear with glucose administration.

Focal seizures occur when the cerebrum suffers structural damage. Chemotherapy-related causes of focal brain lesions include methotrexate-induced leukoencephalopathy causing focal necrosis; L-asparaginase-induced coagulopathy causing regional

ischemia and stroke [20]; and cisplatin-induced vasospasm and transient ischemia [21].

Cerebellar Dysfunction

Cerebellar dysfunction in patients with cancer is most commonly seen with metastatic spread to the cerebellum or brainstem. Meningeal carcinoma will occasionally cause cerebellar signs by infiltrating cerebellar pathways. Structural cerebellar lesions often show asymmetric dysfunction, which may be useful in differentiating this from drug-induced cerebellar toxicity.

Cytosine arabinoside and 5-fluorouracil can cause cerebellar toxicity from specific, irreversible damage to the cerebellar Purkinje cells, resulting in truncal ataxia, unsteady gait, dysarthria, and nystagmus [22–24]. The dysfunction is generally symmetric. MR imaging is normal acutely, but cerebellar atrophy is often detected on MR imaging months later.

Cranial Neuropathy

Cranial neuropathy in cancer patients most commonly indicates meningeal carcinoma, tumor involvement of the bones of the cranial base with encroachment of neural foramina, or rarely, brainstem metastases. Chemotherapy-induced cranial neuropathy is rare. Vincristine can cause cranial nerve palsies; extraocular eye movement abnormalities are most commonly seen [25]. Intraventricular administration of drugs and biologic response modifiers can cause transient cranial nerve palsies, often due to abnormalities in cerebrospinal fluid circulation.

Optic Nerve and Retinal Neuropathy

Optic neuropathy is occasionally seen in patients with meningeal carcinoma with infiltration of the optic nerve. Additionally, compression from cranial base tumors can cause a similar loss of vision. A paraneoplastic syndrome has been described in patients with small cell lung cancer in which optic atrophy is the hallmark feature. Antiretinal antibodies have been found in the serum of these patients. Retinopathy is most commonly associated with intracarotid administration of nitrosoureas and cisplatin [26]. High concentrations of drug flow into the ophthalmic artery, which supplies the retina, causing severe pain and often complete loss of vision. Newer techniques, allowing administration above the ophthalmic artery, have eliminated this local toxicity.

Intravenous cisplatin administration has been associated with optic disc swelling and optic neuropathy. This is an idiosyncratic reaction and the mechanism is not known [27].

Spinal Cord Toxicity

The most common cause of spinal cord dysfunction in patients is epidural cord compression, either from direct extension from bone metastases or from paravertebral spread through the intervertebral foramina. Lumbar intrathecal administration of methotrexate and cytosine arabinoside can cause focal myelopathy [28,29]. Symptoms appear hours to days after treatment and include sensory loss, upper and lower motor neuron dysfunction, radiating pain (similar to Lhermittes' syndrome), and bowel and bladder incontinence. The myelopathy may be transient or progressive; complete, irreversible paraplegia is usually seen with progressive dysfunction.

Peripheral Neuropathy

Peripheral neuropathy occurs frequently in patients with cancer (estimated 10–20% of patients). Paraneoplastic sensorimotor neuropathy and cachexia-associated neuropathy are the most common causes. Other important causes include extrapment neuropathy associated with cachexia and meningeal carcinoma. Several chemotherapy agents cause a dose-related peripheral neuropathy.

Vincristine causes disruption of microtubules, thus affecting both small and large peripheral nerve fibers [30]. Small caliber nerve fibers are more severely affected resulting in a stocking-glove neuropathy. Vincristine also causes autonomic neuropathy, presenting as orthostatic hypotension or intestinal dysmotility [25].

Cisplatin causes aggregation of neurofilaments, therefore large caliber nerve fibers are more severely involved. Hence, sensory loss in cisplatin neuropathy is characterized by loss of vibration and proprioceptive function. Cisplatin occasionally causes autonomic neuropathy [31].

Taxol promotes microtubule polymerization and aggregation, causing a mixed sensory motor neuropathy similar to that seen with vincristine [1]. Procarbazine causes a stocking-glove sensory motor polyneuropathy; autonomic neuropathy has also been described with this drug [32]. Misomidazole and metronidazole (radiation sensitizers) cause dose-limiting peripheral neuropathy [33].

Myopathy

Myopathy is a rare symptom in cancer. When it does occur, it usually is a consequence of treatment. Although rare, myopathy has been described in association with taxol and vincristine [34]. Signs and symptoms suggest a myositis with these drugs. Interferon and other biologic agents can cause myalgias but show no evidence of producing muscular dysfunction or breakdown. Cisplatin, as well as other agents that cause electrolyte abnormalities (*eg*, hypomagnesemia), can produce muscle cramping.

PREVENTATIVE MANAGEMENT

Effective treatment is not available for most neurotoxicities. Therefore, optimal management includes strategies to prevent these toxicities from developing.

Observation and Early Cessation

Comprehensive observation and monitoring of patients who are at risk of developing neurotoxicity, with early cessation of treatment, may reduce the severity of the toxicity. For example, systemic vincristine administration is known to produce fatal neurotoxicity on rare occasions by causing intestinal dysmotility. Patients with gastrointestinal symptoms who are taking this drug should be closely monitored and may require cessation of treatment.

Lumbar administration of chemotherapy can result in a progressive, often irreversible, myelopathy. Patients often complain of radicular back pain, or Lhermittes' sign, early in the course of chemotherapy-induced myelopathy. Early toxicity is confirmed by an elevated CSF level of myelin basic protein [35].

Optimal Scheduling of Therapy

An optimal treatment schedule should be devised to reduce synergistic neurotoxicity. Leukoencephalopathy is a more frequent occurrence when intrathecal chemotherapy is administered after radiation treatment to the brain or spinal cord. Therefore, when possible, intrathecal chemotherapy should be completed before radiation therapy is undertaken [36]. A similar synergy exists when high-dose chemotherapy (*eg*, methotrexate) or chemotherapy that crosses the blood–brain barrier (nitrosoureas) are used after cranial irradiation.

Chemotherapy with similar effects on the nervous system will likely cause more severe neurotoxicity. For example, the combination of taxol and vincristine can cause severe peripheral neuropathy.

It is important to consider pre-existing neurologic dysfunctions when selecting treatment regimens. Patients with pre-existing peripheral neuropathy are at higher risk of developing vincristine-induced gastrointestinal dysfunction than are patients without an underlying neuropathy [36]. Patients with underlying hearing loss will have more profound ototoxicity with cisplatin than patients with normal hearing initially.

Prior to intraventricular chemotherapy administration [111]Indium-DTPA CSF flow studies are required with the tracer injected into the reservoir systems and observation of tracer clearance. Reduced flow of the tracer over the cortical convexities indicates that communicating hydrocephalus is present. Therefore, intraventricular treatment will result in retention of drugs in high concentration in the lateral ventricules, accelerating the development of leukoencephalopathy [37].

Localized back pain associated with lumbar intrathecal chemotherapy administration may indicate early myelopathy and may require the discontinuation of therapy.

PHARMACOLOGIC TREATMENT
Seizures

Most seizures associated with cancer chemotherapy administration are self-limiting, requiring no treatment or short-term treatment with an anticonvulsant. *Phenytoin* is usually the first-line anticonvulsant for chemotherapy-induced seizures. Most patients require a loading dose of 18 mg/kg. If the patient is having frequent seizures, the loading dose should be administered intravenously, at a rate not to exceed 50 mg/min. Continuous ECG monitoring and frequent blood pressure monitoring are mandatory. If cardiac rhythm abnormalities or decreases in blood pressure are noted, the infusion rate should be lowered. Oral loading, dividing the dose over 8 to 12 hours, is not associated with cardiac side effects and is indicated for the patient who is not actively seizing. Daily maintenance doses for adults are generally 300 to 400 mg. Serum levels should be monitored weekly until a suitable dose is determined.

Other anticonvulsants can be administered for chemotherapy-induced seizures but are not as easily used. *Benzodiazepines* are primarily used for status epilepticus. Lorazepam is currently the first-line drug used for status epilepticus. Long-term use of benzodiazepams is generally reserved for unusual seizure disorders. *Phenobarbital* can be administered intravenously, orally, or rectally. In the patient with frequent seizures, intravenous loading (15 mg/kg) can cause severe respiratory depression, requiring intubation and hypotension. Intravenous loading of phenobarbital should only be done in an intensive care unit. Oral loading should be done over several days to reduce the lethargy and somnolence associated with barbiturate use.

Carbamazepine cannot be given as a loading dose and therefore is not useful in status epilepticus, but it is very effective in controlling most seizure types including focal seizures. In general, the patient is started on a low dose (200 mg BID), which is gradually increased over several days. Most patients require 800 to 1000 mg/day for results. Blood levels should be carefully monitored, the first generally 1 week after initiating therapy. A complete blood count, electrolytes and liver function tests should also be obtained 1 week and 1 month after carbamazepine therapy has begun. Carbamazepine can also cause mild myelosuppression and may exacerbate the effects of chemotherapy on bone marrow cells.

Peripheral Neuropathy

Although there are no proven agents to prevent neuropathy, there are strategies to ameliorate the pain that often accompanies the peripheral neuropathy caused by chemotherapy. Most patients note improvement with the use of tricyclic antidepressants, such as nortriptyline and amitriptyline. Both are generally started at 25 mg qhs, gradually increasing the dose over several weeks to a maximum of 100 to 150 mg. This treatment may take several weeks to produce an effect. If tricyclic therapy is not beneficial, the anticonvulsants phenytoin and carbamazepine can occasionally decrease neuropathic pain. The dosing is the same as described for seizures, although rapid intravenous loading of phenytoin is never indicated for the treatment of neuropathy because of the increased risk associated with this method.

REFERENCES

1. Lipton RB, Apfel SC, Dutcher JP, *et al.*: Taxol produces a predominantly sensory neuropathy. *Neurology* 1989, 39:368–373.

2. Price RA, Jamieson PA: The central nervous system in childhood leukemia II. Subacute leukoencephalopathy. *Cancer* 1975, 35:306–318.

3. Bleyer WA: Neurologic sequelae of methotrexate and ionizing radiation: A new classification. *Cancer Treat Rep* 1981, 65(suppl 1):89–98.

4. Pazdur R, Redman BG, Corbett T, *et al.*: Phase I trial of spiromustine (NSC 172112) and evaluation of toxicity and schedule in a murine model. *Cancer Res* 1987, 47:4213–4217.

5. Gilbert MR, Grossman SA: The incidence and nature of neurologic problems in patients with solid tumors. *Am J Med* 1986, 81:951–954.

6. Kay HEM, Knapton PJ, O'Sullivan JP, *et al.*: Encephalopathy in acute leukemia associated with methotrexate therapy. *Arch Dis Child* 1972, 47:344–354.

7. Ch'ien LT, Aur RJA, Stagner S, *et al.*: Progression of methotrexate-induced leukoencephalopathy in children with leukemia. *Med Pediatr Oncol* 1981, 9:133–141.

8. Suzuki K, Takemura T, Okeda R, Hatakeyama S: Vascular changes of methotrexate-related disseminated necrotizing leukoencephalopathy. *Acta Neuropathol* 1984, 65:145–149.

9. Nakazato Y, Ishida Y, Morimatsu M: Disseminated necrotizing leukoencephalopathy. *Acta Pathol Jpn* 1980, 30:659–670.

10. Liu HM, Maurer HS, Vongsvivut S, Conway JJ: Methotrexate leukoencephalopathy. *Human Pathol* 1978, 9:635–648.

11. Nand S, Messmore HL Jr, Patel R, *et al.*: Neurotoxicity associated with systemic high-dose cytosine arabinoside. *J Clin Oncol* 1986, 4:571–575.

12. Barnett MJ, Richards MA, Ganesan TS, *et al.*: Central nervous system toxicity of high-dose cytosine arabinoside. *Semin Oncol* 1985, 12:227–232.

13. Grossman L, Baker MA, Sutton DMC, Deck JHN: Central nervous system toxicity of high-dose cytosine arabinoside. *Med Pediatr Oncol* 1983, 11:246–250.

14. Rosenblum MK, Delattre J-Y, Walker RW, Shapiro WR: Fatal necrotising encephalopathy complicating treatment of malignant gliomas with intra-arterial BCNU and irradiation: A pathological study. *J Neurooncol* 1989, 7:269–281.

15. Walker RW, Allen JC, Rosen G, Caparros B: Transient cerebral dysfunction secondary to high-dose methotrexate. *J Clin Oncol* 1986, 4:1845–1850.

16. Priest JR, Ramsay KC, Steinhrz PG, *et al.*: A syndrome of thrombosis and hemorrhage complicating L-asparaginase therapy for childhood acute lymphoblastic leukemia. *J Pediatr* 1982, 100:984–989.

17. Hook CC, Kimmel DW, Kvols LK, *et al.*: Multifocal inflammatory leukoencephalopathy with 5-fluorouracil and levamisole. *Ann Neurol* 1992, 31:262–267.

18. Somers SS, Reynolds JV, Guillou PJ: Multifocal neurotoxicity during interleukin-2 therapy for malignant melanoma. *Clin Oncol* 1992, 4:135–136.

19. Adams F, Quesada JR, Gutterman JU: Neuropsychiatric manifestations of human leukocyte interferon therapy in patients with cancer. *JAMA* 1984, 252:938–941.

20. Feinberg WM, Swenson MR: Cerebrovascular complications of L-asparaginase therapy. *Neurology* 1988, 38:127–133.

21. Berman IJ, Mann MP: Seizures and transient cortical blindness associated with cis-platinum (II) diamminedichloride (PDD) therapy in a thirty-year-old man. *Cancer* 1980, 45:764–766.

22. Dworkin LA, Goldman RD, Zivin LS, Fuchs SG: Cerebellar toxicity following high-dose cytosine arabinoside. *J Clin Oncol* 1985, 3:613–616.

23. Winkelman MD, Hines JD: Cerebellar degeneration caused by high-dose cytosine arabinoside: A clinicopathological study. *Ann Neurol* 1983, 14:520–527.

24. Moertel CG, Reitemeier RJ, Bolton CF, Shorter RG: Cerebellar ataxia associated with fluorinated pyrimidine therapy. *Cancer Chemother Rep* 1964, 41:15–18.

25. Sandler SG, Tobin W, Henderson ES: Vincristine-induced neuropathy: A clinical study of fifty leukemia patients. *Neurology* 1969, 19:367–374.

26. Defer G, Fanchon F, Schaison M, *et al.*: Visual toxicity following intra-arterial chemotherapy with hydroxyethyl-CNU in patients with malignant glioma. *Neuroradiology* 1991, 33:432–437.

27. Walsh TJ, Clark AW, Parhad IM, Green WR: Neurotoxic effects of cisplatin therapy. *Arch Neurol* 1982, 39:719–720.

28. Brener AL, Pitman SW, Dawson DM, Schoene WC: Paraparesis following intrathecal cytosine arabinoside: A case report with neuropathologic findings. *Cancer* 1977, 40:2871–2822.

29. Galiano RG, Costeinzi JJ: Paraplegia following intrathecal methotrexate: Report of a case and reveiw of the literature. *Cancer* 1976, 37:1663–1668.

30. Sahenk Z, Brady ST, Mendell JR: Studies on the pathogenesis of vincristine-induced neuropathy. *Muscle Nerve* 1987, 10:80–84.

31. Boogerd W, ten Bokkel Huinink WW, Dalesio O, *et al.*: Cisplatin-induced neuropathy: Central, peripheral and autonomin nerve involvement. *J Neurooncol* 1990, 9:255–263.

32. Kaplan RS, Wiernik PH: Neurotoxicity of antineoplastic drugs. *Semin Oncol* 1982, 9:103–130.

33. Rose GP, Dewar AJ, Stratford IJ: A Biochemical neurotoxicity study relating the neurotoxic potential of metronidazole and nitrofurantoin with misonidazole. *Int J Rad Oncol Biol Phys* 1982, 8:781–785.

34. Slotwiner P, Song SK, Anderson PJ: Spheromembranous degeneration of muscle induced by vincristine. *Arch Neurol* 1966, 15:172–176.

35. Clark AW, Cohen SR, Nissenblatt MJ, Wilson SK: Paraplegia following intrathecal chemotherapy. Neuropathologic findings and elevation of myelin basic protein. *Cancer* 1982, 50:42–47.

36. Rosenthal S, Kaufman S: Vincristine neurotoxicity. *Ann Int Med* 1974, 80:733–737.

37. Chamberlain MC, Corey-Bloom J: Leptomeningeal metastases: [111]Indium-DTPA CSF flow studies. *Neurology* 1991, 41:1765–1769.

38. Gilbert MR, Friemer ML: Neurotoxicity of cytoxic agents. In Johnson RT, Griffin JW (eds): *Current Therapy in Neurologic Disease*, 3rd ed. 1993, St. Louis: Mosby-Year Book. pp. 312–316.

ACUTE ENCEPHALOPATHY

Acute encephalopathy has been frequently associated with chemotherapy administration. Acute, reversible encephalopathy is most often caused by high intravenous doses of drugs, particularly methotrexate and cytosine arabinoside. Other agents, such as L-asparaginase, levamisole, vincristine, ifosphamide, procarbazine, interferon, and interleukin can cause temporary cognitive dysfunction, although this is generally thought to be an idiosyncratic reaction. There are no known diagnostic tests; the diagnosis is made after all other structural and metabolic causes of encephalopathy are excluded. For most agents there is no specific treatment other than supportive measures and withholding further treatment. There are some reports of folinic acid (leukovorin) protecting against or reducing the severity of methotrexate-induced encephalopathy. The prognosis in most cases of acute encephalopathy is good, with most patients making a gradual, but complete recovery.

CAUSATIVE FACTORS

Dose-related: methotrexate, cytosine arabinoside, interferon, interleukin; **Idiosyncratic:** L-asparaginase, levamisole, vincristine, ifosfamide procarbazine

PATHOLOGIC PROCESS

Unknown for most agents; animal studies suggest that high-dose methotrexate alters brain metabolism, which is evident by decreased glucose utilization

DIFFERENTIAL DIAGNOSES

Metabolic derangement: hepatic dysfunction, renal dysfunction, hyponatremia, hypomagnesemia, hypernatremia, hypermagnesemia, hypocalcemia, hypercalcemia, hypoxia, hyperamonemia; **Infection:** encephalitis, meningitis, cerebral abscess, systemic infection; **Toxic:** drug-induced (*eg*, narcotic, antidepressant); **Structural CNS lesion:** brain metastases, meningeal carcinoma, cerebrovascular accident, intracranial hemorrhage, subarachnoid hemorrhage; **Seizures**

PATIENT ASSESSMENT

Metabolic survey: electrolytes, serum magnesium and calcium, renal function tests, liver function tests, serum ammonia, arterial blood gas; CT scan or MR imaging of the brain, lumbar puncture, electroencephalogram, toxicology screening

TOXICITY GRADING

0	1	2	3	4
None	Mild somnolence or agitation	Moderate somnolence or agitation	Severe somnolence, agitation, confusion, disorientation, or hallucinations	Coma, seizures, toxic psychosis

CHRONIC DEMENTIA

Progressive loss of cognitive function is often a late treatment complication of cancer in the nervous system. The combination of intrathecal chemotherapy with cranial irradiation is the most common predisposing factor. Intrathecal chemotherapy, especially when it follows cranial radiotherapy, is associated with the highest risk of neurotoxicity. Similar neurotoxicity has been seen with high-dose intravenous chemotherapy and intracarotid intra-arterial chemotherapy. Pathologicially, the lesions are characterized by axonal swelling and loss of myelin, with a predilection for the white matter, hence the name leukoencephalopathy. Narrowing and calcification of small blood vessels, a calcific angiitis, have also been reported in association with this syndrome.

The first signs of cognitive loss are generally noted 1 to 2 years after treatment. MR scans of the brain show attenuation of signal in white matter, which is best visualized on T2 images. Prognosis for patients with significant cognitive loss is poor, with little chance of recovery; some patients progress to intractable seizures, coma, or death. Other patients show only mild loss of intellect, often detectable only by sophisticated cognitive function testing.

INTERVENTIONS

There is no known treatment for leukoencephalopathy, but several measures can be taken to reduce the risk of its development.

1. Intrathecal chemotherapy should be administered prior to cranial irradiation.
2. When an Ommaya reservoir or other intraventricular catheter is used for injection of chemotherapy, a [111]Indium-labeled albumin scan should be obtained. The tracer is injected into the lateral ventricle, using the reservoir system. Scans should be obtained at 6, 24, and 48 hr to confirm flow out of the ventricular system and reuptake of tracer along the cortical convexities through the arachnoid granulations into the systemic circulation. Failure of normal flow will greatly increase the exposure of the brain to chemotherapy and accelerate the development of leukoencephalopathy.

CAUSATIVE FACTORS

Intrathecal chemotherapy: methotrexate, cytosine arabinoside, thiotepa; **Intravenous chemotherapy:** methotrexate, cytosine arabinoside, thiotepa; **Intra-arterial chemotherapy:** nitrosoureas (*eg*, BCNU, PCNU), cisplatin

PATHOLOGIC PROCESS

Unknown, although methotrexate has been shown to cause primary axonal damage in an *in vitro* model of the central nervous system

DIFFERENTIAL DIAGNOSES

Structural brain lesions: brain metastases, meningeal carcinoma, indolent infection (chronic meningitis, cerebral abscess), encephalitis (Creutzfeld–Jacob, progressive multifocal leukoencephalopathy, HIV, toxoplasmosis), subdural hematoma, Alzheimer's dementia, multi-infarct dementia; **Chronic nonchemotherapeutic drug toxicity:** narcotics, antidepressants, antiemetics, H_2 blockers; **Metabolic derangements:** renal failure, hepatic failure, chronic hypoxia

PATIENT ASSESSMENT

CT scan or MR imaging of the brain; lumbar puncture; electroencephalogram; toxicology screening; metabolic survey including renal function tests, liver function tests, serum ammonia, arterial blood gas (O_2 saturation)

Over 70% of patients with cancer have moderate-to-severe pain that requires treatment with opiates. There is broad consensus that over 85% of these patients can be well-palliated using knowledge, medications, and techniques that are readily available. Most patients can expect excellent analgesia with conventional oral approaches to pain relief. However, despite the effective therapies available and the obvious need to ensure that patients with serious illnesses be made as comfortable as possible, only a small proportion of patients with cancer pain receive adequate analgesia. At a recent National Cancer Institute Workshop on cancer pain, it was concluded that cancer pain management remains grossly inadequate and little different from what it was two decades ago. As a result, it is important to understand 1) the major obstacles that complicate the delivery of appropriate analgesia, 2) the different types of pain and common pain syndromes in cancer patients, and 3) the appropriate use of available pharmacologic, anesthetic, neurosurgical, and adjunctive treatment approaches.

OBSTACLES TO THE DELIVERY OF APPROPRIATE ANALGESIA

Some explanations for the failure to provide adequate pain relief are patient-related. Because pain is entirely subjective, the patient must communicate its intensity to health care providers before it can be appropriately managed. This communication is often nonexistent or suboptimal because many patients are hesitant to complain, to appear weak or frail, or to divert the physician's attention from the tumor. In addition, many patients are concerned that increasing pain signifies progressive cancer and that discussions with their physician may confirm this. Frequently, patients are reluctant to take opioids fearing addiction, tolerance, and the potential toxicities. These fears can be magnified by the "Just say NO to drugs" mentality that currently prevails.

Health care providers also contribute to inadequate pain treatment for patients with cancer. Physicians and nurses receive little formal instruction on cancer pain during training, appropriate role models in this area are scarce in academic institutions, and textbooks emphasize disease-oriented therapy, often overlooking pain issues. As a result, studies demonstrate that physicians and nurses neglect pain control issues, fail to evaluate the underlying causes of cancer pain, and are overly concerned about the differences between opioid addiction, tolerance, and toxicities (Table 1). They also lack essential

opioid prescribing skills and have little understanding of the intensity of cancer pain in patients [1,2]. In addition, regulatory efforts to control opioid diversion may discourage physicians from prescribing these important drugs.

TYPES OF CANCER PAIN

Recognition of the type of pain experienced by the patient with cancer can help direct the diagnostic evaluation and therapeutic decisions. The three types of cancer pain include 1) *nociceptive pain*, which occurs with the activation of somatic or visceral peripheral nociceptors, 2) *neuropathic pain*, which is a consequence of direct injury to peripheral or central nervous system (CNS) structures, and 3) *sympathetically maintained pain* (SMP), which results from involvement of the sympathetic nervous system (Table 2). Painful bone metastases, which are thought to be mediated through elevated prostaglandin levels in the periosteum, are a common example of somatic nociceptive pain. Visceral nociceptive pain is experienced with organ distension and may be referred to cutaneous sites, confusing the examiner. The burning discomfort or shocklike paroxysms typical of a brachial plexopathy are characteristic of neuropathic pain. This pain does not respond readily to opioids, but agents that affect spontaneous discharges in nerves may be useful. SMP, which is much less prevalent than nociceptive or neuropathic pain in patients with cancer, is characterized by a burning quality, allodynia, hyperpathia, brawny edema, and osteoporosis. Prompt sympathetic blockade and physical therapy are critical to successful SMP management.

CAUSES OF CANCER PAIN

Pain in patients with cancer may occur as a result of direct tumor involvement, diagnostic tests, antineoplastic therapy, or illnesses that are unrelated to the tumor (Table 3). Approximately two thirds of all pain results from tumor involvement of soft tissue, bone, or neural structures. The common chronic cancer pain syndromes are well described in the literature [3–5]. Establishing the cause of pain in patients is critical to optimal pain management and preservation of quality of life. This is especially true in patients with back pain. Over 60% of patients with cancer, back pain, abnormal spine roentgenograms, and completely normal neurologic examinations have epidural metastases on computer tomographic (CT) scan or magnetic resonance imaging (MRI). Epidural metastases may also develop

Table 1. Important Opioid-related Terminology

Physical dependence
  Physiologic response to chronic opioid administration characterized by development of the abstinence syndrome on abrupt withdrawal of opioids
  A potential problem in virtually all patients receiving moderate-to-high doses of opiates
Tolerance
  Normal pharmacologic response to chronic opioid therapy characterized by the development of resistence to analgesic and other effects of the drug
  Overcome by increasing the dose administered
Psychological dependence (addiction)
  Abnormal behavior pattern characterized by an all-consuming desire to obtain opioids for reasons other than pain relief, often occurring at the expense of the patient's physical, social, and environmental well-being
  Extraordinarily rare in patients with cancer pain
  Not to be confused with "pseudo-addiction," which is commonly seen in patients who are undertreated and in pain and are attempting to obtain analgesia

Table 2. Types of Cancer Pain

Nociceptive pain
  Somatic, *eg*, bone metastases
  Visceral, *eg*, organ distention
  Results from activation of somatic or visceral peripheral nociceptors
Neuropathic (deafferentation) pain
  Burning discomfort or shock-like paroxysms (*eg*, brachial plexopathy)
  Resistant to opioid therapy
  Results from a direct injury to peripheral or central nervous system structures
Sympathetically maintained pain
  Burning quality associated with allodynia, hyperpathia, edema, and osteoporosis
  Responds to sympathetic blockade and physical therapy
  Results from involvement of the sympathetic nervous system

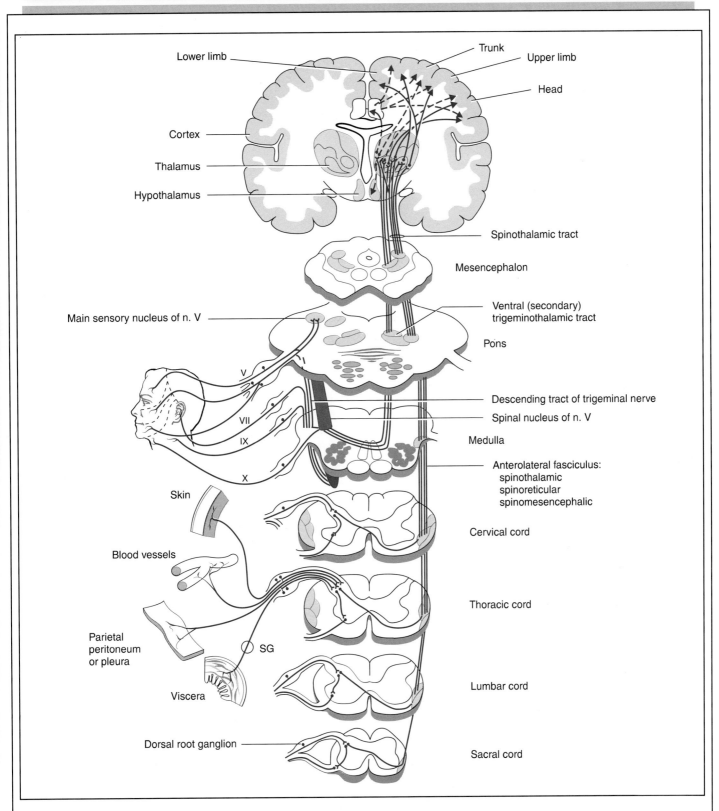

FIGURE 1

Primary neural pathways for transmission of nociceptive information from various body structures to the brain. (*Redrawn from* Bonica [5]; with permission.)

when a paravertebral mass extends through the intervertebral foramina. This can occur without bone destruction. Patients with back pain and undiagnosed, untreated epidural metastases will develop sudden, and usually irreversible, paralysis with loss of bowel and bladder function. Furthermore, pain from epidural metastases is resistant to opioids but usually is dramatically relieved by the administration of glucocorticoids and radiation therapy.

The appropriate treatment of headache in patients with cancer also depends on a precise and timely diagnosis. Herniation and death can result from untreated brain metastases, progressive pain and irreversible cranial nerve palsies occur when metastases to the base of the skull are not suspected, and progressive multifocal neurologic signs and symptoms that result in a rapid demise occur in patients with untreated leptomeningeal metastases. Specific therapy for each of these diagnoses will usually lead to a far superior outcome. Common examples of serious and preventable problems that may develop without careful diagnostic evaluations and appropriate therapy include the development of pathologic fractures in weight-bearing bones and the extension of tumor from painful brachial or lumbar plexus lesions into the epidural space.

Pain can occur as a consequence of antineoplastic therapy. Approximately 10% of women who undergo surgery for breast cancer develop a tight, burning pain in the posterior arm, axilla, or anterior chest immediately or months following surgery. This postmastectomy syndrome must be differentiated from brachial plexus involvement by tumor (rapid progression, Horner's syndrome, involvement of lower plexus), a transient inflammatory plexopathy, radiation fibrosis (less painful, more gradual, and involving the upper plexus), or an injury related to surgical positioning. Postthoracotomy syndromes are also common in this patient population. Radiation therapy and chemotherapy can cause a painful mucositis that responds to opioids. Chemotherapeutic agents, most notably cisplatin and vincristine, can result in a painful peripheral neuropathy. In addition, nearly 10% of patients with cancer have pain from illnesses, such as osteoarthritis, that are entirely unrelated to their neoplasm.

ASSESSMENT

Treatment of the pain should be initiated while the cause of the pain is being evaluated. This allows patients to undergo diagnostic studies more comfortably, provides insight into the sensitivity of the pain to an initial therapeutic trial, and reassures patients that their pain complaints are being seriously addressed. A careful history is essential. Pain intensity should be formally assessed using a validated pain assessment scale, and the results should be recorded serially on a flowsheet in the medical record. This facilitates assessment of the efficacy of therapeutic interventions. A thorough physical examination with emphasis on the neurologic system is crucial. Appropriate laboratory tests are then ordered based on the clinical findings.

MANAGEMENT
Pharmacologic Therapy

Pharmacologic approaches are the primary therapy for most patients with cancer pain as they are usually effective, work rapidly, and are low risk and inexpensive [6–8]. Aspirin, acetaminophen, or another nonsteroidal anti-inflammatory agent (NSAID) should be consid-

Table 3. Common Cancer Pain Syndromes

I. Pain syndromes associated with tumor infiltration
  A. Base of skull
    1. Orbital
    2. Middle fossa
    3. Clivius metastases
    4. Odontoid fracture
    5. Parasagittal
    6. Jugular foramen
    7. Sphenoid sinus metastases
  B. Cranial nerve
    1. Glossopharyngeal neuralgia
    2. Trigeminal neuralgia
  C. Peripheral nerve
    1. Intercostal neuropathy
    2. Peripheral neuropathy
  D. Plexus
    1. Cervical plexopathy
    2. Brachial plexopathy
    3. Lumbosacral plexopathy
  E. Epidural space
    1. Epidural cord dompression
    2. Epidural metastases
  F. Subarachnoid space
    1. Neoplastic meningitis
  G. Intraparenchymal CNS
    1. Brain metastases
    2. Spinal cord metastases
  H. Visceral involvement
    1. Obstruction of hollow viscus or ducts
    2. Rapid growth in solid organs

I. Other
  1. Vascular compromise
  2. Necrosis or ulceration of mucous membrane
  3. Pleural/pericardial involvement

II. Pain syndromes associated with cancer therapy
  A. Post-surgical pain syndromes
    1. Postmastectomy
    2. Post-thoracotomy
    3. Post-radical neck dissection
    4. Phantom limb and stump pain
  B. Postradiation pain syndromes
    1. Fibrosis or brachial or lumbosacral plexus
    2. Acute radiation dermatitis or mucositis
    3. Radiation-induced peripheral nerve tumors
    4. Radiation myelopathy
  C. Postchemotherapy pain syndromes
    1. Peripheral neuropathy
    2. Steroid pseudorheumatism
    3. Mucositis
  D. Acute herpetic and postherpetic neuralgia

III. Examples of common pain syndromes unrelated to cancer
  A. Lumbar or cervical disk disease
  B. Migraine

Table 4. Non-opioid Analgesics for Mild Pain

Drug	Initial dose (mg)	Maximum daily dose (mg)	Comments*
Acetaminophen	650, q 6 h	6000	Not anti-inflammatory; hepatotoxicity at high doses; no effect on platelet aggregation; no GI toxicity
Aspirin	650, q 6 h	6000	GI intolerance common, platlet disaggregation
Choline magnesium trisalicylate	500, q 12 h	3000	No platelet effect, fewer GI effects than other NSAIDs
Salsalate	500, q 12 h	3000	
Ibuprofen	600, q 6 h	4200	Available over-the-counter
Naproxen	250, bid	500	Twice daily dosing
Indomethacin	25, tid	200	Available in sustained-release and suppository forms, but has higher incidence of side effects
Piroxicam	20, q d	40	Once daily dosing, but high incidence of GI effects if given chronically
Ketorolac	30, q 6 h	120	Parental form available; no studies in treating chronic pain

*These agent are effective in bone and musculoskelatal pain. In addition, tolerance, physical dependence, and addiction are not issues in their use. Their major disadvantages include a ceiling effect to analgesia, known platelet and GI toxicities, and a lack of effectiveness in most severe pain syndromes.

ered for mild-to-moderate pain (Table 4). If pain persists, the addition of codeine, oxycodone, or hydrocodone will frequently provide pain relief (Table 5). For persistent or severe pain, the codeine (or its congener) is replaced by a potent opioid such as morphine (see Table 8). For unknown reasons, patients frequently tolerate one NSAID or opioid much better than another. Thus, drug substitution should be attempted before abandoning an entire class of agents.

The vast majority of patients can be managed with oral opioids, which are much more convenient and far less costly for patients. These are best given "around the clock," in an effort to keep pain under control rather than attempting to intermittently treat excruciating pain. Although tolerance to these agents occurs, tumor progres-

sion is the most common reason for increasing opioid requirements. If tolerance becomes a clinical problem, the doses of these drugs can be increased as sedation and respiratory depression become less of a factor in management. Addiction is extremely rare in patients with cancer taking opiates for pain relief. Constipation should be anticipated and treated prophylactically. Other opioid side effects can be managed without excessive difficulty (Table 6).

Adjuvant drugs to manage pain can be extremely helpful (Table 7). Steroids are effective anti-inflammatory agents and reduce the edema

Table 5. Weak Opioids for Moderate Pain

Drug	Route	Equianal-gesic dose (mg)*	Peak effect (hr)	Duration of effect (hr)	Comments
Codeine	PO	200	0.5	3–6	Ceiling for analgesia reached at doses > 240 mg/d PO; metabolized to morphine
	IV, IM	130	0.5	3–6	
Oxycodone	PO	30	0.5	3–6	Parental formulation not available
Hydrocodone	PO	NA	0.5	4–6	Only available as fixed combination with acetaminophen or aspirin
Propoxyphene	PO	NA	1.0	4–6	100 mg napsylate = 65 mg hydrochloride salt
Pentazocine	PO	NA	2.0	3	Oral form also available in combination with naloxone; not recommended for treatment of cancer pain
	IV		0.25	1	

*Approximate potency relative to 10 mg of parental morphine.

Table 6. Opioid Toxicities and Their Management

Side effect	Management	Specific agents
Constipation	Begin bowel program when initiating therapy; combinations of agents may be useful	Stool softeners Irritants Bulk laxatives Lubricants Enemas
Nausea and vomiting	Treat with antiemetics (esp. phenothiazine and anticholinergic agents); switch to another opiate	Promethazine Prochlorperazine Scopolamine Hydroxyzine
Sedation	Use of stimulants	Dextramphetamine Methylphenidate
Pruritis	Treat with antihistamines; consider another opiate, but avoid morphine	Hydroxyzine Diphenhydramine
Myoclonus	Switch to another opiate or lower dose; avoid meperidine, especially in patients with impaired renal function	
Withdrawal symptoms	Taper dose by 50% every other day when discontinuing	Clonidine

Table 7. Important Adjuvant Pain Medications

Drugs	Initial oral dose (mg)	Indication for use	Comments
Antipsychotics			
Halperidol	2, q 6 h	Delirium, agitation, neuropathic pain	Little available data of efficacy for pain relief
Chlorpromazine	10, q 6 h		
Tricyclic antidepressants			
Imipramine	75, qhs	Burning, deafferentation pain, pain complicated by insomnia or depression	Pain relief not seen for 7–10 days after initiating therapy; monitor serum levels
Amitriptyline	75, qhs		
Desipramine	25, tid		
Doxepin	10, tid		
Anticonvulsants			
Carbamazepine	100, bid	Lancinating neuropathic, postherpetic, or phantom limb pain	Monitor serum levels; dose titration may be necessary
Phenytoin	100, tid		
Benzodiazepines			
Clonazepam	0.5, bid	Muscle relaxation, neuropathic pain	Avoid abrupt withdrawal; other benzodiazepines are not indicated for neuropathic pain
Phenothiazines			
Methotrimeprazine	10, q 4–6 h*	Only methotrimeprazine is an analgesic	Avoid promazine and prochlorperazine—may be antianalgesic
Steroids			
Dexamethasone	20 × 1, then q 6 h	Pain due to tumor infiltration of neural structures, bone pain, cord compression	Higher doses may be needed for cord compression

*IV dose recommended since not available in oral formulation.

associated with brain and epidural metastases. Antidepressants may elevate mood, help with insomnia, and alleviate neuropathic pain. Some anxiolytic agents are indicated in select patients and may potentiate the effect of opiates. Anticonvulsants, such as carbamazepine and phenytoin, may be effective against neuropathic pain, and amphetamines can decrease opioid-induced sedation. Caution must be exercised in the use of adjuvant drugs with sedative properties, as the dose of opioids, which are the mainstay of therapy, should not be compromised by the toxicities of these secondary agents.

Patients who present with severe pain should be treated aggressively with analgesics (Table 8). In general, short-acting opioids should be used to permit rapid oral or intravenous dose escalations.

In patients with a normal mental status examination, patient-controlled analgesia can be very useful to titrate opioid doses and balance drug toxicities. Serial pain intensity measurements should be used to judge the efficacy of analgesic therapy. Once the pain is well-controlled, opiate requirements frequently drop significantly even without other intervention. It may then be appropriate to convert the patient to a standard or controlled release oral preparation using a narcotic equivalency table (Table 9). Patients with substantial pain who are unable to take oral medications may benefit from parenteral infusions or transdermal opioids. Long-term rectal or repeated subcutaneous or intramuscular injections are usually unnecessary and unacceptable to patients.

Table 8. Strong Opiates for Severe Cancer Pain

Drug	Route	Equianalgesic dose (mg)*	Peak effect (hr)	Duration of effect (hr)	Comments
Morphine	PO	30–60	1.5–2.0	4–6	Preferred opiate for cancer pain
	PO (SR)	30–60	2.0–3.0	8–12	
	IV, IM	10	0.5–1.0	3–6	
Hydromorphone	PO, PR	7.5	1.0–2.0	3–4	Good choice for SQ due to potency
	IV, IM	1.5	0.5–1.0	3–4	
Meperidine	PO	300	1.0–2.0	3–6	Not preferred due to CNS toxic metabolite that accumulates in renal failure
	IV, IM	75	0.5–1.0	2–3	
Levorphanol	PO	4	1.0–2.0	6–8	Terminal half-life of 11 hr necessitates slow dose titration; drug accumulation may occur
	IV,IM	2	1.0–1.5	6–8	
Fentanyl	TD	0.1 (?)	72	≥ 12	Terminal half-life of < 1 hr makes IV only suitable for continuous infusion: long duration of TD effect makes dose titration difficult
	IV, IM	0.1	< 1.0	0.5–1.0	
Methadone	PO	20	?	4–6	Terminal half-life of 15–150+ hr, but duration of effect is not prolonged; however, drug accumulation can occur making dose titration difficult
	IV, IM	10	0.5–1.5	4–6	
Butorphanol	IN	2	1.0	3–4	Mixed agonist-antagonist may precipitate withdrawal in patient previously receiving a pure agonist; thus not generally recommended for cancer pain
	IV, IM	2	0.5–1.0	3–4	

*Approximate potency relative to 10 mg of parental morphine.
IN—intranasal; SR—sustained release; TD—transdermal.

Table 9. Routes of Administration for Opioid Analgesics

Route of administration	Comments	Cost considerations
Oral	Preferred route for cancer pain management	$ D
Buccal/sublingual	Avoids first pass through the liver; no other advantage over oral; unavailable in US	$ D
Rectal	Available for morphine, oxymorphine and hydromorphone administration, dosing is equivalent to oral, but absorption may be erratic and incomplete	$ D
Transdermal	Available for fentanyl administration; absorption may be affected by subcutaneous fat stores, hypo- or hyperthermia, placement in a radiation port, and ambient temperature; controversial conversion recommendation	$ D
Intranasal	Available for buprenorphine, but not evaluated for management of chronic pain	$ D
Subcutaneous	Bioavailability similar to IV; infection, bleeding, and irritation at injection site may occur	$$$ D,(P),S,Ph,RN,C
Intramuscular	Contraindicated for management of chronic pain	$$ D,S,RN
Intravenous	Indicated only when other routes fail	$$$ D,P,S,Ph,RN,(SF),C
Epidural/intrathecal	May be useful for avoiding systemic side effects of opiates; usually not effective if systemic treatment has failed	$$$$ D,P,S,Ph,RN,SF,C

C—risk of costly complications; D—drug; P—pump rental; Ph—pharmacy services; RN—nursing services; S—supplies (tubing, filters, batteries, tape, heparin); SF—surgical fee; ( )may or may not be necessary. Approximate costs: $—< $500/mo; $$—< $1000/mo; $$$—< $3000/mo; $$$$—< $5000/mo.

Antineoplastic Therapy

As most cancer pain results from tumor invading or compressing normal tissues, if the responsible lesions are reduced in size by antineoplastic therapies, the pain is usually well-palliated. Surgery is particularly effective in relieving pain from intestinal obstruction, pathologic fractures, and obstructive hydrocephalus. Radiation therapy is the treatment of choice for most patients with local pain from tumor progression. It is most frequently administered to patients with symptomatic bone metastases, epidural cord compressions, brachial and lumbar plexus involvement, and brain metastases, and in other situations where local tumor expansion, compression, or infiltration cause pain or ulceration. Certain malignancies respond to chemotherapy with a high (lymphomas, germ cell tumors, leukemias) or moderate (breast, ovarian, small cell lung cancer) degree of certainty. In these neoplasms, chemotherapy may provide substantial tumor regression and pain relief.

Nonpharmacologic Therapy

Nonpharmacologic approaches such as progressive muscle relaxation, massage, guided imagery, biofeedback, and hypnosis have also been found to be useful adjuncts to pain management. Although psychotherapy can be useful for an associated depression, unrelieved pain is reason enough to be depressed, and optimal pain relief, by itself, may result in substantial alleviation of the depression.

Neurostimulatory techniques, such as transcutaneous electrical nerve stimulation (TENS), peripheral nerve stimulation, dorsal column stimulation, and deep brain stimulation, have been used in treating cancer pain. TENS is safe, noninvasive, relatively inexpensive, and easily added to other analgesic approaches. It can provide short-term benefits in patients with cancer and a 2- to 4-week trial will often determine its clinical utility. Peripheral nerve stimulation requires an implanted stimulator and the direct application of an electrode around a peripheral nerve. Because it can be used only in peripheral nerves in the arms or legs and provides short-term benefits, its use in cancer pain is very limited. Dorsal column stimulation is usually performed with an epidural electrode that is introduced

with a Tuohy needle. It may be helpful in mild-to-moderate neuropathic pain. Deep brain stimulation is rarely used as it requires placement of stimulating electrodes into the internal capsule, thalamus, or hypothalamus. It can provide good, but incomplete, pain relief in patients with nociceptive pain, but is ineffective in deafferentation pain.

Regional Analgesics

Injection of local anesthetics or neurolytic agents in or around nerves or nerve roots has been used in patients with cancer for over 75 years. This approach remains a primary treatment modality in many countries where opioids are unavailable. Regional analgesia can be achieved with three types of agents: 1) long-acting local anesthetics (such as bupivacaine), which provide pain relief for 3 to 12 hours, 2) opioids injected into the epidural or subarachnoid space, and 3) neurolytic agents (alcohol or phenol), which produce analgesia that can last for weeks to months (Table 10).

Anesthetic blocks can be used as a diagnostic tool to ascertain the cause of the pain. For example, abdominal visceral pain may be differentiated from abdominal or chest wall discomfort with celiac plexus and intercostal nerve blocks. These techniques can also be useful to predict the efficacy and side effects of neurolytic blocks or neurosurgical operations, allowing the patient to experience temporarily the numbness and other associated symptoms that can result from a permanent procedure. Anesthetic blocks can also be useful on trigger points in patients with myofascial pain syndromes. Local administration of anesthetic agents are occasionally complicated by hypotension, toxic reactions from accidental intravenous or subarachnoid administration, or pneumothorax following needle placement.

Intraspinal opioids produce analgesia without blocking other sensory, motor, or sympathetic functions. The primary benefit of intraspinal administration is the marked reduction in the total daily dose of opioid required to give similar analgesia by the oral or parenteral route. Chronic epidural or intrathecal opioids are invasive, expensive, and usually ineffective in patients requiring high doses of systemic opioids. They can be complicated by tolerance,

Table 10. Regional Anesthetic Techniques for Cancer Pain

Types of blocks	Examples	Indications	Comments
Local anesthetic blocks			
Diagnostic	Intercostal nerve block	Determine cause and response and side effects following local therapies	Analgesic effect is brief
Treatment of sympathetically maintained pain	Stellate ganglion block	Sympathetically maintained pain	Repeated blocks may be needed
Trigger point injections	Trigger point injection	Myofascial pain syndrome	Repeated blocks may be needed
Neurolytic (alcohol or phenol) blocks			
Peripheral	Intercostal nerve block	Chest wall tumor	Pain relief usually lasts several months
Visceral	Celiac plexus block	Pancreatic cancer	Pain relief usually lasts several months
Neuraxial	Epidural intrathecal neurolysis	Pain localized to two or three dermatomes	Pain relief usually lasts several months
Regional opioids			
Epidural	Long-term epidural catheter for infusions	Uncontrolled pain or side effects on systemic therapies; < 3 mo life expectancy	Addition of local anesthetics may be effective in neuropathic pain
Intrathecal	Surgically implanted catheter and pump for infusions	Uncontrolled pain or side effects on systemic therapies; > 3 mo life expectancy	Addition of local anesthetics may be effective in neuropathic pain
Intraventricular	Ommaya reservoir and pump for infusion	Invasive and rarely indicated	Efficacy similar to intrathecal opioids

From Grossman, Staats [6]; with permission.

diffuse pruritus (20% of patients), urinary retention (15%), and nausea and vomiting (20%). Respiratory depression is unusual and is most commonly seen in the postoperative setting. Intrathecal and epidural combinations of opioids and low-dose anesthetics may be more efficacious.

Neurolytic blocks are primarily indicated in patients with localized or regional pain. Subarachnoid and extradural phenol and alcohol destroy nociceptive fibers in the dorsal rootlets simulating a surgical rhizotomy. This can be particularly useful in thoracic pain where few motor effects are noted. However, in cervical and lumbar regions, nearly 20% of patients develop transient motor and/or sphincter dysfunction, which may be permanent in 5% of patients. Celiac plexus blocks can relieve pain originating in the pancreas, stomach, gallbladder, or other upper abdominal viscera. Intercostal blocks are helpful in chest or abdominal wall pain. Less commonly used blocks include Gasserian ganglion neurolysis (advanced cancer pain in the anterior two thirds of the head) and brachial plexus blocks (for patients with preexisting limb paralysis). Because a chemical neuropathy frequently follows neurolytic injections, they are usually reserved for patients with advanced disease.

Neuroablation

Neuroablative procedures are infrequently performed on patients with cancer because of the success of more conservative therapeutic options. Three procedures that are occasionally used are the open unilateral anterolateral cordotomy, the percutaneous cordotomy, and the commissural myelotomy. An open cordotomy is performed through a T2 or T3 laminectomy and produces excellent pain relief in the lower part of the body in 80% of patients. However, this procedure is complicated by a mortality rate of 5 to 10% and significant morbidity in 15% of patients. Hemiparesis, urinary retention, sexual impotence, unmasking pain on the opposite side of the body, and late sensory abnormalities are not infrequent. Bilateral cordotomies are associated with even higher complication rates. Percutaneous cordotomy has a much lower complication rate and provides excellent pain relief. However, pain generally recurs in 50% of patients within 3 months following the procedure. A commissural myelotomy can be considered in select patients with bilateral pelvic and perineal pain. This involves a laminectomy and surgical division of the crossing fibers of the spinal cord. Although it may result in good pain relief with sphincter sparing, there are few neurosurgeons with the extensive expertise necessary to perform this procedure safely.

REFERENCES

1. Grossman SA, Sheidler VR, Swedeen K, *et al*.: Correlations of patient and caregivers ratings of cancer pain. *J Pain Symp Manage* 1991, 6:53–57.

2. Grossman SA: Undertreatment of cancer pain: Barriers and remedies. *Support Care Cancer* 1993, 1:74–78.

3. Portenoy RK: Cancer pain: Epidemiology and syndromes. *Cancer* 1989, 63:2298–2307.

4. Foley KM: The treatment of cancer pain. *New Engl J Med* 1985, 313:84–95.

5. Bonica JJ: The Management of Pain, 2nd ed. 1990, Philadelphia: Lea & Febiger.

6. Grossman SA, Staats PS: The current management of pain in patients with cancer. *Oncology*, in press.

7. Agency for Health Care Policy and Research: Clinical Practice Guidelines: Acute Pain Management: Operative or Medical Procedures and Trauma. AHCPR Publication No. 92-0032, February 1992.

8. Agency for Health Care Policy and Research: Clinical Practice Guidelines: Cancer Pain Management. AHCPR Publication, in press.

CANCER PAIN

The majority of patients with cancer experience some degree of pain that requires management with analgesics, including nonsteroidal anti-inflammatory agents, opioids, and/or regional blocks. Most patients (85%) can expect pain control with conventional oral approaches. However, an appreciation of the obstacles to analgesia delivery and an understanding of the appropriate use of the various approaches to pain treatment are essential to successful management.

MANAGEMENT OR INTERVENTION

1. Pharmacologic approaches
   a. Nonopioid agents (*eg*, aspirin, acetaminophen, NSAIDs) for mild-to-moderate pain
   b. Weak opioids (*eg*, codeine) for moderate, persistent pain
   c. Strong opioids (*eg*, morphine) for severe pain
   d. Adjuvant drugs (*eg*, antidepressants, anticonvulsants) as secondary agents to reduce associated pain syndromes
2. Antineoplastic therapy to reduce size of tumor
   a. Surgery
   b. Radiation
   c. Chemotherapy
3. Nonpharmacologic therapy
   a. Psychotherapy and other suggestive approaches (*eg*, biofeedback, guided imagery, relaxation techniques)
   b. Neurostimulatory techniques (*eg*, TENS)
4. Regional analgesia
   a. Long-acting local anesthetics
   b. Opioids and/or anesthetic agents injected into the epidural or subarachnoid space
   c. Neurolytic agents
5. Neuroablative procedures
   a. Open unilateral anterolateral cordotomy
   b. Percutaneous cordotomy
   c. Commissural myelotomy

CAUSATIVE FACTORS

Tumor infiltration at base of skull, cranial nerve, peripheral nerve, plexus, epidural space, subarachnoid space, intraparenchymal CNS, visceral involvement; **cancer therapy**: postsurgical pain, postradiation pain, post chemotherapy, acute or post-heptic neuralgia; **unrelated to cancer**

PATHOLOGIC PROCESS

Nociceptive pain: results from activation of somatic or visceral peripheral nociceptors; **neuropathic pain**: results from direct injury to peripheral or CNS structures; **sympathetically maintained pain**: results from involvement of the sympathetic nervous system

OBTAINING THE DIAGNOSIS

Determine the cause of the pain to facilitate optimal treatment; treat pain aggressively during evaluation process to ensure patient comfort and optimal work-up

PATIENT ASSESSMENT

History: oncologic issues, current pain problem, prior pain experiences, prior drug reactions and sensitivities, psychiatric illness, substance abuse, therapeutic goals; pain assessment: use validated pain intensity scale, record results on flowsheet; physical examination: complete exam required with special attention to neurologic system; selected laboratory studies: blood tests, radiographs, bone scan, CT scan or MR imaging (brain, spine, chest, abdomen, pelvis, brachial plexus), myelography, lumbar puncture, EMG, nerve conduction tests

PAIN INTENSITY ASSESSMENT TOOLS

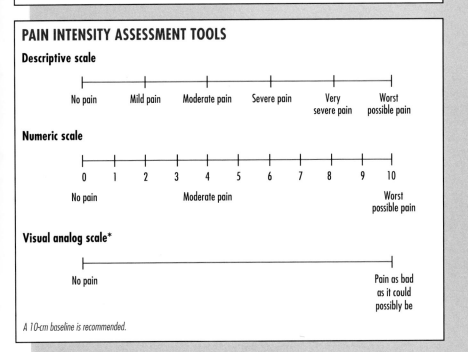

Descriptive scale

No pain — Mild pain — Moderate pain — Severe pain — Very severe pain — Worst possible pain

Numeric scale

0 1 2 3 4 5 6 7 8 9 10
No pain — Moderate pain — Worst possible pain

Visual analog scale*

No pain — Pain as bad as it could possibly be

A 10-cm baseline is recommended.

Cutaneous manifestations in cancer patients present a diagnostic and therapeutic challenge. Skin lesions may represent a direct toxic effect of an antineoplastic agent, an allergic reaction to an antibiotic, a manifestation of bone marrow toxicity, a sign of sepsis or underlying opportunistic infection, or an unrelated skin disease. Mucocutaneous complications of chemotherapy and biologic response modifiers (colony-stimulating factors, interferons, interleukins, etc.) are variable in presentation. While some skin manifestations are benign and self-limited, others can be life-threatening. This chapter provides a practical approach to the diagnosis and management of patients who have selected mucocutaneous manifestations of chemotherapy and biologic response modifiers (BRMs).

CUTANEOUS REACTION PATTERNS

TOXIC ERYTHEMA

In toxic erythema, vasodilation of the dermal vasculature occurs. It is usually associated with dermal edema. Scaling and serous crusting may be present, depending on the extent and duration of the reaction and its effects on epidermal integrity. Vasodilation is usually blanchable with pressure. Lack of complete blanchability may represent erythrocyte extravasation. Numerous chemotherapeutic agents and biological response modifiers are capable of inducing toxic erythema

[1–3] (Table 1). The condition is believed to be induced by direct injury to the superficial dermal microvasculature.

The differential diagnoses and management of the toxic erythema are presented in Tables 2 and 3.

Generalized Erythema
Generalized Toxic Erythema

Generalized toxic erythema is a reaction pattern characterized by generalized redness and edema. Fever and lymphadenopathy may be associated with the condition. This reaction pattern begins as a diffuse papular erythema, with extension to confluence, usually over 12 to 48 hours. This initial stage is often followed by desquamation 2 to 6 days later. The mucous membranes are usually spared.

Toxic Epidermal Necrolysis

Toxic epidermal necrolysis (TEN) is a potentially life-threatening condition characterized by erythema and tenderness of the skin and mucous membranes followed within days by epidermal necrosis exposing the unprotected "raw" superficial dermis. This reaction pattern most often is drug-induced. Other etiologic considerations, particularly in the oncologic setting, include sepsis, leukemia, graft-versus-host disease, and lymphoma. The mortality rate of TEN approaches 20 to 30%, with morbid complications related to fluid and electrolyte imbalance, gastrointestinal hemorrhage, and bacterial or fungal sepsis. The tumor antibiotic mithramycin has been associated with TEN [4].

Table 1. Chemotherapy and Biologic Response Modifiers that Induce Toxic Erythema

Generalized	Acral	Infusion and injection site	Pressure point	Neutrophilic eccrine hidradenitis	Mucositis
Broxuridine	Ara-C*	*Linear erythema*	Bleomycin	Bleomycin*	Actinomycin D
Cyclosporin A	combination—ara-C plus	Broxuridine	Methotrexate	Ara-C*	Bleomycin
GM-CSF	doxorubicin plus	Doxorubicin (approx 3%)†		combination—bleomycin plus	Busulfan
IFNß	vincristine	IL-2		doxorubicin plus dacarbazine	Ara-C
IL-2	Bleomycin	IL-2 + LAK cells		plus vincristine	Cyclophosphamide
IL-2 + TIL	Cyclophosphamide	IL-2 + TIL			5-Fluorouracil
IL-2 + LAK cells	Doxorubicin	TNF			Daunomycin
	5-Fluorouracil				Daunorubicin
Toxic epidermal necrosis	Hydroxyurea	*Toxic chemical phlebitis*			Doxorubicin
Mithramycin	Methotrexate	BCNU			Methotrexate
	Mitotane	Daunomycin			IL-2 + LAK cells
	Combination:—6-mercap-	Doxorubicin			IL-2 + TIL
	topurine and allopurinol	5-Fluorouracil			IL-2 + LAK + TIL
		Mechlorethamine			
		Thrombophlebitis			
		Acidinylanside			
		BCNU			
		Dacarbazine			
		GM-CSF			
		Mechlorethamine			
		Erythema, edema, and pain			
		IL-2			
		IL-3			
		TNF/IFN δ			
		GM-CSF			

*Most common agents.
† Adriamycin flare.
Ara-C—cytosine arabinoside; GM-CSF—granulocyte-monocyte–colony-stimulating factor; IFN—interferon; IL-2—interleukin-2; LAK—lymphocyte activated killer; TIL—tumor infiltrating lymphocytes; TNF—tumor necrosis factor.

Table 2. Differential Diagnoses of Toxic Erythema

Generalized toxic erythema	Toxic epidermal necrolysis	Acral erythema	Infusion and injection site erythema	Pressure point erythema and erosions	Neutrophilic eccrine hidradenitis	Mucositis
Exfoliative dermatitis-drug reactions Allopurinol, barbiturates, NSAIDs, penicillins, sulfonamides, phenytoin	*Drug reactions** Antibiotics, barbiturates, phenylbutazone, phenytoin, sulfonamides, sulfones	*Bacterial cellulitis* *Bone marrow transplantation* *Erythema multiforme*	Cellulitis Extravasation injury	Pressure blisters Decubitus ulcers Friction blisters	Bacterial sepsis Disseminated fungal infection Erythema multiforme	*Infections* Bacterial, candida, fungal, viral
Exofilative dermatitis secondary to dermatoses Atopic dermatitis, contact dermatitis, pityriasis, rubra, pilaris, psoriasis	*Idiopathic* Bacterial infections (clostridium, *Escheria coli*, klebsiella, pseudomonas, streptococcus, fungal (aspergillus), viral (hepatitis A, herpes simplex/zoster, varicella)	*Erythromelalgia* CML, myelofibrosis, polycythemia vera, thrombocytopenia, medications (nifedipine, nicardipine, bromocriptine) SLE, idiopathic			Leukemia cutis Metastatic cancer	*Radiation therapy*
Idiopathic exfoliative dermatitis (10–20% of all cases)		Graft-vs-host disease (acute)				
Interleukin-2†	*Graft-vs-host reaction* Malignancies: leukemia, lymphoma					
Exfoliative dermatitis secondary to malignancies Leukemia, lymphoma, Sezary's syndrome	*Vaccinations* Influenza, measles, smallpox *Staphylococcal scalded skin syndrome*					

*Most common agents.
†Reported to cause erythrodermic flares of psoriasis.
CML—chronic myelogenous leukemia; NSAIDs—nonsteroidal anti-inflammatory drugs; SLE—systemic lupus erythematosis.

Table 3. Supportive Care and Management of Toxic Erythema

Reaction pattern	Complication(s)	Supportive care	Laboratory	Topical therapy	Systemic therapy
Generalized toxic erythema	Dehydration, electrolyte imbalance, hypothermia, high-output cardiac failure, pruritus, sepsis	Remove drug; cardiac precautions; electrolyte, fluids and protein replacement; warm blankets	Skin and blood cultures, serum albumin (low), BUN/creatinine, hematocrit	Powdered oatmeal baths tid-qid, midpotency topical corticosteroids (triamcinolone 0.1%, betamethasone valerate 0.1%, etc.) bid, petrolatum USP tid-qid	Diphenhydramine or hydroxyzine 25–50 mg q 6–8 hr, prednisone 1 mg/kg/24 hr (severe cases)
Toxic epidermal necrolysis	Acute renal failure, electrolyte and fluid imbalance, GI bleeding, sepsis	Remove drug, burn unit care (if available), electrolyte and fluids, oropharnygeal suction, ophthalmologic care	Blood/urine/sputum cultures with early signs of infection	Silver nitrate 0.25% or acetic acid 0.1% soaks tid-qid, debridement, "burn" care in burn unit, cadaver skin grafts	Prednisone 1 mg/kg/24 hr during very early phase of drug-induced toxic epidermal necrolysis, but not once necrosis reaction has occurred, antibiotics for superinfection
Acral erythema	Pain, pruritus, bullae	Reassurance, spontaneous resolution in 5–7 d with drug discontinuation	None	Cool water compresses, petrolatum USP	Patient-controlled analgesia oral narcotic, analgesics, oral diphenhydramine or hydroxyzine (25–50 mg q 6–8 hr PRN) for pruritus
Infusion and injection site erythema	Pain, pruritus	Reassurance, spontaneous resolution in 24–48 hr after infusion	Skin culture if signs of infection present (persistent and expanding erythema, pus, etc.)	Cool water compresses	Nonsteroidal anti-inflammatory drugs, diphenhydramine or hydroxyzine for pruritus, antibiotic for infection
Pressure point erythema and erosions	Pain, infection	Remove source of pressure	Skin culture if signs of infection present	Sterile saline compresses, topical antibiotic to erosions bid-tid	None
Neutrophilic eccrine hidradentitis	Asymptomatic or tenderness	Reassurance, spontaneous resolution in 1–2 wk	Leukocytosis	Potent topical corticosteroid	None
Mucositis	Dehydration, infection, pain, weight loss	Bland soft diet, hydration, pain control, reassurance, healing expected in 5–7 d	Bacterial, fungal, or viral culture if suspected or if healing delayed	Mouthwash q 2–4 hr PRN using lidocaine, diphenhydramine, or dyclonine elixer, tetracycline rinses q 4 hr	Narcotic and non-narcotic analgesics for severe pain

The information here is provided as guidance only. Prescribers should always consult the manufacturer's current prescribing information.

Localized Erythema

Acral Erythema

Acral erythema is a reaction pattern not uncommonly associated with chemotherapy [5]. Patients treated for acute myelogenous leukemia with high-dose or continuous-infusion chemotherapy are at highest risk for the condition. Acral erythema is usually preceded by a tingling sensation for 3 to 4 days, followed by a well-defined patchy macular erythema on the palms, soles, digital joints, and interarticular spaces. The erythema is often tender to palpation, and occurs with or without edema, bullae, and desquamation. The mechanism of acral erythema is poorly understood but is thought to be a direct toxic effect of the chemotherapy on endothelium or a localized leukocytoclastic vasculitis. Localized chemotherapy-induced acral erythema usually resolves in 3 to 7 days once the chemotherapeutic agent has been discontinued. Most patients experience recurrence of this reaction pattern with rechallenge of the causative chemotherapeutic agent using similar or modified dosage schedules.

Erythematous Flare of Actinic Keratoses

Inflammation, crusting, and weeping of actinic (solar) keratoses commonly follows topical or systemic 5-fluorouracil therapy. Actinic keratoses are potentially premalignant tumors of the skin representing atypical hyperplasia of epidermal keratinocytes induced by ultraviolet radiation. They may be discrete or confluent, rough and scaling patches, usually measuring 0.5 to 1 cm in diameter. Distribution of lesions on areas exposed to sunlight, and their gross morphologic features, help to establish the diagnosis.

Infusion and Injection Site Erythema

Infusion and injection site erythema as a result of chemotherapy and BRMs may be due to local capillary dilation, an axon flare–mediated hypersensitivity reaction pattern, or chemically induced toxic effect on blood vessels. The linearity of the erythema, often along the vein of delivery, is an important diagnostic clue. Infusion site thrombophlebitis manifests as linear erythema and a tender, palpable cord. Local injections of GM-CSF may cause inflammation at previously noninflamed injections sites [6]. The mechanism of this local or systemic reaction is unclear but appears to be immunologically mediated. Localized infections (19% incidence), necessitating antibiotic therapy, have been reported to occur with subcutaneous IL-2 injections [7]. The recurrence risk upon rechallenge is not well described.

Erythema on Pressure Points

Toxic erythema and ulcerations localized to pressure point areas, and unrelated to infiltration or extravasation, may occur as a result of chemotherapy. High-dose methotrexate and bleomycin have been associated with this reaction pattern. It is not known if this reaction pattern will worsen with continued infusion of the offending agent. The recurrence risk upon reexposure is not well described.

Neutrophilic Eccrine Hidradenitis

A unique reaction pattern induced by chemotherapy, neutrophilic eccrine hidradenitis (NEH) manifests as erythematous and purpuric nodules and plaques occurring on the face, neck, axillae, back, chest, abdomen, and dorsum of the hands and legs. It usually begins about 2 weeks after the initiation of therapy. Histopathologically, the most important features are necrosis of the eccrine glands and neutrophilic infiltration. Patients at highest risk for NEH are often febrile, male, and on high-dose chemotherapy. They are often being treated for leukemia, Hodgkin's or non-Hodgkin's lymphoma, testicular cancer,

or osteosarcoma. The mechanism of NEH is unclear but may be related to the preferential secretion of these chemotherapeutic agents by eccrine ducts. NEH usually resolves spontaneously in 1 to 2 weeks. Recurrence of NEH with retreatment, especially cytarabine, has been reported in some patients [8].

Mucositis

The systemic administration of chemotherapy may cause mucositis [9,10]. Mucositis also occurs with BMR use. Inflammation and erosion of buccal, tongue, nasal, esophageal, intestinal, rectal, and vulvovaginal mucosa may occur, generally beginning 4 to 10 days after administration of the offending agent. The mechanism of mucositis is believed to be direct cellular toxicity to rapidly growing epithelium. The severity of mucositis is variable, often depending on the dosage and frequency of administration and use of concurrent medication, which may alter renal tubular secretion of the offending agent. Healing generally begins within 5 to 7 days after cessation of the causative agent. Mucositis commonly recurs upon reexposure, often necessitating a reduction in dosage and scheduling or discontinuation of the offending agent altogether.

HYPERSENSITIVITY REACTIONS

Fortunately, hypersensitivity reactions induced by chemotherapy and BRMs are rare. Hypersensitivity reaction patterns can be generalized or localized and can be the result of systemic or topical therapy. Severity can range from mild pruritus without a rash, to diffuse erythema, urticaria, and anaphylaxis. Deciding which agent is responsible for a given reaction can be difficult, particularly when numerous other medications are being administered concurrently. Chemotherapeutic agents and BRMs can elicit types I, II, and IV hypersensitivity reactions [11–13] (Table 4).

Immediate or Type I Reactions

Type I hypersensitivity reactions (anaphylactic type) are dependent upon antigen cross-linking IgE and the binding of activated IgE to

Table 4. Chemotherapy and Biologic Response Modifiers that Induce Hypersensitivity Reactions

Type I hypersensitivity*	Type III hypersensitivity*	Type IV hypersensitivity
l-Asparaginase	l-Asparaginase	Topical†
Azathioprine	Azthioprine	BCNU
Cisplatin	Busulfan	5-Fluorouracil
Chlorambucil	Chlorambucil	Mechlorethamine
Cyclophosphamide	Hydroxyurea	
Cyclosporin	Mechlorethamine	Systemic*
Daunomycin	Thiotepa	Morbilliform or papular
Doxorubicin		drug reaction†
Mechlorethamine		Mitomycin C
Melphalan		
Methotrexate		
Teniposide/etoposide		
Thiotepa		
Zinostatin		

*Induced by systemic therapy.
†Induced by topical therapy.
‡Not reported for chemotherapeutic agents.

mast cells (Fc receptor), stimulating the release of vasoactive amines and producing inflammation. Type I reactions manifest as urticaria, angioedema, pruritus, and anaphylaxis. Type I reactions related to chemotherapy most commonly are caused by l-asparaginase, cisplatin, and cyclophosphamide. Localized urticaria, edema, and pruritus along the proximal vein of infusion or injection, usually transient, may occur with the tumor antibiotic adriamycin. Other systemically administered chemotherapeutic agents and BRMs associated with type I reactions are listed in Table 4.

Antibody-Mediated or Type II Reactions

Type II hypersensitivity reactions are believed to be caused by the binding of antibodies to cell surface antigens, resulting in antibody-dependent cell-mediated cytotoxicity and/or complement-mediated lysis. Transfusion hypersensitivity, acquired hemolytic anemia and thrombocytopenia, connective tissue disorders (SLE, rheumatoid arthritis, and autoimmune thyroiditis), myasthenia gravis, and certain types of cutaneous blistering diseases are clinical examples of type II reactions. To date, chemotherapeutic agents and BRMs have not been reported to elicit this cutaneous reaction pattern. A generalized, pruritic vesicular eruption has been reported to occur with combination mitomycin C and doxorubicin therapy, but it is not known whether this cutaneous reaction represents a true type II reaction.

Immune Complex-Mediated or Type III Reactions

Type III hypersensitivity reactions are believed to be caused by the deposition of antigen–antibody complexes in blood vessels, activation of the complement cascade, and inflammation and tissue damage. Type III reactions are manifested by urticaria, erythema multiforme, and pink or purple papules showing necrotizing vasculitis. Erythema multiforme is a reaction pattern involving skin and/or mucous membranes characterized by iris- or target-shaped erythematous plaques and/or vesicobullous lesions. Hypersensitivity vasculitis appears as urticaria, purpuric papules, or papulovesicles/blisters, manifested histopathologically as segmental neutrophilic inflammation and fibrinoid necrosis of postcapillary venules. The vasculitis commonly presents on the lower legs or ankles, buttocks, and distal arms.

Delayed or Type IV Reactions

Type IV hypersensitivity reactions are believed to be T-cell mediated. Antigen-sensitized T cells, upon reexposure to the offending agent after 24 to 48 hours, release lymphokines that recruit inflammatory cells (T cells, macrophages, neutrophils) and produce inflammation. Allergic contact dermatitis, morbilliform drug reactions, granulomatous disease such as tuberculosis and sarcoidosis, and graft-versus-host disease are the prototypical clinical examples. Type IV cutaneous systemic reactions present as erythema and edema, with or without vesiculation. Topical applications of some chemotherapeutic agents, used in the treatment of mycosis fungoides and actinic (solar) keratosis, can induce type IV contact hypersensitivity reactions (Table 4).

Assessment and Management of Hypersensitivity Reactions

Urticaria and angioedema may occur not only from chemotherapy and BRMs but also from whole blood and immunoglobulin transfusions, radiocontrast media, antibiotics, narcotic analgesics, and other medications. Urticarial wheals generally last less than 24 hours in a single location before fading (and often appearing elsewhere). If urticarial wheals last longer than 72 to 96 hours in the same location, a skin biopsy should be considered to exclude urticarial necrotizing vasculitis. Angioedema may be associated

with laryngeal and intestinal wall edema, manifesting as respiratory distress and abdominal pain, respectively.

A diagnosis of erythema multiforme is based on the gross morphologic features (lesions are target or iris shaped) and distribution (skin and/or mucous membranes), with a typical histopathologic appearance. Radiation therapy can induce generalized erythema multiforme. Hypersensitivity vasculitis should be differentiated from isolated bacterial or fungal septic infarcts, particularly because both can present with acute constitutional symptoms (fever, chills, etc.) and purpuric papules. Necrotizing vasculitis may also be a manifestation of sepsis. In immunocompromised patients, antibiotic coverage should be initiated immediately until blood culture results have been obtained.

Type IV cutaneous hypersensitivity reactions that are the acute contact allergic type may be confused clinically with cellulitis. Allergic contact dermatitis is a pruritic eczematous dermatitis with asymmetry and artificial patterning, whereas cellulitis is noneczematous and manifested by confluent redness, induration, and tenderness. Typical morbilliform cutaneous reactions in the patient with cancer often occur as a result of transfusion reactions, underlying viral infections, or medications. Morbilliform cutaneous eruptions have not been well described for the most commonly used chemotherapeutic agents.

The differential diagnoses and management of hypersensitivity reactions are presented in Tables 5 and 6.

Table 5. Diffential Diagnoses of Hypersensitivity Reactions Induced by Chemotherapy and Biologic Response Modifiers

Urticaria and angioedema	Erythema multiforme	Necrotizing vasculitis
C_1-inhibitor deficiency Hereditary angioedema	Connective tissue disease SLE	Connective tissue disease Inherited C2 deficiency, SLE, polyarteritis nodosa, rheumatoid arthritis (adult), Sjögren's syndrome
Drug reactions Barbiturates, dextran, therapeutic enzymes, hydralazine, mercurials, penicillin, sulfonamides	Idiopathic (approx 50%) Infections Herpes simplex*, histoplasmosis, mycoplasma*, mononucleosis, tuberculosis, tularemia, vaccinia	Cryoglobulinemia Paraproteinemia
Food additives Azo dyes, benzoates and tartrazine	Drug reactions Barbiturates, hydantoin, NSAIDs, penicillin, phenothiazines, rifampin, sulfonamides and sulfonylureas	Drug reactions (other than chemotherapy) Aspirin, indomethocin and phenylbutazone, chloroquine and quinidine, penicillin and sulfonamides, phenothiazines, thiazides
Histamine-releasing agents Acetylcholine, aspirin, codeine, epinephrine, ethanol, isoproterenol, procainamide, penicillin, sulfonamides, polymyxin B, D-tubocurarine	Radiation therapy	Idiopathic Henoch–Schönlein purpura
Medical disorders Hypo- or hyperthyroidism, mastocytosis		Infections CMV, hepatitis B, HIV, SBE
Physical factors Cholinergic, cold, solar, heat, and vibration		Serum sickness
Radiocontrast media		Transfusion reactions Whole blood, immunoglobulins
		Other Cystic fibrosis, lymphoma, ulcerative colitis

*Most common infections.
CMV—cytomegalovirus; HIV—human immunodeficiency virus; NSAIDs—nonsteroidal anti-inflammatory drugs; SBE—subacute bacterial endocarditis; SLE—systemic lupus erythematosis.

FLUSHING

The exact mechanism of cutaneous flushing is poorly understood. The condition results from capillary dilation secondary to emotional, neural, and biochemical (histamine) influences [14] (Table 7). Flushing can be wet (neural-mediated) from eccrine sweating, or dry (vascular smooth muscle) depending upon the inciting factor(s). It may also be a prodromal sign to an impending anaphylactic reaction. Identification of the underlying cause (Table 8) and patient reassurance is often sufficient. Antihistamines may provide relief of associated pruritus.

RADIATION RECALL

Radiation recall in the skin is a reaction pattern characterized by erythema and desquamation occurring at the site of prior radiation following the administration of chemotherapy. This reaction generally takes place within 7 days after delivery of the offending chemotherapeutic agent, months to many years (as long as 15 years) following radiation therapy. Severity varies from mild erythema and desquamation to vesiculation, oozing, and full-thickness cutaneous necrosis with persistent and painful ulceration. Radiation recall reactions can involve not only the skin but also the esophagus, intestine,

Table 6. Supportive Care and Management of Hypersensitivity Reactions

Hypersensitivity reaction pattern	Manifestation	Supportive care	Laboratory	Topical therapy	Systemic therapy*
Type I	Pruritus, urticaria, angioedema, anaphylaxis	Withdraw offending agent if severe; secure airway for respiratory compromise	Skin biopsy if individual lesions last > 72 hr to exclude vasculitis	Cool water compresses, midpotency topical steroid bid-tid (eg, fluocinolone, betamethasone)	Hydroxyzine or diphenhydramine 25–50 mg PO q 4–6 hr PRN; prednisone 1 mg/kg/d w/rapid taper over 10–14 d; epinephrine (1:1000) 0.3–0.5 ml SC q 20–30 min X 3 for anaphylaxis†
Type III	Urticaria, pruritus, erythema multiforme, vasculitis	*Urticaria* (same as Type I) *Erythema multiforme and vasculitis* Withdraw offending agent or treat underlying disease; ophthalmologic evaluation for ocular involvement	*Urticaria* (same as Type I) *Erythema multiforme* Viral culture if herpes simplex virus suspected; CBC w/diff, eosinophilia suggests drug *Vasculitis* Serum complement level (decreased), urinalysis (erythrocytes/albumin), skin biopsy, blood cultures	*Urticaria* (same as Type I) *Erythema multiforme* Mild: midpotent topical steroid bid-tid; viscous lidocaine 2%, diphenhydramine 2% or dyclonine 1% swish q 4–6 hr PRN pain for oral lesions *Vasculitis* Compressive bandages to lower extremities	*Urticaria* (same as Type I) *Erythema multiforme and vasculitis* Mild: antihistamines q 4–6 hr PRN for pruritus; severe: prednidsone 60–80 mg/d bid, analgesics PRN pain; topical antibiotic tid to eroded lesions†
Type IV	*Localized lesions* Pruritus, secondary bacterial infection, hypo- or hyper-pigmentation *Systemic reaction* Morbilliform or papular rash	Discontinue topical agent Discontinue systemic agent if severe	Skin culture for purulent drainage	Saline or aluminum acetate (1:20 dilution) soaks tid-qid; high potency topical steroid (eg fluocinonide 0.05%) bid-tid for 7–10 d	*Severe cases* Prednisone taper (15 d); 40–30–20 mg/d QAM X 5 d; hydroxyzine or diphenhydramine 25–50 mg q 6 hr PRN; antibiotics if skin culture positive†

*Adult doses
†Pediatric doses: diphenhydramine 5 mg/kg/24 hr; hydroxyzine in children < 6 yr, 50 mg/24 hr in tid-qid dosing; > 6 yr, 50–100 mg/24 hr in tid-qid dosing; prednisone 1 mg/kg/24 hr (AM dosing) initially, then 50% dosage reduction every 4–7 d.

Table 7. Agents Causing Flushing Reactions

Chemotherapy	Biologic response modifiers	Hormonal therapy	Other
BCNU	Interferon alpha-2a	Tamoxifen	*Antiemetics*
Cisplatin	Interleukin-2	Leuprolide acetate	Alizapride
Dacarbazine	GM-CSF		Metoclopramide
Doxorubicin	TNF		
Mithramycin*	Interleukin-2/lymphocyte		*Immunosuppressive*
Procarbazine†	activated killer cell immunotherapy		Tacrolimus (FK506)

*Most common agents.
†"Antabuse (disulfiram) effect" by inhibiting aldehyde dehydrogenase.

Table 8. Differential Diagnoses of Flushing Reactions

Medications/drugs	Tumors	Procedures	Medical disorders
Alcohol intolerance with: Cephalosporins, hypoglycemic agents (chlorpropramide), metronidazole, Hodgkin's disease (with or without bone pain), calcium channel blockers Cyclosporin Rifampin Vanocomycin	Carcinoid syndrome Central nervous system tumors Chronic granulocytic leukemia (basophilic) Medullary carcinoma of the thyroid Pheochromocytoma	Hormonal stimulation tests Ovine corticotropin Mesenteric traction Radiographic contrast media Orchiectomy	Dumping syndrome (following gastric surgery) Horseshoe kidney (Rovsing's syndrome) Menopause Rosacea

heart, and lungs [15]. The precise mechanism is not well understood. Radiation recall reactions are less likely to occur if delivery of high-risk agents is delayed 7 to 10 days following radiation treatment.

The causes, differential diagnoses, and management of radiation recall are presented in Table 9.

PHOTOSENSITIVITY

Drug-induced phototoxicity is a cutaneous reaction pattern characterized as an exaggerated sunburn (erythema, edema, vesiculation, and scales) in response to the simultaneous administration of an offending agent and exposure to ultraviolet radiation therapy. Any individual may be susceptible. Several chemotherapeutic agents have been reported to elicit phototoxic reactions (Table 10). Drug-induced photoallergic reactions, a unique individual susceptibility, occur much less frequently. Photoallergy occurs when a drug acts as an antigen (photo product) in the skin, and an immunologic response occurs, manifesting as a rash. To date, chemotherapeutic agents and BRMs have been associated with photosensitivity of the phototoxic type but not with photoallergic reactions.

PIGMENTARY ALTERATIONS

Cutaneous pigmentary alterations can occur as a result of cancer chemotherapeutic agents. Hyperpigmentation is much more common than hypopigmentation. Although a benign reaction pattern, pigmentary alterations often cause great anxiety to patients and those administering medical care. Pigmentary changes related to cancer chemotherapy may be localized or diffuse and can involve the mucous membranes. Histopathologically, hyperpigmentation is represented by increased melanin deposition in the basal cell layer of the epidermis and/or superficial papillary dermis. Previously, the mechanism of action was hypothesized to involve altered ACTH and MSH levels. Support for this mechanism is lacking. The chemotherapeutic agent may be acting as a nonspecific stimulator of melanin production by susceptible melanocytes. Common offending drugs include alkylating agents and the tumor antibiotics [16,17] (Table 11).

Chemotherapy-induced cutaneous hyperpigmentation usually lasts several weeks to 6 months. For persistent localized areas of hyperpigmentation that are of cosmetic concern, a combination of topical tretinoin 0.025%, hydrocortisone 1% cream, and hydroquinone over several weeks of daily therapy (3 to 4%) may be helpful in lightening the areas but only if the melanin pigmentation is localized to the epidermis. A total sunblock should also be worn during the treatment process. Hydroquinone may cause contact irritant and allergic reactions.

PRURITUS

The pathophysiology of pruritus is poorly understood, and therapy is difficult to administer. Studies suggest that the sensation of itch is carried to the central nervous system via unmyelinated C fibers in the skin [18]. Many different peripheral chemical mediators have been implicated in the sensation of pruritus, including histamine, proteases, substance P and prostaglandins. Pruritus may be caused by primary skin diseases, medications, metabolic disorders, underlying malignancy, and malnutrition (Table 12). Pruritus also may be an early sign of an impending hypersensitivity reaction. In the patient with cancer, multiple causes for generalized pruritus other than chemotherapeutic agents and BRMs need to be considered (Table 13).

Management of pruritus is directed toward treatment of the underlying cause if identified. Symptomatic supportive care includes

Table 9. Radiation Recall Reactions

Associated chemotherapeutic agents	Differential diagnoses	Supportive care
Actinomycin D Bleomycin BCNU Cytosine arabinoside Cyclophosphamide Doxorubicin 5-Fluorouracil Hydroxyurea Interleukin-2* Methotrexate Vinblastine Vincristine	*Acute radiation dermatitis* 3000–4000 cGy: erythema and edema 4500–6000 cGy: wet or dry desquamation following vesicles and bullae *Chronic radiation dermatitis* > 6000 cGy: epidermal atrophy (± hyperkeratosis), telangiectasias, hypo- and hyperpigmentation, dermal sclerosis and appendageal loss; chronic painful ulcerations	*Radiation recall reactions and acute radiation dermatitis* Tepid wet compresses and topical corticosteroid preparations improve pain, erythema, and edema; avoidance of trauma, friction, temperature extremes, and rubbing; suspected infections should be cultured and appropriate antibiotic therapy directed toward sensitivity results *Chronic radiation dermatitis* Periodic observation for the development of basal cell and squamous cell carcinoma for as long as 40 years; topical antibiotics (eg, silver sulfadiazine, bacitracin, mupirocin) for ulceration

*"Recall" of fever, chills, nausea, and hypotension with concurrent IV contrast dye administration.

Table 10. Drug-induced Photosensitivity

Associated chemotherapeutic agents	Differential diagnoses	Management
Actinomycin D Bleomycin Dacarbazine Doxorubicin 5-Fluorouracil* Nafoxidine (anti-estrogen) Mitomycin-C‡ 6-Mercaptopurine* Methotrexate† Procarbazine Triazinate (folate antagonist)† Vinblastine	*Pellegra-like syndrome** Isoniazid, carcinoid syndrome, Hartnup disease, malnutrition (niacin/tryptophan) *Photodermatoses* Polymorphous light eruption, lupus erythematosis, solar urticaria, porphyrias, xeroderma pigmentosum *Phototoxic reactions* Antibiotics: demethylchlortetracycline, oxytetracycline, doxycycline, sulfonamides; coal tar and derivatives; diuretics: aminodarone, furosemide, thiazides; griseofulvin; nonsteroidal anti-inflammatory drugs (piroxicam); phenothiazines, psoralens *Photoallergic reactions* Aftershave lotion (musk ambrette), benzocaine (topical), bezophenones (sunscreens), neomycin, para-aminobenzoic acid esters, phenothiazines, sulfonamides, sunscreens (6-methyl coumarin), whiteners (stilbenes)	Cool wet compresses Triamcinolone 0.1% cream twice daily for 7–10 d to decrease pain, erythema, and edema Avoidance of midday sun in spring and summer, double layer clothing, topical sunscreens (SPF approx 30) applied to all exposed sites during sunny months while receiving chemotherapy

*"Pellagra-like" syndrome with an acute sunburn-type dermatitis in a photodistribution followed by skin thickening and hyperpigmentation.
†Most common photosensitizing chemotherapeutic agents.
‡Photo-induced recall ulceration following an extravasation injury 3 mo earlier.

colloidal oatmeal powder baths bid, topical water-trapping agents (eg, petrolatum), menthol lotions, and oral antihistamines (eg, diphenhydramine 25–50 mg, hydroxyzine, 25-50 mg q 4–6 hr/PRN, and doxepin, 10 mg q 4–6 hr/PRN). Ultraviolet B (290–320 nm) phototherapy is effective in treating uremic pruritus. Activated charcoal may be useful in treating cholestatic pruritus. Intravenous naloxone may be useful in intractable cases of pruritus.

PURPURA AND PETECHIAE

Hemorrhages in the skin, or purpura, may be macular or papular. Small purpuric macules, termed *petechiae*, represent pinpoint, nonblanchable submucosal, intraepidermal, or intradermal hemor-

rhage. Chemotherapy-induced petechiae are usually secondary to bone marrow suppression and thrombocytopenia (often in association with leukopenia). Spontaneous bleeding generally occurs when the platelet count falls below 20,000 and often first manifests in the skin. Cutaneous petechiae provide clinicians with an early warning to imminent bleeding at mucosal sites, as well as in the kidney and brain. Other causes of petechiae include capillary fragility, platelet autoantibodies, and vasculitis (purpuric papules). BRM therapies have also been reported to induce petechiae (Table 14). Any chemotherapeutic agent or BRM that can cause bone marrow depression may be associated with the development of petechiae. Large purpuric macules, termed *ecchymosis*, usually represent intradermal hemorrhage secondary to reduction of clotting factors.

Table 11. Chemotherapy-induced Mucosal and Cutaneous Hyperpigmentation and Hypopigmentation

Mucosal pigmentation	Diffuse cutaneous pigmentation	Localized cutaneous pigmentation	Linear/"flagellate" cutaneous pigmentation††	Solar distribution of pigmentation
Buccal mucosa Adriamycin, busulfan, cisplatin, cyclophosphamide, 5-FU *Tongue* Adriamycin, hydroxyurea *Gingiva/teeth* Cyclophosphamide	*Most common* Bleomycin, busulfan*, cyclophosphamide, hydroxyurea, thiotepa† *Other agents* Actinomycin D, daunorubicin, 5-FU, methotrexate, mithramycin, procarbazine	*Acral* Doxorubicin, tegafur (5-FU analogue) *Acanthosis nigricans-like‡* Triazinate *Occlusive bandage/EKG pad sites* Thiotepa *Poikiloderma§* Hydroxyurea *Pressure points* Bleomycin, hydroxyurea *"Serpetine" supravenous¶ (following infusion)* Bleomycin, daunorubicin, 5-FU, mitomycin C, triazinate *Topical therapy*** BCNU, mechlorethamine, 5-FU	Bleomycin	Cyclophosphamide, daunorubicin, 5-FU, methotrexate

*Addisonian pigmentation pattern without anorexia, weight loss, weakness, or biochemical evidence of adrenocortical insufficiency.
†Also reported to cause hypopigmentation (leukoderma) following topical administration.
‡Verrucous, hyperpigmented, velvety plaques occurring in the axillae, groin, inframmary and popliteal fossae areas.
§Hypo- and hyperpigmentation, atrophy, and telangectasia localized to the dorsal hands, fingers, and toes.
¶Along the vein of infusion.
**Used for treatment of mycosis fungoides (BCNU, mechlorethamine) and solar keratoses (5-FU).
††A unique linear reaction pattern consisting of grouped hyperpigmented streaks; mechanism unknown.
5-FU—5-fluorouracil.

Table 12. Pruritus Secondary to Chemotherapy and Biologic Response Modifiers*

Adriamycin†
Cytarabine and daunorubicin combination therapy
GM-CSF (E. coli derived)
Interleukin-2 (with or without LAK cells)‡
Mechlorethamine
Methotrexate
Thiotepa

*Any chemotherapeutic agent or BRM that can induce a Type I, II, or IV hypersensitivity reaction may also be associated with either localized or generalized pruritus.
†Particularly along the vein of infusion.
‡Approximately 48% incidence of capillary leak syndrome, associated with generalized pruritus.

Table 13. Differential Diagnoses of Generalized Pruritus

Drugs	Endocrine disturbances	Hematologic disease	Hepatic disease	Malignancies	Renal disease
Aspirin, codeine, dextran, morphine	Carcinoid syndrome, diabetes mellitus, hypo- or hyperthyroidism, secondary hyperparathyroidism (chronic renal failure)	Anemia, paraproteinemia, polycythemia vera	Hepatitis, obstructive jaundice (intra- or extrahepatic)	Adenocarcinoma, central nervous system tumors, leukemia, lymphoma, myeloma, mycosis fungoides	Chronic renal failure (uremia)

Purpura fulminans is a purpuric reaction that may be secondary to thrombosis and infarctive necrosis of deep blood vessels in the skin, often on the basis of bacterial, fungal, or viral infection.

Management of patients who have purpura involves identifying and eliminating or treating the underlying cause (Table 15). Treatment of chemotherapy-induced thrombocytopenia becomes necessary when the platelet count falls below 20,000/ml because the risk of spontaneous bleeding is high. Platelet transfusion should be initiated two to three times weekly to maintain counts between 20,000 and 50,000. Platelet counts should then be monitored every 2 days to determine if the bone marrow is recovering. All medications that can adversely affect platelet function should be withheld (if possible) during bone marrow depression and recovery phases.

RAYNAUD'S PHENOMENON AND DIGITAL GANGRENE

Raynaud's phenomenon is characterized by blanching of the skin followed by cyanosis and hyperemia as a consequence of vasospasm. It commonly occurs on the fingers and toes with exposure to cold or stressful events. Sclerodactyly may follow repeated or persistent vasospasm. Rarely, gangrene may occur following severe digital ischemia. The mechanism of Raynaud's phenomenon induced by chemotherapy or BRMs is unknown, but may occur as a result of concomitant vasospasm and endothelial injury. Table 16 provides a list of agents responsible for inducing Raynaud's phenomenon [19].

After the assessment and differential diagnosis have been concluded (Table 17), management of Raynaud's phenomenon induced by chemotherapy and BRM involves dosage reduction or

Table 14. Chemotherapy and Biologic Response Modifiers that Induce Macular and Papular Purpura

Agent	Mechanism	Location	Presentation
Bleomycin	Thrombocytopenia, platelet aggregation, vascular endothelial damage	Generalized and acral	Petechiae and papular purpura
Hydroxyurea	Cutaneous necrotizing vasculitis	Lower extremities	Papular purpura
Interferon alpha	Thrombocytopenia, idiopathic autoimmune thrombocytopenia (2% incidence of platelet autoantibodies)	Generalized and acral	Petechiae
Interleukin-2/LAK cell infusions	(?) Capillary leak syndrome	Ankles	Papular purpura (vaculitis)
G-CSF	Leukocytoclastic vasculitis	Thighs	Papular purpura
GM-CSF	Unknown	Generalized	Macular purpura following GM-CSF–induced toxic erythema
Prednisone	Capillary fragility	Generalized, particularly at sites of trauma	Large macular purpura (ecchymosis)

Table 15. Differential Diagnoses of Purpura

Papular purpura (vasculitis)	Purpuric macules (petechiae and ecchymosis)
Carcinoma GI, leukemia, lymphoma, lung	*Benign lymphocytic capillaritis* (pigmentary purpuras)
Collagen vascular diseases Dermatomyositis, inflammatory bowel disease, polyarteritis nodosa, rheumatoid arthritis, Sjögren's syndrome, SLE	*Coagulopathies* Coumadin, DIC, heparin, liver disease
Hyperviscosity Cryoglobulinemia (hepatitis, leukemia, myeloma, metastatic disease, SBE), cryofibrinogens (hepatitis), cold agglutinins (lymphoma)	*Infections* Bacteremia, SBE, viremia (esp. CMV) *Medications* NSAIDs, corticosteroids
Infections SBE, HIV, streptococcal, TB, viral hepatitis B (serum sickness reaction—usually urticarial, but may be purpuric papules)	*Resolution phase of toxic erythemas* *Systemic diseases* Diabetes mellitus, uremia
Lymphomatoid granulomatosis *Medications* NSAIDs, penicillin, phenothiazines, quinidine, sulfonamides, thiazides	*Senile skin and venous stasis* *Thrombocytopenia* Bone marrow depression, idiopathic and thrombotic, thrombocytopenic purpura
Polyarteritis nodosa and granulomatous arteritides	*Thrombocythemia (> 100,000)* *Trauma*

CMV—cytomegalovirus; DIC—disseminated intravascular coagulation; HIV—human immunodeficiency virus; NSAIDs—nonsteroidal anti-inflammatory drugs; SBE—subacute bacterial endocarditis; SLE—systemic lupus erythematosis; TB—tuberculosis.

Table 16. Agents Associated with Raynaud's Phenomenon and Digital Gangrene

Raynaud's phenomenon	Digital gangrene
Bleomycin	Bleomycin
Cyclosporin (high dose of 10 mg/kg/d)	Combination bleomycin and vincristine
Combination bleomycin and vinblastine	Combination bleomycin, doxorubicin and vincristine*
Vinblastine	

*Reported in two patients treated for AIDS-related Kaposi's sarcoma.

Table 17. Differential Diagnoses of Raynaud's Phenomenon

Connective tissue disorders	Compression (local)	Hyperviscosity states	Medications	Vascular diseases
Dermatomyositis Lupus erythematosis Rheumatoid arthritis Scleroderma Sjögren's syndrome	Carpel tunnel syndrome	Cold agglutinins Macroglobulins	Beta-blockers Interferon alpha and beta* Nicotine	Arteriosclerosis "Blue toe syndrome"† Thromboangiitis obliterans

*Digital numbness and paresthesias preceding development of digital vasculitis.
†Cholesterol microembolization and digital ischemia may follow instrumentation of an atheromatous aorta.

discontinuation of the offending agent. Cold exposure and cigarette smoking should be avoided. Nifedipine and reserpine may be used for severe symptomatic cases. Prostacyclin infusions (3 times weekly for 5 hours) have been reported to provide symptomatic relief.

ACNEIFORM ERUPTIONS

Acneiform (ie, acnelike) eruptions generally occur on the face, shoulders, back, and chest and manifest as erythematous follicular papules and papulopustules. This reaction pattern was first reported to occur with actinomycin D [20]. Azathioprine, high-dose methotrexate and cyclosporin infusions can also cause acneiform eruptions. Steroid acne, following long-term administration of corticosteroids or corticotropin, is a true folliculitis that presents as an acneiform eruption. Steroid acne presents as numerous (often uncountable), stable and chronic monomorphous red papules and papulopustules involving the shoulders, trunk, and upper arms. In contrast to acne vulgaris, steroid acne usually spares the face and lacks the presence of comedones.

The primary differential diagnoses of acneiform eruption include cutaneous septic emboli and gram-negative folliculitis. Monomorphous appearance, chronicity, uncountable number, and fixed nature suggest the diagnosis of steroid acne. Acneiform eruptions generally clear following discontinuation of the offending agent. Topical tretinoin cream (0.025% bid) combined with a 5 to 10% benzoyl peroxide creme may be useful.

EXTRAVASATION INJURIES

Chemotherapy extravasation may lead to local skin, tendon, and muscle necrosis. The agents that cause injury from extravasation are listed in Table 18. Early recognition and withdrawal of the offending agent are necessary to abort further tissue damage. To date, no BRMs have been reported to cause extravasation injuries. High-risk extravasation areas include joint spaces, underlying tendons, and neurovascular bundles, particularly because these areas lack thick subcutaneous fat layers. Once the chemotherapeutic agent has leaked out of the vein of delivery, it binds to DNA in the surrounding tissues causing cell death. Continued release of the vesicant drug leads to progressive ulceration. The most common mechanisms of extravasation from venous access ports include needle dislodgment, catheter tip thrombosis, separation of the catheter tip from the access port, and leakage through defective catheters.

In the differential diagnosis, an agent that can cause a chemical phlebitis may simulate an early extravasation injury. The "adriamycin-flare" reaction may also be confused with early extravasation. Management of extravasation injuries is empirical. Immediate discontinuation of the infusion and withdrawal of the delivery needle is necessary. Ice should be applied as much as tolerated to decrease drug diffusion and tissue edema. Surgical

consultation should be obtained within 72 hours if pain persists in the area of extravasation. Extensive debridement may be necessary [21]. Specific antidotes for adriamycin and mechlorethamine extravasation include locally injected sodium bicarbonate and (0.17 M) sodium thiosulfate, respectively [22]. Beneficial effects of local hydrocortisone (50–100 mg) and hyaluronidase injections following vincristine and adriamycin extravasation, respectively, have been reported.

HAIR AND NAIL REACTION PATTERNS

ALOPECIA AND OTHER HAIR DISORDERS

Alopecia (hair loss) is a common manifestation of chemotherapy toxicity and can occur following BRM and radiation therapy [23] (Table 19). In a normal state, about 85% of scalp follicles are in an *anagen* (actively growing) *phase* and the remaining 10 to 15% are in a *telogen* (resting) *phase*. The resting phase lasts 6 to 12 weeks, followed by shedding of the hair. Less than 5% of scalp hair is in transitory resting phase between anagen and telogen, termed *catagen phase*. The rate of hair growth of the scalp is normally 0.3 mm per day.

Chemotherapy-induced alopecia represents an anagen effluvium. The degree of alopecia depends upon the route of administration (higher with intravenous dosing), the particular drug, the schedule of delivery, and the use of the drug in combination. Chemotherapy-induced anagen hair loss usually begins 2 to 4 weeks after the offending agent and becomes noticeable when 50% or more of the hair is shed. Chemotherapy and BRMs can also induce a telogen effluvium. In telogen effluvium, shedding of resting hairs increases secondary to an accelerated shift of the growing phase to the resting phase. Hair

Table 18. High-Risk Agents for Extravasation Injury

Actinomycin D	Mechlorethamine	Streptozotocin
Daunomycin	Mithramycin	Vinblastine
Doxorubicin*	Mitomycin C*	Vincristine*

*May cause severe chemical cellulitis followed by full-thickness cutaneous necrosis, as well as injury and/or necrosis of the underlying muscles, nerves, and tendons.

Table 19. Hair Disorders Caused by Chemotherapy and Biologic Response Modifiers

Anagen effluvium*	Telogen effluvium	Hirsutism and hypertrichosis	Special signs
Actinomycin D	Interleukin-2/LAK	Cyclosporin A	*Flag sign*
Bleomycin	cell immunother-	Interferon alpha§	Horizontal, pigmented
Cyclophosphamide†	apathy		scalp; hair banding
Daunomycin	Any major stressor,		following methotrex-
Doxorubicin†	including		ate; similar to hair
Etoposide	chemotherapy		changes seen in
5-Fluorouracil			kwashiorkor
Hydroxyurea			
Ifosfamide			*Tic-tac sign*
Mechlorethamine			Spiny follicular projec-
Melphalen			tions on the under-
Methotrexate			surface of detached
Mitomycin C			scalp scale following
Mitoxanthrone‡			radiation therapy
Vincristine†			
VP-213			

*Most common agents.
†Reported to induce a selective loss of white scalp hair in two patients.
§Reported to stimulate growth of long, thick, curly eyelashes.
LAK—lymphocyte activated killer.

loss in telogen effluvium occurs 6 to 12 weeks after the inciting agent. A decrease in scalp hair density is experienced without concomitant scalp skin pathology in both anagen and telogen effluvium.

Hair breakage from a structurally altered and weakened shaft can also occur following chemotherapy-induced toxicity to actively growing hair follicles. There is also a 10 to 20% incidence of changes in hair density, pigmentation, and texture after hair regrowth following chemotherapy-induced alopecia. Hirsutism (excessive androgen-dependent hair growth) and hypertrichosis (increase in nonsexual- and nonandrogen-dependent hair growth) have been reported to occur following BRM therapies.

In the patient with cancer, radiation-induced alopecia is the main differential consideration of an acute anagen effluvium. Temporary hair loss occurs with radiation doses less than 3000 to 3500 cGy. Regrowth begins within 1 month. If the radiation dose exceeds 4000 cGy, permanent alopecia may result due to follicular destruction [24]. As previously noted, any major systemic stressor can cause a telogen effluvium. Other causes of a telogen effluvium include major surgical procedures, general anesthesia, acute blood loss, hypo- or hyperthyroidism, medications (heparin, propanolol, vitamin A derivatives), significant weight loss, high fever, and malnutrition [25]. The precipitating event usually takes place about 6 to 16 weeks prior to the telogen effluvium. The management of alopecia is indicated in Table 20.

HYPERPIGMENTATION OF THE NAILS

Nail hyperpigmentation is the result of increased melanin deposition in the nail plate, bed, or matrix. The stimulus for increased melanin

Table 20. Management of Alopecia

1. Supportive: reassurance that full regrowth is expected, but with temporarily altered color and texture
2. Avoidance (pre-chemotherapy) of scalp tourniquets and hypothermia caps because the scalp may act as a reservoir for malignant cells in leukemia and lymphoma
3. Minoxidil (twice daily application) may be useful in stimulating regrowth but supporting data are not available.

synthesis in chemotherapy-induced hyperpigmentation is unknown but may be related to a direct toxic effect (stimulatory) on the nail (bed and matrix) melanocytes. Nail hyperpigmentation (brown-black color) can diffusely involve the nail plate or present as horizontal (transverse) or longitudinal bands. Transverse banding is more common than longitudinal banding. Some chemotherapeutic agents can cause more than one reaction pattern (Table 21). Nail hyperpigmentation can involve both the fingernails and toenails and has been reported to follow both systemic and topical chemotherapy. Generally, nail hyperpigmentation begins 1 to 3 months after chemotherapy initiation and resolves spontaneously within 2 to 3 months after discontinuation. To date, nail hyperpigmentation has not been reported to occur with any of the BRMs previously mentioned. Fingernails require 3 to 4 months to grow out completely in a normal state but will grow more slowly in a diseased state. Toenails normally take 5 to 6 months to grow out completely.

OTHER NAIL DISORDERS

Diffuse *blue discoloration* of the nail plates has been reported following 5-fluorouracil administration. It appears that this reaction pattern is environmentally mediated because the pigment may be scraped off the nail plate. Mitoxantrone, a tumor antibiotic, has been noted to cause blue discoloration of the fingernails, sclerae, and urine. The mechanism is unknown (Table 21).

Onychodystrophy is malformation of a nail. The nail clinically becomes brittle and atrophic. In *onycholysis*, a separation of the nail plate from the nail bed occurs. The separated nail usually appears white and opaque.

In *Beau's line* linear depressions transverse the nail plate. The lines are caused by an acute transient arrest in nail growth. Any stressful systemic event, including high fever, weight loss, or chemotherapy administration, may elicit this reaction pattern. *Muehrcke's lines* are characterized by paired transverse white lines on the nail plate, separated by normal (pink) color. The lines remain fixed and grow out as the nail grows. They usually appear in patients with severe chronic hypoalbuminemia (< 1.8 g/dl for 4 months) and nephrotic syndrome. The mechanism for development of Muehrcke's nails is unknown.

Table 21. Causes of Nail Reaction Patterns in the Patient with Cancer

Hyperpigmentation	Onychodystrophy	Onycholysis	Beau's lines	Muehrcke's lines	Blue discoloration
Diffuse (nail bed and plate) Adriamycin, cyclophosphamide, melphalan, methotrexate, tegafur	Hydroxyurea	*Chemotherapy* Adriamycin, bleomycin (painful), 5-FU, hydroxyurea	Chemotherapy Circulatory shock High fever Myocardial infarction Pulmonary embolism Sepsis	Combination cisplatin, doxorubicin, CCNU, and vincristine* Severe chronic hypoalbuminemia Liver disease	Doxorubicin, 5-FU, mitoxantrone
Transverse banding Actinomycin D, bleomycin, cyclophosphamide, daunorubicin, doxorubicin, 5-FU (topical), hydroxyurea		*Infections* *White*: candida albicans, dermatophyte; *green*: pseudomonas, proteus			
Longitudinal banding Cyclophosphamide, doxorubicin, hydroxyurea, melphalan		*Medical disorders* Primary or secondary thyroid disease (mainly hyperthyroid)			
		Other Phototoxic drug reaction (tetracyclines)			

Reported in a patient with normoalbuminemia being treated for bronchial squamous cell carcinoma.

REFERENCES

1. Adrian R, Hood A, Skarin A: Mucocutaneous reactions to antineoplastic agents. *CA—Cancer J Clin* 1980, 30:143–157.

2. Nixon D, Pirozzi D, York R, *et al.*: Dermatologic changes after systemic cancer therapy. *Cutis* 1981, 27:181–194.

3. Conrad K, Dexter L: Cutaneous reactions related to treatment with BMRs. In Yasko J, Dudjak L (eds): *Biological Response Modifier Therapy—Symptom Management*. Emeryville, CA: Cetus, 1990; 129–134.

4. Purpora D, Ahern M, Silverman N: Toxic epidermal necrolysis after mithramycin. *N Engl J Med* 1978, 299:1412.

5. Baack B, Burgdorf W: Chemotherapy-induced acral erythema. *J Am Acad Dermatol* 1991, 24:457–461.

6. Lieschke G, Maher D, Cebon J: Effects of bacterially synthesized recombinant human granulocyte-macrophage colony-stimulating factor in patients with advanced malignancy. *Ann Intern Med* 1989, 110:357–364.

7. Syndman DR, Sullivan B, Gill M, *et al.*: Nosocomial sepsis associated with interleukin-2. *Ann Intern Med* 1990, 112:102–107.

8. Margolis D, Gross P: Neutrophilic eccrine hidradenitis: A case report and review of the literature. *Cutis* 1991, 48:198–200.

9. Hood A: Cutaneous side effects of cancer chemotherapy. *Med Clin North Am* 1986, 70:187–208.

10. Lenhard R, Sarah R: Acute complications of chemotherapy. In Martin D, Abeloff M (eds): *Complications of Cancer*. Baltimore: Johns Hopkins University Press, 1979; 361–366.

11. Weiss R, Bruno S: Hypersensitivity reactions to cancer chemotherapeutic agents. *Ann Intern Med* 1981, 94:66–72.

12. Wawrzyncak E: Systemic immunotoxin therapy of cancer: Advances and prospects. *Br J Cancer* 1991, 64:624–630.

13. Pastan I, Fitzgerald D: Recombinant toxins for cancer treatment. *Science* 1991, 254:1173–1177.

14. Wilkin J: Flushing reactions in the cancer chemotherapy patient. *Arch Dermatol* 1992, 128:1387–1389.

15. Aristizabal S, Miller R, Schlichtemeier A, Jones S: Adriamycin-irradiation cutaneous complications. *Int J Radiat Oncol Biol Phys* 1977, 2:325–331.

16. Bronner A, Hood A: Cutaneous complications of chemotherapeutic agents. *J Am Acad Dermatol* 1983, 9:645–662.

17. Hendrix J, Greer K: Cutaneous hyperpigmentation caused by systemic drugs. *Intern J Dermatol* 1992, 31:458–466.

18. Denman S: A review of pruritus. *J Am Acad Dermatol* 1978, 17:761–767.

19. Dorsk B: Raynaud's phenomenon and cancer chemotherapy. *Ann Intern Med* 1981, 95:652–653.

20. Epstein E, Lutzner M: Folliculitis induced by actinomycin D. *N Engl J Med* 1969, 281:1094–1096.

21. Larson D: Treatment of tissue extravasation by antitumor agents. *Cancer* 1982, 49:1796–1799.

22. Dunagin W: Dermatologic toxicity. In: Perry M, Yarbro J (ed.) *Toxicity of Chemotherapy*. New York: Grune and Stratton, 1984; 125–153.

23. Joss R, Kiser J, Weston S, Brunner K: Fighting alopecia in cancer chemotherapy. *Recent Results in Cancer Research* 1988, 108:117–125.

24. Baird S, McCorkle R, Grant M: *Cancer Nursing*. Philadelphia: WB Saunders, 1991; 256–257,337,351,858.

25. Fitzpatrick T, Johnson R, Polano M, *et al.* (eds): Telogen effluvium. *Color Atlas and Synopsis of Clinical Dermatology*, 2nd ed. New York: McGraw-Hill, 1992; 196.

DRUG-RELATED CUTANEOUS REACTIONS

Cutaneous reaction patterns induced by chemotherapeutic agents are variable in presentation and clinical outcome. Most reaction patterns are benign and self-limited and do not require discontinuation of the offending agent: however, some may be severe and life-threatening. Early recognition of drug-related skin (including hair and nail) eruptions may save the patient with cancer considerable morbid complications.

Severe cutaneous reaction patterns (grading 4) generally involve 40 to 60% of body surface. Patients with these eruptions are febrile and are at high risk for development of high-output heart failure, tachycardia, peripheral edema, and sepsis, particularly if there is skin breakdown. Severe reactions may also be localized and may cause the patient with cancer significant pain or pruritus.

MANAGEMENT OR INTERVENTION

1. Mild reactions
   a. Reassure patient that condition is benign and self-limiting
   b. Analgesics for pain
   c. Antihistamines for pruritus
   d. Tretinoin cream for acneiform eruptions
   e. Topical corticosteroids for hypersensitivity and photosensitive reactions
2. Severe reactions
   a. Withdrawal of offending agent for life-threatening generalized reactions and dosage reduction or agent substitution for localized reactions
   b. Correction of electrolyte and protein imbalances
   c. Hydration
   d. Systemic corticosteroids
   e. Antihistamines for pruritus
   f. Antibiotics for infection
   g. Narcotic analgesics for pain
   h. Plastic surgery evaluation for extravasation injuries

CAUSATIVE AGENTS

Mild: bleomycin, busulfan, cisplatin, cyclophosphamide, cyclosporin, cytosine arabinoside, daunorubicin, doxorubicin, GM-CSF, 5-fluorouracil, interleukin-2, hydroxyurea, mechlorethamine, melphalan, methotrexate, mithramycin, prednisone, procarbazine, thiotepa, vinblastine, vincristine;
Severe: actinomycin D, bleomycin, busulfan, cisplatin, cyclophosphamide, cytosine arabinoside, doxorubicin, 5-fluorouracil, GM-CSF, hydroxyurea, interleukin-2, l-asparaginase, methotrexate, mechlorethamine, mithramycin, vinblastine, vincristine

PATHOLOGIC PROCESS

Direct toxic injury to superficial dermal endothelium and microvasulature; direct cellular toxicity to growing epithelium or surrounding tissues (in extravasation injuries); cessation of actively growing tissues (hair and nails) secondarily to direct cellular cytotoxicity; bone marrow suppression

PATIENT ASSESSMENT

Complete medical and dermatologic history and evaluation; review of medications and associated therapies (*eg*, radiation therapy); determine percentage of body surface involved (one palm is approximately 1.2 % of total body surface) and distrubution; constitutional symptoms (fever, malaise); skin biopsy to rule out other causes of erythroderma; skin cultures for secondary infections

PREVENTION

Complete drug sensitivity (allergy) history; complete dermatologic (*eg*, eczema, psoriasis) history; dosage reduction or drug substitution with known history of drug reactions; sunscreens for photosynthesizing agents and prior radiation therapy

TOXICITY GRADING

1	2	3	4
Acneiform eruptions	Photosensitivity	Extravasation injuries	Erythroderma
Alopecia	Pruritus	Acral erythema	Toxic epidermal necrolysis
Flushing	Purpura (grades 2–3)	Raynaud's disease	Raynaud's disease with digital gangrene
Type IV hypersensitivity (grades 1–2)	Radiation recall (grades 2–3)	Mucositis	
Nail dystrophy	Type I and III hypersensitivity (grades 2–3)		
Pigmentation abnormalities			

Surgery, radiation therapy, and chemotherapy are the traditional modalities used for the treatment of cancer. These treatments, used either alone or in combination, can cure approximately 50% of all cancers. The other 50%, that is, those patients who are not cured by these traditional modalities and eventually succumb to their diseases, represent greater than 500,000 patients annually in the United States. These sobering statistics have prompted the continued search for new treatment approaches.

Over the past decade, there has been a revolution in biotechnology and immunology that has led to the development of numerous potential biologic response modifiers suitable for testing as cancer therapy. These have included nonspecific immunostimulants such as vaccines, monoclonal or polyclonal antibodies, adoptively transferred cells, specific immunostimulatory cytokines, and growth factors. Currently, only granulocyte colony-stimulating factor (G-CSF), granulocyte-macrophage colony-stimulating factor (GM-CSF), interleukin-2 (IL-2), interferon α, levamisole, and bacillus Calmette-Guérin (BCG) are approved for cancer therapy.

In this section, many of the complications associated with the biologic therapy for malignancy are discussed. In general, discussions focus on complications observed with Food and Drug Administration (FDA)–approved agents used at approved doses and schedules (Table 1). Many other biologic agents currently under investigation, as well as some chemotherapeutic agents, have produced similar side effects and, therefore, some of these discussions may be more generally applicable.

CONSTITUTIONAL EFFECTS: FLU-LIKE SYNDROME

Constitutional effects, often described as an influenza-like syndrome including fever, chills, malaise, myalgias, arthralgias, headache, and occasionally nausea, vomiting, diarrhea, nasal congestion, dizziness, and light-headedness were described in reports from early human interferon α trials that used crude preparations of interferon. These effects were initially thought to be related to contaminants in the interferon preparations. When these symptoms persisted with highly purified interferon preparations and later with recombinant interferon, they were believed to be directly related to interferon. Subsequent studies have demonstrated that interferon α is intrinsically pyrogenic—*ie*, capable of inducing prostaglandin E_2 (PGE_2) synthesis (in the rat hypothalamus)—and a direct role for interferon in producing constitutional symptoms has been postulated [1]. With the use of other recombinant proteins such as IL-2 and GM-CSF, the flu-like syndrome was again observed, suggesting that a common mechanism was involved. IL-2 and GM-CSF stimulate lymphocytes or monocytes to release or generate the secondary cytokines interleukin-1 (IL-1), tumor necrosis factor (TNF), interleukin-6 (IL-6), and interferon γ, which are believed to mediate the fever and many of the constitutional effects associated with IL-2 or GM-CSF administration. The PGE_2 released in response to various pyrogenic primary or secondary cytokines is believed to be the ultimate mediator of many of the flu-like symptoms.

All patients receiving standard high-dose IL-2 therapy, most patients receiving interferon therapy, and some patients receiving GM-CSF therapy develop the flu-like syndrome. These side effects are dose related, occur 1 to 6 hours after a dose, are more common with bolus administration, and resolve spontaneously within 24 hours of a single dose administration. When administered repeatedly, tachyphylaxis often develops, with symptoms subsiding over time. Pretreatment with nonsteroidal anti-inflammatory agents appears to lessen the febrile response, and with symptomatic therapy, this or other constitutional effects are rarely dose limiting. High fevers occur-

Table 1. FDA-approved Biologic Agents for Cancer Treatment

Agent	Dose	Route	Schedule	Approved Indications
Interferon alpha (IFN α-2a or 2b)	2 million IU/m^2	IM or SC	3 X/wk	Hairy cell leukemia
	30 million IU/m^2	IM or SC	3 X/wk	AIDS-related Kaposi's sarcoma
Bacillus Calmette-Guérin (BCG)	One ampule (1–8 X 10^8 colony forming units of TICE BCG or 50 mg wet weight) in 50 ml saline	Bladder installation for 2 hr	Weekly X 6 wk then monthly for 6–12 mo	Carcinoma in situ of the bladder
G-CSF	5 μg/kg/d	SC or IV	Daily for up to 2 wk or until absolute neutrophil count (ANC) has reached 10,000/mm^3	Febrile neutropenia in patients with nonmyeloid malignancies receiving myelosuppressive chemotherapy
GM-CSF	250 μg/m^2/d	IV as a 2-hr infusion	Daily for 21 days beginning 2–4 hr after the autologous marrow infusion and not less than 24 hr after the last dose of chemotherapy and 12 hr after the last dose of radiation therapy until ANC > 20,000 cells/mm^3	Myeloid reconstitution after autologous bone marrow transplantation for non-Hodgkin's lymphoma, acute lymphoblastic leukemia, and Hodgkin's disease
Levamisole hydrochloride	50 mg	PO	Q 8 hr for 3 d with initiation of 5-FU therapy, then 50 mg PO q 8 hr for 3 d every 2 wk X 1 yr	Adjuvant treatment in combination with 5-FU after surgical resection for Dukes' stage C colon cancer
Interleukin-2	600,000 IU/kg (0.037 mg/kg)	IV over 15 min	Q 8 hr X 14 doses. Following 9 d of rest, the schedule is repeated for another 14 doses for a maximum of 28 doses/course. If there is a response to the first course of treatment, a second course may be given after at least a 7-wk rest period	Adults with metastatic renal cell carcinoma

ring after several days of treatment or recurring after resolution of the early fevers are unusual and should prompt a search for an infectious source and, if indicated, institution of appropriate antibiotic therapy.

Constitutional effects occur in up to 33% of patients receiving levamisole. Symptoms generally occur on the day of treatment, range from mild and transient to severe and progressive, and necessitate discontinuation of therapy in up to 2% of patients [2,3]. Intravesical administration of BCG causes a flu-like syndrome in up to 60% of patients. Symptoms usually begin 6 to 12 hours after a dose, may persist for 1 to 2 days, and typically parallel the severity of the associated cystitis. Unlike IL-2, GM-CSF, and interferon α, symptoms are far more common after several doses of BCG than after the initial dose. Symptoms persisting beyond 2 days often indicate systemic BCG infection and warrant prompt institution of antituberculous therapy [4,5]. The etiologic mechanisms for the constitutional effects produced by levamisole and BCG administration are unclear but may also be related to secondary cytokine release.

A flu-like syndrome may also occur with the administration of systemic chemotherapy, especially high-dose dacarbazine (DTIC) therapy or combination chemotherapy with cytosine arabinoside (ara-C) and cisplatin (CDDP). Up to 50% of patients receiving dacarbazine develop flu-like symptoms, which typically last for several days and often recur with successive treatments [6,7]. Although the mechanism of this toxicity is unknown, it is tempting to hypothesize cytokine release as an important mediator.

FATIGUE

Chronic fatigue is the most important dose-limiting toxicity of interferon-α therapy, and can also be dose limiting in patients receiving IL-2 and GM-CSF therapy. Fatigue usually begins with the initial constitutional effects; however, tachyphylaxis to fatigue does not occur. Instead, with repeated doses, the fatigue may persist or increase in severity, ultimately resulting in a decrease in the patient's performance status. Although there is wide individual variation in tolerance, most patients can tolerate interferon at 3 to 10 MU/d for prolonged periods. With intermittent schedules two to three times per week, tolerance is better and fatigue may be mild or even unnoticed. At doses higher than 20 MU, most patients require a 50% or greater dose reduction during the first 2 to 4 weeks of daily therapy or the first 8 to 12 weeks of intermittent therapy. Doses of more than 100 MU are rarely tolerated for more than 1 to 2 weeks, if given daily, or 4 to 8 weeks, if given intermittently. Fatigue is most severe at doses of greater than 20 MU/d, in elderly patients, and in patients with a poor performance status. In some patients, evening administration of interferon improves tolerance [1].

Fatigue, weakness, and malaise occur in up to 50% of patients receiving high dose IL-2 therapy. Unlike many of the other toxic manifestations of IL-2 therapy that resolve quickly after discontinuation of IL-2 therapy, the fatigue may persist for several weeks after administration of the last dose.

Fatigue occurring with GM-CSF has been reported infrequently (< 5%), perhaps because it is difficult to distinguish from the fatigue associated with high-dose chemotherapy, bone marrow transplantation, or other intercurrent illnesses common to most clinical settings in which GM-CSF is used. Rosenfeld *et al.* [8] reported fatigue in patients with myelodysplasia receiving yeast-derived GM-CSF at doses of 60 to 250 µg/m²/d subcutaneously or by 2-hour intravenous infusion for 14 days. One of 18 patients treated by the intravenous route and 4 of 19 patients treated by the subcutaneous route had a

decrease in ECOG performance status of two grades. One patient receiving 125 µg/m²/d subcutaneously required a dose reduction because of fatigue. Physicians should thus be aware that some patients receiving GM-CSF (especially at doses > 250 µg/m²d may develop significant fatigue requiring dose modification. Fatigue has also been reported in less than 5% of patients treated with levamisole, 7 to 33% of patients treated with BCG (in association with the flu-like syndrome), and rarely, if ever, with G-CSF. With none of these agents was fatigue dose limiting.

The pathogenesis of the fatigue associated with biologic therapy is unclear but may be part of the broad constellation of central nervous system (CNS) toxicity observed with these agents. Dinarello [9] suggests that fatigue may be related to the direct effects of either IL-1 or secondarily released PGE_2 from paraventricular endothelial cells on neurons and glial cells exposed to systemic circulation in the organ vasculosum laminar terminalis (OVLT) of the hypothalamus. In experimental systems, IL-1 administration rapidly induces fever, sleep, and the release of a variety of neuropeptides. Although IL-1 does not cross the blood–brain barrier, glial and possibly neural cells synthesize IL-1 and other neurotransmitters, which then may interact with receptors distributed throughout the brain, including the sleep center where a rapid change from REM to slow-wave activity occurs. IL-1 may also act as a cofactor in synaptic transmission with low concentrations of IL-1 actually augmenting γ-aminobutyric acid-a (GABAa) receptor function. To what extent these effects of IL-1 or unknown effects of other secondary cytokines contribute to the fatigue associated with biologic response modifier therapy remains to be elucidated.

INFECTIOUS COMPLICATIONS

Bacteremia and sepsis have occurred with unusual frequency in patients receiving recombinant IL-2 therapy. In clinical trials with high-dose bolus IL-2, bacteremia occurred in 10 to 20% of treatment courses and was often related to central intravenous catheters. *Staphylococcus aureus* was the most common pathogen isolated, accounting for 65% of cases, followed by *Staphylococcus epidermidis*, *Escherichia coli*, and polymicrobial infection. Patients at highest risk for infection included those with grade 2 or greater skin toxicity with skin desquamation, skin colonization at the catheter site with *S. aureus*, and an indwelling central venous catheter. The bacteremias were often severe, with a large number of positive blood cultures, persistent bacteremia for an average of 2.5 days after institution of appropriate antibiotic therapy, and significant clinical sequelae. Of 20 patients with bacteremia described by Klempner and Snydman [10] two died of sepsis, three developed thrombophlebitis, one developed probable septic arthritis, one had a septic arterial aneurysm at an arterial line site, and one had peritonitis and probable meningitis. Other types of nosocomial infections, such as pneumonia, decubital ulcer, or urinary tract infections, were only rarely seen in these IL-2 recipients.

The management of bacteremia and sepsis associated with IL-2 therapy requires prompt recognition and initiation of appropriate antibiotic therapy. Optimal intravenous catheter care should be practiced to decrease the risk for infection, with catheters being removed after each 5-day course of therapy. Surveillance cultures of the catheter site should be performed twice per week. Prophylactic antibiotic therapy with oxacillin, cephalosporins, or quinolones has decreased the incidence of bacteremia significantly, and thus should be used in all patients with central venous catheters. When sepsis is suspected, blood samples should be obtained from both catheter and peripheral sites and empiric intravenous antibiotic therapy instituted while culture results are awaited. Vancomycin is the antibiotic of choice because gram-positive bacteremia is very common; however, about 10% of infection may be due to gram-negative organisms and thus broader coverage may be indicated in some patients. If the infection is catheter related, the catheter should be removed as soon as possible. Klempner and Snydman [10] suggested that the unusually high incidence of bacterial infections associated with IL-2 administration is related to a severe IL-2–induced impairment in neutrophil chemotaxis.

Brosman and Lamm [4] recently reviewed complications of intravesical BCG therapy in 1254 patient treated over 15 years. The majority of patients had been treated with the Tice strain, although patients were also treated with the Connaught, Pasteur (Armand Frappier), and Glaxo strains. The strains appeared similar in toxicity. Overall, granulomatous involvement of various organs occurred in less than 5% of patients. Granulomatous prostatitis was reported in 1.3% of patients, although if routine prostate biopsy specimens were obtained in asymptomatic patients, the incidence might have been as high as 25% [5]. In most cases, cultures for active BCG infections were negative. Epididymitis–orchitis occurred in 0.2%, renal granulomas in 0.1%, BCG pneumonitis or hepatitis in 0.9%, BCG bone marrow involvement with subsequent cytopenia in 0.1%, and sepsis in 0.4%. Death from disseminated BCG infections, "BCGosis," occurred in seven patients (0.6%). Most patients who developed sepsis or BCGosis showed signs of increasingly severe reactions, with each dose of BCG manifested by higher and more prolonged fevers. In all fatal cases and in most septic cases, intravascular dissemination of BCG was believed to have occurred as a result of traumatic catherization or absorption through an inflamed, friable, bleeding urothelium. The use of isoniazid alone appears ineffective in preventing death from BCG sepsis. Two patients treated with multiple antituberculous agents, including cycloserine, have survived.

In general, there is a much higher incidence of systemic BCG infections in patients treated with intralesional BCG or immunosuppressed patients treated with intradermal BCG. One patient who had a history of intradermal BCG therapy developed activation of dormant BCG infection after immunosuppression with systemic chemotherapy. Because similar activation has not been reported in patients who have received intravesical BCG, routine antituberculous prophylaxis is not recommended for patients treated with intravesical BCG who later require systemic chemotherapy. Finally, not all granulomatous lesions are infectious. Orihuela *et al.* [5] reported several cases of culture-negative pelvic lymphadenitis, hepatic granulomas, and pulmonary lesions, which were believed to be immune in origin.

Interferon therapy has been associated with reactivation of herpes simplex infections in up to 10% of patients within the first several days of treatment. These infections generally clear within 10 days even while patients continue receiving interferon. Disseminated herpes has not been reported [11]. Because interferon has antiviral properties and has been used to treat herpetic infections, this reactivation of herpes simplex is difficult to explain.

Levamisole has only been associated with infections in patients who develop levamisole-induced neutropenia or agranulocytosis, which occurs in less than 2% of patients.

HEMODYNAMIC COMPLICATIONS

Although hypotension is the most frequent dose-limiting side effect of IL-2 therapy, it is uncommonly observed with GM-CSF and interferon therapy, and rarely, if ever, with G-CSF, BCG, and levamisole therapy. Nearly all patients receiving high-dose IL-2 ther-apy by intermittent bolus injection for 5 days develop hypotension. Approximately 75% of these patients require pressure support to continue IL-2 therapy safely. Within 2 to 4 hours after the initial dose of IL-2, vasodilation occurs, with a decrease in systemic vascular resistance and mean arterial pressure, and a compensatory increase in heart rate and cardiac index. The increase in cardiac index is not fully compensated, as evidenced by renal hypoperfusion, resulting in a prerenal state. These changes are identical to the changes observed during the early phases of septic shock. With IL-2 therapy, the lowered systemic vascular resistance does not return to baseline until up to 5 days after the completion of therapy. In addition to the effects on vascular resistance, IL-2 induces a capillary leak syndrome, resulting in third-space accumulation of fluid and worsening of the hypotension. The exact pathway by which IL-2 exerts an effect on vascular smooth muscle remains to be defined, although nitric oxide is believed to be the final and pivotal mediator in this process. In most patients, the hypotension can be safely managed without disruption of IL-2 therapy by the judicious use of intravenous fluids and the institution of pressor support with dopamine or phenylephrine [12].

Hemodynamic complictions of GM-CSF are much less frequent and less carefully studied. The first dose of GM-CSF may be followed in 1 to 4 hours by a "first-dose reaction," characterized by hypotension, hypoxemia, flushing, tachycardia, musculoskeletal pain, dyspnea, nausea, and vomiting. This reaction appears to be more common with doses of 3 µg/kg/d or higher, high-peak serum GM-CSF levels, intravenous administration, and nonglycosylated, bacterially synthesized GM-CSF. Continuous infusion of GM-CSF may decrease the frequency and severity of this reaction. Fortunately, this reaction is limited to the first dose of each treatment cycle and thus is not dose limiting. The mechanism of the first-dose GM-CSF reaction is unclear but appears to be unrelated to TNF [13]. Hypotension may also occur later during a course of therapy and be related to vasodilation and the capillary leak syndrome similar to what has been reported with IL-2, especially with high doses of GM-CSF (< 250 µg/m^2/d or < 10 µg/kg/d) [13,14].

Hypotension has occurred in up to 6% of patients with cancer treated with interferon α. It is generally mild and easily managed with intravenous fluids. Rarely, dose modifications are required [15].

CAPILLARY LEAK SYNDROME

The capillary leak (or vascular leak) syndrome was initially described in trials that used high-dose IL-2 and lymphokine-activated killer (LAK) cells but has subsequently been observed in most patients receiving high-dose IL-2 and in approximately 10% of patients receiving GM-CSF at a dosage of 250 µg/m^2/d by 2-hour infusion. This syndrome is a common dose-limiting side effect of IL-2 and GM-CSF therapy and consists of a generalized increase in vascular permeability, with fluid extravasation into the tissues. Clinical manifestations usually begin within 24 hours of the initiation of IL-2 therapy and progress from mild facial and ankle edema to anasarca with weight gain in excess of 5 to 10% of baseline body weight due to fluid retention. Ascites occurs in some patients, especially those with extensive hepatic metastases, whereas pleural or pericardial effusions occur in approximately 50% of IL-2 recipients. In patients with preexisting pleural or pericardial effusions, IL-2 or GM-CSF may aggravate localized fluid retention. Because of the high risk for cerebral edema when there is disruption of the blood–brain barrier, patients with brain metastases should not receive IL-2 or GM-CSF therapy [16,17].

Diffuse or focal pulmonary infiltrates, observed in 40% of patients treated with IL-2, may result in significant dyspnea, hypoxia, and, in less than 5% of cases, the need for short-term ventilatory support. The development of pulmonary edema is more common in patients with marginal pulmonary reserve (ie, patients with pretreatment FEV_1 of $\leq$ 2.0 1) and in those whose treatment is complicated by bacteremia. The extent of peripheral edema or the amount of weight gain does not correlate with or predict the development of pulmonary infiltrates. Because the extravasation of fluid into the alveoli occurs in the setting of a normal pulmonary capillary wedge pressure, the pulmonary infiltrates are most likely caused by an increased capillary permeability rather than fluid overload or left ventricular dysfunction [18]. A similar syndrome has been reported in the setting of bone marrow transplantation with the use of high-dose cytosine arabinoside or a combination of high-dose busulfan, etoposide, and carmustine [19,20].

The management of the capillary leak syndrome is often complicated by other treatment side effects, especially hypotension. Symptomatic fluid retention limits the amount of fluid that can be administered to support the blood pressure, and hypotension precludes the use of diuretics to reverse fluid retention. Severe cardiovascular or pulmonary toxicity is an indication to withhold doses of IL-2 or GM-CSF, or to decrease the dose of GM-CSF. Diuretics can be safely administered and are indicated, once therapy has been completed and blood pressure has normalized, to assist in the clearance of excess retained fluid. Side effects resolve rapidly after the discontinuation of therapy, with most patients reverting to their baseline weight in 4 to 5 days after completing a course of treatment.

Although the pathogenesis of the capillary leak syndrome is uncertain, most likely a combination of factors are involved. Direct endothelial injury is mediated by IL-2–activated leukocytes (natural killer (NK) or LAK cells in particular) or their oxidative products. Both IL-2 and GM-CSF activate peripheral blood mononuclear cells to release secondary cytokines, including TNF and IL-1. These secondary cytokines may worsen the process by inducing various adhesion molecules necessary for the attachment of activated leukocytes to the endothelium. On the other hand, these cytokines, especially IL-1, may at the same time render the endothelium less susceptible to cell-mediated injury. Finally, IL-2 treatment is associated with systemic complement activation and high plasma concentrations of anaphylatoxins such as C3a, which have potent effects on vascular permeability [16].

ALLERGIC AND IMMUNE-MEDIATED COMPLICATIONS

Biologic therapy alters the immune system in a variety of ways, including alteration of tumor antigen expression, stimulation of immune effector cells, enhancement of humoral immunity, and the release of secondary cytokines. This immunomodulation is most likely responsible for both the beneficial effects and toxic effects of biologic therapy. Not surprisingly, a number of allergic and immune-mediated side effects have been observed in patients treated with IL-2, interferon, and, less commonly, with GM-CSF, G-CSF, BCG, and levamisole.

Allergic reactions are common and frequently occur at the local site of administration. When IL-2, interferon, GM-CSF, or G-CSF are administered subcutaneously, self-limited erythematous cutaneous reactions occur at the injection site. Similarly, when BCG is administered intravesically, a self-limited cystitis occurs in 60 to 90% of patients [5,21]. Acute serious hypersensitivity reactions such as urticaria, angioedema, bronchoconstriction, and anaphylaxis have rarely been observed with IL-2, interferon α, GM-CSF, G-CSF, levamisole, and BCG.

A "recall reaction" to iodinated radiographic contrast medium occurs in approximately 10% of patients undergoing routine intravenous contrast studies for follow-up of previous IL-2 therapy. Reactions usually occur at least 1 month after initial exposure to IL-2 and contrast medium. Typical reactions begin 1 to 4 hours after reexposure to radiographic contrast medium and consist of fever, chills, rash, diarrhea, nausea, vomiting, urticaria, dyspnea, weakness, and hypotension. Reactions appear to be more common in patients receiving intra-arterial rather than systemic IL-2 therapy or concomitant administration of IL-2 and radiographic contrast material. This "recall reaction" may be related to enhancement by IL-2 of an immune response to radiographic contrast material, followed by an anamnestic response on reexposure to the contrast material [22].

Each of these agents, but especially IL-2 and interferon, has been associated with the development or exacerbation of preexisting autoimmune or chronic inflammatory diseases. Both IL-2 and interferon have been associated with the development or exacerbation of preexisting autoimmune thyroiditis, hemolytic anemia, immune thrombocytopenia purpura (ITP), rheumatoid arthritis, psoriasis, vasculitis, inflammatory bowel disease, and nephritis [1,22]. GM-CSF has been associated with reactivation of ITP, autoimmune thyroiditis, rheumatoid arthritis, and hemolysis, whereas G-CSF has been associated with the development of vasculitis in two patients treated for chronic neutropenia and in one patient treated for hairy cell leukemia [17]. Although BCG vaccination and intralesional BCG administration have been associated with erythema nodosum, cutaneous vasculitis, and generalized Shwartzman reaction, these side effects have not been reported with intravesical BCG treatment [5]. Symoens et al. [23] reported a higher frequency of levamisole-induced leukopenia and agranulocytosis in patients with rheumatic diseases (4.9%) when compared with patients with cancer (2%). However, these results are difficult to interpret because leukopenia and agranulocytosis occur frequently in patients with rheumatic diseases in the absence of levamisole therapy. The agranulocytosis appears to be related to anti-granulocyte antibodies and circulating immune complexes [2]. A cutaneous necrotizing vasculitis has also been reported with levamisole therapy [23]. The mechanisms involved in the development of autoimmune and inflammatory diseases with biologic therapy are complex and as yet poorly defined. In some cases the administered cytokine may play a direct role in the pathogenesis of disease.

Enhanced production of autoantibodies to insulin, thyrotropin, platelets, and other antigens has been reported after biologic therapy, and it is likely that, as our experience with biologic agents grows, numerous other autoantibodies will be detected. Many of these autoantibodies may be associated with the development of autoimmune disease. For example, after high-dose IL-2 therapy, 10 to 20% of patients develop a thyroiditis that is often associated with increased serum titers of antithyroid antibodies. Patients typically present with hypothyroidism approximately 8 to 10 weeks after the initiation of treatment. Frequently, a transient period of hyperthyroidism or even thyrotoxicosis precedes the hypothyroidism. Thyroid dysfunction is more frequent in women, in patients with antithyroid antibodies or subclinical evidence of thyroiditis pretreatment, and in patients receiving prolonged and repeated courses of IL-2, particularly in association with interferon α. The thyroid abnormalities resolve spontaneously 4 to 10 months after treatment is completed. Similarly, patients treated with interferon α may develop antithyroid antibodies and associated thyroid abnormalities. Treatment should be discontinued in patients whose thyroid function cannot be normalized with drug therapy [1,24]. IL-2 and interferon α–related thyroid dysfunction may be related to a direct toxic effect of activated NK or LAK cells on thyrocytes, an inhibition of thyroglobulin production by secondary cytokines such as IL-1 and TNF, a direct or indirect stimulation of humoral immunity to thyroid autoantigens, or reactivation of preexisting T-cell clones directed against thyroid autoantigens, resulting in autoimmune thyroiditis [22].

Both neutralizing and nonneutralizing antibodies against IL-2, GM-CSF, and interferon have been observed. The clinical significance of these antibodies remains unclear, but in several cases the development of neutralizing antibodies to interferon was associated with disease relapse [1]. Many factors influence the frequency, magnitude, and importance of antibody induction, including underlying disease, treatment schedule, cumulative dose, treatment duration,

route of administration, blood sampling time, source of protein, and assay methods. For interferon α, the underlying disease plays an important role in frequency of antibody formation, with the highest incidence occurring in patients treated for Kaposi's sarcoma (5%) and renal cell carcinoma (32–38%) [25]. In addition, interferon-neutralizing antibodies occur more frequently with interferon α-2a than with interferon α-2b perhaps because of different purification techniques. Despite numerous systemic IL-2 trials, neutralizing antibodies to IL-2 develop uncommonly. The low incidence of IL-2 antibodies may be related to the short duration of standard high-dose IL-2 therapy. As new studies with long-term administration of low-dose IL-2 therapy are now underway, the incidence and clinical significance of IL-2 antibody formation may become significant. In addition, a case report and *in vitro* studies suggest that interferon may act synergistically with IL-2 in inducing a humoral response, with the resultant production of high titers of anti–IL-2 antibodies [26].

REFERENCES

1. Quesada JR, Talpaz M, Rios A, *et al.*: Clinical toxicity of interferons in cancer patients: A review. *J Clin Oncol* 1988, 4:234–243.
2. Parkinson DR, Jerry LM, Shibata HR, *et al.*: Complications of cancer immunotherapy with levamisole. *Lancet* 1977, 1:1129–1132.
3. Quirt IC, Shelly WE, Pater JL, *et al.*: Improved survival in patients with poor-prognosis malignant melanoma treated with adjuvant levamisole: A phase III study by the National Cancer Institute of Canada Clinical Trials Group. *J Clin Oncol* 1991, 9:729–735.
4. Brosman SA, Lamm DL: The preparation, handling and use of intravesical bacillus Calmette-guérin for the management of stage Ta, T1, carcinoma *in situ* and transitional cell cancer. *J Urol* 1990, 144:313–315.
5. Orihuela E, Herr HW, Pinsky CM, Whitmore WF: Toxicity of intravesical BCG and its management in patients with superficial bladder tumors. *Cancer* 1987, 60:326–333.
6. Beusa JM, Mouridsen HT, van-Oosterom AT, *et al.*: High-dose DTIC in advanced soft-tissue sarcomas in the adult: A phase II study of the E.O.R.T.C. Soft Tissue and Bone Sarcoma Group. *Ann Oncol* 1991, 2:307–309.
7. Margolin K, Doroshow J, Leong L, *et al.*: Combination chemotherapy with cytosine arabinoside (ara-C) and cis-diamminedichloroplatinum (CDDP) for squamous cancers of the upper aerodigestive tract. *Am J Clin Oncol* 1989, 12:494–497.
8. Rosenfeld CS, Sulecki M, Evans C, Shadduck RK: Comparison of intravenous versus subcutaneous recombinant human granulocyte-macrophage colony-stimulating factor in patients with myelodysplasia. *Exp Hematol* 1991, 19:273–277.
9. Dinarello CA: Interleukin-1 and interleukin-1 antagonism. *Blood* 1992, 77:1627–1652.
10. Klempner MS, Snydman DR: Infectious complication associated with interleukin-2. In Atkins MB, Mier JW (eds): *Therapeutic Applications of Interleukin-2.* 1993: New York: Marcel Deker, 409–424.
11. Sherwin SA, Knost JA, Fein S, *et al.*: A multiple-dose phase I trial of recombinant leukocyte A interferon in cancer patients. *JAMA* 1982, 248:2461–2466.
12. Gaynor ER, Fisher RI: Hemodynamic and cardiovascular effects of IL-2. In Atkins MB, Mier JW, (eds) *Therapeutic Applications of Interleukin-2.* 1993: New York: Marcel Deker, 381–387.
13. Cebon J, Lieschke GJ, Bury RW, Morstyn G: The dissociation of GM-CSF efficacy from toxicity according to route of administration: A pharmacodynamic study. *Br J Haematol* 1992, 80:144–150.
14. Lieschke GJ, Cebon J, Morstyn G: Characterization of the clinical effects after the first dose of bacterially synthesized recombinant human granulocyte-macrophage colony-stimulating factor. *Blood* 1989, 74:2634–2643.
15. Jones GJ, Itri LM: Safety and tolerance of recombinant interferon alpha-2a (Roferon-A) in cancer patients. *Cancer* 1986, 57:1709–1715.
16. Mier JW: Pathogenesis of the IL-2-induced vascular leak syndrome. In Atkins MB, Mier JW (eds): *Therapeutic Applications of Interleukin-2.* 1993: New York: Marcel Deker, 363–380.
17. Lieschke GJ, Burgess AW: Granulocyte colony-stimulating factor and granulocyte-macrophage colony-stimulating factor. *N Engl J Med* 1992, 327:28–35.
18. Margolin KA: The clinical toxicities of high-dose IL-2. In Atkins MB, Mier JW (eds): *Therapeutic Applications of Interleukin-2.* 1993, Marcel Deker, New York: 331–362.
19. Woods WG, Ramsay NK, Weisdorf DJ, *et al.*: Bone marrow transplantation for acute lymphoblastic leukemia utilizing total body irradiation followed by high doses of cytosine arabinoside: Lack of superiority over cyclophosphamide-containing conditioning regimens. *Bone Marrow Transplant* 1990, 6:9–16.
20. Takahashi H, Sekiguchi H, Kai S, *et al.*: Recurrent pulmonary edema in a patient with acute lymphoblastic leukemia after syngeneic bone marrow transplantation. *Rinsho Ketsueki* 1992, 33:354–359.
21. Lamm DL, Stogdill VD, Stogdill BJ, Crispen RG: Complications of bacillus Calmette-guérin immunotherapy in 1,278 patients with bladder cancer. *J Urol* 1986, 135:272–274.
22. Atkins MB: Autoimmune disorders induced by interleukin-2 therapy. In Atkins MB, Mier JW, (eds): *Therapeutic Applications of Interleukin-2.* 1993, New York: Marcel Deker, 389–408.
23. Symoens J, Veys E, Mielants M, Pinals R: Adverse reactions to levamisole. *Cancer Treat Rep* 1978, 62:1721–1730.
24. Schultz M, Muller R, von zur Muhlen A, Brabant G: Induction of hyperthyrodism by interferon-alpha-2b. *Lancet* 1989, 1:1452.
25. Figlin RA: Biotherapy in clinical practice. *Semin Hematol* 1989, 26(suppl 3):15–24.
26. Kirchner H, Korfer A, Evers P, *et al.*: The development of neutralizing antibodies in a patient receiving subcutaneous recombinant and natural interleukin-2. *Cancer* 1990, 67:1862–1864.

FLU-LIKE SYNDROME

Patients undergoing biologic therapy with IL-2, interferon alpha, GM-CSF, and, less frequently, BCG and levamisole, develop a flu-like syndrome consisting of fever, chills, malaise, myalgias, arthralgias, headache, and occasionally nausea, vomiting, diarrhea, nasal congestion, dizziness, and light-headedness. For IL-2, interferon alpha, and GM-CSF, these side effects are dose-related, occur 1 to 6 hours after a dose, are more common with bolus administration, and resolve spontaneously within 24 hours of administration of a single dose. With repeated daily doses (q 8 hr for IL-2, daily for interferon alpha and GM-CSF) there is a tendency to tachyphylaxis, with symptoms subsiding over time; however, with intermittent treatment, tachyphylaxis usually does not occur. With BCG, these side effects occur 6 to 12 hours after intravesical administration, and resolve within 1 to 2 days. The severity tends to parallel the intensity of the local reaction. With levamisole, side effects typically occur on the days of treatment. With any of these agents, fevers that occur after several days of therapy or that recur after resolution of early fevers are unusual and an infectious cause should be sought. Rarely are these constitutional symptoms dose-limiting [1,3,4,17,18].

CAUSATIVE AGENTS

Interferon α, IL-2, GM-CSF, BCG, levamisole, occasionally cytotoxic chemotherapy

PATHOLOGIC PROCESS

Release or generation of secondary cytokines (eg IL-1, TNF, IL-6) by lymphocytes or monocytes in response to IL-2 and GM-CSF; PGE_2 probably directly responsible for interferon-related constitutional symptoms; mechanism of levamisole and BCG toxicity is unclear, but may also be related to secondary cytokine release

DIFFERENTIAL DIAGNOSES

Co-existing viral, bacterial, or fungal infection, paraneoplastic syndromes

PATIENT ASSESSMENT

Rule out infections or neoplastic causes, especially if symptoms progress and are not closely related to administration of above agents

TOXICITY GRADING

	0	1	2	3	4
Fever in absence of infection	None	37.1–38.0°C 98.7–100.4°F	38.1–40.0°F 100.5–104.0°F	> 40.0°C > 104.0°F for < 24 h	> 40.0°C > 104.0°F for 24 h or accompanied by hypotension
Nausea	None	Able to eat reasonable intake	Intake significantly decreased but can eat	No significant intake	—
Vomiting	None	1 episode in 24 h	2–5 episodes in 24 h	6–10 episodes in 24 h	> 10 episodes in 24 h or requiring parenteral support
Diarrhea	None	Increase of 2–3 stools/day over pretreatment	Increase of 4–6 stools/day, nocturnal stools, moderate cramping	Increase of 7–9 stools/day, incontinence, or severe cramping	Increase of ≥ 10 stools/day, grossly bloody diarrhea, or need for parenteral support
Headache	None	Mild, no treatment required	Moderate non-narcotic treatment	Severe narcotics required	—
Sinus congestion	None	Mild, no treatment required	Moderate	—	—
Chills, rigors	None	Mild, < 30 min, resolves spontaneously	Moderate, < 30 min, requires intervention	—	—
Myalgia, arthralgia	None	Mild	Moderate	Severe	Intractable

MANAGEMENT OR INTERVENTION

Agent	Route	Dose (mg)	Action	Schedule	Guidelines
Acetaminophen	PO or PR	650	Antipyretic—inhibits prostaglandin synthesis	q 4 hr	Begin before first dose of IL-2 or IFN and continue until completion
Indomethacin	PO or PR	25	Antipyretic—inhibits prostaglandin synthesis	q 6 hr	Begin before first dose of IL-2 and continue until completion; treat fever with acetaminophen PRN
Diphenhydramine	PO or IV	25–50	Antihistamine—H_1 receptor antagonist	q 8 hr PRN	For fever, malaise, chills secondary to hypersensitivity reaction (especially with BCG)
Prochlorperazine	PO or IV or PR	10 PO or IV, 25 PR	Antiemetic—dopamine receptor antagonist; affects the chemoreceptor trigger zone and vomiting center	q 8 hr PRN	For nausea and vomiting
Meperidine	IM or IV	25–50	Analgesic—CNS opioid agonist	1 q 3–4 hr PRN	For severe chills and rigors
Loperamide hydrochloride	PO	2–4 (max 16 mg/d)	Antidiarrheal—slows intestinal motility	4 mg followed by 2 mg after each unformed stool PRN	For diarrhea
Diphenoxylate hydrochloride with atropine sulfate	PO	2.5– (max 20 mg/d)	Antidiarrheal— slows intestinal motility	2 tablets q 6hr, 10 ml q 6 hr PRN	For severe diarrhea

CHRONIC FATIGUE

The fatigue syndrome accompanying interferon, IL-2, and GM-CSF therapy varies considerably from mild to severe and, in some cases, defines the maximum tolerated dose. Fatigue is dose-related and is often less when intermittent schedules and lower doses are used. Although individual variation in tolerance is wide, fatigue is often more profound in older patients or those with poor performance status.

MANAGEMENT OR INTERVENTION

1. Evening administration of interferon may reduce fatigue or improve tolerance
2. Moderate or severe fatigue with decreased performance status often improves with a 50% dose reduction of interferon alpha or GM-CSF; if no improvement, reduce drug doses an additional 10% of starting dose or discontinue therapy until fatigue resolves

TOXICITY GRADING SCALE

0	1	2	3	4
Asymptomatic	Symptomatic	Symptomatic, in bed < 50% of day	Symptomatic, in bed > 50% of day but not bedridden	Bedridden

CAUSATIVE AGENTS

Interleukin-2, interferon alpha, GM-CSF

PATHOLOGIC PROCESS

Unclear, but may be part of the broad constellation of CNS toxicity observed with these agents; may be related to IL-1 release [9]

DIFFERENTIAL DIAGNOSES

Anemia; comorbid illness, especially chronic infections, thyroid dysfunction, hepatitis, renal dysfunction; tumor progression; other medications, particularly antiemetics, analgesics, sedatives, cytotoxic chemotherapy

PATIENT ASSESSMENT

Obtain hemoglobin, hematocrit, liver function tests, serum electrolytes (calcium), thyroid function tests, TSH, BUN, and creatinine; review other medications; assess for tumor progression

INFECTIOUS COMPLICATIONS

In patients receiving IL-2 therapy bacteremia occurs in 10 to 20%. The majority of these infections are related to the use of an indwelling intravenous catheter and occur toward the end of a course of IL-2 treatment. If unrecognized or if institution of appropriate antibiotic therapy is delayed, these infections can be fatal. Antibiotic prophylaxis with several agents has greatly reduced both the incidence and severity of infections. Although uncommon, systemic BCG infections do occur and in rare cases have been fatal. Most septic and fatal cases are related to intravasation of intravesically instilled BCG, often from traumatic catheterization or instrumentation [4,21].

Interferon therapy has been associated with reactivation of herpes simplex infections in up to 10% of patients within the first several days of treatment. These infections generally clear within 10 days even while interferon therapy continues. Disseminated herpes has not been reported [11]. Levamisole has only been associated with infections in patients who develop levamisole-induced agranulocytosis or neutropenia.

CAUSATIVE AGENTS

IL-2, interferon α, BCG

PATHOLOGIC PROCESS

IL-2 infections: probably related to severely impaired neutrophil chemotaxis, resulting either directly or indirectly from IL-2 administration; **Systemic BCG infections**: most likely related to intravascular dissemination of BCG through an inflamed, friable, or bleeding urothelium; **IFN therapy**: mechanism involved with reactivation of herpes simplex infections is unclear

DIFFERENTIAL DIAGNOSES

Flu-like syndrome associated with biologic agents, unrelated infectious process, drug reaction, paraneoplastic syndrome

PATIENT ASSESSMENT

IL-2: obtain blood cultures from central venous catheter site and peripherally, examine central venous catheter site and skin for generalized reactions, check for lapse in antipyretic administration, assess fever pattern with prior doses; **Interferon alpha**: evaluate lesions, obtain herpes virus culture; **BCG**: rule out other infections causes, culture bacterial strains and biopsy of affected sites

MANAGEMENT OR INTERVENTION

IL-2

1. Optimal intravenous catheter management; remove after ≤ 7 days
2. Surveillance cultures of intravenous catheter twice weekly
3. Prophylactic antibiotics (ciprofloxacin, 250 mg PO BID; cefazolin sodium, 250–500 mg IV q 8 hr; or oxacillin, 500 mg IV q 6 hr for patients requiring central venous catheters
4. Prompt recognition of infections and initiation of appropriate antibiotics after obtaining cultures. Because of high risk for *S. aureus*, vancomycin hydrochloride, 1 g 12 hr (dose adjusted for impaired renal failure) is empiric drug of choice; broader coverage may be indicated in some patients—particularly those with a history of urinary tract infections, biliary colic, abdominal discomfort, or neutropenia
5. Removal of intravenous catheter once infection is suspected or confirmed

IFN

Acyclovir, 200 mg PO 5 ×/d to manage pain associated with herpes labialis infection

BCG

1. Avoid use of BCG in immunosuppressed patients because of risk of systemic infection
2. Postpone BCG treatment until concurrent febrile illness, urinary tract infection, or gross hematuria resolves
3. Delay BCG dose for 7–14 days after traumatic catherization, biopsy, or transurethral resection
4. For fevers greater than 100°F or bladder-irritive symptoms lasting longer than 24 hr and gross hematuria, administer isoniazid, 300 mg PO X 3 d; repeat isoniazid with subsequent administrations
5. Discontinue BCG if patient continues to have fevers while receiving isoniazid, recurrent elevations in liver function tests (related to isoniazid), or signs of prostatitis, orchitis, etc.
6. For systemic BCG infection, therapy should include: isoniazid 300 mg PO daily, rifampin 600 mg PO daily, and ethambutol 1200 mg PO daily for at least 6 mo. For patients with life-threatening BCG sepsis or "BCGosis," administer cycloserine 250–500 mg PO bid for first 3 days of treatment

TOXICITY GRADING

0	1	2	3	4
None	Minor, localized, antibiotics not required	Minor, antibiotics required	Severe, major organ infection	Disseminated, life-threatening

HEMODYNAMIC COMPLICATIONS

Hypotension is the most frequent dose-limiting side effect of high-dose IL-2 therapy, particularly when administered by intermittent intravenous bolus. The sequence of hemodynamic effects is characterized by an initial vasodilatory phase occurring 2 to 4 hours after a dose of IL-2, during which the systemic vascular resistance falls but vascular integrity is maintained. Subsequently, the capillary leak syndrome with third-space accumulation of fluid often develops. The decreased systemic vascular resistance persists until the completion of therapy [12].

The hemodynamic complications of GM-CSF are much less frequent and less carefully studied. The first dose of GM-CSF may be followed in 1 to 4 hours by a first-dose reaction characterized by hypotension, hypoxemia, flushing, tachycardia, musculoskeletal pain, dyspnea, nausea, and vomiting. Fortunately, this reaction is limited to the first dose of each treatment cycle and thus is not dose limiting. Hypotension may also occur later during a course of therapy and be related to vasodilation and the capillary leak syndrome similar to what has been reported with IL-2, especially with high doses of GM-CSF (> 250 µg/m²/d or > 10 µg/kg/d) [13,14].

Hypotension has occurred in up to 6% of patients with cancer treated with interferon alpha. It is generally mild and easily managed with intravenous fluids. Rarely are dose modifications required [15].

CAUSATIVE AGENTS
IL-2, GM-CSF, interferon α

PATHOLOGIC PROCESS
Decreased systemic vascular resistance and consequent hypotension are most likely related to a release of the secondary cytokine TNF; TNF is also responsible for the similar hemodynamic changes observed in early septic shock—may exert its effect on vascular smooth muscle through the synthesis of nitric oxide; mechanism of the first dose GM-CSF reaction is unclear, but appears to be unrelated to TNF [13].

DIFFERENTIAL DIAGNOSES
Bacterial sepsis; hypovolemia secondary to over-aggressive diuresis; vomiting, diarrhea, or bleeding; cardiac dysfunction; concomitant medications

PATIENT ASSESSMENT
Hemoglobin, hematocrit, EKG, BUN/creatinine; evaluate for infection, review daily weight

MANAGEMENT OR INTERVENTION

IL-2
1. Administer normal saline for a weight gain of between 5–10% of baseline weight over the 5-day course of IL-2 therapy
2. In patients with preexisting essential hypertension, therapy with antihypertensive agents should be stopped
3. For hypotension, administer up to 3 normal saline fluid boluses (250 ml each); once weight reaches > 5% of baseline, initiate pressors rather than continue fluid boluses
4. If hypotension persists despite adequate fluid replacement, begin dopamine hydrochloride, 2–8 µg/kg/min; titrate dose to maintain a systolic BP 80–100 mm Hg; monitor for occurrence of atrial tachyarrhythmias—if they occur, and hypotension persists, change to phenylephrine hydrochloride
5. Phenylephrine hydrochloride, 0.1–2.0 µg/kg/min, may be used alone or with dopamine for persistent hypotension
6. Hold dose of IL-2 if patient remains hypotensive despite pressors or if high doses of pressors are required to maintain blood pressure

GM-CSF
1. Symptomatic management of first-dose effect includes oxygen therapy, intravenous fluids for hypotension, NSAIDs for musculoskeletal pains, and morphine sulfate reserved for severe pain;
2. Prehydration may decrease incidence and severity of hypotension

TOXICITY GRADING

0	1	2	3	4
None or no change	Changes requiring no therapy (including transient orthostatic hypotension)	Requires fluid replacement only	Requires pressors, resolves within 48 hours of stopping the agent	Requires pressors for > 48 hours after stopping the agent

CAPILLARY LEAK SYNDROME

The capillary leak (vascular leak) syndrome is a common dose-limiting side effect of IL-2 and GM-CSF therapy. The administration of high-dose IL-2 and, less frequently, GM-CSF results in a generalized increase in vascular permeability and fluid extravasation into the tissues. The capillary leak syndrome is often first manifested as mild facial and ankle edema within 24 hours of the initiation of treatment. It may subsequently progress to anasarca during the course of treatment. Weight gain equivalent to 5 to 10% of baseline body weight due to fluid retention, ascites (especially in patients with extensive hepatic metastases), pulmonary edema, and pleural and pericardial effusions are commonly observed. The development of pulmonary edema is more frequent in patients with marginal pulmonary reserve (ie, in patients with a pretreatment FEV_1 of ≤ 2.0 l) and in those whose treatment is complicated by bacteremia. Edema of the CNS occurs as well and can be fatal in patients with brain metastases. The capillary leak syndrome occurs to some degree in all patients receiving standard high-dose IL-2 therapy, but only rarely in patients receiving GM-CSF in doses ≤ 250 μg/m^2/d or 6 μg/kg/d. The development of these potentially life-threatening side effects often contributes to decisions to withhold IL-2 doses or otherwise limit the intensity or duration of a course of immunotherapy. Side effects resolve rapidly after the discontinuation of therapy, with most patients reverting to their baseline weight in 4 to 5 days after completion of a course of therapy [16,17].

CAUSATIVE AGENTS

IL-2, GM-CSF

PATHOLOGIC PROCESS

Uncertain, but most likely a combination of several factors; direct endothelial injury mediated by IL-2 activated leukocytes (NK and LAK cells, in particular), or their oxidative products; secondary cytokine release, TNF, and IL-1, which may induce various adhesion molecules necessary for attachment of activated leukocytes to endothelium; and/or systemic complement activation with resultant high plasma concentrations of anaphylatoxins such as C3a, which have potent effects on vascular permeability

DIFFERENTIAL DIAGNOSES

Bacterial sepsis; tumor progression with malignant effusions; IVC compression or thrombosis; hepatic dysfunction; congestive heart failure

PATIENT ASSESSMENT

Rule out infection; check radiograph, EKG, LFTs, albumin; evaluate for tumor progression with IVC compression; rule out IVC or other deep vein thrombosis

MANAGEMENT OR INTERVENTION

IL-2

1. Select patients carefully. Patients should have no evidence of cardiac disease or brain metastases, adequate pulmonary reserve ($FEV_1 \geq 2.0$ l or $\geq 75\%$ of predicted for height and age), no significant pleural or pericardial effusions, and ECOG performance status of 0–1
2. Administer normal saline intravenously to limit weight gain to 5–10% of baseline weight over 5-day course of IL-2
3. Give oxygen therapy for symptomatic pleural effusions or pulmonary edema
4. For severe cardiovascular or pulmonary compromise, hold IL-2 until symptoms have resolved; for life-threatening complications, dexamethasone, 10 mg IV q 6 hr may be given
5. Once treatment has been completed and blood pressure is normal off pressors, begin diuresis with furosemide, 20–40 mg PO or IV daily until edema has resolved and patient has returned to baseline weight

GM-CSF

1. Select patients carefully. Patients should have no evidence of cardiac disease or brain metastases, adequate ($FEV_1 \geq 2.0$ l or $\geq 75\%$ of predicted for height and age), and no significant pleural or pericardial effusions
2. Give oxygen therapy for symptomatic pleural effusions or pulmonary edema
3. Reduce dose for moderate cardiovascular or pulmonary compromise
4. For severe cardiovascular or pulmonary compromise, hold GM-CSF therapy until symptoms have resolved; for life-threatening complications, dexamethasone, 10 mg IV q 6 hr may be given

TOXICITY GRADING

	0	1	2	3	4
Weight gain	< 5%	5–9.9%	10.0–19.9%	20–29.9%	≥ 30%
Pulmonary	None or no change	Asymptomatic, with abnormality in PFTs	Dyspnea on exertion	Dyspnea at rest	Severe symptoms not responsive to treatment, requiring intubation
Pericardial	None	Asymptomatic effusion, no intervention required	Pericarditis (rub, chest pain, ECG changes)	Symptomatic effusion; drainage required	Tamponade; drainage urgently required

ALLERGIC AND IMMUNE-MEDIATED COMPLICATIONS

Patients treated with IL-2 and interferon alpha, and less commonly with GM-CSF, G-CSF, levamisole, and BCG may develop a variety of allergic and immune-mediated side effects. Although relatively common, local injection site reactions (cystitis with BCG, erythematous skin lesions at SC injection sites with the other agents) are generally self-limited. Acute serious hypersensitivity reactions, such as urticaria, angioedema, bronchoconstriction, and anaphylaxis have rarely been observed with these agents. Each of these agents has been associated with the development or exacerbation of preexisting autoimmune or chronic inflammatory diseases (eg, immune thrombocytopenia purpura, autoimmune hemolytic anemia, psoriasis, rheumatoid arthritis, vasculitis, thyroiditis, inflammatory bowel disease). In most cases, therapy must be discontinued.

Both neutralizing and nonneutralizing antibodies against IL-2, GM-CSF, and interferon have been observed. The clinical significance of these antibodies remains unclear, but in several cases the development of neutralizing antibodies to interferon was associated with disease relapse [1,25]. The development of autoantibodies to insulin, thyroid peroxidase, platelets, and other antigens has been described and many of these autoantibodies may be associated with the development of autoimmune disease. For example, thyroiditis, which is seen in 10 to 20% of patients undergoing high-dose IL-2 therapy, is frequently associated with the development of antithyroid antibodies.

An unusual "recall reaction" to iodinated contrast medium has occurred in as many as 10% of patients undergoing routine IV contrast studies during follow-up for previous IL-2 therapy. Reactions usually occur at least 1 month after initial exposure to IL-2 and contrast medium. Typical reactions begin 1 to 4 hours after reexposure to radiographic contrast medium, consist of fever, chills, rash, diarrhea, nausea, vomiting, urticaria, dyspnea, weakness, and hypotension, and resolve within 24 hours. Reactions appear to be more common in patients who receive IL-2 and radiographic contrast medium simultaneously (ie, as with intra-arterial therapy) [22].

CAUSATIVE AGENTS
IL-2, interferon α, BCG, levamisole, GM-CSF, G-CSF

PATHOLOGIC PROCESS
Poorly defined: release of secondary cytokines may induce expression of HLA-DR antigens on cells, eg, thyrocytes. These cells are then rendered competent to present cell-specific antigens, eg, thyroglobulin, to autoreactive T lymphocytes already present in the host. In some cases, administered cytokine may play a direct role in pathogenesis. "Recall reaction" may be related to enhancement by IL-2 of an immune response to radiographic contrast material, followed by an anamnestic response on reexposure to the contrast material.

DIFFERENTIAL DIAGNOSES
Allergic reactions or side effects of other medications, comorbid illnesses

PATIENT ASSESSMENT
Varies according to problem

MANAGEMENT OR INTERVENTION
1. Avoid biologic therapy or administer with great caution in patients with history of autoimmune or chronic inflammatory disease
2. Manage acute serious allergic reactions in a standard way with antihistamines, epinephrine, and, in some cases, corticosteroids
3. Discontinue therapy if severe reactions develop
4. Avoid or significantly decrease "recall reaction" to iodinated contrast medium by pretreatment with antipyretics and antihistamines
5. Because of the relatively high frequency of thyroiditis, monitor thyroid function for patients on IL-2 or interferon therapy
6. BCG cystitis may be treated symptomatically with phenazopyridine hydrochloride, 200 mg PO TID, propantheline bromide, 15 mg PO before meals and 30 mg PO QHS, oxbutynin hydrochloride, 5 mg PO tid

TOXICITY GRADING

0	1	2	3	4
None	Transient rash, drug fever < 38°C, 100.4°F	Urticaria, drug fever > 38°C, 100.4°F, mild bronchospasm	Serum sickness, bronchospasm, requires parenteral meds	Anaphylaxis

Immune-mediated complications may be graded using standard toxicity grading criteria for the affected organ or organs.

CAUSES

The mechanisms by which certain factors produce malnutrition in patients with cancer are well known. Gastrointestinal obstruction from tumor, perioperative gastrointestinal tract dysfunction, or the oral or esophageal mucositis that often complicates chemotherapy or radiation therapy represent physical impediments to nutrient intake. In addition, anorexia or a decreased desire for food is a common finding in cancer-bearing states. The causes of the anorexia may be direct actions of tumor-related mediators on the hypothalamic satiety centers, or result indirectly from depression, nausea, or vomiting. Gastrointestinal fistula formation, as well as diarrhea and malabsorption, may result not only from direct influences of certain tumors but may also complicate surgical, chemotherapeutic, or radiation treatment plans. The effects of such malabsorption on nutritional status are obvious.

Even without clear physical reasons, and often even at low tumor burdens, the cancer-bearing state may be associated with a syndrome of anorexia, weight loss, anemia, and severe lean tissue wasting. Although the mechanisms underlying this syndrome of "cancer cachexia" remain elusive, the alterations in substrate handling that characterize this syndrome are well described [1] (Table 1) and are briefly summarized.

Glucose

Carbohydrate-related changes of the tumor-bearing state can be characterized as 1) increased glycolysis, 2) increased anaerobic glycolysis by the tumor and certain host tissues, and 3) increased insulin resistance. The increased glycolysis results in host glycogen depletion and is accompanied by an increase in liver gluconeogenesis. The resultant drain on body energy store is postulated to be, in part, responsible for wasting of peripheral tissues.

Protein

The protein-specific changes associated with cancer cachexia are characterized by an increased peripheral skeletal muscle breakdown, decreased skeletal muscle protein synthesis, as well as an increased hepatic acute-phase protein synthesis. The net result is also an increased peripheral wasting. These protein metabolic changes often occur in spite of decreased food intake, indicating an aberration in the normal mechanisms of protein preservation during starvation in these patients.

Fat

Central to the lipid-related changes in cancer is a decreased activity of lipoprotein lipase, which is a membrane-bound enzyme pivotal in triglyceride uptake by the peripheral adipocytes. The result is poor disposal of circulating triglycerides, peripheral lipid depletion, and hypertriglyceridemia. There may also be increased lipolysis, with the cumulative effect of loss of peripheral lipid stores that is characteristic of the tumor-bearing state.

ASSESSMENT

The simplest and most frequently used measures of nutritional status are the anthropometric measurements of weight, weight loss, arm circumference, and tricep skinfold thickness. Of these, weight loss has been found to be the most useful, with weight loss of more than 5% correlating with poor outcome. Arm circumference or tricep skinfold thickness are not good independent predictors of morbidity or mortality and thus have limited utility.

Circulating levels of serum proteins decrease with malnutrition and therefore have been proposed as clinical markers of malnutrition. The most useful serum protein has been albumin, levels of which have been found to correlate inversely to complications. Because this protein has a circulating half-life of approximately 30 days, decreased circulating levels of this protein are a good index of persistent malnutrition but may not reflect acute changes. Measurements of pre-albumin (half-life, 2–3 d) have been advocated as a better reflection of acute changes in nutritional status. However, costs of measuring proteins other than albumin are still too high to consider using them as routine markers in assessment of the patient with cancer.

Urinary creatinine excretion has also been advocated as a parameter of nutritional status because creatinine excretion in normal persons is related to lean tissue mass. Patients with a creatinine-to-height ratio of less than 60% ideal as determined by standard tables are usually considered severely malnourished. In cancer-bearing states, however, nitrogen excretion often does not correlate with lean tissue mass. Nitrogen excretion has been found to persist at high levels even as wasting progresses, indicating persistent catabolic influences and rendering the creatinine-height ratio of little use in assessing nutrition reserve in this population. Nitrogen excretion is indicative of the level of catabolism and may guide efforts in repletion.

Immune variables have also been touted as a criterion for malnutrition and include delayed-hypersensitivity skin testing or determination of total lymphocyte counts. Three problems exist for using such variables in patients with cancer, however. First, immunosuppression can be a primary consequence of malignancy. Second, host immune function may be altered by other disease-related conditions such as infection, hemorrhage, or cirrhosis. Third, iatrogenic factors such as chemotherapeutic agents or surgical procedures may also alter host immune function.

More sophisticated assessments of nutritional status such as isotopic measurements of body composition or protein metabolism are much too costly and complicated to be used routinely in the assessment of patients with cancer and are relegated to the research arena. Of the previously mentioned variables, the major correlates to

Table 1. Changes in Substrate Handling in Patients with Cancer	
	Energy
Energy expenditure	↑
	Glucose
Glycogen stores	↓
Glucose utilization	↑
Anaerobic glycolysis	↑
Cori cycle	↑
Insulin resistance	↑
	Lipid
Peripheral lipid stores	↓
Lipoprotein lipase activity	↓
Circulating triglyceride levels	↑
	Protein
Skeletal muscle protein stores	↓
Skeletal muscle protein synthesis	↓
Hepatic protein synthesis	↑

outcome are weight loss [2] and albumin level. In fact, studies have shown that a clinical history and clinical assessment are as good as any laboratory or physical variables in predicting outcome [3]. Nevertheless, certain clinical findings should alert the clinician to significant malnutrition and need for repletion, particularly if major surgical or chemotherapeutic intervention is planned. These findings include 1) weight loss of greater than 10%, weight loss of greater than 0.5 kg/wk, evidence of muscular weakness, and serum albumin levels of less than 3.2 g/dl [4].

MANAGEMENT

Strategies with the aim to treat the malnutrition associated with cancer-bearing states must be directed at repleting lean tissue losses that have already occurred and at preventing further loss of vital tissues. Such strategies have to overcome two basic obstacles: First are the physical factors that prevent intake or absorption of nutrients, and second are the alterations in host metabolic substrate handling that predispose to tissue wasting. To date, clinical and experimental strategies that have been devised and practiced can be divided into four main categories: 1) elimination of tumor, 2) increasing of nutrient intake, 3) use of growth factors, and 4) use of pharmacologic agents. Elimination of tumor, whether by surgery, chemotherapy, or radiation therapy, is of paramount importance, and may reverse many of the derangements associated with cancer cachexia.

Total Parenteral Nutrition

In Patients Undergoing Surgery

Since the landmark works of Dudrick showing that high-caloric intravenous feeding alone can provide long-term sustenance for patients, total parenteral nutrition (TPN) has become a widely used part of our clinical armamentarium. In patients with cancer, at least 19 studies examining this modality have been published and reviewed [5]. Even though the majority of the studies do not show improvements in outcome parameters even when aggressive feeding is used, most study designs are flawed by poor control groups, small sample sizes, and heterogeneity of patient populations. These shortcomings are discussed at length in the meta-analysis of this literature by Detsky *et al.* [5]. Two of these studies show positive findings and are sufficiently well executed to deserve further discussion. Muller *et al.* [6] examined patients receiving TPN who were undergoing gastric or esophageal surgery and found that parenteral feedings for 10 days (*n* = 66) significantly reduced the rate of mortality and major postoperative complications when compared with control patients undergoing customary oral feedings (*n* = 59). A subsequent study by the Veterans Administration Study Group [7] examined patients (*n* = 395) undergoing abdominal or thoracic surgery. Although no overall differences existed between the groups in terms of morbidity or mortality in this study of 7 to 10 days of preoperative TPN, in subset analysis, for patients with severe malnutrition as defined by clinical parameters (weight loss >20%, serum albumin level <2.9), there was an advantage to the use of preoperative TPN. Lacking further evidence, a reasonable recommendation is that in patients with a greater than 10% weight loss, preoperative aggressive nutritional supplementation is reasonable, whether by enteral route or parenteral. If the decision is to use the parenteral route, at least a 7- to 10-day course of TPN is warranted. There is no evidence that any shorter course has clinical efficacy, and TPN is certainly not without complications (Table 2). Typical orders for initiating TPN are outlined in Table 3.

In Patients Receiving Chemotherapy

Common adverse effects of chemotherapy include anorexia, emesis, diarrhea, and intestinal mucosal sloughing that leads to malabsorption. These effects and the fact that patients receiving chemotherapy tend to have more advanced disease and larger tumor burdens make this group a theoretically attractive group to treat with parenteral nutrition. However, despite our clinical prejudice that supplemental nutrient administration should improve the clinical status of these patients and animal experimental data suggesting that TPN improves outcome from chemotherapy, no clinical data exist to support this prejudice. A multitude of studies have been performed and are summarized by McGeer *et al.* [8]. The conclusions of this position paper by the American College of Physicians were that TPN in the mildly malnourished patients on the medical oncology ward may be more harmful than helpful, likely due to catheter sepsis in this immunosuppressed population. Furthermore, in the severely malnourished, more data need to be gathered before the risk-benefit ratio of TPN could be determined.

In Patients Undergoing Radiation Therapy

To date, there have been relatively few studies examining the efficacy of nutritional supplementation and results of radiation therapy for cancer. These studies can be described as small, poorly controlled, and inconclusive, and they have recently been reviewed [9]. Based on current clinical data, no conclusion with regard to intravenous nutritional supplementation in this population can be made.

Table 2. Common Complications of TPN

Complication	Frequency (%)
Central line—related	
Pneumothorax	1–3
Thrombophlebitis*	1–2
Brachial plexus injury	0.5–1
Carotid or subclavian artery injuries	0.25–0.5
Overall	4–15
Infectious	
Line sepsis	2–10
Metabolic	
Electrolyte abnormalities	
Hyperglycemia (including hyperglycemic hyper-osmotic coma)	
Hyperkalemia	
Hypomagnesemia	
Hypophosphatemia	
Acid-base disturbances	
Most commonly: hyperchloremic metabolic acidosis	
Congestive heart failure	
Altered liver function	
Total	5–10

*Clinically apparent thrombophlebitis; angiographically evident thrombophlebitis may be 25–30% in select populations.

Enteral Nutrition

The majority of studies concerning aggressive nutritional supplementation in patients with cancer are performed using parenteral nutrition. Certainly, in patients with nonfunctional gastrointestinal tracts, the intravenous route represents the only option. When the enteral route is an option, however, there is clear evidence that this route is preferable from an immunologic and metabolic standpoint. Recent animal and human data indicate that feeding by the intravenous route particularly suppresses host immunologic function. Only one prospective study of adequate sample size has examined the utility of enteral feedings in the treatment of patients with cancer. In a study of 192 patients with unresectable colorectal or lung cancer, patients were randomly assigned to three groups consisting of 1) ad lib nutritional intake, 2) dietary counseling, and 3) dietary counseling and enteral defined formula supplementation if goals of 1.7 to 1.95 times resting energy expenditure were not reached [10]. No difference in clinical outcome could be discerned among the groups in this study. It must be noted, however, that aggressive tube feedings were not pursued in this study. Studies examining aggressive enteral feeding protocols for preoperative patients, patients undergoing chemotherapy, or patients undergoing radiation therapy are still largely lacking, and are a fertile and active area of current research. There is certainly a large selection of enteral supplements available for nutritional treatment for patients with cancer (Table 4).

Table 3. Typical Orders for Total Parenteral Nutrition

Makeup of typical TPN solution (per 1000 ml)	
Nutrients	
Mixed amino acid	50 g
Dextrose	250 g
Electrolytes	
Calcium gluconate	4.6 mEq
Magnesium sulfate	8 mEq
Potassium chloride	22.4 mEq
Potassium phosphate	12 mM
Sodium acetate	18 mEq
Sodium chloride	33.5 mEq
Trace elements (per day)	
Zinc	5 mg
Copper	2 mg
Manganese	0.5 mg
Chromium	10 µg
Multivitamins (per day)	
Vitamin A	1 mg
Ergocalciferol (vitamin D)	5 µg
Vitamin E	10 mg
Thiamine	3 mg
Riboflavin	3.6 mg
Niacinamide	40 mg
Dexpanthenol	15 mg
Pyridoxine HCl	4 mg
Biotin	60 µg
Cyanocobalamin	5 µg
Folic acid	400 mg
Ascorbic acid	100 mg
Fat emulsions	500 ml of 10% solution 2X/wk (4% of total non-protein calories)
Medical orders relating to start of TPN	
Start infusion at 40 ml/hr	
Maximum incremental increase should be 40 ml/hr	
Routine catheter care	
Infuse TPN via pump	
Vital signs q 6 hr	
Urine sugars by dipstick q 6 hr	
Stat glucose for > 2+ and call house officer	
Strict I/O	
Weight 3X/wk	
Routine blood tests	
Three times per week: electrolytes, liver function tests, glucose	
Once weekly: prothrombin time, CBC, platelet count, cholesterol, triglyceride, transferrin	

Potential Adjunctive Methods

In addition to strategies that improve total caloric and nitrogen intake, there are also strategies aimed at delivering specific nutrients at high concentrations to the patients. These clinical strategies are based on experimental studies that demonstrate certain nutrients to have particularly potent trophic or stimulatory effects on components of the host defense mechanism. All of these strategies must currently be considered experimental.

Nucleotides

Nucleotides are essential components of cellular RNA and DNA. Dietary deficiency of nucleic acids alters host cellular immunity, as measured by natural killer cell activity, T-cell response to mitogens, and macrophage cytokine release. Exogenous administration of polynucleotides enhances natural killer cell activity and release of cytokines. To date, one randomized trial on the utility of nucleic acids in patients with cancer has been performed. In a placebo-controlled trial of patients undergoing resection for breast cancer, there was enhanced survival in polyadenylic acid–polyuridylic acid–treated postmenopausal patients [11]. Further studies will have to be performed to verify these results and to examine whether similar effects on patients with other tumor types exist. Even before such studies are performed, however, tube feedings supplemented with nucleotides are already commercially available (Table 4).

Amino Acids

The amino acid, glutamine, has been found to be a primary nitrogenous substrate used by the gastrointestinal tract. As such, it appears to be a particularly potent trophic factor for intestinal mucosa. Specific use of this amino acid has two goals: improvement of gut barrier function and improvement of intestinal absorptive capacity. For this reason, trials are underway to examine the efficacy of adding this amino acid to parenteral and enteral feedings. Preliminary studies in patients undergoing bone marrow transplantation have not shown a major beneficial role for this amino acid in protecting against complications [12]. Trials in other cancer populations are underway.

Arginine is another amino acid with established immunostimulatory effects. Administration of high doses of this amino acid to patients with cancer enhances in vitro parameters of lymphocyte function, including natural killer cell activity, lymphocyte response to stimulation, and increases in T-helper cell numbers [13]. Whether this enhancement will translate to improved outcome during cancer therapy is uncertain. Active trials examining the utility of this amino acid in the treatment of patients with cancer are in progress.

Polyunsaturated Free Fatty Acids

Composition of the dietary fat also seems to have a major effect on host immune function. In particular, the contents of unsaturated free fatty acids appear to be a major determinant on lymphocyte function and macrophage cytokine production. Experimental studies have documented that diets containing fish oils that are high in omega-3 fatty acids may not only enhance measured host immune function but may protect against infection and sepsis. The effects of fish oils, or the manipulations of the dietary fats on tumor-bearing states remain largely unexplored. The findings from studies on sepsis and infection as well as the prevalence of infection in the cancer-bearing populations certainly encourage these lines of investigation.

Growth Factors

Advances during the last century have uncovered the important roles that peptide growth factors and steroids play in growth and development. It was not until recently, however, with widespread application of molecular biologic techniques, that large-scale production of many growth factors was possible. Currently, peptide hormones, such as insulin, growth hormone, and insulin-like growth factor, are available in large quantities and, along with anabolic steroids, represent potential therapeutic modalities for cancer cachexia. Even though many studies have been performed examining the potential roles of growth factors in patients with cancer, their role in the clinical treatment of this population is still poorly defined.

The pancreatic hormone *insulin* has major anabolic as well as catabolic effects. It promotes amino acid and carbohydrate uptake by many tissues, increases use of glucose for glycogen synthesis and lipogenesis, decreases gluconeogenesis, decreases lipolysis, and increases protein synthesis. In these ways, insulin is a major determinant of normal metabolism and growth. Clinicians have long attempted to harness the tissue-sparing effects of this polypeptide in

the treatment of catabolic disease. The three major clinical studies in the injured population all involved either burn or trauma patients. In these populations, infusions of high doses of insulin along with high-dose glucose intravenous feedings produced laboratory measures of protein sparing such as decreased urinary nitrogen excretion, or decreased 3-methylhistidine excretion. These studies were difficult to interpret because the treatment populations had significantly higher caloric intakes than did the control populations. In addition, two possible complications associated with high-dose insulin infusions have deterred clinical use. First, when high doses of insulin are used, life-threatening hypoglycemia is a possible complication. In some studies, monitoring of serum glucose levels has been as frequent as every hour [14]. Second, high-dose insulin and glucose infusions may produce marked increases in lipogenesis. Such an increase in lipogenesis may manifest in sufficient increases of CO_2 production to overcome pulmonary reserve and produce respiratory compromise and failure. An increased lipogenesis may also lead to fatty liver formation and hepatic dysfunction. Thus, the use of high-dose insulin alone is unlikely to be a clinically useful adjunct to nutritional supplementation.

Growth hormone is a 191-amino acid polypeptide secreted by the anterior pituitary gland and is a prime stimulus for growth during puberty. In adults, this hormone is also released in an intermittent pulsatile pattern that may be important in normal homeostasis. The actions of this hormone are complex, but can be briefly summarized as protein anabolic, lipolytic, and gluconeogenic. It appears that this hormone redirects the body to use lipids as fuel in preference to proteins and is thus an attractive agent in the treatment of the catabolic patient. Despite these clear theoretical advantages, proving clinical utility of growth hormone in the injured patient has been difficult.

The majority of clinical nutritional studies performed before the availability of synthetic human growth hormone in the mid-1980s were performed with orthopedic or burn patients. Since then, numerous preclinical studies and three clinical studies in patients with cancer have been performed. A most impressive clinical testimony to the potent influences of growth hormone on nitrogen accrual is the study by Jiang *et al.* [15] demonstrating that, even in

Table 4. Common Oral Nutritional Supplements

Product	Cal/ml	Non-prot cal:gN	Osmolality	Tube/Oral	Taste	Cost	Advantage
Isocal	1.06	167:1	300	Both	Fair	+	Isotonic, tolerated well orally, inexpensive
Isocal HCN	2.00	145:1	690	Both	Fair	++	Useful in fluid restriction
Ensure	1.06	153:1	470	Both	Good	+	Taste suitable for oral supplement, inexpensive, low residue; can be used for bowel prep
Ensure plus	1.50	146:1	690	Both	Fair	++	Useful in fluid restriction, low residue
Sustacal HC	1.50	134:1	650	Both	Good	++	Low sodium content
Isosource HN	1.20	116:1	330	Both	Fair	++	Low residue
Specialty formulas							
Pulmocare	1.50	125:1	520	Tube	Poor	+++++	Low non-protein caloric content may be beneficial for patients with pulmonary compromise
Impact	1.00	71:1	375	Tube	Poor	+++++	Contains arginine, fish oils, nucleotides; suggested to improve immune function
Elemental formulas							
Vivonex TEN	1.00	149:1	630	Tube	Poor	+++++	Elemental; predigested, low fat, low residue
Criticare HN	1.06	148:1	650	Tube	Poor	++++	Elemental; predigested, low fat, low residue

the setting of hypocaloric feedings, growth hormone can produce positive nitrogen balance in patients who have undergone surgery for intra-abdominal tumor. Although these studies in patients with cancer, as well as a majority of studies in other clinical populations, provided evidence for improved nitrogen retention with growth hormone administration, none have as yet provided evidence that this retention is accompanied by improved clinical outcome. This inability is likely due to the small sample sizes in all studies performed to date, and the short follow-up in these studies. A large randomized trial of this hormone in patients with cancer is imperative because the cost of this hormone is not inconsequential.

More recently, combination therapy consisting of growth hormone and insulin has been studied as an adjunct to nutritional supplementation. Preliminary studies in patients with cancer [16] have shown that daily injections of growth hormone for 3 days followed by a constant infusion of insulin acutely promotes skeletal muscle and whole body nitrogen retention at doses of insulin that are of a log magnitude less than the previously discussed clinical studies of insulin alone. The mechanisms of the hormone interaction and whether this or other combinations of growth factors will be clinically useful await future studies.

Insulin-like growth factor-1 (IGF-1), originally isolated and called somatomedin-C, is an intermediary hormone that mediates many of the actions of growth hormone. IGF-1 exerts many of the effects of insulin, including hypoglycemia and inhibition of lipolysis. In vitro, IGF-1 stimulates protein synthesis and in vivo this hormone inhibits proteolysis. Because of the recent synthesis of this molecule by recombinant techniques, potentially limitless quantities are now available, facilitating in vivo studies and making large-scale clinical trials possible. Studies of this hormone as a nutritional adjunct in animals have been encouraging. Results of initial clinical studies should be available in the near future.

Androgenic steroids have long been known to have potent anabolic activities. Pharmacologic modifications of the natural androgens have been performed with the aim of reducing their androgenic actions, increasing the ease of administration, and enhancing their anabolic actions. Such efforts have resulted in production of a class of synthetic compounds referred to as *anabolic steroids*.

These compounds have been tested in the clinical setting for a long time. As early as 1944, Abels *et al.* [17] found that testosterone propionate enhanced nitrogen balance in three patients with gastric cancer. Since then, the clinical utility of anabolic steroids has been examined in diverse clinical populations, including at least three other studies in patients with cancer. The study of Hansell *et al.* [18] deserves particular mention, as it is the only study of even moderate size. In this study, 60 patients undergoing colorectal surgery were randomly assigned to receive or not receive stanozolol along with either hypocaloric or eucaloric supplementation. Improved nitrogen balance was noted only in the group with hypocaloric nutrition. Even though several studies have shown an improvement in serum or urine parameters of nitrogen retention, no study to date has shown an improvement in any clinical outcome parameter, which may again be the result of inadequate sample sizes in the studies. Additionally, the varied nutritional regimens and the steroid preparations used make this literature particularly difficult to decipher. One must conclude that the question of whether anabolic steroids have any role as an adjunct to clinical nutrition remains unanswered. Certainly, a large trial, possibly in a multicenter fashion, is necessary to evaluate utility of these compounds as measured by clinical outcome.

Another major obstacle to the use of anabolic steroids in the clinical setting is the significant side effects of these compounds. Virilization is a potential side effect, often manifested by hirsutism, acne, clitoral hypertrophy, voice coarsening, and male-pattern baldness. Alternatively, peripheral conversion of testosterone and androstenedione to estradiol and estrone may result in feminizing effects such as gynecomastia. Other potential detrimental effects include hypogonadism, lipoprotein abnormalities—including increased low-density lipoprotein levels—sleep apnea, and hepatic complications, including development of hepatocellular carcinoma.

The Role of Growth Factors in Oncology

A major goal of aggressive nutritional support is growth of normal tissues. A commonly voiced concern in nutritional support of the patients with cancer, however, is disproportional growth of the neoplastic tissues. Such concerns are fueled by animal studies that have documented disproportionately enhanced tumor growth due to nutritional support. No clinical study in patients collaborate these animal models, however. When using stable isotope methods, Mullen *et al.* [19] could not demonstrate an increased synthetic rate in tumor tissues compared with normal tissues.

A major theoretical obstacle to routine usage of growth factors in the clinical setting is fear that growth factors may stimulate cancer growth. Animal and in vitro studies have linked growth hormone to the development of certain lymphoid malignancies [20]. IGF-1 has also been shown to be a stimulus for the in vitro growth of breast tumors [21] and lung tumors [22]. However, data also have shown that growth hormone administration in rats actually decreased the number of tumor metastases in a transplantable adenocarcinoma model [23]. The relative influences of the mitogenic effects of growth factors as compared with their beneficial influence on host cancer surveillance through improvements in immunocompetence remain to be determined. Further, if certain growth factors are capable of shifting tumors into the proliferative phase, such action may render tumors more sensitive to radiation therapy or chemotherapy. Therapeutic investigations involving this treatment strategy are currently underway in myeloid leukemia where colony-stimulating factors are being administered as priming agents to stimulate acute myeloid leukemic blast cells to become more sensitive to cell cycle–specific chemotherapy. No human study to date has examined the effects of growth factors on cancer appearance or growth. These studies will not only be interesting but will also be necessary before growth factor therapy can be accepted as a routine clinical modality. Trials of growth factors as adjuncts to chemotherapy or radiation therapy will undoubtedly be an area of fruitful future investigations.

Pharmacologic Agents

In addition to the various growth factors and anabolic steroids, many pharmacologic agents have been proposed as potential agents for enhancing weight gain during the treatment for malignancy. The following are three agents that have undergone the most extensive trials.

Megestrol Acetate

Megestrol acetate is a synthetic progestational agent used in the therapy for advanced breast cancer. In this population, the clinical observation was made that this agent improved appetite and weight gain. Although the relative importance of the central nervous system appetite-stimulating effects of this compound versus the metabolic effects of megestrol on peripheral tissue metabolism is still being debated, clinical trials of this compound as a nutritional adjunct in patients with cancer have already begun. In a recent study, 89 patients with various tumor types were evaluated in a randomized placebo-controlled study [24]. The patients receiving megestrol had a significantly improved appetite and food intake. Whereas clinical utility of this medication as a modality in the treatment of disease-related malnutrition is far from proven, megestrol certainly holds promise in such a capacity and is currently under investigation for a variety of disease states [25].

Cyproheptadine

This antihistamine was tested in the cancer population because of the observation that this compound enhances appetite in non–cancer bearing humans. Early trials had suggested that cyproheptadine might increase appetite in tumor-bearing humans, but more recent studies have failed to verify this. In a randomized, blinded, placebo trial involving 295 patients with advanced malignancy, there was no improvement in anorexia or weight gain [26]. There is currently no role for this drug in the clinical treatment of cancer cachexia.

Metoclopramide

Primary effects of tumor-bearing states as well as effects of treatment may produce alterations in intestinal motility. Of the treatment-related factors, the most prominent are postsurgical ileus and intestinal dysmotility associated with narcotic administration. Metoclopramide has been proposed as an agent to be used to alleviate intestinal dysmotility in these and other cancer-related situations. Although it is clear that metoclopramide clearly improves gastric emptying after gastrointestinal surgery and in select cancer-bearing states, whether administration of this drug can affect any clinically measurable nutritional parameter remains undetermined. Future prospective trials with defined nutritional endpoints will be necessary to ascertain the utility of this agent in clinical practice.

Dronabinol

Whether effects of disease or treatment, nausea and vomiting are a significant part of the clinical course of patients with cancer. Certainly, nausea and vomiting can be a prime reason for reduced food intake. Strategies for improving nutritional status have therefore been directed at mitigating nausea and vomiting. Dronabinol, the major active ingredient of the marijuana plant, is an effective agent in the treatment of otherwise refractory nausea and vomiting. This reduction in nausea is likely the mechanism of improved appetite that was noted in early studies that used this drug. A small ($n = 42$) single-arm trial evaluating this agent with appetite and weight loss as clinical parameters has been performed. Administration of dronabinol improved appetite and reduced the rate of weight loss [27]. Further controlled trials will be needed to ascertain the efficacy of this drug in the nutritional treatment of patients with cancer.

Other Agents

As the mechanisms of the anorexia and altered substrate cycles associated with cancer-bearing states are better understood, many other agents have emerged as potential therapeutic modalities for cancer cachexia. For example, as the causative roles of cytokines such as tumor necrosis factor and interleukin-1 in mediating the anorexia and metabolic changes in cancer are elucidated, agents such as specific antibodies against these cytokines or pharmacologic agents such as pentoxyphylline, which block the effects of these cytokines, may emerge as useful modalities in the clinical treatment of cachexia. At present, however, these must be regarded as experimental agents.

CONCLUSIONS

It is agreed that progressive nutritional depletion is often a major clinical feature of patients with cancer, at times dominating the clinical manifestations of the disease. Many strategies have been investigated in efforts to improve the nutritional status of these cancer patients. TPN can clearly improve caloric intake and nitrogen balance, particularly in those with dysfunctional gastrointestinal tracts. Pharmacologic agents may improve gastrointestinal tract dysmotility and attenuate nausea. Growth factors may also improve nitrogen and protein balance. Except in the severely malnourished, however, none of these modalities alone has thus far been shown to improve clinical outcome.

A combination of the previously mentioned strategies will likely prove most fruitful in the treatment of the patients with cancer; therefore, studies combining the various modalities are necessary. Areas holding potentially the greatest promise for future research include studies of the multitude of recombinant growth factors that are becoming available and studies of the gastrointestinal tract as the primary route of aggressive nutritional supplementation. In the meantime, a practical strategy can still be recommended from available data (Table 5). Elimination of tumor is still of paramount importance, and effective responses to therapy are clearly associated with more dramatic response to nutritional support. Patients with greater than 10% weight loss will likely benefit from 7 to 10 days of aggressive intravenous nutritional support before major therapy. Narcotic usage should be minimized and drugs that attenuate nausea and gastrointestinal dysmotility as supplemental agents in the nutritional therapy for patients with cancer should be considered.

Table 5. Current Recommendations for Nutritional Support in Patients with Cancer

Eliminate tumor

Maintain adequate oral intake, as possible

Consider total parenteral nutrition or tube feedings for patients with > 10% weight loss

In patients with > 10% weight loss, consider 7–10 days of TPN prior to surgery

Minimize narcotic usage

Consider drugs that attenuate nausea and GI dysmotility as supplemental agents in nutritional therapy

REFERENCES

1. van Eys J: Nutrition and cancer: Physiological interrelationships. *Ann Rev Nutr* 1985, 5:435–461.

2. Dewys WD, Begg C, Lavin PT, *et al.*: Prognostic effect of weight loss prior to chemotherapy in cancer patients. Eastern Cooperative Oncology Group. *Am J Med* 1980, 69:491–497.

3. Baker JP, Detsky AS, Wesson DE, *et al.*: Nutritional assessment: A comparison of clinical judgement and objective measurements. *N Engl J Med* 1982, 306:969–972.

4. Hill GL: Malnutrition and surgical risk: Guidelines for nutritional therapy. *Ann R Coll Surg Engl* 1987, 69:263–265.

5. Detsky AS, Baker JP, ORourke K, Goel V: Perioperative parenteral nutrition: A meta-analysis. *Ann Intern Med* 1987, 107:195–203.

6. Muller JM, Brenner U, Dienst C, Pichlmaier H: Preoperative parenteral feeding in patients with gastrointestinal carcinoma. *Lancet* 1982, 1:68–71.

7. Perioperative total parenteral nutrition in surgical patients: The Veterans Affairs Total Parenteral Nutrition Cooperative Study Group. *N Engl J Med* 1991, 325:525–532.

8. McGeer XX: American College of Physicians. Parenteral nutrition in patients receiving cancer chemotherapy. *Ann Intern Med* 1989, 110:734–736.

9. Heys SD, Park KG, Garlick PJ, Eremin O: Nutrition and malignant disease: Implications for surgical practice. *Br J Surg* 1992, 79:614–623.

10. Chlebowski RT: Nutritional support of the medical oncology patient. *Hematol Oncol Clin North Am* 1991, 5:147–160.

11. Lacour J: Clinical trials using polyadenylic-polyuridylic acid as an adjuvant to surgery in treating different human tumors. *J Biol Resp Modif* 1985, 4:538–543.

12. Ziegler TR, Young LS, Benfell K, *et al.*: Clinical and metabolic efficacy of glutamine-supplemented parenteral nutrition after bone marrow transplantation. A randomized, double-blind, controlled study. *Ann Intern Med* 1992, 116:821–828.

13. Daly JM, Reynolds J, Thom A, *et al.*: Immune and metabolic effects of arginine in the surgical patient. *Ann Surg* 1988, 208:512–523.

14. Hinton P, Allison SP, Littlejohn S, Lloyd J: Insulin and glucose to reduce catabolic response to injury in burned patients. *Lancet* 1971, 1:767–769.

15. Jiang ZM, He GZ, Zhang SY, *et al.*: Low-dose growth hormone and hypocaloric nutrition attenuate the protein-catabolic response after major operation. *Ann Surg* 1989, 210:513–524.

16. Wolf RF, Pearlstone DB, Newman E, *et al.*: Growth hormone and insulin reverse net whole body and skeletal protein catabolism in cancer patients. *Ann Surg* 1992, 216:280–290.

17. Abels JC, Young NF, Taylor HC: Effects of testosterone and of testosterone propionate on protein formation in man. *J Clin Endocrinol Metab* 1944, 4:198–201.

18. Hansell DT, Davies JW, Shenkin A, *et al.*: The effects of an anabolic steroid and peripherally administered intravenous nutrition in the early postoperative period. *Jpen* 1989, 13:349–358.

19. Mullen JL, Buzby GP, Gertner MH, *et al.*: Protein synthesis dynamics in human gastrointestinal malignancies. *Surgery* 1980, 87:331–338.

20. Rogers PC, Kemp D, Rogol A, *et al.*: Possible effects of growth hormone on development of acute lymphoblastic leukemia. *Lancet* 1977, 1:434–435.

21. Lippman ME, Dickson RB, Bates S, *et al.*: Autocrine and paracrine growth regulation of human breast cancer. *Breast Cancer Res Treat* 1986, 7:59–70.

22. Nakanishi Y, Mulshine JL, Kasprzyk PG, *et al.*: Insulin-like growth factor can mediate autocrine proliferation of human small cell lung cancer line in vitro. *J Clin Invest* 1988, 82:354–359.

23. Donoway RB, Torosian MH: Growth hormone inhibits tumor metastases. *Surg Forum* 1989, 40:413–415.

24. Tchekmedyian NS, Hickman M, Siau J, *et al.*: Megestrol acetate in cancer anorexia and weight loss. *Cancer* 1992, 69:1268–1274.

25. Tchekmedyian NS, Hickman M, Heber D: Treatment of anorexia and weight loss with megestrol acetate in patients with cancer or acquired immunodeficiency syndrome. *Semin Oncol* 1991, 18:35–42.

26. Kardinal CG, Loprinzi CL, Schaid DJ, *et al.*: A controlled trial of cyproheptadine in cancer patients with anorexia and/or cachexia. *Cancer* 1990, 65:2657–2662.

27. Plasse TF, Gorter RW, Krasnow SH, *et al.*: Recent clinical experience with dronabinol. *Pharmacol Biochem Behav* 1991, 40:695–700.

MALNUTRITION

Tissue wasting is a common and often devastating sequela of the cancer-bearing state. This loss in body mass can result in multi-organ derangements including impaired immune function, impaired locomotive capacity, and, ultimately, impaired respiratory function. As little as a 5% reduction in lean body mass has been associated with increased mortality in patients with cancer. Numerous factors contribute to produce wasting and malnutrition in patients with cancer. Recent advances in our understanding of these factors, as well as improvements in nutrient delivery methods and availability of immunostimulatory nutrients and growth factors offer exciting potential modalities for specific treatment of cancer-related wasting.

MANAGEMENT

1. Eradication of tumor
2. Increasing nutrient intake
   a. Enteral supplementation
   b. Intravenous supplementation
   c. Specific nutrient administration
      i. Nucleotides
      ii. Specific amino acids
      iii. Polyunsaturated free fatty acids
3. Growth factors
   a. Anabolic steroids
   b. Insulin
   c. Growth hormone
   d. Insulin-like growth factors
4. Pharmacologic agents
   a. Megestrol
   b. Cyproheptadine
   b. Metoclopramide
   c. Dronabinol

CAUSATIVE FACTORS

Poor intake: anorexia, gastrointestinal dysfunction (blockage, diarrhea, malabsorption); altered substrate cycles; stress of surgery, chemotherapy, or radiation therapy: peri-operative intestinal dysfunction, diarrhea, vomiting, anorexia, malabsorption

PATHOLOGIC PROCESS

Gastrointestinal obstruction from tumor, perioperative gastrointestinal tract dysfunction, oral or esophageal mucositis complicating chemotherapy or radiation therapy, anorexia, depression, nausea, vomiting, gastrointestinal fistula formation, diarrhea, malabsorption

PATIENT ASSESSMENT

Absolute indicators of malnutrition: weight loss >10%, weight loss of 0.5 kg/wk, clinically evident muscular weakness, serum albumin < 3.2 g/dl; *Relative indicators of malnutrition*: immune parameters—anergy in delayed hypersensitivity testing, T-cell numbers < 1500 /ml, decreased complement levels; hypoproteinemia—thyroxine-binding pre-albumin, transferrin, retinol-binding protein; creatinine-height ratio < 60% ideal; negative nitrogen balance; clinical—stomatitis, GI dysfunction

TOXICITY GRADING

	0	1	2	3
Degree of malnutrition	None	Mild	Moderate	Severe
Clinical findings	No weight loss	Weight loss < 5%	5–10% weight loss	> 10% weight loss, muscular weakness
Laboratory findings	Normal albumin, normal transferrin level, reactive delayed hypersensitivity skin test	Albumin < 3.5, decreased transferrin level, < 5 mm reactivity on skin test	Albumin < 3.2, nonreactive skin test	Albumin < 2.7

PATIENT CARE DOCUMENTATION

DIAGNOSIS

ALLERGY HISTORY

PROTOCOL NAME/NUMBER

STATUS	DATE						
	ECOG PERFORMANCE						
	KARNOFSKY STATUS						
	TEMPERATURE						
	PULSE/RESP						
	BP						
	HEIGHT/CM						
	WEIGHT/KG						

TREATMENT CYCLE							
C/HEMMO							

PREMEDICATIONS							

CONCURRENT MEDICATIONS							

BLOOD PRODUCT	PRBC's							
	PLATELETS							
	OTHER							

INITIALS		1	2	3	4	5	6

LABORATORY DATA	DATE						
	WBC						
	HGB						
	HCT						
	PLATELETS						
	POLYS						
	BANDS						
	ANC						
	PT						
	PTT						
	SGOT						
	SGPT						
	BILI						
	ALK PHOS						
	GGTP						
	LDH						
	GLUCOSE						
	NA						
	K						
	CL						
	CO2						
	BUN						
	CREAT						
	CREAT CLEAR						
	CALCIUM						
	MAGNESIUM						
	PHOSPHORUS						
	URIC ACID						

INITIALS	1	2	3	4	5	6

TUMOR MARKERS						

Eq: CEA, CA-125, AFP/BHCG, PSA, PAP

TUMOR MSRMT	1					
	2					
	3					

SIGNATURE/DATE		SIGNATURE/DATE	
1		4	
2		5	
3		6	

PATIENT CARE DOCUMENTATION

COMMON TOXICITY GRADING SCALE						
DATE						
1-NEURO/SENSORY CHANGES						
2-VISION CHANGES						
3-HEARING CHANGES						
4-NEURO/MOTOR CHANGES						
5-CONSTIPATION						
6-NEURO/CORTICAL CHANGES						
7-NEURO/CEREBELLAR						
8-HEADACHE						
9-PAIN (OTHER THAN HEAD)						
10-CARDIAC CHANGES						
11-EDEMA						
12-PULMONARY CHANGES						
13-NAUSEA						
14-VOMITING						
15-DIARRHEA						
16-MUCOSA(ORAL)CHANGES						
17-TASTE CHANGES						
18-HEMATURIA						
19-PROTEINURIA						
20-SKIN CHANGES						
21-ALOPECIA						
22-BLEEDING						
23-INFECTION						
24-FEVER						
25-MYALGIAS/ARTHRALGIAS						
26-CHILLS						
27-FACIAL FLUSHING						
28-NASAL CONGESTION						
29-FATIGUE						
30-SLEEP DISTURBANCE(S)						
OTHER						

Left margin: COMMON TOXICITY GRADING SCALE

BEHAVIORAL CHANGES						
CHANGES IN:						
31-NUTRITIONAL STATUS						
32-COGNITIVE FUNCTION						
33-COPING						
34-MOOD						
35-SOCIAL SUPPORT						
36-RELATIONSHIPS						
37-SEXUAL ACTIVITY						
INITIALS	1	2	3	4	5	6

Left margin: NUTRITIONAL AND

Right margin of toxicity table: REFERRAL NEEDS

DATE						
RATE HOW PATIENT FEELS TODAY ON 1-10 SCALE						
PATIENT'S PRIORITIZATION 1 OF PROBLEMS 2 3						
INITIALS	1	2	3	4	5	6

REFERRAL NEEDS	DATE	REFERRED TO
HOME CARE		
HOSPICE CARE		
HOME INFUSION		
PSYCHOLOGICAL NEEDS		
FINANCIAL NEEDS		

PROGRESS NOTES/REMARKS

PROGRESS NOTES CONTINUED ON BACK

ECOG COMMON TOXICITY GRADING SCALE

			0	1	2	3	4
NEURO	1	neuro/sensory	none or no change	mild paresthesis loss of deep tendon reflexes	mild or moderate objective sensory loss; moderate paraesthesia	severe objective sensory loss or paresthesis that interfere with function	-----
	2	vision changes	none or no change from baseline	transient blurring	persistent or frequent blurring, double vision	partial loss of vision	blindness
	3	hearing changes	no change from baseline	asymptomatic, hearing loss on audiometry tests only	tinnitus and/or mild symptomatic hearing loss	hearing loss interfering with ADLs; correctable with hearing aid	deaf, not correctable
	4	neuro/motor	none or no change	subjective weakness, no objective findings	mild objective weakness without significant impairment of function	objective weakness with impairment of function	paralysis
	5	constipation	normal, no change from baseline	BM delayed 1-2 days from norm, not disruptive to lifestyle, corrected with diet, fluid, exercise	continued delay in BM 1-2 days from norm, disruptive to lifestyle, bowel prescription implemented	increased cramping, abd distention, flatus, straining, no BM for ≥ 2-3 days from norm, enemas required	interventions ineffective, fecal impaction, incontinence, ileus
	6	neuro/cortical	none	mild somnolence or agitation	moderate somnolence or agitation	severe somnolence, agitation, confusion, disorientation or hallucinations	coma, seizures, toxic psychosis
	7	neuro/cerebellar	none	slight uncoordination, dysdiadokinesis	intention tremor, dysmetria, slurred speech, nystagmus	locomotor ataxia	cerebellar necrosis
	8	headache	none	mild	moderate to severe but transient	unrelenting and severe	-----
	9	pain	no pain	mild, no analgesics	mild, non-narcotic interventions	moderate, short acting narcotics	severe, long-acting narcotics
CARDIAC	10	cardiac status	none	ST-T changes sinus tachy > 110 at rest	Atrial arrhythmias Unifocal PVCs	mild CHF multifocal PVCs pericarditis	severe or refract CHF tamponade
	11	edema	none	mild/restricted to lower extremities; relieved by elevation	mild, to lower extremities; weight gain of ≥ 5 lbs	edema extends beyond lower extremities; weight gain ≥ 10 lbs; pitting edema	gross generalized edema, system failure
PULMONARY	12	pulmonary	none or no change	asymptomatic with abnormality in PFTs	dyspnea on significant exertion	dyspnea at normal level of activity	dyspnea at rest
GI	13	nausea	none	able to eat reasonable intake	intake significantly decreased, but can eat	no significant intake	-----
	14	vomiting	none	1 episode in 24°	2-5 episodes in 24°	8-10 episodes in 24°	> 10 episodes in 24° or requiring parenteral support
	15	diarrhea	absence of diarrhea	2-3 stools/day	4-6 stools/day, or nocturnal stools, or moderate cramping	7-9 stools/day or incontinence or severe cramping	≥ 10 stools/day or grossly bloody diarrhea, or need for parenteral support
	16	mucosa (oral) status	none	painless ulcers, erythema, or mild soreness	painful erythema, edema, or ulcers, but can eat	painful erythema, edema, or ulcers and cannot eat	requires parenteral or enteral support
	17	taste changes	no change	slight alteration, metallic	markedly altered	-----	-----
GU	18	hematuria	negative	micro only	gross, no clots	gross + clots	requires transfusion
	19	proteinuria	no change	1 + or <0.3 g% or < 3 g/l	2-3 + or 0.3-1.0 g% or 3-10 g/l	4+ or >1.0 g% or <10 g/l	nephrotic syndrome
SKIN	20	skin status	none or no change	scattered macular or papular eruption or erythema that is asymptomatic	scattered macular or papular eruptions or erythema with pruritus or other associated symptoms	generalized, symptomatic macular, papular, or vesicular eruption	exfoliative dermatitis or ulcerating dermatitis
ALOPECIA	21	alopecia	no loss	mild hair loss	pronounced or total hair loss	-----	-----
BLEEDING	22	bleeding	none	bruising, petechiae, visible bleeding site, stable H/H	1-2 unit transfusion episode	3-4 unit transfusion episode	greater than 4 unit transfusion episode
INFECTION	23	infection	none	mild, no active rx	moderate, localized infection requires active rx	severe systemic infection requires active rx, specify site	life-threatening, sepsis, specify site
FEVER	24	fever	none	37.1°-38.0°C or 98.7°-100.4°F	38.1°-40.0°C or 100.5°-104.0°F	> 40.0°C or > 104.0°F for less than 24 hours	> 40.0°C (104.0°F) for > than 24 hours or fever with hypotension
FLU LIKE SYNDROME	25	myalgias/ arthralgias	none, no change from baseline	mild, transient, no interventions	moderate, frequent, relieved by medical interventions	severe, continuous, relieved by medical interventions	severe, continuous, not relieved by medical interventions
	26	chills	no chills	feels cold	chills, rigors; no drug intervention	rigors; relieved with drug intervention	rigors; not relieved with drug intervention
	27	facial flushing	none	yes	-----	-----	-----
	28	nasal congestion	none	mild	moderate	severe	-----
FATIGUE	29	fatigue	normal, no change from baseline	mild/ noticeable but no change in ADLs	moderate; some change in ADLs	severe; requires assistance to perform ADLs	continuous fatigue, unable to perform ADLs with assistance; bed ridden
SLEEP	30	sleep disturbance	no problem, no change from baseline	changes in sleep patterns; medical intervention not necessary	changes in sleep patterns; medical intervention effective	changes in sleep patterns; medical intervention somewhat effective	totally unable to sleep at night; medical intervention ineffective

ECOG PERFORMANCE STATUS
0 = ASYMPTOMATIC
1 = SYMPTOMATIC, FULLY AMBULATORY
2 = SYMPTOMATIC, IN BED < 50% OF DAY
3 = SYMPTOMATIC, IN BED > 50% OF DAY, BUT NOT BEDRIDDEN
4 = BEDRIDDEN

KARNOFSKY
100 = ASYMPTOMATIC
80-90 = SYMPTOMATIC, FULLY AMBULATORY
60-70 = SYMPTOMATIC, IN BED < 50% OF DAY
40-50 = SYMPTOMATIC, IN BED > 50% OF DAY, BUT NOT BEDRIDDEN
20-30 = BEDRIDDEN

NOMOGRAM FOR BODY SURFACE AREA

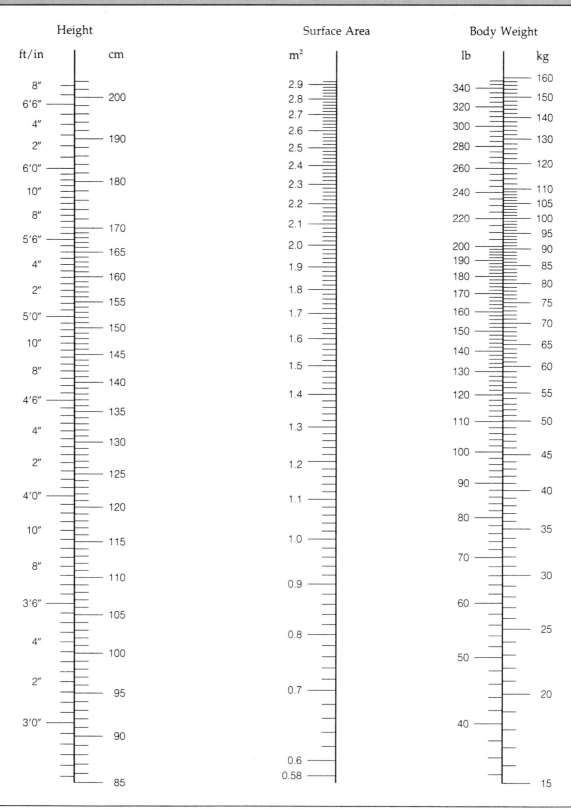

Height		Surface Area	Body Weight	
ft/in	cm	m²	lb	kg

Note: an estimate of a patient's surface area can be obtained by marking the patient's height and weight and drawing a line between these two points; the point at which this line intersects the middle scale represents the patient's surface area.

From "Normal laboratory values," in *Scientific American Medicine* (1991), with permission.

CANCER CENTER DIRECTORY

COOPERATIVE CANCER TREATMENT CENTERS

ECOG Member Institutions

Albany Medical College
47 New Scotland Avenue
Albany, NY 12208-3479
518-459-0731
Scot C. Remick, MD

Albert Einstein College
Albert Einstein Cancer Center
Van Etten Hospital
Medical Oncology, Room 2C14
1300 Morris Park Avenue
Bronx, NY 10461
212-904-2754
Peter Wiernik, MD

Case Western Reserve University
MetroHealth Medical Center
Cancer Care Pavilion
2500 MetroHealth Drive
Cleveland, OH 44109-1998
216-398-6000
Edward G. Mansour, MD

Emory University
Emory Clinic—Central
Leukemia Research Laboratories
P.O. Box AE
1024 Woodruff Building
Emory University
Atlanta, GA 30322-0463
404-727-5839
W. Ralph Vogler, MD

University of Florida
University of Florida—Gainsville
Division of Medical Oncology
Box 100277
Gainsville, FL 32610-0277
904-392-4611
David J. Oblon, MD

Fox Chase Cancer Center
Central & Shelmire Avenues
Philadelphia, PA 19111-2497
215-728-2626
Robert L. Comis, MD

Indiana University
Indiana University Medical Center
Section of Hematology/Oncology
University Hospital & Outpatient
  Center, Room 1730
550 North University Boulevard
Indianapolis, IN 46202-5265
317-274-0920
Lawrence H. Einhorn, MD

The Johns Hopkins University
Johns Hopkins Oncology Center
Johns Hopkins Hospital
600 North Wolfe Street
Baltimore, MD 21205
410-955-3300
David S. Ettinger, MD

Mayo Clinic/Ncctg
Mayo Clinic/Rochester
Mayo Building, East 12 B
Rochester, MN 55905
507-284-2511
John H. Edmonson, MD

University of Miami
P.O. Box 016960 (D8-4)
Miami, FL 33101
305-547-6826
Peter A. Cassileth, MD

Moffitt Cancer Center
P.O. Box 280179
Tampa, Fl 33682-0179
813-972-4673
John C. Ruckdeschel, MD

New York University
New York University Medical Center
School of Medicine
550 First Avenue
New York, NY 10016-6451
212-263-6485
Ronald H. Blum, MD

Northwestern University
Northwestern University Medical School
Section of Medical Oncology
303 East Chicago Avenue, Olson Pavilion
Chicago, IL 60611-3008
312-908-5284
Al Bowen Benson III, MD

Medical College of Ohio
P.O. Box 10008
3000 Arlington Avenue
Toledo, OH 43699-0008
419-381-4172
Ronald T. Skeel, MD

University of Pennsylvania
University of Pennsylvania Cancer Center
6 Penn Tower 3400 Spruce Street
Philadelphia, PA 19104-4283
215-662-4000
John H. Glick, MD

University of Pittsburgh
University of Pittsburgh Medical Center
MUH, 7 Main North
3459 Fifth Avenue
Pittsburgh, PA 15213-3583
412-648-6575 or 6570
John M. Kirkwood, MD

University of Rochester
University of Rochester Cancer Center
Strong Memorial Hospital
601 Elmwood Avenue, Box 704
Rochester, NY 14642-0001
716-275-2121
John M. Bennett, MD

Rush-Presbyterian-St. Luke's Medical Center
Professional Building, Suite 809
Section of Oncology/Department of Medicine
1725 West Harrison Street Chicago, IL
  60612-3897
312-942-5904
Jules E. Harris, MD
Janet M. Wolter, MD
South Africa

H.F. Verowerd Hospital and University of
  Pretoria
Department of Medical Oncology
Private Bag X169
Pretoria 0001
Republic of South Africa
21-3211 Ext. 2332
Geoffrey Falkson, MD

Stanford University
Stanford University Medical Center
300 Pasteur Drive
Stanford, CA 94305-5216
415-723-4000
Branimir I. Sikic, MD

Tufts University
New England Medical Center Hospital
  ECOG Studies Office, P.O. Box 452
750 Washington Street
Boston, MA 02111-1854
617-956-5000
Daniel D. Karp, MD

Vanderbilt University
Division of Medical Oncology
1956 The Vanderbilt Clinic
Nashville, TN 37232-5536
615-322-4967
David H. Johnson, MD

Vermont Regional Cancer Center
University of Vermont
1 South Prospect Street
Burlington, VT 05401-3498
802-656-4414
John D. Roberts, MD

Medical College of Wisconsin
Milwaukee County Hospital
Milwaukee County Medical Complex
Department of Medicine
Section of Hematology/Oncology
8700 West Wisconsin Avenue
Milwuakee, WI 53226-3595
414-257-6246
Ernest C. Borden, MD

University of Wisconsin
Clinical Science Center
Wisconsin Clinical Cancer Center
600 Highland Avenue, K4/666
Madison, WI 53792-0001
608-263-8600
James A. Stewart, MD

ECOG Participating Consultants

Memorial Sloan-Kettering Cancer Center
Department of Radiation Oncology
1275 York Avenue
New York, NY 10021
212-639-6817
Bruce D. Minsky, MD

M.D. Anderson Cancer Center
Department of General Surgery
1515 Holcombe Boulevard, Box 106
Houston, TX 77030
713-792-7217
Merrick I. Ross, MD

SWOG Member Institutions
University of Arizona
Arizona Cancer Center
Hematology/Oncology, Room 1957
1501 North Campbell Avenue
Tucson, AZ 85724-0001
602-626-2667
Thomas P. Miller, MD

University of Arkansas
Arkansas Cancer Research Center, Slot 724
4301 West Markham
Little Rock, AR 72205-7101
501-686-5222
Bart Barlogie, MD

Brook Army Medical Center
Hematology-Oncology Service
Box 517, Beach Pavilion
Ft. Sam Houston, TX 78234-6200
521-221-2287
Timothy O'Rourke, MD

Boston University Medical Center
University Hospital
88 East Newton Street
Boston, MA 12118-2393
617-638-8473
Maureen T. Kavanah, MD

University of Cincinnati
Barrett Cancer Center
University Hospital
234 Goodman Street
Cincinnati, OH 45267-0501
513-558-7625
Louis E. Schroder, MD

City of Hope National Medical Center
Department of Medical Oncology/Ther Res
1500 East Duarte Road
Duarte, CA 91010-0269
818-359-8111
James H. Doroshow, MD

Cleveland Clinic Florida
3000 West Cypress Creek Road
Ft. Lauderdale, FL 33309
305-978-5192
James K. Weick, MD

University of Colorado
Medical Oncology, Box B-171
Health Science Center
4200 East 9th Avenue
Denver, CO 80262-0001
303-270-3007
Paul A. Bunn, MD

University of California, Davis
Division of Hematology/Oncology
UC Davis Cancer Center
4501 X Street
Sacramento, CA 95817
916-734-3772
Frederick J. Meyers, MD

University of Texas, Galveston
Division of Hematology/Oncology
University of Texas Medical Branch
RT E-65
Galveston, TX 77550
409-772-1164
Suzanne McClure, MD, PhD

University of Hawaii
Cancer Research Center of Hawaii
1236 Lauhala Street
Room 406
Honolulu, HI 96813
808-433-5394
Jeffrey L. Berenberg, MD

Henry Ford Hospital
Oncology Division K-13
2799 West Grand Boulevard
Detroit, MI 48202-2689
313-876-1850
Robert A. Chapman, MD

University of California, Irvine
UC Irvine Cancer Center
101 The City Drive
Building 44, Route 81
Orange, CA 92668
714-456-6310
Frank L. Meyskens, MD

University of Kansas
Division of Clinical Oncology
University of Kansas Medical Center
3901 Rainbow Boulevard
Kansas City, KS 66160
913-588-6029
Ronald L. Stephens, MD

University of Kentucky
Lucille P. Markey Cancer Center
800 Rose Street
Lexington, KY 40536-0001
606-233-8043
Michael A. Doukas, MD

University of California, Los Angeles
Oncology
200 UCLA Medical Plaza, Suite 510
Los Angeles, CA 90024-7050
310-825-3706
Robert A. Figlin, MD

Louisiana State University
School of Medicine
1542 Tulane Avenue
New Orleans, LA 70112-2865
504-568-5843
John N. Bickers, MD

Loyola University
Section of Hematology/Oncology
Building 54, Suite 067A
2160 South 1st Avenue
Maywood, IL 60153-5500
708-216-3336
Richard I. Fisher, MD

University of Michigan
Upjohn Center, Room 4701
Box 0504
1301 East Catherine
Ann Arbor, MI 48109-0504
313-747-1417
Ronald B. Natale, MD

University of Mississippi
Division of Oncology
University of Mississippi Medical Center
2500 North State Street
Jackson, MS 39216-4505
601-984-1095
James Tate Thigpen, MD

University of New Mexico
University of New Mexico Cancer Center
900 Camino de Salud, NE
Albuquerque, NM 87131-5636
505-277-2151
James A. Neidhart, MD

Ohio State University
Ohio State University Hospital
Room N1021, Doan Hall
410 West 10th Avenue
Columbus, OH 43210-1240
614-293-8858
Stanley P. Balcerzak, MD

University of Oklahoma
OU Health Sciences Center
920 Stanton L. Young Boulevard
Room 4 SP 100
Oklahoma City, OK 73104-5028
405-271-8920
Dilip L. Solanki, MD

Oregon Health Sciences University
Division of Surgical Oncology, L224A
3181 SW Sam Jackson Park Road
Portland, OR 97201-3098
503-494-8478
William S. Fletcher, MD

Providence Hospital
Medical Oncology, 3rd Floor
22301 Foster Winter Drive
Southfield, MI 48075-3707
313-552-0620
Anibal Drelichman, MD

CANCER CENTER DIRECTORY

SHMC Tumor Institute
  Puget Sound
  1221 Madison
  Seattle, WA 98104-1387
  206-386-2929
  Saul E. Rivkin, MD

University of Texas, San Antonio
  Department of Medicine/Oncology
  University of Texas Health Science Center
  7703 Floyd Curl Drive
  San Antonio, TX 78284-7884
  512-617-5186
  Geoffrey R. Weiss, MD

Scott & White/Texas A & M
  Texas A & M College of Medicine
  Division of Hematology/Medical Oncology
  Scott & White Clinic
  2401 South 31st Street
  Temple, TX 76508-0001
  817-774-5590
  John J. Rinehart, MD

University of Southern California
  Kenneth Norris Hospital
  1441 Eastlake Avenue, Room 162
  Los Angeles, CA 90033-0804
  213-224-6677
  Franco Mario Muggia, MD

St. Louis University
  Department of Medical Oncology
  3635 Vista Avenue at Grand Boulevard
  P.O. Box 15250
  St. Louis, MO 63110-0250
  314-577-8854
  William S. Velasquez, MD

Temple University
  Comprehensive Cancer Center
  3322 North Broad Street
  Philadelphia, PA 19140-5102
  215-221-8030
  John S. MacDonald, MD

University of Utah
  Medical Service (111)
  VA Medical Center
  500 Foothill Boulevard
  Salt Lake City, UT 84148
  801-584-1234
  Harmon J. Eyre, MD

Wayne State University
  Harper-Grace Hospital
  Division of Medical Oncology
  P.O. Box 02188
  Detroit, MI 48201
  313-745-8910
  Manuel Valdivieso, MD

NCI-DESIGNATED CANCER CENTERS

Alabama
University of Alabama Comprehensive
    Cancer Center*
  1918 University Boulevard
  Basic Health Sciences Building, Room 108
  Birmingham, AL 35294
  205-934-6612

Arizona
Universtiy of Arizona Cancer Center
  1501 North Campbell Avenue
  Tucson, AZ 85724
  602-626-6372

California
Jonsson Comprehensive Center (UCLA)*
  200 Medical Plaza
  Los Angeles, CA 90027
  213-206-0278
  The Kenneth Norris Jr. Comprehensive
    Cancer Center

University of Southern California
  1441 Eastlake Avenue
  Los Angeles, CA 90033-0804
  213-226-2370

City of Hope National Medical Center†
  Beckman Research Institute 1500 East
    Duarte Road
  Duarte, CA 91010
  818-359-8111

University of California at San Diego
    Cancer Center †
  225 Dickinson Street
  San Diego, CA 92103
  619-543-6178

Charles R. Drew University of Medicine
    and Science (consortium)
  12714 South Avalon Boulevard, Suite 301
  213-754-2961

Calorado
University of Colorado Cancer Center†
  4200 East 9th Avenue, Box B190
  Denver, CO 80262
  303-270-7235

Connecticut
Yale University Comprehensive Cancer
    Center*
  333 Cedar Street
  New Haven, CT 06510
  203-785-6338

District of Columbia
Lombardi Cancer Research Center*
  Georgetown University Medical Center
  3800 Reservoir Road, NW
  Washington, DC 20007
  202-687-2192

Florida
Sylvester Comprehensive Cancer Center*
  University of Miami Medical School
  1475 Northwest 12th Avenue
  Miami, FL 33136
  305-548-4800

Illinois
Illnois Cancer Council*
  200 South Michigan Avenue
  Chicago, IL 60604
  312-986-9980

University of Chicago Cancer Research Center †
  5841 South Maryland Avenue
  Chicago, IL 60637
  312-702-9200

Maryland
The Johns Hopkins Oncology Center*
  600 North Walfe Street
  Baltimore, MD 21205
  301-955-8638

Massachusetts
Dana-Farber Cancer Institute
  44 Binney Street
  Boston, MA 02115
  617-732-3214

Michigan
Meyer I. Prentis Comprehensive Caner Center
    of Metropolitan Detaoit*
  110 East Warren Avenue
  Detroit, MI 48201
  313-745-4329

University of Michigan Cancer Center*
  101 Simpson Drive
  Ann Arbor, MI 48109-0752
  313-936-9583

Minnesota
Mayo Comprehensive Cancer Center*
  200 First Street Southwest
  Fochester, MN 55905
  507-284-3413

New Hampshire
Norris Cotton Cancer Center*
  Dartmouth-Hitchcock Medical Center
  2 Maynard Street
  Hanover, NH 03756
  603-616-5505

New York
Columbia University Comprehensive Cancer
    Center*
  College of Physicians & Surgeons
  630 West 168th Street
  New York, NY 10032
  212-305-6905

CANCER CENTER DIRECTORY

Memorial Sloan-Kettering Cancer Center*
1275 York Avenue
New York, NY 10021
1-800-525-2225

New York University Cancer Center*
462 First Avenue
New York NY 10016-9103
212-263-6485

Roswell Park Cancer Institute*
Elm and Carlton Streets
Buffalo, NY 14263
716-845-4400

Albert Einstein College of Medicine†
1300 Morris Park Avenue
Bronx, NY 10461
212-920-4826

University of Rochester Cancer Center†
601 Elmwood Avenue, Box 704
Rochester, NY 14642
716-275-4911

North Carolina

Cancer Center of Wake Forest University at
the Bowman Gray School Medicine*
300 South Hawthorne Road
Winston Salem, NC 27103
919-748-4354

Duke Comprehensive Cancer Center*
P.O. Box 3843
Durham, NC 27710
919-286-5515

Lineberger Cancer Research Center*
University of North Carolina School of
Medicine
Chapel Hill, NC 27599
919-966-4431

Ohio

Ohio State University Comprehensive Cancer
Center*
410 West 10th Avenue
Columbus, OH 43210
614-293-8619

Case Western Reserve University†
University Hospitals of Cleveland
Ireland Cancer Center
2074 Abington Road
Cleveland, OH 44106
216-844-5432

Pennsylvania

Fox Chase Cancer Center*
7701 Burholme Avenue
Philadelphia, PA 19111
215-728-2570

Pittsburgh Cancer Institute*
200 Meyran Avenue
Pittsburgh, PA 15213-2592
1-800-537-4063

University of Pennsylvania Cancer Center*
3400 Spruce Street
Philadelphia, PA 19104
215-662-6364

Rhode Island

Roger Williams Cancer Center†
825 Chalkstone Avenue
Providence, RI 02908
401-456-2071

Tennessee

St. Jude Children's Research Hospital†
332 North Lauderdale Street
Memphis, TN 38101-0318
901-522-0306

Texas

The University of Texas M.M. Anderson
Cancer Center*
1515 Holcombe Boulevard
Houston, TX 77030
713-792-3245

The institute of Cancer Research and Care†
8122 Datapoint Drive, Suite 600
San Antonio, TX 78229
52-616-5900

Utah

Utah Regional Cancer Center†
University of Utah Medical Center
50 North Medical Drive, Room C210
Salt Lake City, UT 84132
801-581-5052

Vermont

Vermont Regional Cancer Center*
University of Vermont
1 South Prospect Street
Burlington, VA 05401
802-656-4580

Virginia

Massey Cancer Center†
Medical College of Virginia
Virginia Commonwealth University
1200 East Broad Street
Richmond, VA 23298
804-786-9641

Washington

Fred Hutchinson Center Research Center*
1124 Columbia Street
Seattle, WA 98104
206-467-4675

Wisconsin

Wisconsin Clinical Cancer Center*
University of Wisconsin
600 Highland Avenue
Madison, WI 53792
608-263-8098

*Comprehensive cancer centers.
†Clinical cancer centers.

COMMUNITY CLINICAL ONCOLOGY PROGRAM

Alabama

University of South Alabama Minority-Based
CCOP
USA Cancer Center
Room 414
307 University Boulevard
Mobile, AL 36688
205-460-7194

Alaska

Virginian Mason Medical Center CCOP
1100 9th Avenue
Seattle, WA 98111
206-223-6945

Arizona

Greater Phoenix CCOP
2nd Floor
925 East McDowell Road
Phoenix, AZ 85006-2726
602-239-2413

California

Bay Area Tumor Institute CCOP
Suite 204
2844 Summit Street
Oakland, CA 94609
510-540-1591

California Healthcare System CCOP
Suite 206
2340 Clay Street
San Francisco, CA 94115
415-457-1150

Florida

Mount Sinai CCOP
Mount Sinai Medical Center
4300 Alton Road
Miami Beach, FL 33140
305-535-3310

Florida Pediatric CCOP
Florida Association of Pediatric Tumor
Programs, INC.
P.O. Box 13372
Gainesville, FL 32604-1372
904-375-6848

Georgia

Atlanta Regional CCOP
St. Joseph's Hospital
5665 Peachtree Dunwoody Road NE
Atlanta, GA 30342-1701
404-252-9639

Southeast Cancer Contral Consortium CCOP
2062 Beach Street
Winston-Salem, NC 27103-2614
919-777-3036

Grady Hospital Minority-Based CCOP
P.O. Box 26042
Atlanta, GA 30335-3801
404-616-4885

CANCER CENTER DIRECTORY

Illinois
Carle Cancer Center CCOP
  Carele Clinic Association
  602 West University Avnue
  Urbana, IL 61801
  217-383-3010

Iowa
Cedar Rapids Oncology Project CCOP
  788 8th Avenue SE
  Cedar Rapids, IA 52401
  319-363-8303

Iowa Oncology Research Association CCOP
  1044 Seventh Street
  Des Moines, IA 50314
  515-244-7586

Sioux Community Cancer Consortium CCOP
  Central Plains Clinic, Ltd.
  Suite 2000
  1000 East 21st Street
  Sioux Falls, SD 57105
  605-331-3160

Kansas
Wichita CCOP
  P.O. Box 1358
  929 North Saint Francis Street
  Wichita KS 67201
  316-262-4467

Lousiana
Oschner CCOP
  Ochsner Cancer Institute
  1514 Jefferson Highway
  New Orleans, LA 70121
  504-838-3708

Tulane University Minority-Based CCOP
  1430 Tulane Avenue
  New Orleans, LA 70112
  504-588-5482

Missouri
Kansas City CCOP
  Baptist Medical Center
  6602 Rockhill Road
  Kansas City, MO 64131
  816-276-7834

Ozarks Regional CCOP
  Suite 450
  1000 East Primrose
  Springfield, MO 65807
  417-883-7422

St. Louis-Cape Girardeau CCOP
  Suite 3018
  Tower B
  Mercy Doctors Building
  621 South New Ballas Road
  St. Louis, MO 63141
  314-569-6959

Nevada
Southern Nevada Cancer Research
    Foundation CCOP
  Suite C-14
  501 South Rancho Drive
  Las Vegas, NV 89106
  702-384-0013

New Jersey
Bergen-Passaic CCOP
  Hackensack Medical Center
  30 Prospect Avenue
  Hackensack, NJ 07601
  201-441-2363

Newark Inner City Minority-Based CCOP
  Center for Medicine and Immunology
  1 Bruce Street
  Newark, NJ 07103
  201-456-4600

North Dakota
St. Luke's Hospitals CCOP
  Roger Maris Cancer Center
  820 4th Street North
  Fargo, ND 58122
  701-234-2397

Ohio
Allegheny CCOP
  Allegheny-Singer Research Institute
  320 East North Avenue
  Pittsburgh, PA 15212-9986
  412-359-3630

Columbus CCOP
  1151 South High Street
  Columbus, OH 43206
  614-846-0044

Dayton CCOP
  Cox Heart Institute
  3525 Southern Boulevard
  Kettering, OH 45429
  513-296-7278

Toledo CCOP
  3314 Collingwood Boulevard
  Toledo, OH 43610
  419-255-5433

Oklahoma
Saint Francis Hospital/Natalie Warren
    Bryant CCOP
  6161 South Yale Avenue
  Tulsa, OK 74136
  918-494-1243

Puerto Rico
Florida Pediatric CCOP
  Florida Association of Pediatric Tumor
    Programs, Inc.
  P.O. Box 13372
  Gainesville, FL 32604-1372
  904-375-6848

San Juan City Minority Based CCOP
  G.P.O. Box 70344
  Centro Medico Mail Station 54
  San Juan PR 00928
  809-758-9217

South Carolina
Southeast Cancer Control Consortium CCOP
  2062 Beach Street
  Winston-Salem, NC 27103-2614
  919-777-3036

Spartanburg CCOP
  Spartanburg Regional Medical Center
  101 East Wood Street
  Spartansburg, SC 29303
  803-560-6812

South Dakota
Rapid City Regional CCOP
  Rapid City Medical Center
  P.O. Box 4097
  Rapid City, SD 57709
  605-341-8901

Sioux Community Cancer Consortium CCOP
  Central Plains Clinic, Ltd.
  Suite 2000
  1000 East 21st Street
  Sioux Falls, SD 57105
  605-331-3160

Washington
Columbia River CCOP
  Room B6-10
  4805 Northeast Glisan Road
  Portland, OR 97213
  503-239-7767

Northwest CCOP
  Tacoma General Hospital
  Suite 204
  314 South K Street
  Tacoma WA 98405-0986
  206-594-1461

Virginia Mason Medical Center CCOP
  1100 9th Avenue
  Seattle, WA 98111
  206-223-6945

Wisconsin
Marshfield Medical Research Foundation
    CCOP
  Marshfiled Clinic
  1000 North Oak Avenue
  Marshfield, WI 54449
  715-387-5134

Milwukee CCOP
  Suite 516
  2901 West Kinnickinnic River Parkway
  Milwaukee, WI 53215-3690
  414-672-1892

FREE POSTAGE! No stamp required if you live in the following countries:

AUSTRALIA, BELGIUM, BERMUDA, CYPRUS, DENMARK, FINLAND, FRANCE, GERMANY, HONG KONG, ICELAND, ISRAEL, ITALY, LUXEMBOURG, MONACO, THE NETHERLANDS, NEW ZEALAND, NORWAY, PORTUGAL, REPUBLIC OF IRELAND, SINGAPORE, SPAIN, SWEDEN, SWITZERLAND, THE UNITED ARAB EMIRATES, UNITED KINGDOM, UNITED STATES.

BUSINESS REPLY MAIL
FIRST CLASS MAIL PERMIT NO. 33925 PHILADELPHIA, PA

Postage Will Be Paid By Addressee

CURRENT SCIENCE
SUBSCRIPTIONS
20 N THIRD ST
PHILADELPHIA, PA 19106-9815

By air mail
Par avion

IBRS/CCRI NUMBER: PHQ-D/453/W

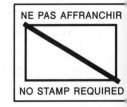

NE PAS AFFRANCHIR

NO STAMP REQUIRED

REPONSE PAYEE
GRANDE-BRETAGNE

CURRENT SCIENCE
34-42 CLEVELAND STREET
LONDON W1E 4QZ
GREAT BRITAIN

BUSINESS REPLY MAIL
FIRST CLASS PERMIT NO. 33925 PHILADELPHIA, PA

Postage Will Be Paid By Addressee

CURRENT SCIENCE
SUBSCRIPTIONS
20 N THIRD ST
PHILADELPHIA, PA 19106-9815

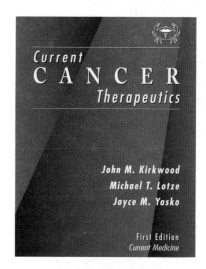